*Books by David S. Sobel, M.D.*

An Everyday Guide to Your Health
Ways of Health *(editor)*
The People's Book of Medical Tests


*Books by Tom Ferguson, M.D.*

Medical Self-Care: Access to Health Tools *(editor)*
The People's Book of Medical Tests

# The People's Book of Medical Tests

## David S. Sobel, M.D., and Tom Ferguson, M.D.

A Medical Self-Care Book
Summit Books
NEW YORK

Designed by Barbara M. Marks
Manufactured in the United States of America

10   9   8   7   6   5   4   3   2

Library of Congress Cataloging in Publication Data

Sobel, David S. (David Stuart)
    The people's book of medical tests.

    Bibliography: p.
    Includes index.
    1. Diagnosis.   2. Diagnosis, Laboratory.
3. Consumer education.   4. Medicine, Popular.
I. Ferguson, Tom, 1943–     . II. Title.
[DNLM: 1. Diagnosis, Laboratory—popular works.
QY 4 S6767p]
RC71.3.S57   1985   616.07'5   85-2841
ISBN: 0-671-44172-8
ISBN: 0-671-55377-1 Pbk.

*To Judy and Meredith,*
*for their love and support,*
*and for reminding us*
*that there was more to life*
*than "The Book"*

# Acknowledgments

This book would simply not have been possible without the generous advice and support of many people. Our reviewers and advisors included Janeth Adelson, M.D., Linda Adler, M.P.H., Charles Aring, M.D., Paula Arriaga, A.R.R.T., John M. Barry, M.D., Raj Bhandari, M.D., Katherine Boyle, R.N., N.P., Bethea W. Brindley, M.D., Jay Brodsky, M.D., Charles Bruhn, M.D., Barbara Carroll, M.D., Paul Cheeseman, M.D., Gregory Culberson, M.D., Judith L. Dethlefs, M.D., Erlinda Dizon, M.D., Joseph R. Ferrito, M.A., Robert G. Filpi, M.D., Julie Friberg, R.N., N.P., Peter Friend, M.D., John Fuentes, C.R.T.T., Steven Goetsch, Ph.D., Michael M. Gold, M.D., Phoebe Goodwin, R.N., Calvin Gordon, M.D., Sadja Greenwood, M.D., Frank Hadlock, M.D., Elizabeth M. Hatfield, M.P.H., Austin Hayes, M.P.H., Edward Hayhurst, M.D., William Hendee, Ph.D., Stephen Henry, M.D., Gary Hughes, M.D., Stephen Hulley, M.D., M.P.H., Ellen Hvistendahl, R.N., N.P., Magnus 'T. ibn Ale, M.D., Karen Johnson, M.D., Steven Johnson, M.D., Ada Koransky, M.D., Thomas A. Kula, Jr., M.D., Priscilla W. Laws, Ph.D., Peter Lee, M.D., Wayne Leong, M.D., Fred LeRocker, Judith Leverah, M.S., Lynne Lewis, Martin Little, M.D., Peter Long, M.D., William Lonsdale, M.D., Jeffrey Lou, M.D., John Mann, M.D., Joseph Mason, M.D., Ronald Miller, M.D., Bijan Moridani, M.D., Pius Morozumi, M.D., Rod Moser, P.A., Andrew Neal, M.D., Jerry Newman, M.B.A., John Pacuilli, M.D., Naomi Pless, Lee S. Portnoff, M.D., Dorothy Duffy Price, B.A., C.N.M.T., Sandra Procter, M.D., Leo Ramek, M.D., Jay Raman, M.D., Robert C. Rock, M.D., Jonathan Rompf, M.D., Shelly Roth, M.D., Mary E. Schaaf, M.D., Philip E. Sheldon, M.D., Michael J. Sheridan, M.D., Jack Siegel, M.D., Neal Smith, D.D.S., Gary Stein, M.D., Edward Talberth, M.D., William Thurston, M.D., Barbara Toohey, Robert L. Stiller, M.D., Ann Von Gehr, M.D., H. David Watts, M.D., Karen Wcislo, M.S., Linda Weinman Wolf, M.D., Stanley Wong, D.D.S., Newell E. Wood, M.D., and Peter E. Wood, Ph.D.

A few of our reviewers, Mary Barnett, M.P.H., Richard Dorsay, M.D., Bruce Ettinger, M.D., and James Vaudagna, M.D., deserve additional thanks for their heroic efforts and generous contributions to this project.

To Adelaide Townsend, a resourceful

medical librarian who was able on more than one occasion to track down key references, we offer our gratitude.

As part of this project several hundred patients who had undergone various diagnostic tests were interviewed to obtain a better understanding of the tests from a patient's perspective. First our thanks to the patients who freely shared their sensations, experiences, and advice. And we thank the many people who helped with these interviews, including the nursing students at San Jose State University and their supervisor Kathy Rose Grippa, R.N., Ph.D., Sebajooe Mohammad, R.N., Vivian Low, R.N., and our very special thanks to Polly Ann Cator, who with great sensitivity and skill did the lion's share of the interviews.

We have listed a number of our most important printed resources in our *For Further Reading* section, but we would like to especially acknowledge five ground-breaking books which we found particularly useful: *Diagnostics*, edited by Helen Klusek Hamilton (Intermed Communications, Springhouse, Pennsylvania, 1981); *The Patient's Guide to Medical Tests*, by Cathey Pinckney and Edward R. Pinckney (Facts on File, New York, 1978, 1982); *Do-It-Yourself Medical Testing*, also by Cathey Pinckney and Edward R. Pinckney (Facts on File, New York, 1983); *The Complete Book of Medical Tests*, by Mark A. Moskowitz and Michael E. Osband (W. W. Norton & Co., New York, 1984); and *It's Your Body: Know What the Doctor Ordered*, by Marion Laffey Fox and Truman G. Schnabel (The Charles Press, Bowie, Maryland, 1979). We are grateful to these authors for their pioneering efforts in making important medical information accessible.

Joe Graedon, who has been down this path several times before, was a great source of inspiration and support.

Jim Silberman, our publisher at Summit Books, first suggested that such a book was needed and then waited patiently and supportively while we wrote it. John Brockman, of John Brockman Associates, got us started on the project, and Ileene Smith of Summit Books stood behind us.

We would also like to thank our copy editor, Phil James, who made sure that every sentence was clear and consistent, and our illustrator, Karen Nagareda, whose imaginative drawings help bring the book alive.

Finally, we are deeply indebted to our editor, Kate Edgar. Her painstaking editing and insightful queries continually challenged us to communicate clearly. And her enthusiasm was unflagging.

# Foreword

**H**ere at last is a book to unlock the mysteries of medical testing. *The People's Book of Medical Tests* will help you understand any commonly performed test, and will help you decide whether a test ordered by your doctor is really needed—you'd be amazed at how often tests are performed when the results won't affect your treatment in any way.

Going to the doctor used to be simple; he looked you over, probed and tapped a little, listened to your heart, asked a few questions, and may have ordered a test or two. Finally, out came the prescription pad, and you were given some medicine. You weren't expected to ask too many questions—after all, doctor knew best.

Times have changed. Today's patients are more likely to ask questions, participate in treatment decisions, request second opinions, and check up on the drugs their doctors prescribe. But one aspect of medicine has remained largely inaccessible to consumers, up to now—the area of diagnostic testing. Most people still accept without question any test their doctor orders.

Medical testing itself has changed a great deal over the past few years. New technologies such as fiberoptics, computer imaging, and ultrasound now allow physicians to look into virtually every part of the human body. At the same time, though, diagnostic tests have become far more numerous, complicated, expensive, and sometimes even more dangerous than ever before. The responsible medical consumer is now faced with decisions about a long and bewildering list of tests: CAT scans, liver scans, blood cultures, urine cultures, cardiac catheterization, stress ECGs, biopsies, taps, electronic fetal monitoring, complicated scoping procedures, x-rays, ultrasound, and dozens of other supersophisticated diagnostic procedures—not to mention dozens of commonly performed blood and urine tests, which have themselves become vastly more complex.

*The People's Book of Medical Tests* gives the concerned reader a full description of the procedure for each of these tests, as well as any discomfort, risks, side effects, or aftercare that might be involved, the approximate cost, and guidelines for understanding the results.

In addition, an excellent section on home medical testing gives step-by-step instructions for performing more than twenty tests which can now be done safely and effectively at home without professional help.

Perhaps most importantly, this book breaks new ground in describing the *patient's* experience of each test, as well as the medical procedures. Too often health books include a wealth of technical information but ignore how the patient will actually feel during and after the test. Very little attention has been paid to this important area of medical care and, in fact, very little research has been done. Frequently, even doctors are unaware of how the tests they order will feel to their patients. But David Sobel, M.D., and Tom Ferguson, M.D., have interviewed hundreds of patients who have undergone diagnostic tests. *The People's Book of Medical Tests* is unique in its full descriptions of the sights, sounds, and sensations a patient is likely to encounter during each test. Armed with this knowledge, one can go into a test with less anxiety, and can participate more fully in one's own health care.

*The People's Book of Medical Tests* is a valuable contribution to the literature of medical self-care. It is the most comprehensive, readable, and useful guide to diagnostic testing that any layperson or health professional could ever ask for, with everything a health consumer might need to know about virtually all commonly performed medical tests. No one should have another medical test without consulting this book.

David Sobel, M.D., and Tom Ferguson, M.D., are members of a new generation of physicians who believe it should be a doctor's chief goal to put tools, information, and power into the hands of the health consumer. This book does exactly that. For all of us, I offer these two caring and committed physicians my heartfelt thanks.

JOE GRAEDON

# Preface

One of us (D.S.) had a personal experience that shows what a powerful effect even a common, relatively safe medical test can have.

It was the first day of his internship, and he was involved in a bewildering new routine—admitting patients, prescribing medications, and ordering tests on his patients. In the midst of this frantic activity, he received an order himself: he was to report to the x-ray department immediately.

When he arrived and asked why, the x-ray technician told him in no uncertain terms that "Everybody in the hospital must have an x-ray and you're no exception." He was led into a small changing room and was told to put on a hospital gown. As he slipped out of his crisp new white doctor's coat, he began to be aware of a distinct loss of power.

His first challenge was to figure out how to put on the gown. Which way was the front? Should he wait in the dressing room or was he expected elsewhere? He decided to sit down and wait, growing more and more anxious with each passing minute. He could feel the drops of sweat trickling down under his arms.

When no one had come after a quarter of an hour, he ventured hesitantly back out to the waiting room. By now the gown was soaked with sweat under the arms. The dozen fully dressed waiting-room patients regarded his partially clothed body with great curiosity.

He finally located the technician and meekly asked what he was supposed to do. "Oh, gee," he was told. "I completely forgot you were in there."

Even though the rest of the procedure went relatively smoothly, he was transformed from an assertive young physician to an exhausted wreck by the time the test was completed. And a chest x-ray is far less intimidating, painful, and dangerous than many of the procedures routinely done in every hospital. If this could happen to an insider, a physician on the hospital staff, how frightening the whole business of medical testing must seem to a layperson to whom the hospital is unknown territory.

Dozens of similar experiences—our own, those of friends, and those of patients we've cared for—convinced us that there was a tragic lack of information and support for people undergoing diagnostic tests, and a real need for a guide through the

11

often frightening, sometimes dangerous world of medical testing.

This book was written for all those who are striving to take more responsibility for their own health care and for all the health professionals who are helping them do so.

The information provided in this book represents, to the best of our knowledge, currently accepted clinical practice. But medical tests can vary depending upon who performs them, where they are done, your particular medical condition, and the latest advances in testing. The information here is designed as a guide to help you discuss with your doctor the need for a test, how you prepare, how it is performed, and what the risks are. If the information differs from your doctor's recommendations, discuss this with your doctor. He or she should be able to clarify your individual situation and provide you with the latest knowledge in the rapidly changing world of medical tests.

DAVID SOBEL
San Jose, California

TOM FERGUSON
Austin, Texas

*January 1985*

# Contents

| | |
|---|---|
| Acknowledgments | 7 |
| Foreword—Joe Graedon | 9 |
| Preface | 11 |

## I. Understanding Medical Tests — 19

## II. Medical Diagnostic Tests — 33

### 1. Testing Your Blood and Urine — 35

| | |
|---|---|
| Testing Your Blood | 35 |
| Collecting a Blood Sample | 36 |
| Testing Your Urine | 37 |
| Collecting a Urine Specimen | 38 |
| *Blood and Urine Tests* | 42 |
| Acid Phosphatase | 42 |
| Adrenocorticotropic Hormone (ACTH) | 43 |
| Alcohol | 44 |
| Aldosterone | 45 |
| Alkaline Phosphatase | 45 |
| Alpha-Fetoprotein | 46 |
| Ammonia | 47 |
| Amylase | 48 |
| Antinuclear Antibodies (ANA) | 50 |
| Arterial Blood Gases | 50 |
| Bicarbonate | 51 |
| Bilirubin | 52 |
| Blood Typing (ABO and Rh) | 53 |
| Calcium | 55 |
| Carbon Dioxide | 56 |
| Carbon Monoxide | 57 |
| Catecholamines | 58 |
| Carcinoembryonic Antigen (CEA) | 59 |
| Chloride | 60 |
| Chromosomal Analysis | 60 |
| Complete Blood Count (CBC) | 61 |
| Hematocrit | 61 |
| Hemoglobin | 62 |
| Red Blood Cell Count | 63 |
| Red Blood Cell Indices | 63 |
| White Blood Cell Count and Differential | 64 |
| Platelet Count | 65 |
| Peripheral Blood Smear | 66 |
| Cortisol | 66 |
| Creatinine and Creatinine Clearance | 67 |
| Dexamethasone Suppression Test | 68 |

| | |
|---|---|
| Drug Monitoring | 69 |
| Antibiotics | 69 |
| Barbiturates | 69 |
| Digoxin | 70 |
| Lithium | 70 |
| Phenytoin (Dilantin) | 71 |
| Quinidine | 71 |
| Salicylates | 71 |
| Theophylline | 72 |
| D-Xylose Absorption Test | 72 |
| Estriol | 73 |
| Estrogens | 73 |
| Ferritin | 74 |
| Folic Acid | 75 |
| Follicle-Stimulating Hormone (FSH) | 76 |
| Galactosemia Screening | 77 |
| Gastrin | 77 |
| Glucose | 78 |
| Glycohemoglobin | 80 |
| Growth Hormone | 81 |
| Hemoglobin Electrophoresis | 81 |
| Histocompatibility Testing (HLA) | 82 |
| Immunoglobulins | 83 |
| Iron | 84 |
| Ketones | 85 |
| Kidney Stone Analysis | 85 |
| Lactic Acid | 86 |
| Lead | 87 |
| Lipase | 88 |
| Luteinizing Hormone (LH) | 88 |
| Magnesium | 89 |
| Parathyroid Hormone | 89 |
| Partial Thromboplastin Time (PTT) | 90 |
| Phenylketonuria (PKU) Screening | 91 |
| Phosphorus | 91 |
| Potassium | 92 |
| Pregnancy Tests | 93 |
| Progesterone | 94 |
| Prolactin | 95 |
| Prothrombin Time (PT) | 96 |
| Renin | 96 |
| Reticulocyte Count | 98 |
| Rheumatoid Factor (RF) | 98 |
| Schilling Test (Vitamin $B_{12}$ Absorption) | 99 |
| Sedimentation Rate (ESR) | 100 |
| Serum Glutamic Oxalacetic Transaminase (SGOT) | 101 |
| Serum Glutamic Pyruvic Transaminase (SGPT) | 102 |
| Serum Osmolality | 103 |
| Serum Protein (Total) | 103 |
| Serum Protein Electrophoresis | 104 |
| Sickle-Cell Test | 105 |
| Sodium | 106 |
| Tay-Sachs Screening | 107 |
| Testosterone | 108 |
| Thyroid Function Tests | 108 |
| Toxicology Screening | 109 |
| Urea Nitrogen (BUN) | 110 |
| Uric Acid | 111 |
| Urinalysis | 112 |
| Volume | 112 |
| Color and Clarity | 113 |
| Odor | 114 |
| Specific Gravity | 115 |
| pH | 116 |
| Glucose | 116 |
| Ketones | 118 |
| Protein | 118 |
| Blood and Hemoglobin | 119 |
| Bilirubin | 120 |
| Urobilinogen | 121 |
| Microscopic Analysis | 121 |
| Cells | 122 |
| Casts | 122 |
| Crystals | 123 |
| Bacteria | 123 |
| Miscellaneous | 123 |
| Vitamin $B_{12}$ | 123 |

## 2. Testing for Infection — 125

*Microscopic Examination and
  Cultures* — 126
Blood Cultures — 127
Sputum Cultures — 128
Stool Cultures — 130
Throat Cultures — 131
Urine Cultures — 131
Skin and Wound Cultures — 132
Viral Cultures — 133
*Other Tests For Infection* — 133
Tuberculin Skin Tests — 133
*Infectious Disease Antibody Tests* — 136
AIDS Antibody Test — 136
Cold Agglutinins — 137
Hepatitis Virus Tests — 137
Mononucleosis Tests — 138
Rubella Tests — 139
Toxoplasmosis Tests — 139
*Sexually Transmitted Disease Tests* — 140
Gonorrhea Tests — 140
Herpes Tests — 143
Syphilis Tests — 144
Chlamydia Trachomatis Tests — 146

## 3. Testing for Heart Disease — 147

Cholesterol and Trigylceride — 148
Heart Attack Enzymes — 151
Electrocardiogram — 153
Exercise Electrocardiogram — 155
Ambulatory Electrocardiogram — 158
Echocardiogram — 160
Cardiac Catheterization and
  Coronary Angiography — 162
Thallium Scan — 167
Infarct Imaging — 170
Cardiac Blood Pool Imaging — 171
Pericardial Tap — 173

## 4. Tests for Women — 175

Vaginal Self-Examination — 175
Test for Vaginitis (Wet Mount) — 177
Pap Smear — 179
Colposcopy and Cervical Biopsy — 183
Endometrial Biopsy — 185
Breast Self-Examination — 187
Mammogram — 189
Breast Ultrasound — 192
Breast Biopsy and Aspiration — 193
Fertility Awareness — 195
Fertility Testing — 201
Hysterosalpingogram — 202
Culdocentesis — 204
Fetal Ultrasound — 205
Amniocentesis — 208
Electronic Fetal Monitoring — 213

## 5. Tests for Men — 218

Testicular Self-Examination — 218
Self-Test for Erection Problems — 219
Semen Analysis — 221
Prostate Biopsy — 223
Testicular Biopsy — 225

## 6. X-Rays — 227

Abdominal X-Ray — 233
Arteriogram—General — 234
Arteriogram—Cerebral/Carotid/
  Vertebral — 237
Arteriogram—Lung — 241
Arthrogram — 243
Barium Enema — 245
Bronchogram — 249
Chest X-Ray — 251
CT Scan—Body — 253
CT Scan—Head — 256
Cystourethrogram — 260
Dental X-Rays — 262

Extremity X-Rays                              264
Gallbladder X-Rays                            266
Intravenous Pyelogram (IVP)                   269
Lymphangiogram                                272
Myelogram                                     275
Skull X-Rays                                  277
Spine X-Rays                                  278
Upper Gastrointestinal (GI) Series            280
Venogram                                      283

**7.  Nuclear Scans**                         286

Bone Scan                                     287
Brain Scan                                    289
Gallbladder and Biliary Tract Scans           290
Gallium Scan                                  292
Liver/Spleen Scan                             293
Lung Scans                                    295
Renal Scans                                   297
Thyroid Scan and Radioactive
   Iodine (RAI) Uptake Test                   299
Other Scans                                   301
   Salivary Gland Scan                        301
   Testicular or Scrotal Scan                 301
   Vein Scan                                  302

**8.  Ultrasound**                            303

Abdominal Ultrasound                          304
   Abdominal Aorta                            304
   Liver                                      305
   Gallbladder                                305
   Spleen                                     305
   Pancreas                                   306
   Kidneys                                    306
Thyroid Ultrasound                            306
Pelvic Ultrasound                             307
Doppler Ultrasound                            309

**9.  Scoping Procedures:
    Looking Inside Your Body**               311

Arthroscopy                                   312
Bronchoscopy                                  315
Colonoscopy                                   319
Cystoscopy                                    322
Laparoscopy                                   325
Laryngoscopy                                  329
Mediastinoscopy                               331
Ophthalmoscopy                                333
Sigmoidoscopy                                 335
Upper Gastrointestinal Endoscopy              338

**10.  Biopsies and Taps**                    343

*Biopsies*                                    343
Bone Biopsy                                   344
Bone Marrow Biopsy and
   Aspiration                                 346
Kidney Biopsy                                 348
Liver Biopsy                                  351
Lung Biopsy                                   353
Lymph Node Biopsy                             356
Skin Biopsy                                   357
Thyroid Biopsy                                359

*Taps*                                        362
Abdominal Tap                                 362
Joint Tap                                     363
Pleural Tap                                   365
Spinal Tap                                    367

**11.  Other Tests**                          371

Allergy Testing                               371
Cystometrogram                                373
Electroencephalogram                          375
Electromyogram and Nerve
   Conduction Studies                         375
Glaucoma Tests                                379

Hair Analysis 381
Hearing Tests (Audiometry) 382
Impedance Plethysmography 384
Magnetic Resonance Imaging 385
Pulmonary Function Tests 387
Sweat Test 389
Vision Tests 390

## III. Home Medical Tests 393

### 1. Self-Examination 396
Body Temperature Measurement 396
Pulse Measurement and Fitness
    Testing 400
Home Vision Tests 403
Home Ear Examination 409
Self-Exam for Dental Plaque 412
Home Blood Pressure Monitoring 413
Self-Testing for Lung Function 418

### 2. Self-Diagnostic Tests 421
Home Urinalysis 421
Self-Testing for Urinary Tract
    Infections 428
Home Pregnancy Tests 431
Home Blood Glucose Monitoring 434
Home Throat Cultures 438
Self-Test for Breath Alcohol 441
Home Screening for Bowel Cancer 443
Self-Test for Bowel Transit Time 446
Home-Test for Pinworms 447

## IV. Medical Tests for Healthy People 449

*Appendices* 464
1. Anesthesia 465
2. Medical Tests: Your Personal
    Record 468
3. Reader Survey 469

*For More Information* 474

Index 477

# Understanding Medical Tests

**D**o I really need this test? Exactly what will they do to me? Will it hurt? What are the risks? How should I prepare myself? What do the results mean?

Sometime, somewhere, you will be confronted with these and other questions regarding medical tests. Each year over 10 billion medical tests are performed in the United States alone: that works out to more than 40 tests per person per year.

For some this will mean a simple blood or urine test. Others will undergo more complex procedures: biopsies, taps, scans, x-rays, catheterizations, electronic monitoring, and various procedures in which scopes are used to peer inside the body. It seems that no orifice or body cavity is beyond the reach of needles or scoping instruments. Automated machines stand ready to analyze every bodily fluid down to the most minute component.

We may be forgiven if we sometimes stand in awe of these medical marvels. But we would be more fools than innocents if we failed to ask responsible questions when doctors suggest one of these powerful, potentially dangerous, and sometimes extremely expensive techniques.

## Informed Choice

You may be surprised to learn that except for life-threatening emergencies, doctors cannot order medical tests without your permission. In practice, most doctors simply order tests without much explanation.

And most patients go along with such "orders," never exercising their right to ask questions or make the final decision. For tests that involve significant risk, your doctor is required by law to obtain a signed statement of your informed consent to perform the test:

> When a given procedure inherently involves a known risk of death or serious bodily harm, a medical doctor has a duty to disclose to his patient the potential of death or serious harm, and to explain in lay terms the complications that might possibly occur. (Cobbs *vs*. Grant, 8 Cal 3rd, 229, 1972.)

Doctors also have a legal requirement to explain to you the potential consequences of refusing to have a recommended diagnostic procedure or screening test.

However, the final decision about having or not having any diagnostic test is always *yours*. This book was written to help you exercise that responsibility.

For some tests you need only assure yourself that the test is necessary and safe. For example, if your doctor recommends a simple blood test, a few brief questions should provide you with all the information you need. However, if the test is complex, expensive, or potentially harmful, you would be well advised to read up on the test in some detail and prepare a list of any unanswered questions.

The following questions are those we think anyone should ask before undergoing a medical test.

# Do I Need This Test?

The first and most important question should be whether you really need the test at all. Before agreeing to any test you should ask your doctor, "What will we do if the test results are abnormal?" and "What will we do if the results are normal?" If the answer to both questions is the same, you probably do not need the test.

Your doctor should be able to explain to your satisfaction how the test results will help diagnose your problem or change the planned therapy. Answers like "Because you need it" or "Because it's a test we usually do in this kind of situation" are not satisfactory. Here's an example of a better explanation: "I'm recommending that you have a barium enema because you've been passing some blood in your stool. We know from a previous test that the blood is not due to hemorrhoids, so we need to find the source of the bleeding. It might be something quite harmless, but it could also be some serious problem which needs prompt and appropriate treatment."

## Avoiding Unnecessary Testing

Unnecessary tests not only are a waste of money but also expose you to unnecessary discomfort, inconvenience, and risk. Some investigators believe that as many as 9% of all tests are performed by doctors to protect themselves from the threat of malpractice suits. An American Medical Association survey revealed that at least three out of every four doctors admitted ordering tests for the sole purpose of having a better defense in the event of a subsequent malpractice trial.[1] Such concerns are not totally unjustified. Some patients and juries expect doctors to do "everything" possible to diagnose a condition. These sometimes unrealistic expectations understandably place doctors under pressure to order tests to protect themselves.

Unnecessary tests may also be ordered because they are profitable. In general, doctors are not paid for their time, but rather for what they *do*. That is, many doctors earn more by ordering tests or performing procedures than by taking the same amount of time to question, examine, counsel, or think about a patient's problem. Further, physicians may be under pressure to order a certain number of tests to help justify or pay for new medical equipment. While such financial considerations may not be in the forefront of the doctor's mind, they still can subtly influence the ordering of tests.

Patient demand, real or presumed, also helps determine how many tests are done. Many patients feel that more tests mean better care. We often hear comments like "My doctor is so thorough, he did nearly every test available." While it is undoubtedly true that having tests done can provide some comfort and reassurance,[2] a diagnosis can most often be made based on asking questions (a history), a physical examination, and the clinical judgment of an experienced physician. In one study a careful history alone allowed a correct diagnosis in over 80% of the patients. Laboratory test results led to a change in diagnosis in only 10% of cases.[3] In another study routine blood and urine tests contributed to less than 1% of all diagnoses.[4]

## Screening Tests

Screening tests are intended to detect disease before symptoms appear. Doctors and patients alike tend to assume that if a few tests are good, more must be better. However, extensive screening can create more problems than it detects.

For example, most normal values for blood and urine tests are designed so that 95% of healthy people will receive normal results. This means that for each test done, 5% of *healthy* people will receive "abnormal" or "borderline" results. So, if you have twelve separate tests performed, you stand about a 50% chance of having an "abnormal" result—even if you are perfectly healthy. Most of these falsely abnormal results will fall within normal limits if you are retested, but retesting can be costly and inconvenient. Also, the falsely abnormal results may produce needless anxiety. Furthermore, studies show that when most doctors are confronted with unexpected abnormal lab results in the absence of symptoms, they tend to ignore them anyway.[5]

Several large scientific studies have failed to show much benefit from this "shotgun" approach to laboratory screening. With few exceptions (see Medical Tests for Healthy People later in the book), routine screening tests, including the panels of tests reflexively ordered when a patient enters a hospital, contribute little—except to medical bills.

### Ask About Alternatives

One way to help avoid unnecessary medical tests is to ask your doctor what alternatives are available. If you have already had a proposed test, ask if the previous results will be sufficient. Every effort should then be made to obtain your previous results. This is one reason it is useful to keep a record of all the diagnostic tests you have had, when and where they were performed, and what the results were (see Appendix, Medical Tests: Your Personal Record).

If a test involves considerable risk, discomfort or inconvenience, ask your doctor if there is an alternative test. For example, ultrasound can now often be used instead of x-rays in certain situations. Home diagnostic tests can sometimes be used instead of or as an adjunct to office or laboratory testing (see later section, Home Medical Tests).

Another alternative to certain tests may be a thorough interview and physical examination by your doctor. And sometimes the best test is the test of time. Waiting and watching the symptoms under a doctor's supervision for a certain period may provide the necessary clue to the diagnosis. Or the symptoms may resolve on their own, making tests unnecessary.

For each of the tests described in this book, we have included a discussion of the situations in which the test is usually performed. This should be taken as a very rough guideline. Discuss your particular case with your doctor.

Remember, the key questions are "Do I need this test?" and "How will the results of this test change my treatment?"

# How Should I Prepare for This Test?

Many medical procedures require that you do certain things before the test begins. This preparation is often critical to the proper performance and interpretation of the test. Some tests cannot be performed at all if you do not prepare properly.

For each of the tests in this book we have included a description of the things you should do before having the test. This includes certain important information you should tell your doctor before the test: Are you taking any medications, prescription or over-the-counter? Do you have allergies to any medications, anesthetics, or x-ray contrast materials? Have you ever had bleeding problems? Is there a possibility that you might be pregnant? If your doctor doesn't ask you about these things, make sure you bring them up.

With some tests you will be given instructions not to eat or drink anything before the test. This is often referred to as "NPO" (*nulla per os*) or "nothing by mouth." If you are taking medications, be sure to ask if you should continue taking them before the test.

Your physician should also tell you when you will need someone to drive you home after a certain type of test, or when you might want to bring along something to occupy yourself during long waiting periods.

The specific preparation instructions for each test depend upon the type of test and where and by whom it is performed. Preparation instructions may vary somewhat from the suggestions listed in the book, so be sure to check with your doctor or the hospital department where the test will be done. If you don't fully understand the preparation procedure, be sure to ask about it.

# How Is the Test Performed?

You should know in advance exactly what will happen during the test. This allows you to ask more specific questions and to be aware of what to expect. It may also help allay some anxiety or concerns about the test.

Understanding the procedure also helps you cooperate during and after the test; this cooperation can be critical to the accuracy and safety of many procedures.

For each procedure you should know where and by whom the test is performed, what happens during the test, how long it

takes, and what you should do after the test. The exact procedure may vary from place to place and doctor to doctor, so be sure to review the planned procedure with your doctor or hospital staff member before the test begins.

# How Will the Test Feel?

When asked if a certain test will hurt, doctors often say, "This won't hurt a bit" or "You won't feel a thing." If you ask patients about the test you may hear a different story. Many doctors simply don't know how the test feels. Others may downplay the discomfort to avoid alarming you or discouraging you from undergoing a necessary procedure.

We disagree with this approach. Studies suggest that if the procedure is discussed with you in advance, including specific information on what physical sensations to expect, you will have less anxiety and discomfort before and during the test.[6,7]

To get a better answer to the question "How will it feel?" we interviewed over 300 patients who underwent various diagnostic tests. We asked them to describe in detail their sensations, anxieties and concerns during and after the test. We include information and comments from these patients in many test descriptions to give you a better sense of what to expect. We also invite you to share your experience of diagnostic tests with us (see Reader Survey in the Appendix).

We learned some fascinating things from these patient interviews. We found that health professionals tend to seriously underestimate the impact of tests on patients. The doctor may observe the patient for only a few minutes during a test and may not be fully aware of the inconvenience or discomfort the patient experiences before and after the procedure.

We also found that patients tend to overestimate the discomfort of most procedures, preparing for the worst. We frequently heard "It wasn't nearly as bad as I thought" or "The anticipation of the test was much worse than the test itself." Sometimes the anxiety was fueled by misinformation about what would happen during the test. The discomfort of many patients is due more to anxiety about the test results ("What will it show?") than to the discomfort of the procedure itself.

With certain tests, particularly those that involve the genital or rectal area, the discomfort may be due more to embarrassment than to pain. During these tests it is helpful to remember that your doctor and the staff are usually quite accustomed to the test and its potential embarrassments. If you are particularly anxious, a brief discussion about your concerns before the exam is often helpful.

Some patients experience discomfort during a test which is not due to the test itself but to their medical condition. For example, if you have back pain you may find it particularly uncomfortable to lie on an x-ray or exam table. You should discuss with your doctor how your particular medical condition may affect the test and how any potential discomfort can be minimized.

The sensation patients experience during many tests varies considerably with the skill, experience, sensitivity, and gentleness of the doctor or technician performing the test. Patients who have a great deal of confidence in their physician are able to relax more during the test and in general experience less discomfort.

During the test it is important that you let the doctor or assistants know what you are feeling. Your sensations may provide a clue to a complication. If you are uncomfortable, there is usually something that can be done to bring relief. But if you don't speak up or signal your doctor, there is no way he or she can help you.

For each of the tests described we have included a section called "How Does It Feel?" This includes the physical sensations (sights, sounds, smells, tastes, and feelings) that patients commonly report during and after the tests. We also mention the symptoms you might experience after the test and when you should notify your doctor.

## What Are the Risks?

The decision to have any test should always include a consideration of the balance between potential benefits and risks.

All tests have risks. Even if the test itself presents no risk, an inaccurate result can lead to a missed diagnosis as well as delayed or inappropriate treatment. Certain test findings can result in "labeling" you as diseased, provoking needless anxiety and even causing problems obtaining employment or insurance. For example, several studies have shown that the misdiagnosis of heart disease in children resulted in significant restriction of activity and intellectual development.[8,9] Even labeling adults as "hypertensive" can lead to increased absenteeism from work over and above the effects of the increased blood pressure itself.[10]

Of course, medical tests can also have direct physical risks. Anytime the body is penetrated by a needle, tube, or viewing instrument there is some risk of infection, bleeding, or damage to vital structures. Even frequent blood drawing, the bane of many hospitalized patients, can result in a significant cumulative blood loss and ane-mia.[11,12] The hazards of radiation exposure, even though modest, must also be considered (see p. 227). Reactions to anesthetics, drugs or contrast materials also produce complications, which on rare occasions can lead to death.

Unfortunately, there is little scientific information available on the frequency and severity of complications due to specific diagnostic tests,[13] but we do know that complications from diagnostic tests are significantly underreported. One study revealed that 14% of patients undergoing such invasive diagnostic procedures as cardiac catheterization, pleural tap, bronchoscopy, and liver biopsy developed at least one complication. Over three fourths of these complications required specific therapy, prolonged hospitalization, or both.[14]

For each of the tests in this book we describe the known risks and complications. When possible we provide estimates of how frequent those complications are (e.g., 1 in 100, 1 in 10,000). Your risks, however, will vary depending upon your age, general state of health, past medical history, the skill and experience of your doctor and the other staff members, and your ability to cooperate. You should discuss with your doctor the likely risks in your specific situation.

# What Do the Results Mean?

The meaning of test results depends on two factors: the accuracy of the test and how the test results relate to other information about your state of health.

## Testing a Test

No test is 100% accurate. The accuracy depends on the nature of the test itself, how it is performed, and how it is interpreted. The purpose of all medical tests is to help distinguish those who are sick from those who are well. How successfully a test is able to achieve this can be described using three terms: *sensitivity*, *specificity*, and *predictive value*. An understanding of these concepts is important to appreciating the usefulness and limits of tests.[15,16]

*Sensitivity* is the ability of a test to correctly detect the disease when it is present. For example, if you have a certain disease, sensitivity refers to the probability that the test will show that you have that abnormality. Suppose a test has a sensitivity of 90%, very good as tests go. This means that if 100 people with the disease are tested, 90 will have abnormal (positive) results. However, this also means that 10% of people with the disease will *not* be detected by the test. In other words, 10% of those with the disease will show a *false-negative* test result—they have the disease but have normal (negative) test results.

*Specificity* refers to the ability of a test to correctly identify those people who do *not* have a disease. Clearly, a test would not be very useful if it was frequently abnormal in those who were healthy. If a test with a specificity of 90% is given to 100 healthy people, 10 healthy people will have *false-positive* results—that is, the test will be positive (abnormal) even though no disease is actually present.

*Predictive value* is defined as the probability that a positive (abnormal) test result will be accurate, meaning that you actually have the disease. This value is regarded as the most meaningful way to measure a test's accuracy. The predictive value is very much influenced by the frequency (prevalence) of the disease being looked for. The rarer the disease, the greater the possibility that an abnormal result will be a false-positive.

An analogy may help. Suppose that you are going fishing for tuna. You obtain a net with holes of a certain size. All fish larger than the holes in the net will be caught while smaller fish will escape. This means that while you will catch all the larger tuna, you may miss some of the smaller ones. This is like a false-negative test—the tuna are present but the "net test" does not detect them.

You may also catch some other large fish, such as dolphin or shark, in your net. This is like a false-positive—you get a positive "net test" result but it is not what you were looking for. You then have to separate the tuna from the other large fish which can be a cumbersome and expensive procedure.

The overall success (predictive value) of your fishing expedition in catching tuna rather than dolphin or shark depends not only on the size of the holes in your net (sensitivity and specificity), but the number of tuna in the water in the first place. If there are few tuna, then most of the fish you catch might be those you don't want. However, if tuna are plentiful you are likely to come away with a good catch. Similarly, an accurate and valuable test is one that "catches" those people who have the condition being tested for, excludes those who do not, and is applied in a situation where sick people are likely to be found.

If all of this is not clear to you, you are not alone. A recent study of doctors in a leading medical center showed that fewer than one in five were able to correctly apply the concept of predictive value.[17] Nevertheless, these concepts are critical to understanding when a certain test should be performed and how to interpret the results.

## "Abnormal" Test Results Do Not Equal "Diseased"

When confronted with an abnormal test result the natural tendency is to assume that you are sick. However, this is often not the case.

First of all the abnormality may be a statistical fluke. Due to limitations in the specificity of the test, a certain percentage of *healthy* people tested will automatically have abnormal results (false-positives). For example, the "normal" or reference values for many blood and urine tests are established by testing healthy volunteers, often young laboratory workers, medical students, or blood donors. The "normal" range of values is then constructed to include 95% of those "healthy" people. However, this means that 5% (one in twenty) healthy people will have abnormal values on any given lab test. A "normal" person has been defined, somewhat in jest, as one who has not been sufficiently investigated.

The range of normal values used may not be appropriate for you. Since these reference values are usually set up by testing young, white, healthy volunteers, the results may not indicate a "healthy" range if you are older, of a different race, obese, or differ in some other significant way from the reference population. Your "abnormal" results may, therefore, mean that you are different from the norms but not necessarily diseased.

Normal values also vary considerably from laboratory to laboratory depending upon the type of equipment, calibration, and methods used. Therefore, test results from one laboratory cannot necessarily be compared with results from another laboratory even on the same test. In this book we give examples of normal values taken from a standard textbook on laboratory medicine.[18] Your results may require a different range of normal values for interpretation. Consult your doctor or laboratory for the appropriate standards.

Several other factors can affect your laboratory test results.

*Diet*: The results of some laboratory tests will vary considerably depending upon when and what you have eaten. For example, blood glucose (sugar) levels vary considerably depending upon how long it has been since you have eaten.

*Drugs*: Nearly every drug—including prescription medications, over-the-counter drugs, illegal drugs, alcohol, and tobacco—can have an effect, sometimes profound, on laboratory tests. This is one reason it is always important to report to your doctor any drugs you are taking, since these may affect the interpretation of test results.

*Activity*: Exercise and even posture (whether you have been lying down or sitting up) can significantly alter certain lab tests. For example, the finding of red blood cells in your urine may be a sign of serious kidney disease, but may also be due to vigorous exercise.

*Stress*: Emotional stress can also influence laboratory tests.

*Time of day*: Many physiological functions, and therefore laboratory values, vary rhythmically. For example, many hormone values will reach peak values at specific times of the day.

*Specimen collection*: Results can also be affected by how the specimen is collected and handled. For example, if the tourniquet is left on your arm too long while a blood sample is being drawn, the results may be altered.

Interfering factors such as these are discussed for each test in this book to alert you to possible sources of variation in the test results.

## Laboratory Error

Test results may also be inaccurate due to laboratory error. A small degree of variation in laboratory instruments and reagents will create some unavoidable variation in test results. However, even in the most carefully managed laboratories 2%–5% of results are erroneous due to clerical errors such as mislabeling or other mistakes such as using inappropriate methods.[19] Further, physician's office laboratories are on average considerably less accurate than government-inspected and -regulated hospital commercial laboratories.[20]

## Disagreements in Interpretation

Many tests require subjective interpretation and are therefore more likely to show variability. For example, in a study of the reading of chest x-rays, over 70% of reports contained disagreements among experienced radiologists. In 25% of the reports important findings were missed.[21] Other researchers have found that radiologists failed to spot 20%–50% of lung cancers visible on chest x-rays. They concluded that an error rate in interpretation of approximately 30% is unavoidable.[22]

It appears that on most tests that require interpretation, physicians will disagree at least 10%–20% of the time.[23] This is one good reason to seek an experienced second opinion on test results, particularly when potentially dangerous therapies or procedures are recommended on the basis of test findings.

## "Normal" Test Results Do Not Equal "Healthy"

Owing to the limitations in the sensitivity of tests, a certain percentage of people will have false-negative results—that is, the test result will be normal (negative) even though the person really is sick. Furthermore, each of us has our own biochemical individuality. Changes in the values of certain lab tests may be a sign of disease even if the results still fall within the normal limits. Therefore, current tests may be understood better when interpreted in light of your previous results.

Another reason why you may be sick and still have normal test results derives from the definition of normal. Normal usually means average—that is, you will be compared with average values characteristic for the population. However, normal doesn't necessarily mean optimal, healthy, or desirable. For example, you might have a "normal" (average) blood pressure or cholesterol level but lower levels may actually be healthier. As one observer commented, "It is 'normal' to die of heart disease in the United States."

Tests don't always provide answers. Even when extensive testing is performed, a specific diagnosis is not always reached. For example, 121 patients were admitted to one hospital for the evaluation of fainting. The list of investigations to which these patients were subjected included ECG monitoring, echocardiograms, cardiac catheterization, EEG, CT scans, brain scans, lumbar punctures, cerebral angiography, and glucose tolerance tests. At the end of this marathon of testing a definitive cause for the fainting was established in only 13 of the 121 patients.[24]

Given the potential for errors and variation in medical tests, repeating most non-invasive abnormal tests is usually advised before taking action. Too often patients are labeled as having a certain disease on the basis of a single test. Repeating the test may well "cure" the "disease."

In interpreting any test result it is essential to remember that medical tests are only one part of the picture, and often not the most important part. Your tests must always be viewed in the context of other information available about you: your past medical history, family, age, sex, habits, use of medications, symptoms, and physical examination. Doctors should treat patients, not test results. All medical tests just provide diagnostic clues. These clues must be put together with other sources of information about you to understand the significance of the results in your case.

Finally, we've mentioned the terms "positive" and "negative" in referring to test results. The meaning of these terms often depends upon context. "Positive" usually refers to the presence of a specific finding, usually an abnormality, and "negative" refers to the absence of such findings. If you are told your chest x-ray is "negative," this means that it is normal. However, with some tests a "positive" result is desirable. For instance, if you have a positive rubella titer on a screening blood test, this means that you are appropriately immunized against German measles. So don't be mislead by "positive" or "negative" results. Find out exactly what the results mean for you.

# What Does the Test Cost?

Our yearly bill for medical tests in the United States includes $30 billion for laboratory tests, $20 billion for x-rays, $50 billion for other diagnostic procedures, and $40 billion in medical visits for diagnostic purposes. The total: a staggering $140 billion per year, or over $600 for every man, woman, and child. Diagnostic tests and evaluations account for nearly one half of our total health care bill.[25]

Even though you may not be paying for all these medical tests directly, all of us end up paying more in higher insurance premiums, membership fees in prepaid health plans, hospital and doctor's charges, and higher taxes. Even low-cost tests such as routine blood and urine tests can add up when performed frequently.[26]

Most people, doctors included, don't know how much tests cost. Studies show that when doctors are asked to estimate the cost of various tests the results are far off the mark.[27] How cost-conscious are you? As an exercise we invite you to test yourself by trying to estimate the cost of some common tests (see table).

---

### Guess How Much These Tests Cost

1. Complete blood count (CBC)   \_\_\_\_\_
2. Complete urinalysis   \_\_\_\_\_
3. Serum cholesterol   \_\_\_\_\_
4. Electrocardiogram   \_\_\_\_\_
5. Bacterial culture with antibiotic sensitivity testing   \_\_\_\_\_
6. Chest x-ray   \_\_\_\_\_
7. CT scan (head)   \_\_\_\_\_
8. Upper GI series x-ray   \_\_\_\_\_
9. Bronchoscopy   \_\_\_\_\_
10. Cardiac catheterization   \_\_\_\_\_

Answers:
1. $10   2. $10   3. $10   4. $40
5. $40   6. $50   7. $300   8. $100
9. $400   10. $2000

---

For each of the tests in this book we provide a range of typical charges. These approximate cost figures are based on a 1985 survey of various doctors and hospitals. Many factors can influence the actual charges. The cost of the same test may vary depending on whether the test is performed in a hospital, commercial labora- tory, or doctor's office. Tests done in hospitals often cost more, as profits from the laboratory are sometimes used to make up for losses in other areas of the hospital. Costs also vary by geographical location, whether the test is performed by a specialist, and whether the person is having the test as an inpatient or an outpatient.

Knowing the cost of a test should not deter you or your physician from recommending it if it is necessary. On the other hand, the dollar cost of the test should be one factor in estimating the costs and risks of a test against which to balance the potential benefits. In the end, we are all paying for the tests, and at a minimum we should know what we are paying for.

■

Medical tests sometimes save lives, but in other cases they may be unnecessary or actually harmful. A frank, informed discussion between you and your doctor is the best way to decide whether tests are needed and what the results might mean. The information provided in this book will help you take an active and informed role in this vital aspect of your health care.

## References

1. Why most MDs practice "defensive medicine." *American Medical News* 1977;20 (March 28):33.
2. Sox HC, Margulies I, Sox CH: Psychologically mediated effects of diagnostic tests. *Annals of Internal Medicine* 1981;95:680–685.
3. Hampton JR, Harrison MJG, Mitchell JRA, et al: Relative contributions of history-taking, physical examination, and laboratory investigation to diagnosis and management of medical

outpatients. *British Medical Journal* 1975;(May 31):486−489.

4. Sandler G: Costs of unnecessary tests. *British Medical Journal* 1979; (July 7):21−24.

5. Schneiderman LJ, DeSalvo L, Baylor S, et al: The "abnormal" screening laboratory results: Its effect on physician and patient. *Archives of Internal Medicine* 1972;129:88−90.

6. McHugh NG, Christman NJ, Johnson JE: Preparatory information: what helps and why. *American Journal of Nursing* 1982;(May):780−782.

7. Anderson KO, Masur FT: Psychological preparation for invasive medical and dental procedures. *Journal of Behavioral Medicine* 1983;6:1−40.

8. Bergman A, Stamm S: The morbidity of cardiac non-disease in schoolchildren. *New England Journal of Medicine* 1967;276:1008.

9. Cayler G, et al: The effect of cardiac "non-disease" on intellectual and perceptual motor development. *British Heart Journal* 1973;35:543.

10. Haynes RB, Sackett DL, Taylor DW, et al: Increased absenteeism from work after detection and labeling of hypertensive patients. *New England Journal of Medicine* 1978;299:741−744.

11. Rosenzweig AL: Iatrogenic anemia. *Archives of Internal Medicine* 1978; 138:1843.

12. Hashimoto F: Bleeding less for diagnostics (letter). *Journal of the American Medical Association* 1982;248:171.

13. Flegel K, Oseasohn R: Adverse effects of diagnostic tests: a study of the quality of reporting. *Archives of Internal Medicine* 1982;142:883−887.

14. Schroeder SA, Marton KI, Strom BL: Frequency and morbidity of invasive procedures. *Archives of Internal Medicine* 1978;138:1809−1811.

15. Riegelman RK: *Studying a Study and Testing a Test*. New York: Little, Brown and Company, 1981.

16. Krieg AF, Gambino R, Galen RS: Why are clinical laboratory tests performed? When are they valid? *Journal of the American Medical Association* 1975;233:76−78.

17. Casscells W, Schoenberger A, Graboys TB: Interpretation by physicians of clinical laboratory results. *New England Journal of Medicine* 1978;299:999−1001.

18. Henry JB (ed.): *Clinical Diagnosis and Management by Laboratory Methods* (17th edition). Philadelphia: W.B. Saunders Co., 1984.

19. Brecher G: Put lab tests to the test. *Physician's Management* 1981;(April): 57−64.

20. Physician-office lab results less accurate than those of licensed labs, study shows. *Medical World News* 1984;(April 9):46−47.

21. Herman PG, Gerson DE, Hessel SJ, et al: Disagreements in chest roentgen interpretation. *Chest* 1975;68:278−282.

22. Forrest JV, Friedman PJ: Radiological errors in patients with lung cancer. *Western Journal of Medicine* 1981; 134;485−490.

23. Koran LM: The reliability of clinical methods, data, and judgments. *New England Journal of Medicine* 1975; 293:642−646, 695−701.

24. Kapoor WN, Karpf M, Maher Y, et al: Syncope of unknown origin. *Journal of the American Medical Association* 1982;247:2687−2691.

25. Pinckney ER: The accuracy and significance of medical testing. *Archives of Internal Medicine* 1983;143:512−514.

26. Fineberg HV: Clinical chemistries: the high cost of low-cost diagnostic tests, in *Medical Technology: The Culprit Be-*

*hind Health Care Costs?* Proceedings of the 1977 Sun Valley Forum on National Health. DHEW Publication No. (PHS)79−3216, 1977.

27. Robertson WO: Costs of diagnostic tests: Estimates by health professionals. *Medical Care* 1980;18:556−559.

# Medical Diagnostic Tests

# 1 Testing Your Blood and Urine

## Testing Your Blood

The blood is a unique organ. It is made up of two parts—the blood cells and the liquid in which the blood cells are carried. About 40%–50% of the volume of whole blood is made up of cells: red blood cells (which carry oxygen to the tissues), white cells (which fight infection), and platelets (which help the blood clot).

The liquid portion of unclotted blood is called *plasma*. It contains hundreds of dissolved substances—minerals and vitamins, gases, sugars, hormones, antibodies, fats, proteins, and traces of foods and drugs. The blood is the body's main transportation system for getting these substances to the cells. When blood has been allowed to clot, some of the dissolved substances become part of the clot. The remaining liquid is called *serum*.

One group of blood tests, *blood chemistries*, includes all the tests of substances dissolved in the blood fluid. Another group, *hematologic tests*, looks at the size, shape, and other characteristics of the blood cells

themselves. *Serologic testing* analyzes your blood for antibodies, immune complexes, antigen-antibody reactions.

Groups of tests frequently ordered together include the following:

*Complete blood count*: red blood cell count, white blood cell count, differential white count, hematocrit, hemoglobin, red cell indices, platelet count.

*Electrolytes*: sodium, potassium, carbon dioxide, chloride.

*Liver function tests*: alkaline phosphatase, lactic dehydrogenase, serum glutamic oxalacetic transaminase (SGOT), serum glutamic pyruvic transaminase (SGPT), bilirubin, $5^1$-nucleotidase, serum leucine aminopeptidase, serum protein, prothrombin time.

*Thyroid function tests*: free thyroxine index (FTI), $T_3$ level, $T_3$ uptake, $T_4$ level, thyroid-stimulating hormone (TSH).

Although a few tests may be performed at the doctor's office, most are sent to a specialized laboratory where the tests are performed by large automatic machines. Since different laboratories sometimes use different testing procedures, it is not always possible to compare results on the same test from two different facilities.

If the laboratory doing the tests is nearby, results on most tests are usually available within 24 hours. If the sample must be sent to a distant lab, results may take longer. A few tests—especially studies of immune function—may take longer.

# Collecting a Blood Sample

Blood samples for laboratory testing are most frequently obtained by means of a needle inserted into a vein—usually one of the veins on the front of the arm, opposite the elbow. This procedure is called *venipuncture.*

Veins rather than arteries are usually used because they are closer to the surface and more easily accessible. Any vein close to the skin can be used. Other commonly used venipuncture sites include the veins on the back of the hands and the veins on the ankles and feet.

A few tests require a sample of blood from an artery. These samples are obtained by an *arterial stick* (see p. 37). In some cases a blood sample is obtained by a *fingerstick* (see p. 37).

Blood may be drawn in a doctor's office, clinic, laboratory, hospital, or at home. Samples are usually collected by a doctor, nurse, lab technician, or blood-drawing technician (phlebotomist). Samples from some home tests can be collected by the person performing the test (see Home Blood Glucose Monitoring, in Part III).

No special preparation is needed for the blood drawing itself. However, some blood tests do require specific preparations on your part, e.g., fasting, avoiding certain foods, or eating certain foods—see the "preparation" sections for individual blood tests.

## Venipuncture

The person drawing blood will wrap an elastic band (tourniquet) around your upper arm tightly enough to stop the flow of blood through the veins. This makes the veins below the tourniquet bulge beneath the skin, making it easier to insert the needle. You may then be asked to make a fist, to open and close your hand repeatedly, or to squeeze a small, cylinder-shaped object. This muscular activity, along with the tourniquet, serves to force blood into the veins, making them larger, more visible, and easier to enter with the needle.

The venipuncture site is cleaned with an antiseptic solution, usually alcohol, and the needle is inserted into the vein.

When the needlepoint is properly placed within the vein, the blood will flow into the syringe or vacuum container attached to the needle. If vacuum containers (vials) are used, the person drawing blood may remove blood-filled vials from the needle holder and replace them with empty vials while the needle is still in place. (The colored tops on the different vials indicate what preservative, if any, is within the container.) Several differently colored vials may be drawn at once so that a separate vial can be sent to different areas of the laboratory; each area performs a different type of test (e.g., chemistry, hematology, serology, etc.).

Once the sample has been collected the tourniquet is released and a gauze pad or cotton ball is placed over the venipuncture site as the needle is withdrawn. You will then be asked to maintain pressure on the gauze for a few minutes to help stop the bleeding. A small bandage is then applied.

It is easier to draw blood on some people than others. If health workers have had difficulty drawing your blood in the past, it's a good idea to say something like, "People have had trouble drawing blood from me before. Last time they found that the veins in the backs of my hands were the easiest place to get it," or whatever applies to your own situation.

If you have ever fainted or nearly fainted during a blood test, let the person drawing your blood know. They will arrange for you to lie down while the sample is collected. This will prevent faintness or lightheadedness. If you feel faint after the test, lower your head for a few minutes.

You may feel nothing at all from the venipuncture, or you may feel a brief pain, frequently described as a "sting" or a "pinch," as the needle goes through the skin. Most people report no pain at all once the needle is in place. Others experience a mild discomfort. The degree of pain felt depends on the skill of the person drawing blood, the condition of your veins, and your sensitivity to pain.

There is very little risk of serious complications of venipuncture, but it is not unusual to experience some bruising at the venipuncture site. You can reduce the risk of bruising by keeping a firm pressure on the site for about five minutes after the needle is withdrawn.

Continued bleeding may be a problem for people with bleeding disorders. If you have bleeding or clotting problems, be sure to let the person drawing your blood know. Very rarely, the vein may become inflamed (phlebitis) after a blood sample is taken. This is usually treated with a warm, moist compress.

There is no separate charge for venipuncture. It is included in the fee for the blood test.

### Fingerstick

In a fingerstick sample, a drop or two of blood is taken from a finger, a heel (in babies), or an earlobe, by lancing the skin of the chosen area with a tiny sterile needle or lancet. This procedure is frequently used for obtaining blood for anemia testing (hematocrit) and for determining your blood type (blood typing). This procedure can also be done at home.

### Arterial Stick

This sample is most frequently taken from the inside of the wrist. You will be asked to sit with your arm extended and your wrist on a small pillow. The examiner will rotate your hand back and forth and will feel for the pulse in your wrist, just below the base of your thumb. He or she will then cleanse the area and may inject a small amount of local anesthetic before inserting the needle into the artery to collect the blood sample. After the needle is removed a bandage will be placed over the puncture site and firm pressure will be applied for five minutes or longer. If an adequate sample is not obtained, the procedure will be repeated. Samples are sometimes taken from the groin.

You will feel a brief, sharp pain as the needle enters the artery. This procedure is more painful than a normal venipuncture because the arteries are deeper and have more nerves than the veins.

Arterial blood samples are used to measure the amount of oxygen, carbon dioxide, and acidity of arterial blood (see p. 50).

## Testing Your Urine

Each time we urinate, we note almost unconsciously any unusual changes in the volume, frequency, color, or odor of the urine. Throughout the ages these and other characteristics of the urine have been used to diagnose illnesses. Thousands of years ago Chinese physicians were said to have poured the urine of patients with suspected diabetes onto the ground. Later they would look to see if ants were attracted by the sugar in the urine.

Today we can perform nearly a hundred different tests on urine. These tests not only tell us about the health of the kidney and urinary system, but also give clues to a wide range of endocrine and metabolic disorders which affect the entire body.

Consider for a moment the extraordinary job your kidneys perform. Each hour the kidneys filter the 5 to 6 quarts of blood in the body approximately 20 times. From the 1500 quarts of blood filtered each day, the kidney produces only about 1 to 2 quarts of urine. The remainder of the filtered blood is returned to the bloodstream. The kidneys must be highly discriminating organs; they must selectively excrete waste products while at the same time preserving vital substances the body needs. Blood cells, antibodies, enzymes, and proteins are normally not excreted in urine. Instead the urine contains a complex solution of certain minerals and metabolic waste products. The composition of this solution varies dramatically depending upon the time of day, posture, exercise, diet, fluid intake, and the metabolic activity of the billions of cells in the body.

# Collecting a Urine Specimen

An accurate urine test begins with proper collection of the specimen. Test results may be inaccurate if the specimen is collected at the wrong time, in the wrong amounts, stored improperly, or contaminated. This not only wastes time and money, but can lead to inappropriate further testing and treatment.

You will almost always be asked to collect the specimen yourself, so you can do a great deal to be sure it is done properly. Make sure you understand which of the following types of specimen are required and exactly how to collect and store it.

*Random specimen*: The random or spot urine specimen is the type most frequently requested. A few ounces (about one-quarter cup) of freshly voided urine are needed. This can be collected at any time of the day, but if the specimen is not taken to the lab within one hour, it should be refrigerated in a covered container. Any plastic or glass container will do, but it must be very clean and dry. Obviously, any residue in the container may contaminate the urine and cause inaccurate results.

*First morning specimen*: The first morning urine is usually more concentrated than specimens collected later in the day. This urine contains a higher concentration of materials excreted by the kidneys, and is thus more likely to reveal abnormalities. A urine pregnancy test, for example, is more accurate when the specimen is a highly concentrated morning specimen. Again, if it will be longer than one hour before the specimen is analyzed, then it should be refrigerated in a covered container.

*Second-voided specimen*: This type of specimen—also sometimes called a "double-voided" specimen—is preferred in testing for sugar and ketones in the urine of diabetics. The bladder is emptied completely and the urine discarded. A glass or two of liquid is consumed, and 30–40 minutes later a second (or double-voided) urine specimen is collected for testing. This second-voided specimen contains freshly produced urine and therefore more accurately reflects the amount of sugar or ketones in the blood at that moment. The first specimen might be misleading since it contains more concentrated urine, which may have been produced hours before.

*Timed specimens*: Since the content of the urine varies throughout the day and night, a single urine specimen may not give an accurate picture of the overall excretion of a given substance. Long-term specimens may be collected for periods of 2 hours, 12 hours, or most commonly 24 hours. A 24-hour urine specimen contains all the urine excreted in a 24-hour period. Instructions for collecting a 24-hour specimen are as follows:

1. The collection period usually starts in the morning. When you first get up, empty your bladder and *discard this first specimen*. Do not include this first specimen in the collection since you want to begin the test period with an empty bladder. Write down the time of this first voiding. This is the time the collection period starts.
2. For the next 24 hours collect, in a large gallon container, *all* the urine you produce. A container with a small amount of preservative in it is usually provided by your doctor or lab. Each time you urinate collect the urine in a small container and add it to the larger one. During the collection period keep the urine refrigerated in the closed container. Empty your bladder for the final collection just at or slightly before the end of the 24-hour collection period. Add this final specimen to the collection and write down the time. *It is essential that you remember to include absolutely all the urine you produce in the 24-hour period.* Put a sign on the toilet, tie a string on your finger, or devise some other type of reminder, but don't forget or the test results will be inaccurate.
3. Try to avoid getting any contaminants such as toilet paper, feces, or menstrual blood into the urine specimen. If you are having your menstrual period, notify your doctor and the test may be postponed.
4. Return the specimen to the laboratory.

Most often the collection of a urine specimen is straightforward. You simply urinate into a clean specimen container, bedpan, or bottle urinal. If you are having a problem obtaining a specimen on demand, try drinking a lot of fluids, listening to the sound of running water, or soaking your hand in warm water.

Sometimes special methods of collection are necessary.

### Clean-Catch Midstream Specimen

Urine specimens can sometimes contain more than urine. Vaginal secretions, menstrual blood, prostatic and urethral fluids, and bacteria from the urethra, vagina, or penis can contaminate the specimen and interfere with interpretation of the results. A special method of cleaning and collection of the urine specimen has been designed to help reduce any possible contamination.

A "clean-catch midstream" urine specimen is required for any urine tests looking for bacteria and infection in the urinary tract. However, since it is relatively easy to perform, it is becoming the standard collection method for most routine urinalyses.

*Procedure for Men*
1. Begin by washing your hands. Then open the lid of the sterile urine container and set the lid down with the inner surface facing up. Be careful not

to touch or contaminate the rim or inner surface of the lid or container by touching it.

2. Retract the foreskin of the penis and clean the head of the penis with two or three antiseptic saturated swabs, cotton balls, or towelettes. Wipe with a circular motion starting at the urinary opening and moving away in enlarging circles. Discard the used swabs and finish the cleaning with a dry swab to remove any excess antiseptic.

3. Begin urinating into the toilet bowl or urinal. After the urine has flowed for several seconds and without interrupting the flow, catch a few ounces of this "midstream" urine to fill the sterile container about two inches deep, and then finish urinating into the toilet bowl or urinal.

4. Replace the lid carefully onto the container and return the specimen to the lab. If it is not possible to deliver the specimen to the lab within one hour, refrigerate it.

*Procedure for Women*

1. Begin by washing your hands. Then open the lid of the sterile urine container and set the lid down with the inner surface facing up. Be careful not to touch or contaminate the rim or inner surface of the lid or container by touching it.

2. With your legs spread to the sides straddle the toilet bowl. Using the fingers of one hand separate and hold open the folds of skin outside the vagina (labia) to expose the urinary opening.

3. Clean the area around the urinary opening using three antiseptic swabs, cotton balls, or towelettes: one for each side of the opening and one for the opening itself. Wipe from *front to back*, using a single downward stroke to avoid

any contamination from the anal area. Discard each swab after one cleansing wipe. Complete the procedure by using a fresh swab to remove any excess antiseptic.

4. With your fingers still separating the labia, begin urinating into the toilet bowl. After the urine has flowed for several seconds and without interrupting the flow, catch a few ounces of this "midstream" urine to fill the sterile container about two inches deep. Avoid touching the rim of the container to the genital area. Then finish urinating into the toilet bowl.

5. Replace the lid carefully onto the container and return the specimen to the lab. If it is not possible to deliver the specimen to the lab within one hour, refrigerate it.

*Note*: If you are menstruating, let your doctor know. It may be advisable to postpone this urine test until after the end of your menstrual period. If it is necessary to do the test immediately, inserting a tampon may help prevent contamination of the specimen with menstrual blood or vaginal discharge.

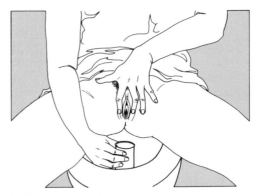

*Collecting a "mid-stream" or "clean-catch" urine specimen.*

## Urinary Catheterization

Sometimes it may be necessary to put a thin rubber tube (catheter) into the bladder in order to obtain a urine specimen. In addition to collecting a specimen for testing, the amount of "residual" urine left in the bladder after voiding can be measured. This method of collection is sometimes used if you are unable to void because of urinary obstruction.

You will be asked to undress from the waist down and to lie on your back. Sterile drapes will be placed around your urethra, and the health professional collecting the specimen will wear gloves to prevent introducing infection into the bladder.

*Men*: The head of the penis is cleansed with an antiseptic. A lubricated rubber tube, as thin as a pencil, is then inserted into the urethral opening. This catheter is slowly and gently advanced some 7–10 inches until the tip reaches the bladder. A specimen of urine is withdrawn through the hollow catheter, and then the catheter is removed.

*Women*: The urethral opening is cleansed. The catheter is then inserted 2 to 3 inches to reach the bladder. A specimen of urine is collected and the catheter withdrawn.

This procedure may be somewhat uncomfortable, particularly in men if there is difficulty moving the catheter past urethral strictures or narrowings. The entire procedure usually takes only a few minutes.

Urinary catheterization is not without risk. The most common complication is the introduction of bacteria into the bladder, resulting in a urinary tract infection which will have to be treated with antibiotics. This occurs in approximately 2%–3% of those undergoing urinary catheterization. In some cases the urinary catheter is left in for days or weeks to continuously drain the bladder. The longer it is left in place, the greater the risk of developing a bladder infection.

## Collecting Urine from Infants

Babies and infants just don't seem to urinate when you want them to (though they often do when you *don't* want them to). There is a urine collection device designed specially to solve this problem. It consists of a plastic bag with adhesive backing around the opening. This opening is fastened around the genital area and the bag then collects the urine whenever it comes. When a sufficient amount has been collected, usually within an hour, the bag is removed. The specimen can be contaminated by feces, powders, or creams used on the baby's skin.

## Bladder or Suprapubic Tap

Sometimes if a sterile urine specimen is required immediately, for example in a very ill infant, a needle may be inserted through the lower abdominal wall directly into the bladder. This method of collection does carry a very slight risk of bleeding, infection, or puncture of the intestines.

# Blood and Urine Tests

## Acid Phosphatase

Acid phosphatase is an enzyme found primarily in the male prostate gland and semen (although traces may be found in other organs). Acid phosphatase is normally present in very small or undetectable levels in the bloodstream. Its presence in significant amounts may indicate prostate cancer.

This test is performed on a venous blood sample (see p. 36).

### Why Performed:

This test is sometimes called the "male PAP test"—an acronym for "prostatic acid phosphatase." It is an important lab test for the detection of prostate cancer. It is also commonly used to follow the response of prostate cancer to treatment. If a digital (finger) exam of the rectum suggests an abnormality (most frequently a lump) in the prostate, this test is often performed to help determine whether cancer of the prostate is present.

### Normal Values:

Values may vary from lab to lab:
0.13 to 0.63 units per liter (U/l)

●*Greater Than Normal Values May Mean*: Significantly elevated values usually indicate prostate cancer which has spread outside the prostate. Very highly elevated values often reflect prostate cancer which has spread to bone. Only about 10% of cancers still confined to the prostate produce an elevated acid phosphatase, so normal levels do not exclude the possibility of prostate cancer.

The following conditions can also produce elevated levels: blockage of blood flow to the prostate, multiple myeloma, Paget's disease (softening and thickening of the bones), anemia, severe infections, thrombophlebitis, Gaucher's disease, hyperparathyroidism, sickle-cell crisis, pulmonary embolism, heart attack, kidney disease, and several other conditions.

Acid phosphatase may also be elevated after prostate exam, prostate massage, enemas, colonoscopies, or other physical stimulation of the prostate—so this test should not be performed for 48 hours after such procedures. A drop in acid phosphatase during treatment for prostate cancer indicates a good response to therapy.

### Interfering Factors:

Fluorides, oxalates, and alcohol can decrease acid phosphatase levels. Clofibrate (Atromid-S) and androgen hormones (in women) can increase them. Rough handling of the blood sample can produce inaccurate results.

### Cost:

$10 to $20

### Special Considerations:

★Most physicians consider an expert rectal exam the most accurate screening test for prostate cancer.

★Since semen contains acid phosphatase, vaginal fluid is sometimes tested for increased levels of acid phosphatase in cases of suspected rape to help determine whether intercourse with ejaculation occurred.

# Adrenocorticotropic Hormone (ACTH) (Adrenocortico-Stimulating Hormone)

Adrenocorticotropic hormone (ACTH) is produced in the pituitary gland. It stimulates the adrenal glands to produce cortisol (see p. 66). When blood cortisol levels increase, the ACTH levels in healthy people normally fall in response; when cortisol levels decrease, ACTH levels normally rise.

There is a normal daily variation in ACTH blood levels: levels are highest between 6 and 8 A.M. and lowest between 6 and 11 P.M. Thus if low ACTH levels are suspected, the blood sample is drawn between 6 and 8 A.M., but if excess secretion is suspected, the sample is drawn between 6 and 11 P.M.

### Why Performed:
This test is usually done when Cushing's disease (in which there is an increased production of ACTH) is suspected. Symptoms of this condition may include a round, reddish face, a heavy trunk with thin arms and legs, and wide purple stretch marks on the abdomen.

### Preparation:
You will be asked to fast and to limit your physical activity for 10–12 hours before the test. At some facilities, you may be asked to eat a high-carbohydrate diet for 2 days before the test. Since stress can increase

ACTH levels, you may be asked to lie quietly for 20–30 minutes before the blood sample is taken. Results of this test are usually available in 4–6 days.

### Normal Values:
Values and units may vary from lab to lab:
> 20–100 picograms per milliliter (pg/ml)

●*Greater Than Normal Values May Mean*: Emotional or physical stress (including surgery, severe pain, insulin-induced hypoglycemia), primary adrenal insufficiency (Addison's disease), Cushing's disease (hypersecretion of ACTH by pituitary adenoma), non-pituitary ACTH-secreting tumor.

●*Less Than Normal Values May Mean*: Decreased adrenal function due to adrenal cortisol-producing tumor or low pituitary function.

### Interfering Factors:
Failure to limit physical activity prior to the test or failure to follow recommended diet may interfere with the results. ACTH levels are decreased by cortisone and other steroid drugs and by drugs that increase cortisone secretion (including estrogens, amphetamines, alcohol, calcium gluconate, spironolactone). Blood lithium levels and pregnancy may also interfere with this test.

### Cost:
$100 to $120

### Special Considerations:
★Since ACTH is rapidly broken down, the sample should be placed in ice and taken to the laboratory immediately.

★ACTH stimulation testing—This test is sometimes used to confirm a diagnosis of adrenal insufficiency. First a baseline blood sample is taken. Next synthetic ACTH (cosyntropin) is injected. Samples are taken after 30 and 60 minutes. Cortisol normally increases after the injection. The absence of such an increase suggests a deficiency of the adrenal gland. (This test is sometimes called the ACTH rapid test.)

# Alcohol (Ethanol)

This test measures your blood alcohol (ethanol) level, and can be used to determine the extent of alcohol intoxication; it can be done for either medical or legal reasons. Highway patrol officers in most states now use devices which measure alcohol levels of the breath. (See Self-Test for Breath Alcohol, p. 441). Urine alcohol levels can also be measured, but the results are less accurate than blood or breath testing.

Alcohol is absorbed into the blood after a person has consumed any alcoholic beverage. Peak blood levels appear 30–70 minutes after the alcohol is consumed. About 90% of alcohol consumed is metabolized in the liver, and 10% is excreted unchanged in the breath and the urine.

If this test is being obtained for medicolegal reasons, a consent form may be required, but refusal to agree to the test may have legal consequences in some states.

**Why Performed:**
This test is done when intoxication is suspected because of coma, disorientation, disequilibrium, or unsafe driving behavior.

**Normal Values:**
0 milligrams per 100 deciliters (mg/dl)

**Cost:**
$25 to $40

## Clinical Effects of Alcohol

| Number of Drinks | Blood Alcohol Level (wt/vol) | (mg/dl) | Clinical Effect |
|---|---|---|---|
| 1–2 | .05% | 25 | relaxation |
| 3 | .10 | 50 | sedation, tranquility |
| 6 | .15 | 100 | slurred speech, poor coordination, thinking slowed |
| 12 | .20 | 200 | difficulty walking, obvious intoxication |
| 18 | .25 | 300 | unconsciousness, tremors, vomiting |
| 24 | .30 | 400 | deep coma, possible death |
| 30 | .35 | 500 | death |

1 drink = one ounce hard liquor = one glass wine = one glass beer

The National Safety Council's Committee on Alcohol and Drugs has provided the following guidelines on alcohol intoxication:
- Below 0.05% (50 mg/dl) a person is not intoxicated.
- Between 0.05% and 0.10% (50 and 100 mg/dl) a person may be judged legally intoxicated, but behavior and circumstances should be considered in making final judgment.
- Over 0.10% (100 mg/dl) conclusively confirms alcohol intoxication.

**Special Considerations:**
★The blood alcohol test measures only the amount of alcohol in a person's blood

at the time the sample is taken. It does not indicate whether the person is an alcoholic.

★A person charged with drunken driving who feels that the breath analysis performed by the police is inaccurate may wish to request a blood alcohol analysis.

★When a blood sample is taken for this test, it is essential that no alcohol be used as an antiseptic to prepare the person's arm for venipuncture; this may cause a falsely elevated result.

# Aldosterone

Aldosterone is a hormone produced by the adrenal glands, located above the kidneys. It makes the kidneys retain more sodium and excrete more potassium. This helps control fluid balance and blood pressure.

Aldosterone secretion is partly controlled by renin, a kidney hormone (see p. 96). Aldosterone is usually measured in a 24-hour urine specimen (see p. 39) but may also be measured in a blood (serum) sample.

**Why Performed:**
To determine the cause of high blood pressure or abnormal blood potassium levels when excessive adrenal gland secretion or an adrenal tumor is suspected. The symptoms that suggest primary hypersecretion of aldosterone include high blood pressure, muscular pains, cramps, and weakness.

**Normal Values:**
May vary from lab to lab:
Urine: 2–26 micrograms (mcg) per 24-hour specimen
Blood: 1–9 nanograms per deciliter (ng/dl)

Levels are significantly affected by whether a person has been standing or lying down for the period immediately before the blood sample is drawn.

●*Greater Than Normal Values May Mean*: Excessive secretion of aldosterone (aldosteronism) may be due to an adrenal tumor (Conn's syndrome), to excess secretion by the adrenal glands, or to a secondary effect of kidney disease, liver disease, or congestive heart failure.

●*Lower Than Normal Values May Mean*: Inadequate secretion of aldosterone may be due to decreased function of the adrenal gland (Addison's disease), salt-losing syndrome, or diabetes.

**Interfering Factors:**
Excessive licorice consumption, progesterone, and certain antihypertensive drugs such as diuretics and hydralazine (Apresoline) can alter aldosterone levels. Ask your doctor whether any of these medications should be stopped before the test. For several weeks before the test do not follow a low-salt diet and for at least 24 hours before the test avoid strenuous exercise or very stressful situations.

**Cost:**
$70 to $120

# Alkaline Phosphatase (Alk Phos)

Alkaline phosphatase is an enzyme found primarily in the liver and in bone. When liver cells are damaged or bone is rapidly growing (either normal or abnormal growth), large amounts of alkaline phosphatase are frequently released into the bloodstream. The chemical structure of the enzyme differs depending upon whether it comes from the liver or from bone. If blood levels of alkaline phosphatase are elevated, further tests may be performed to identify the subfractions (isoenzymes) and thereby, determine the source.

This test is performed on a venous blood specimen (see p. 36).

**Why Performed:**
To help diagnose and monitor the progress of liver disease, which may produce symptoms such as jaundice (yellowing of the skin and eyes), pain in the upper abdomen, nausea, and vomiting. It may also be used to monitor people receiving medications that may be toxic to the liver. This test is often performed along with tests for SGPT (p. 102), SGOT (p. 101), and bilirubin (p. 52) as *liver function tests* (LFTs). Alkaline phosphatase is also measured in certain bone diseases, for example, to evaluate abnormalities found on bone x-rays.

**Normal Values:**
May vary from lab to lab and with age:
    20–90 International Units/liter (IU/l)
    Normal values are considerably higher in children due to rapid bone growth and during pregnancy due to the secretion of large amounts of alkaline phosphatase by the placenta.

●*Greater Than Normal Values May Mean*: Elevated levels of alkaline phosphatase may be found in liver disorders such as hepatitis, cirrhosis, liver cancers, blockage of the bile ducts (obstructive jaundice), or chronic alcohol ingestion. Elevated alkaline phosphatase may also be due to bone diseases such as Paget's disease, osteomalacia, rickets, bone tumors, or conditions with deficient production of parathyroid hormone. Levels may be also increased during the normal healing of a bone fracture.

Many drugs that can cause liver injury may result in elevations of alkaline phosphatase—including antibiotics (penicillins, erythromycin, tetracycline, sulfonamides, isoniazid), narcotics (codeine, morphine, Demerol), methyldopa (Aldomet), propranolol (Inderal), cortisone, allopurinol, tricyclic antidepressants, chlorpromazine, oral contraceptives, antiinflammatory medications (indomethacin, phenylbutazone), and many others.

**Cost:**
$10 to $17

**Special Considerations:**
    ★5'-Nucleotidase: This enzyme (pronounced "five-prime nucleotidase") is released into the bloodstream in large amounts when the liver is damaged or bile ducts obstructed, but not with bone disease. Therefore, this blood test is sometimes used instead of alkaline phosphatase isoenzymes to determine whether an elevated alkaline phosphatase is due to liver or bone disease.

# Alpha-Fetoprotein (AFP)

Alpha-fetoprotein (AFP) is produced by the liver cells of unborn babies and finds its way into the amniotic fluid and the mother's bloodstream. (Either the mother's blood or the amniotic fluid may be tested.) AFP usually drops to very low levels in both the baby's and the mother's blood soon after the baby is born. When levels rise in the blood of adults, it most frequently indicates either pregnancy or liver disease.

## Why Performed:

In adults, to help diagnose suspected cancer of the liver (hepatoma) and to follow its response to treatment. It is also used to diagnose and follow certain tumors of the testicles and the ovaries, to screen patients with testicular cancer for recurrences, and to screen for other cancers.

When done on pregnant women, this test is used to screen the fetus for a number of brain or spine defects, which are known as defects of the neural tube. It is the first of a sequence of tests which can detect about 4 out of 5 cases of fetal spina bifida (a spinal defect) and nearly all brain defects (e.g., anencephaly).

Such defects occur in one to two of every thousand pregnancies. They are not associated with the mother's age, and most women whose babies show such defects had no prior history or family history of similar events. When used to screen for birth defects, this test should be done between the 15th and 18th week of pregnancy.

The benefits of this test are still being hotly debated within the medical profession. At some medical centers, AFP testing is recommended for all pregnant women. About 5% of pregnant women tested have elevated levels on initial testing and about 3% after the test is repeated. For this 3%, fetal ultrasound (p. 205) is then performed. Ultrasound demonstrates a normal cause for elevated levels (most frequently twins or mistaken gestational age) in about half of these cases.

The remaining 1%–2% of women will usually undergo amniocentesis (p. 208). Approximately 9 out of 10 of these will be found to have normal AFP levels in uterine fluid even though abnormal in blood. For approximately 1 of 10 women entering this last phase, amniocentesis results will show strong evidence of a birth defect. Specific results and further plans should then be discussed with your physician or genetic counselor.

## Normal Values:

Units and values may vary from lab to lab: In nonpregnant adults, less than 30 nanograms per milliliter. In pregnancy, values gradually rise until 1–2 months before birth, then gradually decline.

●*Greater Than Normal Values May Mean*: In nonpregnant adults: cancer of the liver, testes, ovaries, bile tract, stomach, pancreas, or some other cancers; cirrhosis; hepatitis. In pregnant woman: fetus with birth defect, interuterine death.

## Cost:

$40 to $50

## Special Considerations:

★In patients with liver cancer, a decrease in AFP indicates a favorable response to therapy.

# Ammonia

Ammonia is one of the end products of protein metabolism. Most of the ammonia in the body is formed by the breakdown of protein by bacteria in the intestines. The liver normally converts ammonia into urea, which is excreted by the kidneys, but in severe liver disease this conversion may be slowed or stopped. If this occurs, blood ammonia levels rise, upsetting the body's acid-base balance and affecting brain function.

This test is performed on a venous blood specimen (see p. 36).

## Why Performed:

To diagnose suspected liver failure.

47

**Normal Values:**

Units and values may vary from lab to lab:
40–80 micrograms per deciliter (mcg/dl).

● *Greater Than Normal Values May Mean*: Severe liver disease (e.g., cirrhosis, hepatic necrosis), severe congestive heart failure, Reye's syndrome, gastrointestinal bleeding, or erythroblastosis fetalis.

**Interfering Factors:**

Ammonia levels are increased by ammonium salts, acetazolamide, thiazide diuretics, furosemide, portacaval shunt, prolonged tube feeding, liver disease, and high-protein diets. Ammonia levels are decreased by neomycin, lactulose, kanamycin, and low-protein diets.

**Cost:**

About $25 to $35

**Special Considerations:**

★Liver disease may produce bleeding problems, so be sure to keep pressure on the venipuncture site until bleeding stops. If bleeding continues, notify your physician.

# Amylase

Amylase is a digestive enzyme which changes starches into sugars. It is produced in the pancreas, salivary glands, fallopian tubes, and liver. Normally very little amylase is found in the blood or urine. However, if the pancreas or salivary glands are inflamed, amylase will be released into blood and urine. The blood levels rise for only a short time, but the amylase excreted in the urine may remain elevated for as long as a week. Serum amylase is measured in a blood sample, while the urine amylase test is performed on a urine specimen collected over 2 hours or 24 hours (see p. 39).

**Why Performed:**

Serum (and sometimes urinary) amylase levels are used to evaluate abdominal pain when pancreatitis (inflammation of the pancreas) is suspected. The tests are also sometimes done to evaluate swelling and inflammation of the salivary glands.

**Normal Values:**

Vary widely from lab to lab:
Serum amylase: 60–160 Somogyi units/deciliter
Urine amylase: 35–260 Somogyi units/deciliter

● *Greater Than Normal Values May Mean*: Inflammation of the pancreas (pancreatitis) or salivary glands (from mumps or obstruction) is usually the cause of increased amylase levels. Cancer of the pancreas with obstruction of the pancreatic duct, intestinal obstruction, perforated ulcer, gallbladder disease, or ruptured tubal pregnancy may also produce elevated amylase.

● *Lower Than Normal Values May Mean*: Severe liver disease (hepatitis and cirrhosis) or such extensive damage to the pancreas that little amylase is produced.

**Interfering Factors:**

Many drugs can raise amylase levels including narcotics (codeine, morphine, Demerol, and Talwin), indomethacin (Indocin), aspirin, thiazide diuretics, and large amounts of alcohol ingested before the test. Saliva contains such large amounts of amylase that coughing, sneezing, or even talking over an uncovered urine or blood specimen can contaminate and artificially increase amylase values.

**Cost:**
$18 to $25 (blood or urine)

# Antibody Screening Tests
## (Direct Coombs Test, Indirect Coombs Test)

Antibodies are molecules produced by the immune system which can bind to foreign substances. Antibodies do not ordinarily attack the body's own tissues, but in certain diseases antibodies to the body's own tissues may be produced. And when a person receives a transfusion, his or her body may produce antibodies against the red blood cells in the blood received.

These tests are used to detect reactions between antibodies and red blood cells: The *indirect Coombs test* checks to see if your blood contains antibodies to the red blood cells in blood you are about to receive as a transfusion. The *direct Coombs test* checks to see if your blood contains antibodies to the red blood cells already in your bloodstream— either your own or those received in a previous transfusion. Both tests can be perfomed on a venous blood specimen (see p. 36).

**Why Performed:**
The indirect Coombs test is used to test the compatibility between your blood and blood you are about to receive in a transfusion. A slightly different form of this test, the *Rh antibody titer*, can be used to detect the presence of anti-Rh antibodies in the mother's blood during pregnancy, so that measures can be taken to protect her baby. This test is frequently done on pregnant women who have blood type Rh-negative when the father of the baby has blood type Rh-positive (see p. 53).

The direct Coombs test is used when hemolytic anemia is suspected. Hemolytic anemia may be due to certain conditions in which a person produces antibodies to his or her own red blood cells (e.g., lupus erythematosus), may result from a transfusion reaction (in which a person has received incompatible blood), or may occur in situations where a mother's anti-Rh antibodies attack her baby's red blood cells (this is called erythroblastosis fetalis).

**Normal Values:**
Indirect Coombs: A negative reaction means that your blood is compatible with the blood to be given by transfusion.

Direct Coombs: A negative reaction means that your blood contains no antibodies to the red blood cells in your bloodstream.

● *Greater Than Normal Values May Mean*: Indirect Coombs: A positive reaction may indicate incompatibility between your blood and the donor's blood—this means you cannot receive blood from that donor. Direct Coombs: A positive reaction suggests that your blood contains antibodies to the red blood cells in your bloodstream. If this test is positive in a pregnant woman, there may be a risk of your body's forming antibodies against your baby's blood cells. This can be prevented by appropriate therapy.

**Interfering Factors:**
Previous blood transfusion or injection with dextran or contrast media can produce false-positive results on both tests. Rough handling of the blood sample may make test results invalid. A large number of drugs— including penicillin and methyldopa (Al-

domet)—can produce a false-positive direct Coombs test.

**Cost:**
$15 to $25

# Antinuclear Antibodies (ANA)

The immune system normally reacts against foreign substances but does not attack the body's own cells. However, in certain conditions (usually called autoimmune or collagen vascular diseases) the immune system can produce antibodies against the body's own tissues. Antinuclear antibodies (ANA) are one type of such antibodies. They may be present in systemic lupus erythematosus (SLE) (an inflammatory disease of the connective tissues), in rheumatoid arthritis, and in other connective tissue diseases. The test for rheumatoid factor (p. 98) is also used to detect antibodies against the body's own tissues. ANA testing is performed on a venous blood sample (see p. 36).

**Why Performed:**
This test is most frequently used to evaluate symptoms such as arthritis or certain skin rashes when systemic lupus erythematosus is suspected.

**Normal Values:**
Values may vary from lab to lab:
    A titer of 1:32 or below
    • *Greater Than Normal Values May Mean*: Systemic lupus erythematosus. However, a positive test does not necessarily mean the person tested has SLE, since moderately elevated levels of ANA may be found in people with such other conditions as viral infections, other collagen vascular diseases, chronic liver disease, and autoimmune disease other than SLE. In addition, some apparently healthy individuals possess antinuclear antibodies. The higher the titer, however, the more likely the person has SLE.

**Interfering Factors:**
A number of drugs can produce positive test results. The most important of these are hydralazine (used to treat hypertension), some antibiotics (including isoniazid, penicillin, and tetracycline), and procainamide (used to treat irregularities of the heartbeat).

**Cost:**
$30 to $40

**Special Considerations:**
    ★*Lupus erythematosus cell test (LE prep)*— This special form of the ANA is sometimes done to confirm a diagnosis of SLE if an ANA test is strongly positive, although some people with SLE do not exhibit a positive LE prep.

# Arterial Blood Gases (ABGs, Blood Gases)

As the blood passes through the lungs, carbon dioxide leaves the blood while oxygen passes into it. Any change in lung or heart function can produce abnormal levels of one or both of these gases. The acidity of the blood may also be affected.

This test measures the concentration of oxygen, carbon dioxide, and hydrogen ions in a blood sample taken from an artery. The oxygen level shows how much oxygen the lungs are delivering to the blood; the carbon dioxide level shows how well the lungs are removing carbon dioxide from the blood; and the hydrogen ion concentration shows how acidic or alkaline the blood is.

Most blood tests are done on samples taken from a vein, but these tests require blood drawn from an artery—usually in the wrist or groin (see p. 37). Arterial blood is needed because the purpose of the test is to measure the levels of substances passing from the lungs to the body's tissues. Venous blood has already passed through the body's tissues—where the oxygen and carbon dioxide levels have been greatly affected—and is on its way back to the lungs.

**Why Performed:**
This test is used to assess the overall acid-base balance of the body. It can be used to evaluate severe breathing problems, to evaluate a person's need for added oxygen, and to monitor respiratory therapy. It is frequently used to evaluate the extent of heart failure, kidney failure, lung disease, uncontrolled diabetes, and drug overdose.

**Normal Values:**
Values may vary from lab to lab:

The amounts of these gases in the blood are measured as partial pressures, expressed in millimeters of mercury (mm Hg).

> Partial pressure of oxygen ($pO_2$)—75 to 100 (mm Hg)
> Partial pressure of carbon dioxide ($pCO_2$)—35 to 45mm Hg
> pH—7.38 to 7.44
> Oxygen content—15% to 23%
> Oxygen saturation—95% to 100%
> Bicarbonate—22 to 25 milliequivalents per liter

Abnormal values will usually indicate one of the following patterns:

*Respiratory acidosis* (pH low, bicarbonate high, $CO_2$ high) may indicate conditions that prevent $CO_2$ from being exhaled, such as asthma, emphysema, heart disease, chest injury, drug overdose, or disorder of the brain or nervous system.

*Respiratory alkalosis* (pH high, bicarbonate low, $CO_2$ low) may indicate hyperventilation or rapid breathing produced by a drug, fever, or high room temperature.

*Metabolic acidosis* (pH low, bicarbonate low, $CO_2$ low) may indicate drug poisoning, especially aspirin and alcohol, severe diarrhea, liver disease, shock, kidney disease, or uncontrolled diabetes.

*Metabolic alkalosis* (pH high, bicarbonate high, $CO_2$ high) may be due to prolonged vomiting or gastric suctioning, diuretic therapy, steroid overdose, or excessive alkali intake.

**Cost:**
$40 to $80

# Bicarbonate

Bicarbonate (which is chemically identical with baking soda) is the most important buffer in the blood, preventing it from becoming too acid.

The body uses inhaled oxygen to oxidize food. One of the by-products of this reaction is carbon dioxide. When carbon dioxide dissolves in the blood it is converted into bicarbonate.

The blood bicarbonate level is regulated by the kidneys: When there is too much bicarbonate, making the blood too alkaline, some is released into the urine. When bicarbonate is needed to reduce the acidity of the blood, the kidney reabsorbs it from the urine.

Much of the bicarbonate formed by the oxidation of food is then carried to the lungs, where carbon dioxide is exchanged for oxygen. If you breathe too rapidly, you can exhale too much carbon dioxide, resulting in a low blood bicarbonate level. This is called *respiratory alkalosis*. (It can result in spasms of the muscles of the hands and feet and a sense of suffocation.)

On the other hand, infrequent, shallow breathing can produce high blood bicarbonate levels, a condition called *respiratory acidosis*. This results from inadequate exchange of carbon dioxide for oxygen in the lungs. Subnormal respiration levels can be caused by carbon monoxide poisoning, drug reactions, head injury, or fluid in the lungs.

This test is performed on a venous blood sample (see p. 36).

## Why Performed:

To diagnose and follow disorders that affect the bicarbonate level in the blood—these include a variety of kidney diseases, toxic coma, and certain disorders of the lungs.

## Normal Values:

Values may vary from lab to lab:

21–28 milliequivalents per liter

●*Greater Than Normal Values May Mean*: Severe vomiting, excessive intake of bicarbonate (especially antacids), diuretic or steroid drugs, difficulty in breathing.

●*Less Than Normal Values May Mean*: Liver disease, rapid breathing, aspirin or other poisoning or overdose, kidney disease, severe diarrhea, shock.

## Interfering Factors:

Increased values may be caused by aldosterone and viomycin.

## Cost:

$8 to $12

## Special Considerations:

★A complete interpretation of acid-base status requires an arterial blood gas study (p. 50).

★Also see carbon dioxide, p. 56, since these two tests are frequently done together.

# Bilirubin

Bilirubin is a brownish-yellow pigment that is a by-product of the breakdown of hemoglobin, the oxygen-carrying substance in red blood cells. The bilirubin is carried in the bloodstream to the liver where it is further metabolized and then excreted through the bile ducts and gallbladder into the intestine. The normal brown color of the stool depends on the presence of this excreted bilirubin.

Bilirubin circulates in the bloodstream in two forms. Before it is acted upon by the liver it is called *indirect (unconjugated) bilirubin*. After being metabolized to a more soluble form by the liver it is called *direct (conjugated) bilirubin*. Total bilirubin (combined direct and indirect) in a blood sample is usually measured first. If this is abnormally high, the direct and indirect components are then determined. Bilirubin may also be measured in the urine (see p. 120).

## Why Performed:

When bilirubin builds up to a certain level in the bloodstream the skin and whites of the eyes may appear yellow, a condition known as jaundice. Bilirubin levels may be checked to determine the presence and cause of jaundice as well as to evaluate anemia, suspected hepatitis, abdominal pain, or very pale-colored stool (which may be a sign of impaired bile excretion). Bilirubin levels may also be monitored to follow the progress of various liver diseases or drugs that may damage the liver.

**Normal Values:**
Values may vary from lab to lab:
> Direct (conjugated) bilirubin: less than 0.3 milligrams/deciliter (mg/dl)
> Indirect (unconjugated) bilirubin: 0.1– 1.0 mg/dl
> Total bilirubin: 0.1–1.2 mg/dl (1–12 mg/dl in newborns)
> ●*Greater Than Normal Values May Mean*: Increased levels of bilirubin in the blood (hyperbilirubinemia) may be due either to increased production of bilirubin or to the inability of the liver to excrete normal amounts of bilirubin. The increased production is most often due to increased destruction of red blood cells (hemolytic anemia). Decreased excretion of bilirubin may result from liver disease (viral, alcoholic, or toxic hepatitis, cirrhosis, infectious mononucleosis) or from blockage of the bile ducts and gallbladder (gallstones or tumor).

The relative proportions of the direct and indirect components of total bilirubin can help determine which of these causes is most likely. For example, excessive breakdown of red blood cells increases indirect, but not direct, bilirubin. Blockage of the bile ducts with a gallstone, however, results in an increased proportion of the total bilirubin which is direct.

**Interfering Factors:**
Numerous drugs can influence bilirubin levels either by affecting the liver directly or by interfering with the chemical test used to measure bilirubin. Increased bilirubin can be caused by many antibiotics, narcotic pain medications, antiinflammatory drugs (indomethacin), anticonvulsants (Dilantin), some oral contraceptives, steroids, diazepam (Valium), flurazepam (Dalmane), and many others. Vitamin C, caffeine, theophylline, and barbiturates may decrease bilirubin levels. Rough handling of the blood specimen or exposure of the specimen to light may also influence the results.

**Cost:**
> Total bilirubin: $10 to $15
> Direct and indirect bilirubin: $10 to $15

# Blood Typing
## (ABO Blood Typing, Rh Blood Typing)

Blood types are determined by the presence or absence of certain genetically influenced proteins, known as antigens, found on the surface of red blood cells. Certain blood tests can be used to characterize the type (A, B, AB, or O) and subtype (Rh-positive or Rh-negative) of your blood. Although there are other ways to type blood, the ABO and Rh types are the most commonly used. They are of special importance for people about to receive a blood transfusion and for pregnant women.

Blood received in a transfusion must be of a compatible type. Otherwise, the body's immunologic system may create antibodies against the transfused blood cells, and this can cause serious illness and even death.

Transfusion of an incompatible blood type is even more dangerous if the immunologic system has previously been exposed to the foreign blood type, since more rapid production of antibodies may produce a more rapid and more extreme rejection of the new blood cells. This would result in large-scale destruction of red cells, severe illness, and possibly death.

Type O blood is called "the universal donor" type, because it can be safely given to anyone, regardless of the recipient's ABO type. This is because type O blood does not possess any of the substances that trigger antibody reactions.

Rh typing is another way of typing your red blood cells. About 80% of the population have Rh proteins on their red blood cells and are called Rh-positive. About 20% do not; they are called Rh-negative. If Rh-positive red blood cells are introduced into the blood of an Rh-negative person, an immunologic reaction usually results. However, the opposite is not true. No harm is done by transfusing Rh-negative cells into a Rh-positive person, since Rh-negative cells do not trigger antibody reactions.

Rh type is of special concern during pregnancy. If an Rh-negative mother has a first child that is Rh-positive, there is a good chance that a few of the baby's blood cells will enter the mother's bloodstream during the baby's birth. There will be no harm done to the newborn or to the mother, but the mother's immune system will begin making antibodies against Rh-positive blood. If the same mother later has another Rh-positive child, the mother's antibodies can pass into the fetal blood and attack the unborn baby's red blood cells, causing injury or death for the fetus (erythroblastosis fetalis).

There is now a treatment that can prevent this from happening. If an Rh-negative mother has an Rh-positive baby, an immunoglobulin (one commonly used brand is RhoGam) is injected into her blood immediately after delivery. It binds with any of the baby's blood cells that may have leaked into the mother's system and prevents the formation of anti-Rh antibodies, which could cause problems during later pregnancies.

In addition to blood typing, blood banks take other precautions to prevent transfusion reactions. Besides checking the ABO type and the Rh type, they also check for antibodies against any of the other protein factors in both donor and recipient blood. This is called crossmatching.

**Why Performed:**

Blood typing is done before a person receives a transfusion, on those who are about to donate blood, and when a woman first learns that she is pregnant.

It may also be done to determine the genetic parents when the identity of the father, mother, or both is uncertain. If the mother and child's ABO, Rh, and other tissue types are checked against those of each of the possible fathers, the candidates can sometimes be narrowed down to one by exclusion. However, it is easier to prove in this way that a person is not the father than it is to prove that he is. Histocompatibility testing (see p. 82) is a more specific test for identifying a person's genetic parents.

**Normal Values:**

Blood may be type A (A antigen present), B (B antigen present), AB (A and B antigens present), or O (neither A nor B antigen is present). In the Rh system, blood may be Rh-positive (Rh antigen present) or Rh-negative (Rh antigen absent). Combining the two systems yields the eight basic blood types of A+, A−, B+, B−, AB+, AB−, O+, and O−. Since blood types are gentically determined, different proportions of the basic blood types appear in different races.

**ABO Blood Type—
Frequency by Population Group**

| Blood Type | Whites | Blacks | Native Americans | Asians |
|---|---|---|---|---|
| A | 40% | 27% | 16% | 28% |
| B | 11% | 20% | 4% | 27% |
| AB | 4% | 4% | 1% | 5% |
| O | 45% | 49% | 79% | 40% |

**Interfering Factors:**
If you have received dextran (a plasma substitute) or any contrast medium (as part of an x-ray procedure), it may interfere with this test.

**Cost:**
ABO typing: $10 to $15
Rh typing: $10 to $15

# Calcium (Ca⁺⁺)

Calcium is the most plentiful mineral in the body. It is essential for the maintenance and repair of bone and teeth, the transmission of nerve impulses, muscle contraction, heart function, and blood clotting. Over 98% of the calcium in the body is stored in bone, while the remaining 1%–2% circulates in the blood. When blood calcium levels fall, calcium is released from the bone reservoir to restore proper levels. If blood calcium levels rise, the excess calcium may be stored in bone or excreted in urine. This complex regulatory mechanism is controlled in part by the dietary intake and intestinal absorption of calcium and vitamin D, the levels of phosphorus (p. 91) in the body, and the secretion of various hormones. Parathyroid hormone (p. 89), secreted from tiny glands embedded in the thyroid gland, causes calcium to be released from bone, increases intestinal absorption of calcium, and causes the kidney to conserve calcium. Calcitonin, a hormone from the thyroid gland, increases calcium excretion by the kidneys. Estrogens promote the deposition of calcium in bone, leaving less to circulate in the blood.

Calcium levels can be measured in the blood (serum) or in the urine. The urine test usually involves collecting a 24-hour urine specimen (see p. 39). You may be asked to follow a special high- or low-calcium diet for several days before the urine test.

**Why Performed:**
To evaluate suspected parathyroid disorders, certain types of cancers and bone diseases, and kidney stones which may form because of excessive amounts of calcium in the urine. The symptoms associated with abnormally low calcium levels in the blood are muscle twitching and spasms (tetany). Higher than normal serum calcium may produce weakness, lethargy, and abdominal discomfort. Blood calcium levels are not a good screening test for inadequate calcium intake or postmenopausal bone loss (osteoporosis), since blood calcium is maintained within normal limits when diet is deficient in calcium even at the expense of significant bone demineralization.

**Normal Values:**
May vary from lab to lab:
Blood (serum) calcium (total): 9.2–11.0 milligrams/deciliter (mg/dl)

Urine calcium:
    average calcium diet: 100–240 mg/ 24 hours
    low-calcium diet: less than 150 mg/ 24 hours
    high calcium diet: 240–300 mg/24 hours

● *Greater Than Normal Values May Mean*: Elevated levels of calcium in the blood (hypercalcemia) and urine (hypercalciuria) may be due to excessive secretion of parathyroid hormone (hyperparathyroidism), cancer (multiple myeloma or cancers which spread to bone), excessive intake of vitamin D or calcium (milk products, calcium-containing antacids), prolonged bed rest, and certain kidney diseases.

● *Lower Than Normal Values May Mean*: Decreased levels of calcium in the blood (hypocalcemia) may be due to low levels of serum protein (albumin). To exclude this possibility, serum protein levels (p. 103) should be measured. Other causes of low serum and urinary calcium include decreased parathyroid gland function (hypoparathyroidism), low dietary intake or absorption of calcium or vitamin D, bone disorders (osteomalacia), certain kidney diseases, and pregnancy.

### Interfering Factors:

Many drugs can influence blood and urine calcium levels. These include thiazide diuretics, acetazolamide (Diamox), hormones (estrogens, oral contraceptives, steroids), and anticonvulsant medications.

### Cost:

Blood (serum) calcium: $10 to $15
Urine calcium: $10 to $15

# Carbon Dioxide
## (Total Carbon Dioxide Content, $CO_2$)

Carbon dioxide and water are end products of the breakdown of food in the body. The blood carries carbon dioxide to the lungs, where it is exhaled. This test measures the adequacy of gas exchange in the lungs.

The test measures all forms of carbon dioxide in the blood—bicarbonate ion, carbonic acid, and dissolved carbon dioxide. As about 90% of carbon dioxide in the serum is bicarbonate, this value is usually fairly close to the bicarbonate level (p. 51).

### Normal Values:

Values may vary from lab to lab. Carbon dioxide can be measured in several ways:
    Carbon dioxide tension ($pCO_2$): 35–45 millimeters of mercury in blood from an artery; 40–45 mm Hg in blood from a vein
    $CO_2$ content: 19–24 millimoles per liter in blood from an artery; 22–38 mM/L in blood from a vein
    $CO_2$ combining power: 24–32 milliequivalents per liter in blood from an artery; 38–50 mEq/L in blood from a vein

● *Greater Than Normal Values May Mean*: The presence of diseases that impair the lung's ability to get rid of carbon dioxide (e.g., emphysema or pneumonia), primary aldosteronism, Cushing's syndrome, excessive acid loss (e.g., through severe vomiting or gastric drainage). High values may occur during anesthesia if the patient rebreathes his own air. Values may also be elevated as the result of excessive antacid use, diuretic drugs, high doses of steroid hormones, vomiting, intestinal obstruction, or starvation.

● *Less Than Normal Values May Mean*: Diabetic acidosis, kidney failure, severe diarrhea, intestinal drainage, hyperventilation, aspirin overdose, overdose of ammonium chloride (a diuretic sold without prescription).

### Interfering Factors:

Test values are increased by high ACTH levels, cortisone, chlorothiazide diuretics, mercury-containing diuretics, excessive intake of alkali, and excessive intake of licorice. Test values are decreased by aspirin, paraldehyde, methicillin, ammonium chloride, dimercaprol, acetazolamide, and accidental consumption of ethylene glycol or methyl alcohol.

### Cost:
$5 to $12

# Carbon Monoxide
## (Carboxyhemoglobin)

Carbon monoxide is a colorless, odorless gas which binds to the hemoglobin in red blood cells much more strongly than oxygen does. Hemoglobin that comes in contact with carbon monoxide (CO) is converted into *carboxyhemoglobin*, a form that is unable to transport either oxygen or carbon dioxide. Thus CO can produce severe toxicity. Carbon monoxide poisoning is probably responsible for more deaths than any other poison.

Carbon monoxide is produced when fuel is burned with insufficient oxygen for complete combustion. The principal sources of this gas are automobile exhaust fumes, heaters or fires burning with insufficient ventilation, and industrial plants.

People with anemia or elevated metabolic rates (e.g., hyperthyroidism), persons with heart or lung diseases, and children are especially sensitive to carbon monoxide poisoning. High blood carbon monoxide levels can precipitate or increase the severity of angina attacks.

Carbon monoxide poisoning is not limited to acute cases, which often end in death. There are also many cases of chronic carbon monoxide poisoning, resulting most frequently from defective gas-burning appliances at home, heavy exposure to auto traffic, or occupational exposure—particularly in garages and poorly ventilated industrial plants.

Chronic carbon monoxide poisoning is much more frequent during the winter among people using unvented gas or kerosene heaters. The principal symptom is usually headache.

This test is performed on a venous blood sample (see p. 36).

### Why Performed:

This test is done when carbon monoxide poisoning is suspected, either because of a history of exposure to the gas or because of such symptoms as headache, dizziness, malaise, sleepiness, unconsciousness, and coma—especially when these symptoms are accompanied by the characteristic "cherry-red" skin color produced by CO poisoning. (This can sometimes be misleading to medical personnel, since persons suffering from insufficient oxygen normally turn a bluish color.)

This test may also be performed to demonstrate one harmful effect of smoking, especially in those with heart or lung disease.

**Normal Values:**

| | |
|---|---|
| Nonsmokers | 0%–3% of total hemoglobin |
| Smokers | 5%–15% |
| Taxi drivers, traffic police | 8%–12% |
| Symptoms develop | 20% |
| Severe poisoning | 30% |
| Unconsciousness | 40% |
| Coma | 50% |
| Death | 60%–80% |

● *Greater Than Normal Values May Mean*: Carbon monoxide poisoning.

**Cost:**
$20 to $35

**Special Considerations:**
★Carbon monoxide is a very powerful poison. One part of CO in 5000 parts of air will produce a 20% hemoglobin saturation in approximately one hour.

# Catecholamines

The two principal catecholamines, adrenaline (epinephrine) and noradrenaline (norepinephrine), are produced in the adrenal glands and are released as part of the body's normal stress reaction. These hormones increase the pulse rate, blood pressure, breath rate, muscle strength, and mental alertness. They reduce the blood supply to the skin and increase blood flow to the muscles and the major organs.

Another catecholamine, dopamine, as well as small quantities of norepinephrine, are produced in the brain. These two sub- stances help transmit nerve impulses within the brain tissue.

Either blood or urine can be tested for catecholamines. When a urine test is used, a 24-hour urine collection (see p. 39) is sometimes required, and levels of VMA (vanillylmandelic acid) and HVA (homovanillic acid) are measured. These substances result from the metabolic breakdown of catecholamines.

**Why Performed:**
This test is most frequently done in cases of hypertension to rule out a suspected pheochromocytoma, a catecholamine-producing tumor of the adrenal glands. (Symptoms of this condition include flushing and episodes of high blood pressure.) This test is also used in the diagnosis of other tumors and in some disorders of the autonomic nervous system.

**Preparation:**
If the urine test is used, you may be asked to follow a special diet for 2–3 days before the test. The diet varies from lab to lab, but the following may be excluded: caffeine (coffee, tea, cocoa, chocolate), aspirin, and vanilla.

If a blood test is done, you will be asked to refrain from smoking for 24 hours before the test and to fast for 10–24 hours before the test. You may be asked to lie down and relax for 45 minutes one hour before the test.

A small indwelling catheter may be placed in a vein in your hand or arm about 30 minutes before the test begins. (The catheter is used because the stress associated with blood-drawing process itself can increase catecholamines.) Be sure to keep warm—ask for a blanket if necessary. Cold can increase catecholamine secretion.

It will take the laboratory about a week to complete the test.

## Normal Values:

Values may differ from lab to lab:

> *Blood:*
> Epinephrine—undetectable to 140 picograms per milliliter (pg/ml)
> Norepinephrine—70–1700 pg/ml
> *Urine:*
> VMA—less than 9 milligrams (mg) per 24 hours
> HVA—less than 15 mg per 24 hours
> Total catecholamines—less than 135 micrograms per 24 hours; less than 18 micrograms per deciliter (single urine sample)
> ● *Greater Than Normal Values May Mean*: Catecholamine-producing tumor, intense stress, or recent electroshock therapy. Catecholamine levels can also be increased in some muscle diseases.

## Interfering Factors:

Failure to follow pretest instructions or having a radioactive scan within a week of this test can interfere with results. A number of drugs can interfere with this test. These include many of high-blood-pressure medications, insulin, alcohol, epinephrine, amphetamines, phenothiazines, decongestants, some antibiotics, and some antidepressants.

## Cost:

> Blood—$50 to $75
> Urine—$30 to $60

## Special Considerations:

★Fractional analysis of a catecholamine sample can help determine its source: different kinds of tumors secrete different kinds of catecholamines.

★Catecholamines are thought to be involved in certain psychiatric problems. However, the biochemical tests for such disorders are still highly experimental.

★Warning: The container used for the 24-hour urine collection contains a strong acid solution. If you are collecting a urine sample at home, you should be extremely careful in handling the container; this acid can produce serious burns.

# Carcinoembryonic Antigen (CEA)

CEA is a protein found in varying amounts in the blood of people with certain types of cancer. It may also exist in people who have certain noncancerous conditions.

This test is performed on a venous blood sample (p. 36).

## Why Performed:

This test is most often used to follow the response of certain cancers, especially cancers of the colon and rectum, to therapy and as an index of whether a cancer is spreading or going into remission. It is also used to look for recurrences of cancer. It should not be used as a screening test and is rarely, if ever, used to diagnose cancer, since CEA may be present from other causes—e.g., smoking, benign tumors, and certain inflammatory disorders. However, very high CEA levels do strongly suggest the presence of cancer.

## Normal Values:

Values may differ from lab to lab:

> Less than 2.5 nanograms per milliliter (ng/ml)
> ● *Greater Than Normal Values May Mean*: Cancers of the colon, rectum, breast, bronchus, ovary, uterus, cervix, and possibly other sites. Values are also frequently in-

creased in 15%–20% of persons with such inflammatory diseases as ulcerative colitis, Crohn's disease, pancreatitis, liver disease, and pulmonary infections. Values in excess of 20 ng/ml are highly suggestive of malignancy.

### Interfering Factors:
Heavy smoking may elevate CEA levels.

### Cost:
$40 to $80

# Chloride (Cl⁻)

Chloride is one of the body's most plentiful minerals. It is an electrolyte (an electrically charged molecule dissolved in body fluids) involved in water balance (the amount of fluid inside and surrounding cells) and the acid-base balance of body fluids. Most body chloride comes from salt (sodium chloride) in the diet. Chloride levels are usually measured in the blood (serum) but may also be determined in a urine specimen collected over 24 hours.

### Why Performed:
To evaluate suspected electrolyte, fluid, kidney, and adrenal gland disorders. Too little chloride in the blood can cause symptoms of muscle twitching, muscle spasms, or shallow breathing. Excessive levels of chloride may produce rapid, deep breathing, weakness, stupor, and coma.

### Normal Values:
May vary from lab to lab:
> Blood (serum) chloride: 95–103 milliequivalents/liter (mEq/L)
> Urine chloride: 140–250 mEq/24 hours
> (varies greatly depending upon dietary intake of salt)

●*Greater Than Normal Values May Mean*: Severe dehydration, excessive adrenal gland function (Cushing's syndrome), certain kidney disorders, hyperventilation, and excessive production of the hormone aldosterone.

●*Lower Than Normal Values May Mean*: Dehydration (due to excessive sweating, vomiting, diarrhea, or severe burns), infections, severe diabetes, intestinal obstruction, kidney failure, and inadequate adrenal gland function (Addison's disease).

### Interfering Factors:
Many drugs can alter chloride levels, including many diuretic medications, blood pressure medications, antiinflammatory drugs, and steroids.

### Cost:
$8 to $12

### Special Considerations:
★In the inherited disorder cystic fibrosis the sweat and mucus produced in the body contains elevated amounts of sodium and chloride. A sweat test (p. 389), which measures chloride concentration in sweat, is used to diagnose this condition.

# Chromosomal Analysis (Karotype)

Chromosomes are tiny coiled strands of genetic material (DNA) found in the nucleus of each cell. The chromosomes carry the genes that determine inherited characteristics.

In this test the chromosomes in a blood

cell are photographed through a microscope. The photograph is then carefully studied, and the photograph of each chromosome is cut out and arranged according to size, shape, and staining pattern. They are then arranged in a standard order and carefully analyzed. A display of chromosome photographs arranged in standard order is called a karotype.

Chromosomal analysis is sometimes done on other cells as well, most frequently on cells obtained by skin biopsy, bone marrow biopsy, or amniocentesis (see p. 208).

### Why Performed:

To help find out whether a chromosomal abnormality might be the cause of a known or suspected disease or developmental problem. It is most frequently done to investigate birth defects, subnormal growth, mental retardation, delayed puberty, abnormal sexual development, infertility, certain inherited disorders, or when a prospective mother is over 35 years of age.

### Normal Results:

A normal human karotype contains 46 chromosomes arranged as 22 matching pairs of autosomal chromosomes and one pair of sex chromosomes. The sex chromosomes determine the sex of the person: females have two X chromosomes, males have one X and one Y chromosome. The size, shape and structure of each chromosome should also be normal.

### Abnormal Results:

Missing, extra, or abnormal chromosomes may indicate any one of a number of genetic disorders. For example, with Down's syndrome there is an extra number 21 chromosome; with Klinefelter's syndrome there is an extra X chromosome; and in Turner's syndrome only one X chromosome is present.

### Cost:

$400 to $500, more if special studies are required.

# Complete Blood Count (CBC)

This is the most frequently performed lab test. It provides a great deal of information about the three kinds of cells in the blood— red blood cells, white blood cells, and platelets. It is most frequently used as a screening test, as an anemia check, and as a test for infection, but it is also used to aid in the diagnosis and treatment of a large number of other conditions.

The CBC is usually done by a machine (called a Coulter counter) which performs seven or more different tests automatically: hematocrit, hemoglobin, red blood cell count, red blood cell indices, white blood cell count, white blood cell differential, and platelet count. One additional test, an examination of a peripheral blood smear under a microscope, is usually done by a technician.

This test is performed on a venous blood sample (p. 36).

### Cost:

$8 to $15

## Hematocrit (HCT, Packed Cell Volume, PCV)

This test measures the portion of blood volume that is made up by red blood cells: A hematocrit of 38 means that 38% of the blood's volume is composed of red cells.

**Why Performed:**

This test is most frequently used to test for anemia. Symptoms of anemia may include pallor, weakness, tiredness, lightheadedness, and shortness of breath, although a person may be severely anemic with essentially no symptoms. The results of this test will tell you whether you are anemic (not enough red blood cells), polycythemic (too many red blood cells), or normal. Blood may be drawn by venipuncture or fingerstick (see pp. 36–37).

Other anemia tests include hemoglobin and red cell count (discussed next).

**Normal Values:**

Values may vary from lab to lab:

Adult men: 40% to 54%

Adult women: 37% to 47%

Children: 31% to 41%

Newborns: 44% to 64%

● *Greater Than Normal Values May Mean*: Polycythemia—this may be due to insufficient oxygen (e.g., high altitude, smoking, carbon monoxide exposure, chronic lung disease), to a decrease in blood fluid volume (low fluid intake, diarrhea, vomiting, profuse sweating, severe burns), to certain diseases (e.g., polycythemia vera), or to trauma (e.g., surgery).

● *Less Than Normal Values May Mean*: Anemia—this may develop as the result of blood loss, increased breakdown of red blood cells, decreased production of red blood cells, or some combination of these processes. Blood loss leading to anemia occurs most frequently from menstrual bleeding or bleeding from the gastrointestinal tract. Anemia produced by bleeding is iron-deficiency anemia, the most common variety.

Decrease in red blood cell production may be due to tumors, toxins, or a lack of the required building blocks, such as iron, folic acid, or vitamin $B_{12}$. Increased break-down of red blood cells (hemolytic anemia) may be due to inherited disorders (e.g., sickle-cell anemia), toxic chemicals, trauma, disease of the liver or spleen, antibodies against red blood cells, or infections (e.g., malaria).

**Interfering Factors:**

When the sample is taken by venipuncture, if the tourniquet is left on too long, it may falsely elevate the hematocrit.

# Hemoglobin (Total Hemoglobin, Hgb)

Hemoglobin is an iron-containing protein found in red blood cells. It forms an easily reversed bond with oxygen molecules, enabling the red cells to carry oxygen from the lungs to the tissues of the body. The hemoglobin level is usually a good index of the blood's oxygen-carrying capacity. Hemoglobin also carries the waste product carbon dioxide from the body tissues to the lungs for excretion.

Abnormal amounts of specific types of hemoglobin can result in disease (see Hemoglobin Electrophoresis, p. 81). Hemoglobin can also be measured in the urine (see Home Urinalysis, p. 119).

**Why Performed:**

To test for anemia (see above).

**Normal Values:**

Values may vary from lab to lab:

Women: 12.0 to 16.0 grams per deciliter (g/dl)

Men: 14.0 to 18.0 g/dl

● *Greater Than Normal Values May Mean*: Polycythemia—see above.

●*Less Than Normal Values May Mean*:
Anemia—see p. 62.

### Interfering Factors:
If the blood-drawing tourniquet is left on too long, it may produce abnormally high hemoglobin values.

## Red Blood Cell Count (RBC Count)

About 40% of the volume of the blood is composed of red blood cells (erythrocytes). It is these cells that make the blood red. The average adult has about 30 trillion red blood cells. These hemoglobin-packed cells carry oxygen from the lungs to all parts of the body. They also carry waste products (principally carbon dioxide) back to the lungs to be exhaled.

This test determines the number of red blood cells in one cubic millimeter of blood. If the red blood cell count is low (anemia), the body may not get the oxygen it needs. If it is too high (polycythemia), the blood cells may be at increased risk of clumping together in the smallest blood vessels (capillaries).

### Why Performed:
To test for anemia (see p. 62) or polycythemia (see p. 62). To evaluate iron-deficiency anemia a special test (reticulocyte count, p. 98) is performed to count the number of immature red blood cells.

### Normal Values:
Values may vary from lab to lab:
> Men: 4.6–6.2 million per cubic millimeter
> Women: 4.2–5.4 million per cubic millimeter

Children: 4.6–4.8 million per cubic millimeter
●*Greater Than Normal Values May Mean*:
Polycythemia—see p. 62.
●*Less Than Normal Values May Mean*:
Anemia—see p. 62.

## Red Blood Cell Indices

Red cell indices are three numbers which describe the size and hemoglobin concentration of red blood cells. These indices are the mean corpuscular volume (MCV), mean corpuscular hemoglobin (MCH), and mean corpuscular hemoglobin concentration (MCHC). The MCV indicates whether the cells are of normal size. The MCH gives the weight of hemoglobin in an average red blood cell. The MCHC is the amount of hemoglobin in an average cell.

### Why Performed:
To help diagnose the cause of anemia (see p. 62), although abnormal indices may also suggest other conditions.

### Normal Values:
Values may vary from lab to lab:
> MCV: 80 to 96 cubic microns (cu $\mu$)
> MCH: 27 to 31 picograms (pg)
> MCHC: 32% to 36%

### Typical RBC Indices in Two Anemias

|  | Iron-Deficiency Anemia | Pernicious Anemia |
|---|---|---|
| MCV | 60 to 80 cu $\mu$ | 95 to 150 cu $\mu$ |
| MCH | 5 to 25 pg | 33 to 53 pg |
| MCHC | 20% to 30% | 33% to 38% |

● *Greater Than Normal Values May Mean*: High MCV values suggest anemia due to deficiency of folic acid or vitamin $B_{12}$ (e.g., pernicious anemia). A high MCV is also found with alcoholism.

● *Less Than Normal Values May Mean*: Low MCV and MCHC values suggest iron-deficiency anemia or thalassemia (an inherited defect of hemoglobin).

# White Blood Cell Count and Differential (WBC, Differential)

The white blood cells (leukocytes) are an important part of the immune system. Their primary role is to fight infection. These cells have the ability to recognize and attack organisms or substances that are foreign to the body. In addition they perform a constant monitoring for newly mutated cancer cells. They are also involved in inflammatory and allergic reactions.

White cells' ability to attack foreign tissues can cause problems in people who have had organ transplants. The recipient's white cells will frequently attack the transplanted organ, producing a rejection reaction. There are now medications that can prevent or reduce the severity of such reactions, but most of them also make the recipient more susceptible to infection.

There is normally only about one white blood cell for every five hundred red blood cells, but if a bacterial infection is present, the number of white cells may increase dramatically. (The white count may or may not increase in viral infections.)

There are several types of white blood cell: neutrophils (polymorphonucleocytes, PMN, "polys"), bands ("stabs," which are immature neutrophils), lymphocytes ("lymphs"), monocytes ("monos"), eosinophils ("eos"), and basophils. Each plays a somewhat different role in the body's immune response.

There are two parts to this test: In the first part (white blood cell count) the total number of white blood cells in a cubic millimeter of blood are determined. In the second part (white blood cell differential) the percentage of each type of white blood cell is measured.

**Why Performed:**
To evaluate suspected infection or inflammation; to evaluate the effects of suspected poisoning by drugs or chemicals; to monitor blood disorders, especially leukemia; to monitor the effects of chemotherapy; and as part of periodic blood screening tests.

**Normal Values:**
Values may vary from lab to lab:

White blood cell count: 4500 to 11,000 per cubic millimeter. May be higher in children.

| | |
|---|---|
| Neutrophils | 47% to 77% |
| Bands | 0% to 3% |
| Lymphocytes | 16% to 43% |
| Monocytes | 0.5% to 10% |
| Eosinophils | 0.3% to 7% |
| Basophils | 0.3% to 2% |

● *Greater Than Normal Values May Mean*: An increased white blood cell count is called leukocytosis and may suggest acute bacterial infection (e.g., pneumonia, tonsillitis, meningitis, septicemia), tissue damage (e.g., heart attack, cancer, cirrhosis of the liver, burns), collagen diseases (e.g., rheumatoid arthritis), smoking, severe stress (fever, surgery, convulsions), or any one of a variety of other diseases (e.g., kidney failure, anemia, parasitic diseases). Very high levels of white blood cells may suggest leukemia. The white count can also be elevated by a large number of drugs (e.g., aspirin, isoniazid, several antibiotics, gold compounds, allopurinol, hydantoin derivatives, primaquine).

White blood cell differential:

> Neutrophils: increased in infection, heart attack, burns, stress response, inflammatory disease.
> Bands: increased in acute bacterial infections.
> Lymphocytes: increased in some viral infections, immune diseases, some leukemias.
> Monocytes: increased in some viral and fungal infections, collagen vascular diseases, some cancers, some leukemias, TB.
> Eosinophils: increased in allergic diseases, parasitic infections, skin diseases, some leukemias, some cancers, autoimmune disease, adrenal insufficiency.
> Basophils: increased in some leukemias, some cancers, hypothyroidism, chronic hypersensitivity states.

When the numbers of neutrophils and bands are increased, as in a bacterial infection, this is often referred to as a *shift to the left*. This is because neutrophils and bands are, by convention, listed in written reports on the far left, while basophils are listed on the right.

●*Less Than Normal Values May Mean*: A decreased white blood cell count is called leukopenia and may indicate a disorder of white cell production (e.g., aplastic anemia, pernicious anemia), viral infections, malaria, agranulocytosis, alcoholism, or uncontrolled diabetes. Decreased values may also be due to certain drugs—antibiotics (e.g., chloramphenicol, penicillin, cephalothin), analgesics (acetaminophen, Tylenol), antithyroid drugs, barbiturates, diazepam (Valium), chlordiazepoxide (Librium), diuretics (e.g., furosemide, Lasix),

indomethacin (Indocin), isoniazid, and agents used in cancer chemotherapy (e.g., methotrexate).

White blood cell differential:

> Neutrophils: decreased by radiation, certain drugs, certain infections, lupus erythematosus, deficiency of vitamin $B_{12}$ or folic acid.
> Lymphocytes: decreased in prolonged severe illness, high steroid levels, immunosuppression, AIDS.
> Monocytes: decrease rarely seen.
> Eosinophils: decreased by drugs, stress response, Cushing's syndrome.
> Basophils: decreased in pregnancy, hyperthyroidism, ovulation, stress.

## Special Considerations:

★The WBC count may vary as much as 2000 per cubic millimeter from day to day as a result of exercise, stress, smoking, digestion, or minor infection.

# Platelet Count (Thrombocyte Count)

This test measures the number of platelets in a cubic millimeter of blood. Platelets (thrombocytes) are tiny cell-like structures which play a major role in blood clotting. When bleeding occurs, the platelets swell, stick together, and form a sticky plug that helps stop the bleeding. Platelets are produced by the bone marrow.

## Why Performed:

This test is used to evaluate prolonged or spontaneous bleeding (from the gastrointestinal tract, urinary tract, vagina, nose, gums, etc.), certain rashes, and easy bruising. It is sometimes done to test clotting before surgery or tooth extraction, to diagnose or monitor a variety of blood diseases, to assess the effects of chemotherapy and radiation treatments on platelet formation. It is also used to monitor treatment with drugs which can have toxic effects on bone marrow.

### Normal Values:

Values may vary from lab to lab: Approximately 150,000–400,000 platelets per cubic millimeter (mm$^3$) of blood.

●*Greater Than Normal Values May Mean*: A greater number of platelets than normal is called thrombocytosis. This may be found in certain types of cancer, leukemia, polycythemia vera, infections, pregnancy, strenuous exercise, iron-deficiency anemia, rheumatoid arthritis and other inflammatory disorders, and after removal of the spleen.

●*Less Than Normal Values May Mean*: This condition is known as thrombocytopenia and can result from either increased platelet destruction (e.g., idiopathic thrombocytopenia purpura, toxic effects of drugs, or other bleeding problems) or decreased platelet production (e.g., bone marrow disease) or anemias caused by vitamin B$_{12}$ or folic acid deficiency. Many drugs can produce a decrease in platelets; these include anticancer drugs, steroids, antiinflammatory medications (phenylbutazone, aspirin), gold, quinidine, thiazide diuretics, meprobamate, antibiotics (sulfonamides, penicillins), and others.

### Peripheral Blood Smear

In this test a technician smears a drop of blood on a glass slide, fixes and stains it, then examines it under a high-power microscope. The size and shape of a large number of red blood cells are examined. The numbers of the different types of white blood cells and the number of platelets are then similarly observed and recorded. Many blood disorders including leukemia and malaria can be detected on the peripheral smear.

# Cortisol

Cortisol is a hormone produced by the adrenal glands in response to the pituitary hormone ACTH (see p. 43). Cortisol is involved in sugar, protein, and fat metabolism as well as preparing the body to fight stress, infections, and inflammation.

Cortisol is normally released in varying amounts throughout the day, reaching a peak level in the early morning and lowest levels in the evening. However, if you sleep during the day and work at night, this pattern may be shifted. The loss of a daily variation in cortisol levels may be one of the first signs of adrenal gland disease.

Cortisol levels are often measured on two blood samples, one drawn at 8:00 A.M. and the other at 4:00 P.M. Urinary free cortisol may also be measured in a 24-hour urine specimen (see p. 39).

### Why Performed:

To diagnose suspected pituitary or adrenal gland problems in patients with symptoms such as alterations in body shape (fat deposits in the face and torso), excessive body hair (hirsutism), impotence or menstrual irregularities, hyperpigmentation of the skin (stretch marks and striae), weakness, or premature sexual development in children (precocious puberty).

**Normal Values:**
May vary from lab to lab:
> Blood (serum) cortisol:
>> 7−10 A.M.: 5−23 micrograms per deciliter (mcg/dl)
>> 4−6 P.M.: 3−13 mcg/dl
>
> Urinary free cortisol: 10−90 mcg/24 hours

● *Greater Than Normal Values May Mean*: Excess secretion by the adrenal gland (Cushing's syndrome and disease).

● *Lower Than Normal Values May Mean*: Decreased activity of the adrenal gland (Addison's disease), decreased pituitary gland function, or congenital adrenal hyperplasia (adrenogenital syndrome).

**Interfering Factors:**
Obesity, extreme stress, pregnancy, and certain medications including oral contraceptives, estrogens, Dilantin, and spironolactone.

**Cost:**
Blood or urine, $40 to $50

**Special Considerations:**
★Additional tests such as ACTH (p. 43) and dexamethasone suppression test (p. 68) may be needed to determine the cause of abnormal cortisol levels.

# Creatinine and Creatinine Clearance

The main job of the kidney is to filter the blood, excreting waste products into the urine while preserving essential elements. One way to measure kidney function is to determine how well the kidney can filter and excrete creatinine, an easily measured waste product of muscle metabolism. Creatinine is normally filtered by the kidney and excreted in the urine. However, in certain types of kidney disease the ability of the kidneys to clear the blood of creatinine decreases and blood levels of creatinine rise.

Creatinine can be measured in the blood (serum) as well as in the urine. While serum creatinine is a rough measure of kidney function, a more precise measure, the creatinine clearance, can be calculated when both serum and urine levels are determined.

No special preparation is necessary for the blood test. However, the creatinine clearance test requires that you collect a 24-hour urine specimen (see p. 39) and that you drink plenty of liquids during the test period. Coffee, tea, large quantities of meat (especially beef) and strenuous exercise should be avoided just before and during the test. Since many medications can interfere with the test, check with your doctor about stopping any medications you may be taking.

**Why Performed:**
To determine the presence and severity of suspected kidney disease and to monitor the progress of known kidney disease. Creatinine and creatinine clearance are also assessed periodically in patients taking certain medications known to be toxic to the kidneys or whose dosages must be altered depending upon kidney function.

**Normal Values:**
> Creatinine: 0.6−1.2 milligrams per deciliter (mg/dl) (varies with the size of the individual)
> Creatinine clearance:
>> Men, 107−139 milliliters (ml) per minute
>> Women, 87−107 milliliters (ml) per minute

The values for creatinine clearance represent the volume of blood cleared of creatinine per minute. The normal values are adjusted for height, weight, sex and age. Creatinine clearance normally decreases with age. Therefore, the normal values usually decrease by 6 ml per minute for each 10 years after the age of 20.

●*Greater Than Normal Values May Mean*: Elevated creatinine in the blood usually indicates significant kidney disease. However, a normal serum creatinine level does not necessarily rule out the presence of kidney disease.

●*Lower Than Normal Values May Mean*: The degree of decline in creatinine clearance usually reflects the degree of kidney damage. This damage may be due to decreased blood flow to the kidneys, due to urinary tract obstruction, or due to infection or inflammation of the kidneys (pyelonephritis or glomerulonephritis). Medications that are toxic to the kidneys (such as many of the cephalosporin antibiotics) can decrease creatinine clearance and increase serum creatinine.

### Interfering Factors:

Thiazide diuretics, ascorbic acid (vitamin C), methyldopa (Aldomet), cephalosporin antibiotics (cefoxitin), and many other drugs can cause false results on these tests.

### Cost:

Serum creatinine: $10 to $14
Creatinine clearance: $18 to $30

# Dexamethasone Suppression Test (DST)

Dexamethasone is a synthetic steroid which normally supresses the secretion of the hormones ACTH (p. 43) and cortisol (p. 66). Dexamethasone usually fails to suppress these hormones in people with Cushing's disease (excess production of ACTH) and in people with certain types of emotional depression caused by biochemical abnormalities (biochemical depression.)

Dexamethasone is usually taken in pill form late in the evening. Several blood samples are collected the next day.

There are two principal problems with this test: it is not very sensitive (that is, many people with biochemical depression do not have a positive test) and there are many conditions and medications that can produce a false-positive result.

### Why Performed:

This test is used to help determine the cause of increased cortisol levels. It may also be performed when serious biochemical depression is suspected and to follow the progress of previously diagnosed depression. The American Psychiatric Association recommends that this test should be used for depression only in selected cases at psychiatric research centers—there are too many other conditions and medications which can produce a positive test when no biochemical depression is present.

### Normal Values:

May vary from lab to lab:

Less than 5 micrograms per deciliter (mcg/dl)

●*Greater Than Normal Values May Mean*: Depressive illness, Cushing's disease, myocardial infarction (heart attack), congestive heart failure, fever, hypertension due to renal artery stenosis, pregnancy, malnutrition, hyperthyroidism, anorexia nervosa, Alzheimer's disease, alcoholism.

### Interfering Factors:
Phenobarbital, phenytoin (diphenylhydantoin, Dilantin), meprobamate (Equanil, Miltown), steroids, estrogens.

### Cost:
$80 to $100

# Drug Monitoring

For some drugs, the dosage level necessary to help you (therapeutic level) is fairly close to that at which toxic effects may occur (toxic level). If you are taking one of these drugs, monitoring of the blood concentration of the drug may be necessary.

Blood levels vary with the time elapsed since the last drug dose was taken. The highest, or peak, levels are usually reached shortly after the drug is taken. Low, or trough, levels are usually reached just before the next dose is due. In some cases both the lowest (trough) and highest (peak) blood levels of a drug are measured.

### Why Performed:
These tests are used to be sure that people taking certain drugs achieve a therapeutic dose while avoiding toxic levels. Drug monitoring is especially useful in people whose ability to metabolize drugs is unpredictable, especially those with decreased function of the liver or the kidneys, since these are the organs that normally eliminate a drug from the body. It is also useful in infants and the elderly, people with congestive heart failure, people taking two or more drugs that may interact, and severely ill patients. This test may also be suggested if the physician suspects that a patient is not taking a recommended medication.

Drug levels may also be measured when an overdose is suspected (see Toxicology Screening, p. 109).

Monitoring can be used for nearly any type of drug, but is most frequently done on people taking certain antibiotics, barbiturates, digoxin, lithium, phenytoin (Dilantin), quinidine, high doses of aspirin or aspirinlike drugs (salicylates), and theophylline.

### Cost:
From $20 to $70, depending on the drug being monitored.

## Antibiotics

Drug monitoring is most frequently done for the aminoglycoside family of antibiotics, because therapeutic levels of these drugs are close to toxic levels. The most frequently used members of this family are gentamicin, tobramycin, and amikacin.

| Drug | Therapeutic Levels | Toxic Levels |
|---|---|---|
| Amikacin | 15–25 micrograms per milliliter | over 25–35 mcg/ml |
| Gentamicin | 4–10 mcg/ml | over 12 mcg/ml |
| Tobramycin | 4–10 mcg/ml | over 12 mcg/ml |

Symptoms of aminoglycoside toxicity include ringing in the ears, hearing loss, other hearing difficulties, dizziness, and blurred vision.

## Barbiturates

Barbiturates are tranquilizing drugs used as anesthetics, sedatives, and sleeping pills. They are also sometimes used to prevent seizures. Barbiturates are the most common cause of drug-induced coma.

Signs of barbiturate toxicity include confusion, headache, slow weak breathing, low blood pressure, low urine output, and soft flabby muscles.

This test is also done on urine, but blood tests give more specific information. It is also sometimes done on the stomach contents of comatose patients. (See Toxicology Screening, p. 109)

Drugs in the salicylate (e.g., aspirin) and sulfonamide (sulfa drug) families can interfere with test results, as can MAO inhibitors, disulfiram, alcohol, rifampin, and primidone.

|  | Therapeutic Levels | Toxic Levels |
|---|---|---|
| Phenobarbital | 15−39 mcg/ml | 40 mcg/ml |
| Amobarbital (Amytal, Tuinal) | 3−12 mcg/ml | 30 mcg/ml |
| Pentobarbital (Nembutal) | 1−5 mcg/ml | 10 mcg/ml |
| Secobarbital | 2−5 mcg/ml | 20 mcg/ml |

## Digoxin

This drug is used in the treatment of heart disease. It increases the force of the heart's contraction, allowing it to operate more effectively.

The blood levels necessary for the desired therapeutic effect are not far from the levels at which toxic symptoms appear. Thus a relatively slight increase in blood levels can produce the symptoms of digoxin toxicity: nausea, vomiting, irregular heartbeats, and hallucinations. In rare cases, digoxin toxicity can cause death.

When digoxin toxicity is suspected it is also important to check blood levels of potassium and creatinine: Low potassium levels increase digoxin toxicity, and high creatinine levels may indicate impaired kidney function, which can reduce the body's ability to metabolize digoxin.

This test is usually done when a person first begins taking digoxin. Once a therapeutic dose has been established, it is important not to change either the dose or the brand of the drug. Research shows that even at the same dose, different brands of the same drug can produce different drug levels.

*Therapeutic levels*: 0.8 to 2.0 nanograms per millileter (ng/ml), but values vary widely from person to person.

*Toxic levels*: Above 2.5 ng/ml, but values vary widely from person to person.

## Lithium

This drug is used to treat extreme mood swings (often referred to as manic-depressive illness) and other disorders. People taking lithium should have their blood levels checked regularly to be sure that they are receiving the right amount of the drug to produce therapeutic but not toxic blood levels.

Lithium blood levels are normally taken the day after treatment begins. Blood levels are measured three times a week until an appropriate level is reached. Blood levels are then tested monthly, more frequently if side effects appear. You must not take lithium for eight hours before this test.

The use of diuretics or a low-salt diet can increase lithium levels. Lithium levels are decreased by aminophylline, sodium bicarbonate, and salt.

Usual side effects of lithium (at therapeutic levels) may include frequent urination, excessive thirst, a slight tremor, and a slightly increased white blood cell count. Symptoms of lithium toxicity include vomiting, weakness, convulsions, markedly increased white blood cell count, and coma.

*Therapeutic levels*: May vary from person to person, but are usually between 0.5 and 1.5 milliequivalents per liter (mEq/L).

*Toxic levels*: Blood levels above 1.5 mEq/L frequently produce toxic symptoms. Blood levels above 4.0 meq/L may cause death.

## Phenytoin (Dilantin)

This anticonvulsant drug is used principally to treat seizure disorders. Its levels fluctuate widely in the body, and a small overdose can cause toxic damage. Toxic symptoms include dizziness and irregular heartbeats.

*Therapeutic levels*: 10 to 20 micrograms per milliliter (mcg/ml).

*Toxic levels*: Above 20–50 mcg/ml, but can vary widely from person to person.

## Quinidine

This drug is frequently used to treat irregularities of the heartbeat. Signs of toxicity include nausea, vomiting, diarrhea, and headache.

*Therapeutic levels*: 2.4 to 5 micrograms per milliliter.

*Toxic levels*: Above 6 micrograms per milliliter.

## Salicylates

The salicylates are the drug family that includes aspirin. Blood levels are monitored in people taking very high doses of these drugs, almost always for arthritis. Aspirin is a common cause of accidental poisoning in children.

Signs of salicylate toxicity include the following:

Mild toxicity—rapid breathing, nausea, burning pain in throat, mouth, or abdomen, ringing in the ears, lethargy, hearing difficulties.

Moderate toxicity—very rapid breathing, sweating, itching, fever, dehydration, blurry vision, loss of coordination, restlessness, delirium.

Severe toxicity—extremely rapid breathing, bluish tinge to skin, decreased urine output, confusion, coma, low body temperature.

*Therapeutic levels*: 2 to 30 milligrams per 100 milliliters (mg/dl).

*Toxic levels*: Toxic symptoms frequently begin to appear above 35 mg/dl, but levels vary from person to person.

### Theophylline

This drug helps to relax the smooth muscle of the bronchi (the tubes through which air passes on its way to and from the lungs). It is frequently used to treat asthma and asthmalike conditions. High blood levels can produce shakiness, abdominal pain, and seizures.

Beverages containing caffeine or caffeinelike substances can produce a slightly elevated test result.

*Therapeutic levels*: 10 to 20 micrograms per milliliter (mcg/ml).

*Toxic levels*: Vary from person to person, but generally over 20 mcg/ml.

# D-Xylose Absorption Test

This test measures the intestines' ability to absorb a simple sugar, D-xylose, in order to determine whether nutrients are being properly absorbed.

### Preparation:

You will be asked to fast overnight before the test. Initial blood and urine samples will then be taken and you will be asked to empty your bladder. Next you will be asked to drink a mixture containing D-xylose. Two hours later, another blood sample will be taken. Five-hour blood samples are also sometimes drawn. All of the urine you produce for a period of five hours (sometimes longer) following the test will be collected and measured. You will be asked to fast and to stay in bed during the test.

### Why Performed:

In cases of suspected malabsorptive disorders of the small intestine, with persistent diarrhea, weight loss, malnutrition, and generalized weakness.

### Normal Values:

Vary with laboratory and amount of D-xylose administered.

●*Less Than Normal Values May Mean*: A malabsorptive disorder of the small intestine. Further tests will be necessary to determine the reason for the malabsorption.

### Interfering Factors:

An excessive number of bacteria within the intestine can cause decreased D-xylose levels in the blood and urine. Kidney disease can cause depressed levels in the urine. The drugs isocarboxazid (Marplan) and phenelzine (Nardil), may reduce D-xylose excretion. Failure to restrict activity may result in inaccurate test results. Aspirin increases D-xylose blood levels; indomethacin decreases blood levels. Conditions in which food remains in the stomach (poor gastric emptying) may produce false-positive test results.

### Cost:

$40 to $80

### Special Considerations:

★You may experience abdominal discomfort, nausea, or mild diarrhea from the large doses of D-xylose. These side effects are uncommon.

★Sometimes, if bacterial overgrowth in the intestine is suspected, antibiotics may be given for a day or two before the test.

# Estriol

Estriol is a female hormone produced in large amounts during pregnancy by the placenta, the tissue that links the fetus to its mother. A steadily increasing estriol production throughout the course of pregnancy reflects a properly functioning placenta and usually means a healthy, growing fetus. Estriol is usually measured in a urine specimen collected over a 24-hour period (see p. 39), although it may also be measured in a blood sample.

**Why Performed:**
Estriol levels may be measured in pregnant women who are at higher risk for complications during pregnancy due to diabetes, high blood pressure, toxemia, a previous history of stillbirth, or other problems. In such high-risk pregnancies estriol measurements are usually performed two or more times per week, starting about the 33rd week of pregnancy. This test may also be performed to determine the health of the fetus if the mother is past her due date.

**Normal Values:**
Vary considerably but should rise steadily throughout the pregnancy.
●*Lower Than Normal Values May Mean*: A decrease in urinary estriol levels (a drop of 40% or more on two successive days or a drop of 20% or more over two successive weeks) strongly suggests that the placenta is not working properly and the baby may be at serious risk. If the estriol is below the expected level, other tests such as fetal monitoring (p. 213) may be performed. Depending upon the results of these tests, the age of the fetus and condition of the

mother, labor may be induced or a cesarean section performed.

Slightly low estriol levels may also be due to fetal adrenal gland insufficiency, congenital abnormalities, maternal hypertension, diabetes, malnutrition, anemia, liver disease, or kidney disease.
●*Greater Than Normal Values May Mean*: Multiple pregnancy (twins, triplets, etc.).

**Interfering Factors:**
The following drugs may influence urine estriol levels: steroid hormones (including estrogens, progesterone, and corticosteroids), phenothiazines, meprobamate, ampicillin, tetracyclines, phenazopyridine hydrochloride, methenamine mandelate, cascara, senna, phenolphthalein, and hydrochlorothiazide.

**Cost:**
$30 to $50

# Estrogens

Estrogens are the female hormones. There are several different types including estriol, estrone, and estradiol (the most potent). Most of the estrogens are produced in the ovaries and in the placenta during pregnancy. Small amounts are also normally secreted by the adrenal glands in men and women as well as by the testicles in men. These hormones are responsible for the development of secondary female sexual characteristics (such as breast enlargement) and normal menstruation. Estrogen secretion, controlled largely by the pituitary gland in the brain, normally varies throughout the menstrual cycle and during the course of pregnancy. Estrogen levels can be measured in a blood sample (p. 36) or in a urine specimen collected over 24 hours (p. 39).

### Why Performed:
To evaluate suspected ovarian disorders and abnormal sexual development. In women this might include early or delayed puberty, excessive menstrual bleeding, or lack of normal menstruation. In men estrogen levels may help explain abnormal sexual development such as breast enlargement.

### Normal Values:
May vary from lab to lab. Total estrogen varies throughout the menstrual cycle.

> Women:
> 22–80 micrograms (mcg) per 24-hour urine specimen or 61–394 picograms per milliliter (pg/ml) of serum during first two weeks of menstrual cycle
> 28–100 mcg per 24-hour urine specimen or 122–437 pg/ml of serum at ovulation
> 4–25 mcg per 24-hour urine specimen or 156–350 pg/ml of serum during menses
> less than 10 mcg per 24-hour urine specimen or less than 40 pg/ml of serum after menopause
> up to 45,000 mcg per 24-hour urine specimen or up to 31,000 pg/ml of serum during pregnancy
> Men:
> 5–18 mcg per 24-hour urine specimen or 40–115 pg/ml of serum

●*Lower Than Normal Values May Mean*: Decreased ovarian function either due to a failure of the ovary to develop and function properly or to a decrease in pituitary gland activity which controls the ovaries.

●*Greater Than Normal Values May Mean*: A tumor or overactivity of the ovaries or adrenal glands, excessive pituitary gland activity, liver disease, or testicular tumors may produce elevated urinary estrogens.

### Interfering Factors:
Pregnancy, steroid medications (estrogens, progesterone, birth control pills, and high-dose corticosteroids), phenothiazine tranquilizers (Compazine, Stelazine, Thorazine), phenazopyridine hydrochloride, tetracyclines, ampicillin, meprobamate, senna, cascara, and hydrochlorothiazide can influence the test results.

### Cost:
$35 to $45

### Special Considerations:
★Estriol, one of the estrogens, rises dramatically during a normal pregnancy and can be used as a measure of the well-being of the fetus (see p. 73).

# Ferritin

Ferritin is a protein which binds to iron. The resulting ferritin-iron complex serves as one of the body's main iron reserves.

Most ferritin is found in the reticuloendothelial cells, but a small amount appears in the blood. Blood ferritin levels usually reflect the amount of available iron stored in the body.

This test is performed on a venous blood sample (p. 36).

### Why Performed:
To screen for iron deficiency or iron overload.

**Normal Values:**

May vary from lab to lab:

Men: 15 to 200 nanograms per milliliter (ng/ml)

Women: 12 to 150 ng/ml

Children: 7 to 600 ng/ml, depending on age

● *Greater Than Normal Values May Mean*: Liver disease, iron overload (hemochromatosis), leukemia, infection, or chronic hemolytic anemia.

● *Less Than Normal Values May Mean*: Chronic iron deficiency.

**Interfering Factors:**

A recent transfusion may produce increased ferritin levels.

**Cost:**

$30 to $50

# Folic Acid (Folates)

Folic acid and folates (closely related compounds) are water-soluble vitamins necessary for the proper formation of blood cells, DNA synthesis, and general body growth. Dietary sources include liver, kidney, beef, nuts, yeast, fruits, green leafy vegetables, eggs, and milk.

The body can store folic acid for only a month or two, so regular consumption is necessary to prevent deficiency. Sometimes, during pregnancy, the growing baby's requirement for folic acid is so great that the mother can develop folic acid deficiency. Folic acid deficiency produces an anemia with enlarged red blood cells (megaloblastic), but deficiency can be diagnosed before symptoms of anemia appear.

This test is performed on a venous blood sample (p. 36).

**Why Performed:**

This test is used to aid in the diagnosis of anemia and to distinguish between folic acid deficiency and vitamin $B_{12}$ deficiency (see p. 123), both of these conditions cause megaloblastic anemia; and to help diagnose folic acid deficiency which may cause symptoms such as a sore tongue and diarrhea.

**Normal Values:**

Vary from lab to lab, but in general, normal levels fall between 5 and 25 nanograms per milliliter (ng/ml).

● *Greater Than Normal Values May Mean*: High dietary intake or supplementation with folic acid, although this vitamin does not appear to be toxic, even in high doses.

● *Less Than Normal Values May Mean*: Inadequate dietary intake or difficulty absorbing folic acid (as the result of such malabsorptive diseases as celiac disease or sprue), alcoholism, inadequate intake of vitamin C, hyperthyroidism, pregnancy, or treatment with medications such as methotrexate, anticonvulsants (Dilantin), and oral contraceptives, which lower folic acid levels. Low levels can cause an anemia characterized by enlarged red blood cells (megaloblastic), leukopenia (not enough white blood cells), or thrombocytopenia (not enough platelets).

**Cost:**

$60 to $80

# Follicle-Stimulating Hormone (FSH)

Follicle-stimulating hormone (FSH) stimulates the activity of the gonads in both sexes: In women, it increases estrogen secretion and prepares the ovary to release its egg. In men, FSH promotes sperm formation. This test may be done on either blood or urine.

FSH is secreted by the pituitary gland. In women, secretion varies with the phase of the menstrual cycle, reaching its highest point at the time of ovulation. In men, FSH production is relatively constant.

FSH measurements are an essential part of a workup for infertility. This test is performed on women more often than on men. Tests for such related hormones as luteinizing hormone (p. 88), estrogen (p. 73), and progesterone (p. 94) are also usually done.

If blood is tested, several samples are usually taken over a 24-hour period. If urine is tested, a 24-hour sample is required.

## Why Performed:

To help diagnose fertility or menstrual disorders, to help determine whether menopause has occurred, to diagnose the cause of early puberty, or to determine the cause of underdevloped sexual organs (hypogonadism).

## Normal Values:

May vary from lab to lab:
   Blood:
      Menstruating women: up to 10 international units per milliliter (IU/ml)
      Menstruating women—midcycle: up to 20 IU/ml
Menopausal women: up to 200 IU/ml
Men: up to 15 IU/ml
Children (prepuberty): up to 12 IU/ml
Urine:
Menstruating women: 4 to 30 IU/ml
Menstruating women—midcycle peak: twice baseline levels.
Menopausal women: 40 to 250 IU/ml
Men: 4 to 25 IU/ml

●*Greater Than Normal Values May Mean*: In women: ovarian failure, Turner's syndrome, polycystic ovaries. Levels are normally high in women who have experienced menopause. In men: testicular damage (from mumps, x-ray exposure, tumor, or trauma), testicular failure, or absence of testicles. In both sexes: precocious puberty, congenital absence of ovaries or testes.

●*Less Than Normal Values May Mean*: Infertility in both men and women, anorexia nervosa, or pituitary failure.

## Interfering Factors:

FSH levels are decreased by steroid hormones (e.g., estrogen, progesterone) and some antipsychotic medications such as chlorpromazine (Thorazine) and other phenothiazines. Radioactive scans done within one week before the test may influence results. Rough handling of the sample may interfere with accurate results.

## Cost:

$40 to $90

## Special Considerations:

★If you are taking medications containing estrogens or progesterone, be sure to discuss their effects on the test with your doctor. You may be asked to discontinue these drugs for a short period prior to the test.

★Be sure that the person drawing your blood notes the phase of your menstrual cycle on the laboratory slip. If you have had a hysterectomy or have experienced menopause, the person drawing your blood should also note that on the lab slip.

# Galactosemia Screening

The enzyme galactose transferase is needed to break down the sugar galactose, which is found in milk and sugar beets. Some babies are born without this enzyme, a condition called galactosemia. Once a diagnosis is made, the treatment is to eliminate foods containing the sugar galactose—especially milk—from the diet. If a child with this disease continues to consume galactose, widespread tissue damage and abnormalities such as cataracts and kidney and liver disease can result.

This test measures the level of galactose transferase in a newborn baby's blood.

**Why Performed:**
All newborn babies must, in most states, be tested for this disease. (In some states the test can be waived if the parents object.)

**Normal Values:**
The enzyme is present.

**Abnormal Values:**
The enzyme is absent. This indicates that the disease is present and that a galactose-free diet should be followed.

**Cost:**
$8 to $12

**Special Considerations:**
★There is a rare form of galactosemia that causes no symptoms and need not be treated.

# Gastrin

Gastrin is a hormone produced by the stomach. When food enters the stomach, it stimulates gastrin secretion. As blood gastrin levels rise, the cells lining the stomach respond by producing gastric acid, which helps digest food. Increasing levels of gastric acid ordinarily inhibit further gastrin production.

Gastrin also stimulates the pancreas to produce insulin and the liver to produce bile—both of which aid in digestion—and stimulates the muscular activity in the intestine walls which moves the food along.

This test is performed on a venous blood sample (p. 36).

**Preparation:**
You must abstain from alcohol for 24 hours before the test and fast for 12 hours before the test. Unlimited water is allowed. Because stress can affect gastrin levels, you will be asked to rest quietly for 30 minutes before the blood sample is drawn.

**Why Performed:**
To help determine the cause of severe ulcer disease of the stomach and/or small intestine, and to help diagnose suspected tumors of the stomach.

**Normal Values:**
Values may vary from lab to lab:
    Less than 300 picograms per milliliter

(pg/ml), although normal values may reach as high as 700 pg per ml in elderly people.

• *Greater Than Normal Values May Mean*: Values above 1000 pg/ml are usually considered diagnostic for Zollinger-Ellison syndrome, in which a tumor (adenoma) of the pancreas, duodenum, or stomach secretes high levels of gastrin, resulting in severe ulcers of the stomach and/or duodenum. Levels as high as 450,000 pg/ml have been reported in this disease. Levels may also be increased in gastric carcinoma, gastric ulcers, pernicious anemia, and end-stage renal disease (because gastrin is normally broken down in the kidney).

### Interfering Factors:

Failure to restrict diet or activity may produce inaccurate test results. Gastrin levels are increased by stress, alcohol, hypoglycemia, amino acids, calcium carbonate, acetycholine, and calcium chloride. Gastrin levels are decreased by atropine, hydrochloric acid, and secretin.

### Cost:

$20 to $50

### Special Considerations:

★*Gastrin Stimulation Test*: For some people with ulcers who have normal gastrin levels, a gastrin stimulation test may be useful. For this test you are asked to eat a protein-rich meal. Blood samples are taken shortly afterward. In people with ulcer disease, gastrin levels increase markedly, while in normal people they increase only slightly.

# Glucose
## (Blood Glucose, Urine Glucose, Fasting Blood Sugar, 2-Hour Postprandial Blood Sugar, Glucose Tolerance Test, Random Blood Sugar)

Glucose is the primary energy source for all body tissues. The sugars and carbohydrates you eat are ordinarily converted into glucose, which can be either used to produce immediate energy or stored as glycogen in the liver or as fat throughout the body. Glycogen and fat thus serve as sources of reserve energy. The body can also manufacture glucose from fats and amino acids.

Glucose can be measured in either the blood or the urine. If your blood is tested, you will either be asked to come in early in the morning to have the blood sample taken after a 12- to 14-hour fast (fasting blood sugar, or FBS), or be asked to eat a meal exactly 2 hours before the blood is to be drawn (2-hour postprandial blood sugar, or 2-hour PP). If neither a fast nor a special meal is observed before the test, it is called a random blood sugar (RBS). It is also possible to measure blood glucose by home testing (p. 434).

Urine normally contains very little sugar. However, when the blood sugar level is very high, as in diabetes, the ability of the kidney to keep sugar out of the urine may be exceeded. (The level of blood glucose at which glucose spills into the urine is called the renal threshold, and is usually between 160 and 180 milligrams per deciliter.) Sugar that spills into the urine carries a large volume of water with it, producing the two classic symptoms of diabetes: excessive urination and thirst.

Urine glucose can be measured by two simple methods: a tablet (reducing) test and a dipstick (enzymatic) test. You can easily perform these tests at home (p. 434). A second-voided urine specimen (p. 38) is required. The results of urine tests should be compared with blood glucose tests. People who have borderline results on this test are sometimes advised to have a glucose tolerance test (see below).

### Why Performed:

To diagnose diabetes or hypoglycemia and to help test for a number of hormonal disorders. Urine testing is performed as part of a routine urinalysis. Both urine and blood may be used as home tests to monitor the effectiveness of diabetic self-care.

### Normal Values:

Fasting blood sugar: 70 to 110 milligrams per deciliter (mg/dl)

2-hour postprandial blood sugar: 120 to 150 mg/dl

Urine: no detectable glucose

● *Greater Than Normal Values May Mean*: Blood sugar—Mild elevations (120 to 150 mg/dl) may be caused by diabetes, pregnancy, hypertension, hyperthyroidism, excessive pituitary function, excessive adrenal function, obesity, thiazide diuretics, or a recent heavy meal.

Moderate elevations (150 to 500 mg/dl) may be caused by diabetes, recent anesthesia, carbon monoxide poisoning, infectious disease, or disease of the central nervous system.

High (greater than 500 mg/dl) levels are always associated with diabetes.

Urine glucose—A positive result suggests that you should have a blood test for glucose.

● *Less Than Normal Values May Mean*:

Hypoglycemia—A below-normal blood glucose accompanied by hypoglycemic symptoms (weakness, nervousness, sweating, nausea, palpitations, irritability, and difficulty thinking clearly) is usually considered diagnostic for hypoglycemia. Decreased levels may also be associated with cold exposure, liver disease, excessive insulin levels, underactive adrenal glands (Addison's disease), underactive pituitary gland (Simmonds' disease), hypothyroidism, prolonged vomiting, prolonged fever, poor nutrition, starvation, severe exercise, Von Gierke's disease (a glycogen storage disorder).

### Interfering Factors:

Infection, illness, or pregnancy can elevate blood glucose levels. Strenuous exercise can reduce blood glucose. Drugs known to increase blood glucose levels include arginine, benzodiazepines, chlorthalidone, corticosteroids, diazoxide, epinephrine, estrogen, ethacrynic acid, furosemide, glucose infusions, lithium, nicotinic acid, oral contraceptives, phenolphthalein, phenothiazides, phenytoin, thiazide diuretics, and triamterene. Drugs known to decrease blood glucose levels include alcohol (ethanol), clofibrate, insulin, oral hypoglycemic drugs, MAO inhibitors, and propranolol.

Drugs that can interfere with the tablet test for urine glucose include vitamin C, many antibiotics, probenecid, methyldopa (Aldomet), and high doses of aspirin. Drugs that can interfere with the dipstick test for urine glucose include vitamin C, levodopa, and phenazopyridine (Pyridium).

### Cost:

$4 to $8

### Special Considerations:

★*Glucose Tolerance Test (GTT)*—This test measures the body's response to a large dose of concentrated sugar. For at least several days before the test, you must eat a diet with plenty of carbohydrates. You will be asked to fast beginning at midnight on the night before the test and to come to the clinic or hospital early in the morning—usually between 7 and 9 A.M. Blood and urine samples will be taken. You will then be asked to drink a concentrated sugar solution. Additional blood samples will be taken at regular intervals over the next 3–5 hours. You will not be allowed to eat anything until the test is completed but will be encouraged to drink lots of water while the test is in process. This will help your body break down the high-sugar drink.

This test is most frequently done to confirm a diagnosis of diabetes or hypoglycemia. If you are being tested for hypoglycemia, you should know that the symptoms you feel during the test may be important evidence in making a diagnosis. Many physicians encourage their hypoglycemic patients to keep a diary of their experiences during the test, so that the patients can have a written record available when discussing their reaction to the test. Symptoms of severe hypoglycemia may include severe weakness, nervousness, restlessness, confusion, hunger, and sweating.

If the health workers conducting the test feel that hypoglycemic symptoms are becoming dangerously severe (e.g., possible unconsciousness), they may discontinue the test and give you a sweet snack or sugar-enriched orange juice to bring your blood sugar back to normal.

The glucose tolerance test is falling into disrepute among some physicians, who feel that one's response to a large dose of concentrated sugar solution may have little to do with one's response to everyday conditions. Many diabetes experts no longer recommend it for the diagnosis of diabetes. Others use it only if the fasting blood sugar

is borderline. When this test is used for hypoglycemia there are many false-positives.

# Glycohemoglobin (Glycosolated Hemoglobin, Hemoglobin $A_{1c}$, Diabetic Control Index)

A blood glucose test (see p. 78) measures the blood glucose at one particular moment and may vary widely from moment to moment, depending upon diet, exercise, and use of insulin or other medications. However, in diabetics it is sometimes useful to get information about the overall control of blood glucose in addition to the momentary measurements. Another blood test, called glycohemoglobin or hemoglobin $A_{1c}$, measures the percentage of hemoglobin molecules that have sugar molecules attached to them. The percentage of the total hemoglobin that has sugar attached to it reflects the blood sugar levels over the preceding 3 to 4 months.

**Why Performed:**
To assess how well a person with diabetes has been able to control his or her blood sugar over the preceding 3 to 4 months.

**Normal Values:**
Values vary from lab to lab:
    3 to 6% of total hemoglobin

●*Greater Than Normal Values May Mean*: Elevated values may indicate diabetes in poor control. Highly elevated values almost always indicate diabetes in poor control.

**Cost:**
$20 to $30

# Growth Hormone
## (HGH, Somatotropin)

Human growth hormone (HGH) regulates growth. Abnormalities in HGH production during childhood can produce gigantism (abnormally tall stature) or dwarfism (abnormally short stature). Both these conditions can be treated if diagnosed early.

When HGH increases in adulthood, growth of the long bones does not occur, but continued growth of other bones can cause protrusion of the jaw, slanting of the forehead, and enlargement of the nose. This condition is called acromegaly. It usually results from a tumor of the pituitary.

This test is performed on a venous blood sample (p. 36).

**Preparation:**
You will be asked to fast for 8–10 hours before the test. You may be asked to lie down and relax in a quiet room for 30 minutes before the blood sample is drawn.

**Why Performed:**
In children, when gigantism or dwarfism is suspected. In adults, to help diagnose suspected tumors of the pituitary.

**Normal Values:**
> Children—up to 15 nanograms per milliliter (ng/ml)
> Women—up to 30 ng/ml
> Men—up to 10 ng/ml

• *Greater Than Normal Values May Mean*: Tumor of the pituitary gland or hypothalamus. Increased HGH levels may also result from diabetes, stress, or intense physical activity.

• *Less Than Normal Values May Mean*: Pituitary insufficiency.

**Interfering Factors:**
HGH levels are increased by amphetamines, arginine, estrogens, glucagon, histamine, insulin, levodopa, methyldopa, nicotinic acid, propranolol and other beta-blocker drugs. HGH levels are decreased by chlorpromazine (Thorazine) and other phenothiazine antipsychotics and by steroids.

A previous radioactive scan can affect results if performed within one week before this test.

**Cost:**
$20 to $35

# Hemoglobin Electrophoresis

Hemoglobin is the complex oxygen-carrying molecule found in red blood cells. It is composed of four long chains of amino acid building blocks. The sequence of these amino acids is determined genetically. Over 300 different types of hemoglobin have been identified, but only three forms (hemoglobin A, $A_2$, and F) are considered normal. Abnormal amounts of these normal hemoglobins or the presence of an abnormal hemoglobin causes a variety of diseases, ranging from mild conditions producing no symptoms to life-threatening anemias.

Hemoglobin electrophoresis is a blood test which separates and measures the different types of hemoglobin in the blood.

## Why Performed:

This test is used to evaluate certain types of anemia when abnormal hemoglobin is suspected. Since the genes that control the manufacture of hemoglobin are inherited, prospective parents with genetic tendencies toward certain types of anemia may be tested and counseled as to the risks to their offspring.

## Normal Values:

Hemoglobin A: greater than 95%
Hemoglobin $A_2$: 1.5 to 3.5%
Hemoglobin F: less than 2%
Abnormal variants: none

## Abnormal Values:

Hundreds of different abnormal hemoglobins (hemoglobinopathies) have been identified. For example, the presence of slightly increased hemoglobin $A_2$ and F suggests thalassemia minor, a harmless condition. However, if both parents have thalassemia minor, then their baby has a chance of developing thalassemia major (Mediterranean anemia), a serious anemia characterized by very low amounts of hemoglobin A and high levels of hemoglobin F. The presence of moderate levels of hemoglobin S indicates sickle-cell trait. High hemoglobin S levels are found in sickle-cell disease, a severe anemia which primarily affects blacks (see p. 105).

## Interfering Factors:

Inaccurate results may be obtained if the person being tested has received a blood transfusion in the past four months from a donor with an abnormal hemoglobin.

## Cost:

$30 to $50

# Histocompatibility Testing
# (Human Leukocyte Antigen, HLA, HL Antigen)

The success of a proposed organ transplant will depend to a large degree on the histocompatibility between the donor and the recipient of the organ. (A high degree of histocompatibility means that the immune system of the recipient does not attack the donor's tissues.) The more cellular histocompatibility sites two people have in common, the more likely a tissue or organ from one can be successfully transplanted to the other. Histocompatibility antigens are present on all human cells, but are most easily tested for on white blood cells.

## Why Performed:

This test is done prior to any skin graft or organ transplant. It is also done before transfusions of platelets or white cells, in some undiagnosed infections, and in cases of disputed parentage. This is a more specific test for a person's genetic parents than blood group typing.

## Normal Values:

No normal values; each HLA is either present or absent.

## Results:

The greater the similarity between donor and recipient, the better the chance the transplanted organ or tissue will survive.

Children inherit one-half of their HLA genes from each parent. Thus, half of a child's HLA antigens will be identical to those of the mother and the other half will be identical to those of the father.

## Cost:

$38 to $50 for single HLA antigens. A panel of four or more HLA sites costs about $300 to $400.

## Special Considerations:

★Some HLA antigens have been found to be associated with certain diseases:

| HLA | Associated Disease |
| --- | --- |
| HLA-A2 | Myasthenia gravis |
| HLA-B7 | Pernicious anemia |
| HLA-B8 | Systemic lupus erythmatosus |
| HLA B-13 & HLA B-17 | Arthritis, psoriasis |
| HLA B-27 | Ankylosing spondylitis |

# Immunoglobulins
## (Gamma Globulins)

Immunoglobulins (gamma globulins) are antibodies which seek out and destroy invading organisms and other substances foreign to the body. Each of these antibodies is usually specific to only one type of invading organism or substance. Immunoglobulins are produced by the lymphocytes (one kind of white blood cell).

There are five major types of immunoglobulin:

IgG (immunoglobulin G) is the most abundant. It responds to any foreign material.

IgA responds to bacterial and viral invasions.

IgM responds to infections and is involved in certain kinds of arthritis.

IgE is involved in allergic reactions.

IgD is still poorly understood.

This test is performed on a venous blood sample (p. 36).

## Why Performed:

To diagnose diseases associated with abnormal immunoglobulin levels—usually frequent bacterial infections.

## Normal Values:

(For adults. Values differ in children.)

IgG: 6.4 to 14.3 milligrams per milliliter (mg/ml)

IgA: 0.3 to 3.0 mg/ml

IgM: 0.2 to 1.4 mg/ml

Approximate proportion of immunoglobulins in healthy people:

IgG 75%

IgA 15%

IgM 5–7%

IgE 2% or less

IgD 1% or less

## Interfering Factors:

Immunoglobulin levels may be decreased by chemotherapy or by radiation therapy.

All immunoglobulin levels are raised by aminophenazone, anticonvulsants, birth control pills, hydralazine, hydantoin derivatives, and phenylbutazone.

All immunoglobulin levels may be decreased by severe BCG (anti-TB vaccine) sensitivity reaction or by methotrexate.

IgG and IgA levels may be decreased by dextrans, methylprednisone, and phenytoin.

IgM levels may be decreased by dextran and methylprednisone.

IgG levels may be increased by methadone.

IgA levels may be increased by alcoholism

IgM levels may be increased by heavy narcotics use.

## Cost:

A panel including IgG, IgA, and IgM costs $10 to $25. Tests for individual immuno-globulins are about $15 to $25.

## Special Considerations:

★People with abnormally low immunoglobulin levels (especially IgG and IgM) may be at increased risk of infection, and should take special care of any respiratory infections or any breaks in the skin and report any signs of infection (e.g., tenderness, swelling, swollen lymph nodes) to their clinician.

# Iron
## (Total Iron-Binding Capacity, TIBC)

Iron is the active component of hemoglobin, the substance in red blood cells that carries oxygen. Iron is essential to life, yet it is present in the blood in amounts much smaller than most other vital substances.

About 78% of the iron in the body is bound to hemoglobin. Some of the remaining iron is bound to a protein (transferrin) in the blood, and some iron is stored in the bone marrow.

The original source of all the body's iron is food. The iron from old blood cells is effectively recycled: It is stored in the protein-bound form in the blood and in the marrow until it is needed to form new red cells.

In healthy adult males dietary iron deficiency is rarely a problem, since men's bodies normally lose such a small amount of iron that they have sufficient iron stores to last for several years, even if no new iron is taken in. But in women of menstruating age, particularly those who are pregnant or breast-feeding, large quantities of iron can be lost. If these women do not eat a diet high in iron, iron deficiency can sometimes be a problem. In some cases, iron supplements may be needed.

This test measures the amount of free iron bound to transferrin in a blood sample. Another test commonly performed at the same time is the total iron-binding capacity (TIBC). This measures the amount of iron it would take to saturate all the transferrin in a given quantity of your blood. By dividing the TIBC by the serum iron, we can obtain the portion of transferrin that is actually saturated.

You should tell your doctor if you are taking vitamins or iron supplements.

## Why Performed:

To help diagnose known or suspected iron-deficiency anemia, and to screen for iron overload (hemochromatosis).

## Normal Values:

|  | Serum Iron (mcg/dl) | TIBC (mcg/dl) | % Saturation |
|---|---|---|---|
| Men | 70 to 150 | 300 to 400 | 20 to 50 |
| Women | 80 to 150 | 300 to 450 | 20 to 50 |

● *Greater Than Normal Values May Mean*: Iron overload (hemochromatosis).

● *Less Than Normal Values May Mean*: Iron deficiency, normal pregnancy, chronic inflammation.

## Cost:

Serum iron: $5 to $10
TIBC: $10 to $15

## Special Considerations:

★*Anemia of chronic disease*—This is a condition in which both iron levels and total iron-binding capacity are low but iron stores in the marrow are normal or high. The chronic disease prevents the body from using the iron effectively.

★Another test of iron stores in the body is measurement of serum ferritin (see p. 74).

# Ketones

The body normally gets its energy from breaking down carbohydrates, principally glucose and glycogen. But if the carbohydrates in your diet are not sufficient for the body's energy needs, it will begin to break down fat.

Fat is broken down in starvation or near-starvation, in very-low-carbohydrate diets, and in diabetes. (In diabetes the body cannot burn carbohydrates because it lacks the necessary insulin.) Ketones are waste products of fat breakdown.

Ketones can be measured in either the blood or the urine. The urine ketone test can be done at home (see p. 426).

## Why Performed:

To detect or monitor uncontrolled diabetes (diabetic ketoacidosis), to evaluate a patient in coma which might be due to uncontrolled diabetes, or to monitor low-carbohydrate diets.

## Normal Values:

Values may vary from lab to lab:
Blood—Usually none, but up to 3 milligrams per deciliter is considered normal.
Urine—None.

• *Greater Than Normal Values May Mean*: Uncontrolled diabetes, starvation, low-carbohydrate diet, prolonged vomiting or diarrhea, severe stress. A small amount of urinary ketones may be produced if a person fasts for a day or longer.

## Interfering Factors:

Levodopa (a medication for Parkinsonism), phenazopyridine (Pyridium, a urinary tract anesthetic), and sulfobromophthalein can cause false-positive results with the dipstick test.

## Cost:

Blood—$10 to $15
Urine—Usually done as part of a complete urinalysis which costs $10 to $20

## Special Considerations:

★Patients in diabetic ketoacidosis will often have a fruity odor to their breath. This is acetone, one type of ketone, which is also excreted through the lungs.

# Kidney Stone Analysis
## (Renal Calculi Analysis)

Urinary stones, also known as calculi, occur in 1%–3% of Americans. They usually form in the kidney, migrate either painlessly or painfully down the ureter into the bladder, and then are passed in the urine. The stones can be collected by carefully straining the urine through a very fine mesh sieve or some fine gauze, and they may range in size from sandlike material to small pellets. A sample of these stones can be sent to the laboratory for chemical analysis. The results of this test can provide important clues to the cause of the stones and can suggest how to treat present stones and prevent others from forming.

### Why Performed:

Kidney stones may be suspected on the basis of X-rays or symptoms including blood in the urine and severe flank pain that sometimes radiates to the groin area.

### Normal Values:

No stones in the urine.

### Abnormal Values:

If a stone or stone fragments are found, the chemical composition can then be determined. About 75% of stones contain calcium oxalate or calcium phosphate. These stones form in urine with an excess of calcium (hypercalciuria). This excess calcium may be due to increased absorption of calcium from the intestine, too much secretion of parathyroid hormone (p. 89), prolonged bed rest (which leaches calcium salts from bone), certain bone diseases and tumors, excessive vitamin D or calcium intake, dehydration, and certain kidney diseases.

Some stones contain uric acid or magnesium ammonium phosphate. Uric acid stones can form in acidic urine or when there is an excess of uric acid in the urine due to gout. Magnesium ammonium phosphate stones can result when bacteria in the urinary tract make the urine too alkaline. Another type of stone, composed of cystine, may be found in a rare inherited metabolic disorder (cystinuria).

### Cost:

$20 to $50

### Special Considerations:

★People with kidney stones are often advised to drink lots of fluids to keep their urine dilute (see home testing for specific gravity, p. 425). A less concentrated urine makes stone formation less likely.

# Lactic Acid

When there is plenty of oxygen in the body's cells, glucose is broken down by oxidation, and the end products are water and carbon dioxide. When there is insufficient oxygen, sugars are broken down by another chemical reaction, and lactic acid is formed. When lactic acid levels rise, the body is said to be in a state of *metabolic acidosis.*

### Why Performed:

When metabolic acidosis is suspected, usually in very ill, hospitalized patients. Symptoms of metabolic acidosis include rapid breathing, sweating, cool clammy skin, sweet-smelling breath, and coma. Metabolic acidosis most frequently occurs in unregulated diabetes.

### Normal Values:

Values may vary from lab to lab:

0.93 to 1.65 milliequivalents per liter (mEq/l)

●*Greater Than Normal Values May Mean*: Lactic acidosis—this can result either from metabolic diseases (e.g., diabetes, anemia, or leukemia), from conditions that prevent sufficient oxygen from reaching the cells (e.g., shock, hemorrhage, infection, heart attack, or pulmonary embolism) or from prolonged strenuous exercise.

### Interfering Factors:

Lactic acidosis can be produced by the following drugs: acetaminophen, alcohol, epinephrine (by IV infusion), glucagon, fructose, and sorbitol.

**Cost:**
$20 to $30

**Special Considerations:**
★The difference between aerobic and anaerobic exercise is that in anaerobic exercise, lactic acid levels are increased, and a person is eventually forced to slow down or stop exercising.

When sprinters push themselves to their physical limits and then gasp and collapse after a race, it is because they are in a state of advanced fatigue due to high lactic acid levels—a very uncomfortable sensation which some highly trained athletes learn to tolerate.

In aerobic exercise, on the other hand, a person does not exceed the level of energy that can be provided by one's aerobic metabolism. In aerobic exercise, the air you breathe contains enough oxygen to oxidize blood sugars completely, without building up a lactic acid debt.

# Lead

The bodies of prehistoric men probably contained no lead at all. Today there is so much of this nonessential mineral in our environment that all of us carry tiny quantities in our bodies. Low body levels are apparently harmless, but high body levels can produce a toxic reaction.

Lead is of medical interest mainly as a hazard to industrial workers, to people exposed to automobile exhaust fumes, and to children. Children who exhibit lead toxicity have most frequently taken it in by mouth as the result of chewing on walls, toys, furniture, or other objects painted with lead-based paint. This type of paint has been off the market for some time, but many objects coated with old paint still remain.

Urine and blood tests are usually done at the same time. A 24-hour sample is required for the urine test. The lead content of hair can also be measured (see Hair Analysis, p. 381).

**Why Performed:**
When lead poisoning is suspected. Symptoms of lead toxicity include vomiting, diarrhea, anemia, headache, a blue line on the gum margin, lethargy, lack of appetite, a metallic taste in the mouth, and weight loss. If lead levels increase, symptoms may include abdominal pain, stupor, and convulsions. This test is used to screen for lead poisoning in children who eat dirt and other foreign material, and as a screening test in workers exposed to lead on the job, especially policemen, service station attendants and others exposed to the exhaust of motor vehicles, and people who work with lead-based paints, plumbing, soldering, manufacturing of some ceramics, insecticides, and lubricants.

**Normal Values:**
Values may vary from lab to lab:
    Blood—up to 50 micrograms per deciliter (mcg/dl)
    Urine—up to 100 micrograms (mcg) per 24 hours
    ●*Greater Than Normal Values May Mean*:
Lead poisoning

**Cost:**
    Blood—$20 to $35
    Urine—$20 to $35

**Special Considerations:**
★*Aminolevulinic Acid* (ALA): Another screening test for lead poisoning is done by measuring the amount of aminolevulinic acid in a 24-hour urine specimen. ALA is

a chemical involved in the production of hemoglobin, the oxygen-carrying molecule in red blood cells. With lead poisoning the production of hemoglobin is blocked, and ALA builds up in the bloodstream and is excreted in urine.

# Lipase

Lipase is an enzyme which helps digest fats. It is produced in the pancreas and released into the small intestine. Increases in blood lipase levels suggest inflammation or other disorder of the pancreas.

This test is usually done together with that for amylase (p. 48), another enzyme produced by the pancreas which breaks down fat. You may be asked to fast overnight before this test.

**Why Performed:**
To help diagnose suspected disease of the pancreas, especially acute pancreatitis. Characteristic symptoms of this condition include nausea, vomiting, and upper abdominal pain.

**Normal Values:**
Values and units vary from lab to lab:
    14 to 280 mIU/ml
    ● *Greater Than Normal Values May Mean:* Inflammation or injury of the pancreas. Very high lipase levels usually indicate acute pancreatitis or obstruction of the pancreatic duct. Levels may also rise in ulcers which break (perforate) through the stomach or intestine wall, releasing digestive juices onto the pancreas; chronic pancreatitis; cancer of the pancreas; or intestinal obstruction. Lipase is normally removed from the blood through the kidneys, so kidney disease may also result in elevated levels.

**Interfering Factors:**
Codeine, meperidine, morphine, and cholinergic drugs cause elevated blood lipase levels, as can bethanechol (Myocholine or Urecholine).

**Cost:**
$10 to $25

# Luteinizing Hormone (LH)

Luteinizing hormone (LH) is produced in the pituitary gland in the brain. Along with follicle-stimulating hormone (see p. 76), it regulates the menstrual cycle in women. In men, LH stimulates the production of the male hormone testosterone by the testes.

This test is performed on a venous blood sample (p. 36).

**Why Performed:**
This test is most frequently done on women, to determine the cause of failure to ovulate as part of the evaluation of infertility.

**Normal Values:**
Values may vary from lab to lab:
Menstruating women:
    Other than at ovulation: 5 to 10 milli-international units per milliliter (mIU/ml)
    At ovulation:           30 to 80 mIU/ml
Postmenopausal women:      30 to 200 mIU/ml
Men:                       6 to 30 mIU/ml
    ● *Less Than Normal Values May Mean:* The absence of a midcycle peak in LH in women suggests absence of ovulation. This may be due to menopause or a pituitary disorder (e.g., Stein-Leventhal syndrome,

Turner's syndrome, or tumor of the pituitary).

**Interfering Factors:**
Steroid drugs (e.g., estrogen, progesterone, testosterone, birth control pills) may produce decreased LH levels.

**Cost:**
$25 to $40

# Magnesium (Mg$^{++}$)

Magnesium is a trace mineral necessary to the proper functioning of certain enzymes in the nerves and muscles. It also helps regulate energy production in the cells and aids in the transport of small molecules across cell membranes. It is one of the most abundant minerals in the body.

Magnesium deficiency can develop as a result of an inadequate diet or long-term treatment with intravenous fluids or tube feeding. It can also be caused by fluid loss from prolonged vomiting or diarrhea.

The first symptom of a developing magnesium deficiency is usually muscle twitches. Severe deficiencies can result in extreme irritability to noise or bright lights. This can progress to coma and even death.

Persons taking diuretics are at increased risk of magnesium deficiency.

This test is performed on a venous blood sample (p. 36).

**Why Performed:**
To evaluate such neuromuscular problems as quivering or twitching muscles, irritability, and weakness. To screen for magnesium deficiency. When a person has blood drawn for a magnesium level, tests will frequently be done for other minerals as well, e.g., calcium, phosphorus, potassium, sodium.

**Normal Values:**
Values may vary from lab to lab:
1.8 to 3.0 milligrams per deciliter (mg/dl)
● *Greater Than Normal Values May Mean*: Kidney failure, dehydration, inactive adrenals.
● *Less Than Normal Values May Mean*: Most commonly chronic alcoholism. Other causes include malnutrition; malabsorption syndrome; severe diarrhea; acute pancreatitis; hyperactive thyroid, parathyroid, or adrenal glands; burns. Low levels are also seen in people taking diuretic drugs.

**Interfering Factors:**
Heavy use of magnesium-containing antacids or magnesium supplements can elevate blood levels. Magnesium levels can be decreased by such diuretics as thiazides and ethacrynic acid and by long-term intravenous feeding that does not include magnesium.

**Cost:**
$10 to $25

# Parathyroid Hormone (PTH, Parathormone)

The parathyroids are four tiny glands that lie behind the thyroid, a butterfly-shaped gland just above the Adam's apple. The parathyroid glands produce parathyroid hormone (PTH).

PTH increases blood calcium levels and decreases blood phosphorus levels. Blood calcium (p. 55) is almost always measured along with PTH.

Both test are performed on a venous blood sample (p. 36).

**Preparation:**
You may be asked to fast and drink only water for 12 hours before this test.

**Why Performed:**
To evaluate suspected disorders of the parathyroids; to determine the cause of abnormal calcium and/or phosphorus levels; to evaluate muscle twitching, muscle pains, and kidney stones; and when certain bone abnormalities are discovered by x-ray.

**Normal Values:**
Values vary from lab to lab:

410 to 1,760 picograms per milliliter (pg/ml)

● *Greater Than Normal Values May Mean*: Pseudohyperparathyroidism, hyperparathyroidism, or PTH-producing tumors of the lung. PTH levels also increase in response to low calcium levels (e.g., in patients with kidney failure or vitamin D deficiency).

● *Less Than Normal Values May Mean*: Hypoparathyroidism (usually resulting from thyroid surgery). PTH levels also decrease in response to high blood calcium levels (e.g., in patients with tumors of the bones or vitamin D overdose).

**Interfering Factors:**
Kidney failure or failure to fast before the test may result in inaccurate results.

**Cost:**
$80 to $100

# Partial Thromboplastin Time (PTT) (Activated Partial Thromboplastin Time, APTT)

This test is used to evaluate blood clotting. If there is a deficiency in the blood's ability to clot, the partial thromboplastin time (PTT) may be longer than normal. This test is also sometimes used to monitor treatment with the blood-thinning (anticoagulant) drug heparin, which prolongs the PTT.

This test has largely replaced the older clotting time test which must be performed immediately at the patient's beside. With the partial thromboplastin time, the blood sample can be sent to the lab and the test performed later.

**Why Performed:**
This test is most often done to evaluate abnormal bleeding, and to monitor the clotting status of people taking the anticoagulant drug heparin. It is also sometimes done before surgical procedures and biopsies to screen for clotting disorders, although its routine use for this purpose is under debate. If a complete history has been taken, this test rarely contributes useful preoperative information except in those taking anticoagulant medications.

People receiving heparin are asked to undergo this test regularly, to determine whether they are getting the right dosage. A physician will usually try to give a heparin dose that will keep the patient's test results at about 1½ to 3 times the normal value.

When activators are added to the PTT test chemicals, the results are called the *activated partial thromboplastin time (APTT)*. The APPT is faster and slightly more sensitive.

Be sure to let your doctor know if you are taking any blood-thinning (anticoagulant) medications.

**Normal Values:**

Values vary considerably from lab to lab. PTT and APTT results are given in seconds along with a time for the control sample. A typical normal value is 25–50 seconds. For people on heparin therapy, the desired range is generally between 60 and 100 seconds; and if the value is less than 60, more heparin is usually indicated. If it is over 100, less heparin is indicated.

●*Greater Than Normal Values May Mean*: Deficiency of certain clotting factors, hemophilia, von Willebrand's disease, presence of an anticoagulant (blood-thinning) medication or other substance which interferes with clotting. This test is used only for screening. If an abnormal result is found, further testing may be necessary.

**Cost:**

$15 to 20

# Phenylketonuria (PKU) Screening (Guthrie Test, Phenylalanine)

Phenylketonuria (PKU) is an inherited condition in which a person is unable to metabolize the amino acid phenylalanine. If not treated early, PKU can result in mental retardation. This condition occurs about once in every 10,000 Caucasian births, and is most common in families of Irish and Scottish descent. This test measures the amount of phenylalanine in the blood.

The blood sample is usually taken from the baby's heel. The test must be performed at least 24 hours after the baby has had its first milk. Babies receiving breast milk should be tested again at one month of age. If the test is positive the child will be put on a special diet to prevent mental retardation.

This test can also be done on urine, but the urine test is not as sensitive.

**Why Performed:**

To screen newborns for PKU. This is routine in most states. The only states in which such testing is not required by law are Delaware, North Carolina, and Vermont. In many states, however, the test can be waived if the parents object.

**Normal Values:**

Values may vary from lab to lab:

Less than 4 milligrams per deciliter (mg/dl)

●*Greater Than Normal Values May Mean*: Phenylketonuria (PKU).

**Cost:**

$8 to 14

# Phosphorus

Phosphorus is required for bone growth and for energy metabolism. Most phosphorus is stored in the bones in the form of calcium phosphate. In a number of disorders (especially kidney disease) there is an inverse relationship between blood levels of phosphorus and calcium (p. 55): if phosphorus blood levels are high, those of calcium are low, and vice versa. Thus phosphorus and calcium levels are frequently measured together. Phosphorus is also closely linked to the many body functions regulated by parathyroid hormone (see p. 89).

This test measures the phosphorus (actually, the phosphate ions) in your blood.

### Why Performed:

In parathyroid disease; in suspected vitamin D deficiency; as an aid to diagnosing some kidney, nerve, and muscle diseases; in suspected phosphorus poisoning.

### Normal Values:

Values may vary from lab to lab:
Adults: 2.3 to 4.7 milligrams per deciliter (mg/dl).
Children: 40 to 70 mg/dl.
• *Greater Than Normal Values May Mean*: Hypoparathyroidism, kidney disease, healing fractures, some bone diseases, phosphorus (phosphate) poisoning, excessive vitamin D intake.
• *Less Than Normal Values May Mean*: Alcoholism, hyperparathyroidism, vitamin D deficiency, some kidney diseases.

### Interfering Factors:

Excessive intake of vitamin D, steroids, androgens, growth hormone, and heparin can elevate phosphorus levels. Vitamin D deficiency, prolonged vomiting and diarrhea, extended intravenous infusions, certain antacids, or treatment with acetazolamide, insulin, or epinephrine can suppress phosphorus levels.

### Cost:

$6 to $12

# Potassium (K⁺)

Potassium is one of the principal minerals in the body's cells. It helps maintain the water balance within each cell and is necessary for proper electrical conduction in nerves and muscles.

Potassium also regulates a number of important enzymes, including those controlling the metabolism of starches and sugars. Potassium levels are normally controlled by the secretion of adrenal hormones and influenced by blood glucose and sodium levels.

Potassium also helps to regulate the function of the heart muscle. Abnormally high or low potassium levels can cause the heart to beat irregularly.

Potassium deficiencies are quite common and can develop rapidly. Such deficiencies are most frequently produced as a side effect of drugs that cause increased urination (diuretics). These drugs are commonly used in the treatment of high blood pressure and in a number of other conditions.

This test is performed on a venous blood sample (p. 36).

### Why Performed:

To check blood potassium levels in people taking diuretic drugs, to determine the cause of irregularities in heart rhythm, and when clinical signs of potassium depletion (muscular weakness, lethargy, abnormalities of heart rhythm) are present. This test is also used to evaluate kidney function and neuromuscular disorders.

### Normal Values:

Values may vary from lab to lab:
3.8 to 5.0 milliequivalents per liter (mEq/l)

• *Greater Than Normal Values May Mean*: A greater than normal blood potassium level is called *hyperkalemia*. It may occur in diabetic ketoacidosis, kidney failure, Addison's disease, or liver disease. Increased levels can also result from severe burns or crush injuries or from excessive intake of potassium supplements.

• *Less Than Normal Values May Mean*: A lower than normal blood potassium level is called *hypokalemia*. It may occur with aldosteronism, Cushing's syndrome, loss of body fluids (through the excessive use of diuretics or laxatives, prolonged vomiting, sweating, or diarrhea), diabetes, or inadequate dietary potassium intake.

### Interfering Factors:

Potassium levels are increased by potassium infusions or supplements, penicillin G, spironolactone, and the toxic effects of some drugs on the kidney. Potassium levels are decreased by insulin, glucose, diuretic therapy (especially thiazides), and intravenous infusions without potassium.

### Cost:

$6 to $20

### Special Considerations:

★The body excretes almost all the potassium it takes in each day; thus it is important to be sure that food intake includes adequate potassium. Foods high in potassium include oranges, bananas, apricots, cantaloupes, figs, orange juice, prune juice, tomato juice, beef, chicken, scallops, veal, dried cooked beans, mushrooms, potatoes, squash, and tomatoes.

★Excess intake of potassium is usually eliminated in the urine, but impaired kidney function can result in a buildup of potassium in the blood. This can produce irregularities of the heartbeat and even death.

★Early signs of excessively high blood potassium levels (hyperkalemia) include nausea, diarrhea, malaise, weakness, muscle twitching, and decreased urine flow. Advanced signs include flaccid paralysis, no urine flow, and slow heartbeat.

★Early signs of low blood potassium (hypokalemia) include rapid, weak, irregular pulse, decreased reflexes, mental confusion, low blood pressure, loss of appetite, and muscular weakness. Extreme or prolonged low blood potassium may produce numbness, respiratory difficulties, ventricular fibrillation, and cardiac arrest.

★Electrocardiography (ECG) tracings are very sensitive indicators of high or low blood potassium levels (see p. 153).

# Pregnancy Tests (Human Chorionic Gonadotropin, HCG)

Within days of conception, a fertilized egg implants in the wall of the womb (uterus), and a lifeline of tissue starts to develop between the egg and uterine lining. This newly formed tissue, the placenta, begins to secrete a hormone, human chorionic gonadotropin (HCG), into the bloodstream. Some of this HCG spills over into the urine. All pregnancy tests are designed to detect HCG in the urine or blood.

In the past, pregnancy tests involved injecting a urine specimen into rabbits, rats, frogs, or toads. The animal was then sacrificed and the tissues examined for signs of the presence of HCG. Fortunately for the animals, immunologic pregnancy tests have been developed which use antibodies, not animals, to detect HCG in urine or blood.

The blood tests for pregnancy (radioimmunoassay or RIA) are more accurate and sensitive than the urine tests. The *blood* test can detect the presence of HCG as early as 7 days after ovulation and fertilization, which is before a missed menstrual period. The older *urine* pregnancy test can accurately detect the presence of HCG (and therefore, pregnancy) by 10 to 14 days after a missed menstrual period. However, the newer urine pregnancy tests are nearly as sensitive as the blood tests, and pregnancy can be detected on or about the day of the missed period. Urine pregnancy tests are performed preferably on a first morning urine specimen, which is likely to contain a higher concentration of HCG. Urine pregnancy tests can also be performed at home (p. 431).

## Why Performed:

To detect pregnancy suggested by a missed menstrual period, breast swelling and tenderness, or morning nausea. Certain types of very rare tumors may also secrete HCG. HCG levels may be measured to detect or follow the progress of treatment of such tumors.

## Normal Values:

No measurable HCG is normally detected in men or nonpregnant women.
  ● *Greater Than Normal Values May Mean*: HCG levels rise rapidly during early pregnancy, peak at about the 10th week, and then taper off. An elevated HCG level ("positive" test) usually means pregnancy. Higher levels of HCG may suggest a multiple pregnancy (i.e., twins, triplets, etc.) HCG-secreting tumors such as hydatidiform mole, choriocarcinoma, and certain testicular tumors may produce elevated levels of HCG.

  ● *Lower Than Normal Values May Mean*: Even though pregnancy tests are highly accurate, the test result may be negative in early pregnancy (false-negative). Therefore, if the test is negative and pregnancy is still suspected, the test should be repeated in one week. Lower than expected levels of HCG for a given stage of pregnancy suggest a pregnancy occurring outside the uterus (ectopic pregnancy) or an impending miscarriage.

## Interfering Factors:

A false-negative pregnancy test may be due to testing too early in pregnancy or too dilute a urine specimen. False-positive urine pregnancy tests can occur with postmenopausal women, and are also caused by excessive blood or protein in the urine specimen, soap residue in the collecting container, and certain medications such as phenothiazines (Compazine, Stelazine, Thorazine), promethazine (Phenergan), or methadone.

## Cost:

  Urine pregnancy test: $5 to $15
  Blood (serum) pregnancy test: $20 to
    $40

# Progesterone

Progesterone is a female hormone secreted by the ovary after ovulation. It stimulates the thickening of the inner layer of the uterus (endometrium), preparing it to receive the fertilized egg. If fertilization does not occur, progesterone levels drop, triggering menstruation. During pregnancy, higher levels of progesterone are produced by the placenta.

This test measures the progesterone in a woman's blood. Progesterone can also be monitored by measuring one of its by-products, pregnanediol, in the urine.

## Why Performed:

As a part of fertility studies, to monitor the function of the placenta during pregnancy, and to confirm ovulation.

## Normal Values:

Values may vary from lab to lab:

At and immediately after ovulation: 10 to 20 nanograms per milliliter (ng/ml)

During the rest of the menstrual cycle: less than 1 ng/ml

● *Greater Than Normal Values May Mean*: Ovulation, cyst or tumor of the ovary, excess secretion of progesterone by adrenal glands.

● *Less Than Normal Values May Mean*: Pituitary disease, absence of ovulation, threatened abortion, toxemia of pregnancy, or fetal death.

## Cost:

$50 to $80

## Special Considerations:

★*Pregnanediol Test*—This urine test is sometimes used to monitor progesterone levels. A 24-hour urine sample is required. No restriction of food or fluids is necessary. Levels normally increase for 10 days after ovulation.

# Prolactin
# (Lactogenic Hormone, HPRL)

Prolactin is a hormone secreted by the pituitary gland. It prepares the breasts to produce milk and stimulates milk production. Although it is secreted in men and in non-pregnant women, its function in such situations is not understood.

Prolactin production normally increases during pregnancy but returns to low levels in mothers who do not breast-feed their babies. In mothers who do breast-feed, prolactin levels continue to rise—the suckling of the baby apparently decreases the brain's production of a substance called prolactin-inhibiting factor which reduces prolactin secretion.

A fasting morning blood sample is required.

## Why Performed:

In suspected pituitary disease. Suspicious symptoms might include menstrual irregularities or infertility in women and breast swelling or decreased sexual desire in men. Also performed to evaluate nipple discharge (galactorrhea).

## Normal Values:

Values may vary from lab to lab and depending on time of day (levels normally highest in the early morning):

Women: 1 to 25 nanograms per deciliter (ng/dl)

Men: 1 to 20 ng/dl

● *Greater Than Normal Values May Mean*: Tumors of the pituitary or hypothalamus, hyperthyroidism.

**Interfering Factors:**
Extreme stress or severe sleep disturbance can elevate values, as can many drugs, including phenothiazines, reserpine, alpha methyldopa, haloperidol, tricyclic antidepressants, and estrogen.

**Cost:**
$40 to $75

# Prothrombin Time
## (PT, Pro Time)

This test is used to measure the blood's ability to clot. Prothrombin is one of a dozen proteins (known as factors) in the blood that are needed to stop bleeding. If there is an insufficient supply of this or other clotting factors, the prothrombin time (PT) will be longer than normal. A prolonged PT can be produced by liver disease, blockage of a bile duct, and use of the blood-thinning drug warfarin (Coumadin).

**Why Performed:**
This test is used to monitor the effects of oral anticoagulant therapy with warfarin or similar drugs, to evaluate bleeding disorders, and as a measure of dietary intake of vitamin K. It is also sometimes done before surgical procedures and biopsies to screen for clotting disorders, although its routine use for this purpose is under debate. If a complete history has been taken, this test rarely contributes useful preoperative information except in people taking anticoagulants.

Let your doctor know if you are taking any medications.

**Normal Values:**
PT results are given in seconds along with a control value. A typical normal range is 11.0–12.5 seconds, but values may vary from lab to lab. Some labs report PT results as a percentage of prothrombin activity. Normal people not taking blood-thinning drugs should have a PT approximately equal to the control value. People receiving warfarin (Coumadin) therapy should have a PT about 1½ to 2 times the control value.

● *Greater Than Normal Values May Mean*: PT values 2½ times or more times the control value suggest severe bleeding problems. This test is used only for screening. If an abnormal result is found, further testing may be necessary. The PT is usually prolonged in people taking anticoagulants.

A number of drugs can interact with warfarin to further prolong the PT. These include aspirin, ACTH, alcohol, steroids, indomethacin, mefenamic acid, para-aminosalicylic acid, methimazole, oxyphenbutazone, phenylbutazone, phenytoin, propylthiouracil, quinidine, quinine, thyroid hormones, and vitamin A.

**Cost:**
$10 to $14

# Renin

Renin is an enzyme produced in the kidney in response to decreased kidney blood flow. It aids in the production of angiotensin, which can increase blood pressure.

This test is used to diagnose high blood pressure (hypertension) due to kidney disease. It may be done in one of two ways: either on a regular blood sample from a vein in the arm, or on samples taken from the renal veins draining each kidney. If renal vein samples are used, separate samples are taken from each vein. The renin levels in the blood from the two kidneys are then compared. (For a description of how the samples are collected, see Special Considerations.)

## Preparation:

You will be asked to observe a "no-added-salt" diet for 3 days before the test and to stay in an upright position for 1–2 hours before the test. You will be asked to abstain from licorice for 2 weeks before the test. Check with your doctor in advance about whether to continue any medications you are taking.

## Why Performed:

To help determine whether hypertension is caused by kidney disease; to determine the cause of low potassium levels or sounds of abnormal blood flow (bruit) in the abdomen. This test is also used to evaluate the function of the adrenal glands.

## Normal Values:

Values may vary from lab to lab:

PRA (plasma renin activity) normally ranges between 0.2 and 4 nanograms per milliliter (ng/ml) per hour. This value varies with body position, amount of salt in diet, and time of day. The ratio of the PRA of the involved kidney to that of the uninvolved kidney should be less than 1.4.

●*Greater Than Normal Values May Mean*: Increased renin production due to kidney disease, following kidney injury, or use of certain diuretics, or some tumors of the adrenals.

●*Less Than Normal Values May Mean*: Extremely high salt intake, abnormally high production of aldosterone by the adrenal glands, use of steroid drugs, or consumption of large amounts of licorice.

## Cost:

Regular blood test: $30 to $50. (Three to six blood samples are usually tested.)

Samples taken via catheter: $75 to $85

## Special Considerations:

★*Obtaining Blood Samples from Renal Veins*—You will be asked to sign a consent form authorizing this procedure. Use this opportunity to discuss with your doctor any concerns you may have about the need for the test, the risks of the test, or how and when it will be performed.

You will receive an injection to help you relax and then will be taken to the x-ray department, where you will be asked to lie on your back on an x-ray table. Your groin (upper thigh) area will be cleansed and the skin will be numbed with an injection of local anesthetic.

A needle will then be inserted into the vein in your groin. A thin, flexible tube (catheter) will be inserted into the vein and threaded into the larger vein (inferior vena cava) which runs down the back of your abdominal cavity. The movement of the catheter will be followed on an x-ray image displayed on a TV screen (fluoroscope). A dye will be injected from time to time to help your doctor locate the tip of the catheter.

The catheter will be advanced into one renal vein and then the other. Samples will be taken from each vein. The catheter is then withdrawn, and the samples are sent to the laboratory for analysis. There is a very slight risk that the catheter might injure or rupture the vein wall. If this should occur, emergency surgery may be necessary.

The blood collection takes about 45 minutes. If you notice any back pain or blood in your urine after the test, let your doctor know.

# Reticulocyte Count

Reticulocytes are red blood cells newly released into the bloodstream from the bone marrow. In this test several hundred of the red blood cells in a sample are counted. The portion of those that are reticulocytes, expressed as a percentage of total red cells, is the reticulocyte count. The reticulocyte count shows how well the marrow is responding to a loss of blood cells by putting new red blood cells into circulation.

This test is performed on a venous blood sample (p. 36).

## Why Performed:
To evaluate the body's response to anemia or to monitor response to treatment for anemia or polycythemia.

## Normal Values:
Values may vary from lab to lab:

0.5% to 1.5%

The "normal" value varies with different hemoglobin levels. After acute blood loss the normal reticulocyte count will be much higher.

●*Greater Than Normal Values May Mean*: Bone marrow is increasing red blood cell production in response to anemia or bleeding. The reticulocyte count should rise dramatically when an iron-deficiency anemia is appropriately treated with iron.

●*Less Than Normal Values May Mean*: Ineffective or diminished red blood cell production as a result of iron-deficiency anemia, pernicious anemia, or other forms of anemia.

## Interfering Factors:
The reticulocyte count may be decreased by drugs that affect the bone marrow; these include many medications used for cancer therapy. It may be elevated by any drugs that cause increased red blood cell destruction (hemolytic anemia).

## Cost:
$5 to $8

## Special Considerations:
★This test cannot distinguish among the various types of anemia. Further testing is usually required for a specific diagnosis.

# Rheumatoid Factor (RF)

The immune system does not ordinarily attack the body's own cells, but most people with rheumatoid arthritis have a "renegade" antibody to the body's own immunoglobulins (large molecules in the blood which help fight infection). This antibody is called the rheumatoid factor (RF). RF can also be elevated in some diseases other than rheumatoid arthritis.

This test is performed on a venous blood sample (p. 36).

## Why Performed:
To help confirm a diagnosis of rheumatoid arthritis.

## Normal Values:
Values may vary from lab to lab:

Negative (RF titer of 1:20 or less)

A negative RF does not necessarily exclude the possibility of rheumatoid arthritis: about 20% of people with the disease do not have elevated RF titers.

●*Greater Than Normal Values May Mean*: RF titers above 1:80 are usually found in people with rheumatoid arthritis. A number of other diseases—including systemic lupus erythematosus, scleroderma, polymyositis, TB, mononucleosis, syphilis, chronic liver disease, and subacute bacterial endocarditis—can cause titers between 1:20 and 1:80. Also about 5% of the population, including up to 25% of the elderly, have positive RF titers without having rheumatoid arthritis.

**Interfering Factors:**
Blood with high lipid or cryoglobulin levels may result in false-positive test results.

**Cost:**
$15 to $35

**Special Considerations:**
★The RF titer frequently does not rise until approximately 6 months after the onset of rheumatoid arthritis. Thus repeating this test at a later date may be useful.

★The results of this test are just one of many criteria for diagnosing rheumatoid arthritis. One set of guidelines suggests that seven of the following criteria must be met before a diagnosis of rheumatoid arthritis is made:

1. Morning stiffness for at least 6 weeks.
2. Tenderness or pain on motion in one or more joints for at least 6 weeks.
3. Swelling of one or more joints for at least 6 weeks.
4. Swelling in at least one additional joint for at least 6 weeks.
5. Joint swelling of symmetrical joints on opposite sides of the body at the same time.
6. Nodules under the skin (subcutaneous nodules).
7. X-ray results which show decalcification of the bone.
8. *A positive blood test for rheumatoid factor.*

9. A poor mucin precipitate in a sample of joint fluid (see Joint Tap, p. 363).
10. Characteristic changes in the joint lining seen on biopsy.
11. Characteristic changes in the subcutaneous nodules seen on biopsy.

# Schilling Test
## (Vitamin $B_{12}$ Absorption)

Vitamin $B_{12}$ is necessary for the production of red blood cells; deficiency of $B_{12}$ can result in anemia. Deficiency may be due to lack of $B_{12}$ in the diet or, more commonly, to a problem with absorbing the vitamin from the intestine. People with pernicious anemia lack sufficient quantities of a protein (referred to as intrinsic factor) which normally binds with $B_{12}$ in the stomach to make its absorption in the intestine possible.

**Preparation:**
You will be asked to fast for 10–12 hours before this test. You will be given an oral dose of radioactively labeled vitamin $B_{12}$, followed in 2 hours by an intramuscular injection of nonradioactive $B_{12}$. You will then be asked to collect a 24-hour urine specimen see (p. 39). This test measures the radioactive $B_{12}$ in that sample.

The injection saturates your body with $B_{12}$, forcing excess $B_{12}$ into the urine. Thus the amount of radioactive $B_{12}$ in the urine sample reflects how well you are absorbing the oral dose of the vitamin. Depending on the results, the test may be repeated in three days. If the repeat test is done, you will be given intrinsic factor along with the radioactive $B_{12}$.

## Why Performed:

To test for pernicious anemia in people who have anemia with larger-than-normal (megaloblastic) red blood cells, or after surgical removal of part or all of the stomach, which may result in a deficiency of intrinsic factor.

## Normal Values:

Values may vary from lab to lab:

Seven percent or more of the radioactively labeled $B_{12}$ is found in the 24-hour urine specimen.

•*Less Than Normal Values May Mean*: If less than 7% of the radioactive $B_{12}$ is found in the urine specimen, it means that you are not absorbing enough $B_{12}$. This poor absorption may be due either to a lack of intrinsic factor in the stomach (pernicious anemia) or to a malabsorption syndrome in the intestine. If you have pernicious anemia, the repeat test with intrinsic factor will result in a significant increase in urinary output of radioactive $B_{12}$. If you have malabsorption syndrome, $B_{12}$ output will be unchanged.

## Interfering Factors:

Decreased kidney function may interfere with this test—a 48- or 72-hour urine collection may be necessary. A radioactive scan or radiation therapy within 10 days of the test may artificially increase results. Laxative use can produce false results.

## Cost:

$150 to $200

## Special Considerations:

★Vitamin $B_{12}$ is principally found in meats, shellfish, eggs, and dairy products; thus strict vegetarian diets may be deficient in $B_{12}$. A special high $B_{12}$ nutritional yeast is available.

★Pernicious anemia cannot be corrected by taking oral vitamin $B_{12}$, since the vitamin cannot be absorbed without intrinsic factor, and intrinsic factor is not available as a pill or injection. Therapy for pernicious anemia requires periodic $B_{12}$ injections.

★Other related tests: Blood $B_{12}$ levels (p. 123) and bone marrow aspiration (p. 346).

# Sedimentation Rate (Sed Rate, Erythrocyte Sedimentation Rate, ESR)

In the early part of the century a Swedish doctor noticed that the red blood cells in the blood of his pregnant patients settled to the bottom of a test tube faster than those of other patients. Further observation showed that this rapid settling was also found in a large number of diseases.

Today the sedimentation rate (erythrocyte sedimentation rate, ESR) is used to screen for and follow a wide variety of inflammations, infections, and cancers. It is useful only as a screening test and can't be used to diagnose any specific disease.

The ESR measures how far the red blood cells settle toward the bottom of a specially calibrated test tube in an hour's time. Inflammations and infections increase the blood's protein content, making the red blood cells stick together. This makes them settle to the bottom of the tube more quickly.

## Why Performed:

Many nonspecific symptoms such as fever, weight loss, joint inflammation, pelvic pain, or headache may suggest the presence of an inflammation, chronic infection, or cancer. The ESR may be used to investigate whether such complaints are due to an underlying disease.

This sensitive but nonspecific screening test frequently gives an early indication that disease is present, even when other tests are negative. But this test reacts to so many different conditions that it is of little use unless a specific disease is suspected. Once a diagnosis has been made, the ESR can sometimes be used to monitor the course of the disease or response to therapy.

**Normal Values:**
Values may vary from lab to lab:
Men:
Under 50 years: 0 to 15 millimeters per hour (mm/hr)
Over 50 years: 0 to 20 mm/hr

Women:
Under 50 years: 0 to 20 mm/hr
Over 50 years: 0 to 30 mm/hr
● *Greater Than Normal Values May Mean*: Acute or chronic infection or inflammation (e.g., pelvic inflammatory disease) tuberculosis, pregnancy, multiple myeloma, rheumatic fever, rheumatoid arthritis, kidney disease, thyroid disease, temporal arteritis, some cancers, many autoimmune diseases.

**Interfering Factors:**
If the blood sample is allowed to stand for more than 3 hours after being drawn, ESR levels may be artificially reduced.

**Cost:**
$8 to $16

# Serum Glutamic Oxalacetic Transaminase (SGOT) (Aspartate Aminotransferase, AST)

Serum glutamic oxalacetic transaminase (SGOT) is an enzyme found mainly in the liver and heart muscle. It is released into the bloodstream when either of these organs is damaged. Thus increased levels are usually associated with liver disease or heart attacks. A newer name for this blood test is aspartate aminotransferase or AST.

**Why Performed:**
To help diagnose and monitor the progress of liver disease which may produce symptoms such as jaundice (yellowing of the skin and eyes), pain in the upper abdomen, nausea, and vomiting. It may also be used to monitor people receiving medications that may be toxic to the liver. This test is often performed along with alkaline phosphatase (p. 45), SGPT (p. 102), LDH (p. 151), and bilirubin (p. 52) as liver function tests (LFTs).

**Normal Values:**
May vary from lab to lab:
10−40 international units per liter (IU/L)
● *Greater Than Normal Values May Mean*: Very high levels are associated with liver damage or inflammation due to viral infections (viral hepatitis, infectious mononucleosis), toxic or alcohol-related injury, blockage of the bile ducts (obstructive jaundice), or cirrhosis. Heart attacks (see p. 151), blood clots in the lungs (pulmonary em-

bolism), excessive breakdown of red blood cells (hemolytic anemia), muscle injury, or inflammation of the pancreas can also increase SGOT levels.

Many drugs can cause liver injury that result in elevations of SGOT. These include antibiotics (penicillins, erythromycin, tetracycline, sulfonamides, isoniazid), narcotics (codeine, morphine, Demerol), methyldopa (Aldomet), propranolol (Inderal), cortisone, allopurinol, tricyclic anti-depressants, chlorpromazine, oral contraceptives, antiinflammatory medications (aspirin, indomethacin, phenylbutazone), and many others.

**Interfering Factors:**
Strenuous exercise or intramuscular injections can raise SGOT levels.

**Cost:**
$10 to $17

# Serum Glutamic Pyruvic Transaminase (SGPT) (Alanine Aminotransferase, ALT)

Serum glutamic pyruvic transaminase (SGPT) is an enzyme found primarily in the liver. It is released into the bloodstream as a result of liver damage. A newer name for this blood test is alanine aminotransferase or ALT.

**Why Performed:**
To help diagnose and monitor the progress of liver disease which may produce symptoms such as jaundice (yellowing of the skin and eyes), pain in the upper abdomen, nausea, and vomiting. It may also be used to monitor people receiving medications that may be toxic to the liver. This test is often performed along with alkaline phosphatase (p. 45), SGOT (p. 101), LDH (p. 151), and bilirubin (p. 52) as liver function tests (LFTs).

**Normal Values:**
May vary from lab to lab:
   10–30 Units per milliliter (U/ml)
   ● *Greater Than Normal Values May Mean*: Very high levels are associated with liver cell damage due to viral hepatitis or drug or chemical toxicity. Moderately elevated levels may be found in infectious mononucleosis, blockage of the bile ducts (obstructive jaundice), cirrhosis, liver cancer, congestive heart failure, or alcohol intoxication. While SGPT levels are often elevated in alcoholism, a normal SGPT does not rule out alcoholism.

Many drugs can cause liver injury that results in elevations of SGPT. These include antibiotics (penicillins, erythromycin, tetracycline, sulfonamides, isoniazid), narcotics (codeine, morphine, Demerol), methyldopa (Aldomet), propranolol (Inderal), cortisone, allopurinol, tricyclic anti-depressants, chlorpromazine, oral contraceptives, antiinflammatory medications (aspirin, indomethacin, phenylbutazone), and many others.

**Cost:**
$10 to $17

# Serum Osmolality

This blood test measures the concentration of particles dissolved in a given quantity of blood serum. Serum osmolality is regulated by antidiuretic hormone (ADH).

If you are not taking in enough water, then as water is constantly filtered out of the blood by the kidneys, the concentration of particles in the remaining blood will increase. In response to this increase, ADH is released from the pituitary gland, and the kidneys respond by excreting less water. This keeps the serum osmolality from increasing even further.

When you drink too much water, the opposite process occurs. Because your serum osmolality is low, ADH is not released. More water is excreted by the kidney, and thus the serum osmolality rises.

**Why Performed:**
To aid in the diagnosis of disorders of water balance and to test the kidney's ability to respond to ADH.

**Normal Values:**
Values may vary from lab to lab:
280 to 295 milliosmols per kilogram (mOsm/kg)
• *Greater Than Normal Values May Mean*: Insufficient water intake, dehydration, insufficient ADH production due to disease of pituitary gland, or kidney disease resulting in the kidneys' inability to respond to ADH.
• *Less Than Normal Values May Mean*: Excessive water intake or excessive ADH production due to pituitary disease.

**Cost:**
$25 to $40

# Serum Protein (Total)
## (Total Blood Protein, Serum Albumin, Serum Globulin, Albumin Globulin Ratio)

More protein is dissolved in the liquid portion of the blood than any other substance. While most other substances in the blood are measured in micrograms, protein is measured in grams.

The two major proteins in the blood are albumin and globulin. Both total protein and separate albumin and globulin levels are usually measured. In addition, the ratio of albumin to globulin can be calculated.

Albumin is the most plentiful protein in the blood. It is produced primarily in the liver and helps keep the fluid portion of the blood within the blood vessels. When albumin levels decrease, fluid may collect in the ankles (pedal edema) or lungs (pulmonary edema or congestive heart failure). Albumin also aids in the transport of many drugs and other substances in the blood.

Some globulins are formed by the liver, some by the immune system. Globulins have many functions, including binding to free hemoglobin, transporting metals, and acting as antibodies to help the body defend itself against invading substances or organisms. Another test, serum protein electrophoresis (p. 104), measures the levels of the specific types of globulin present in the blood.

**Why Performed:**
This test is a part of many routine chemistry screening procedures and is of most use as

a rough indicator of liver function. It is also used to investigate swelling (edema) of the ankles or other parts of the body, the collection of fluid in the lungs, which may cause shortness of breath, and nutritional status.

### Normal Values:
Values may vary from lab to lab:
> Total protein: 6.0 to 7.8 grams per deciliter (g/dl)
> Albumin: 3.2 to 4.5 g/dl
> Globulin: 2.3 to 3.5 g/dl
> Albumin/globulin ratio: 1.5:1 to 2.5:1

●*Greater Than Normal Values May Mean*: An increase in total protein may result from dehydration, vomiting, diarrhea, cancer (multiple myeloma, leukemia), rheumatoid arthritis, and some infections.

If the results of this test are abnormal a more specific test for protein imbalance (serum protein electrophoresis, discussed next) may be done.

●*Less Than Normal Values May Mean*: A decrease in total protein may be due to malnutrition, malabsorption from the intestine, kidney disease, blood loss, or severe burns. Reduced levels may also be due to uncontrolled diabetes, toxemia of pregnancy, shock, certain poisonings, or congestive heart failure. Protein levels may also be low in other prolonged, severe illnesses.

Impaired liver cells lose their ability to produce protein; however, previously produced protein will ordinarily stay in the blood for 12 to 18 days. Thus liver impairment will not usually produce decreased serum protein for approximately 2 weeks.

### Interfering Factors:
Protein levels may be reduced by birth control pills, pregnancy, chronic laxative use, or prolonged recumbency (as in hospitalization or prolonged bed rest). Protein levels may be increased if the tourniquet is left on too long before blood is drawn.

### Cost:
$15 to $20

# Serum Protein Electrophoresis

Proteins (see also Serum Protein, p. 103) are large molecules made of amino acids, some of which carry either positive or negative charges. In this test, a sample of the blood proteins is placed in an electrical field. Each protein molecule will demonstrate a characteristic behavior, depending on its size and its charge—positively charged molecules will move toward the negative pole, and those with a negative charge will move toward the positive pole.

This test is used to separate blood proteins into five types: albumin, alpha-1 globulin, alpha-2 globulin, beta globulin, and gamma globulin. Different proportions of these five subgroups are characteristic of different medical conditions. More sophisticated tests can divide blood proteins into 10 to 12 serum components.

### Why Performed:
To aid in the diagnosis of a number of conditions that affect various blood proteins. These include multiple myeloma, nephrotic syndrome, chronic liver disease, immune deficiencies, and certain inflammatory diseases. This is a useful screening test for abnormalities of serum proteins. If abnormal results are found, more specific tests (e.g., serum quantitative immuno-

globulins, urine protein electrophoresis) may be done.

**Normal Values:**
Values may vary from lab to lab:

| | |
|---|---|
| Albumin | 52%–67% |
| Alpha-1 globulin | 2.5%–5% |
| Alpha-2 globulin | 7%–13% |
| Beta globulin | 8%–14% |
| Gamma globulin | 12%–22% |

●*Greater Than Normal Values May Mean*: Increased alpha-1 globulin may suggest inflammatory disease or cancer. Increased alpha-2 globulin may suggest inflammatory disease, cancer, nephrotic syndrome, or infection. Increased beta globulin may suggest liver disease or lipid disorder. Increased gamma globulin may suggest chronic liver disease, collagen disorder, myeloma, or malignant lymphoma.

●*Less Than Normal Values May Mean*: Decreased albumin levels may suggest liver disease, starvation, nephrotic syndrome, eczema, burns, pregnancy, or hyperthyroidism. Low alpha-1 may suggest emphysema or liver disease. Low alpha-2 may be due to liver damage, trauma, transfusions, or the destruction of red blood cells (hemolysis).

**Cost:**
$25 to $40

# Sickle-Cell Test
## (Hemoglobin S Test)

Sickle-cell disease is an inherited abnormality of the hemoglobin molecule. This condition is found almost exclusively among blacks; 1 in 500 black babies in America is born with sickle-cell disease.

Sickle cells are severely deformed red blood cells which have assumed a sickle shape. These cells cannot pass through the smallest blood vessels, and thus they block blood flow.

Sickling occurs only in red blood cells with abnormal hemoglobin, most commonly hemoglobin S, and only under certain conditions (acidic, low oxygen levels, high temperatures). If these conditions are reversed, the red blood cells will resume their normal shape.

Since each individual has two sets of chromosomes, a person may have either (1) two normal genes for normal hemoglobin, (2) one for normal and one for hemoglobin S, (3) two for hemoglobin S, or (4) one for hemoglobin S and one for some other abnormal hemoglobin. People with only one gene for hemoglobin S are said to have sickle-cell trait, a benign condition. Those with two genes for hemoglobin S are said to have sickle-cell anemia, a serious blood disorder characterized by anemia, organ damage, and painful "sickling crises." About 8% to 10% of the black population have sickle-cell trait.

This test can detect either sickle-cell anemia or sickle-cell trait. The blood sample is usually taken by fingerstick (see p. 37). Tell your doctor if you received a recent blood transfusion, since this may produce inaccurate results.

**Normal Values:**
No sickle cells seen.

●*Greater Than Normal Values May Mean*: A positive test may indicate the presence of sickle cells, but further testing (hemoglobin electrophoresis, p. 81) is required for a definitive diagnosis.

**Interfering Factors:**
A blood transfusion received within the preceding 3 months can cause a false-neg-

ative test result, since the donor's normal hemoglobin may prevent sickling from occurring.

**Cost:**
$25 to $30

**Special Considerations:**

★If you receive positive results on this test and you are considering having children, you should consult a genetic counselor, since there is a significant chance of passing sickle-cell trait or sickle-cell anemia on to your baby.

★While sickle-cell trait is a relatively benign condition, those with sickle-cell anemia should avoid endeavors that might produce sickling of their red blood cells, e.g., strenuous exercise, travel to high altitudes, travel in unpressurized airplanes.

# Sodium (Na⁺)

Sodium is one of the body's principal electrolytes (electronically charged minerals dissolved in body fluids). It is involved in water balance (the amount of fluid inside and surrounding cells), acid-base balance, and the transmission of nerve impulses. Sodium levels can be measured in the blood (serum) or in a urine specimen collected over a 24-hour period (see p. 39). These levels depend on the amount of salt (sodium chloride) and fluid in your diet, fluid losses, and various hormones that help regulate electrolyte and fluid balance. The kidneys play a central role in the excretion of excessive sodium and maintenance of salt balance.

**Why Performed:**
To evaluate suspected abnormalities in electrolyte and fluid balance such as dehydration, excessive accumulation of fluid (edema), suspected kidney and adrenal gland disorders. The symptoms of too much or too little sodium in the blood may be nonspecific, such as agitation, weakness, lethargy, stupor, and coma.

**Normal Values:**
Values may vary from lab to lab:

Blood (serum) sodium: 136–142 milliequivalents/liter (mEq/l)

Urine sodium: 75–200 mEq/24 hours (may vary greatly depending upon dietary intake of salt)

● *Greater Than Normal Values May Mean*: Elevated blood sodium levels (hypernatremia) may be due to dehydration, excessive salt in diet, excessive adrenal gland function (Cushing's disease), kidney disease, and congestive heart failure. Elevated levels of urine sodium may be found in dehydration, excessive salt intake, inadequate adrenal gland function (Addison's disease), severe diabetes, and certain kidney diseases.

● *Lower Than Normal Values May Mean*: Decreased blood sodium levels (hyponatremia) may be due to significant sodium losses (through sweating, vomiting, diarrhea, extensive burns, or kidney disease), excessive fluid intake, or inadequate adrenal gland function (Addison's disease). Low levels of urinary sodium are associated with excessive adrenal gland activity, congestive heart failure, kidney failure, severe lung disease, and very low salt intake.

**Interfering Factors:**
Numerous drugs may alter blood and urine sodium levels, including many diuretic medications, certain blood pressure medications, and steroid drugs.

**Cost:**
$8 to $12

**Special Considerations:**

★In the inherited disorder cystic fibrosis the sweat and mucus produced in the body contain elevated amounts of sodium and chloride. A sweat test (p. 389), which measures the sodium concentration in sweat, is used to diagnose this condition.

# Tay-Sachs Screening
## (Serum Hexosaminidase A and B)

Tay-Sachs disease is an inherited, fatal degenerative disease of the central nervous system. Affected children usually develop normally until the age of 6 months, and then begin to deteriorate physically and mentally. They lose the ability to see, hear, or move. Death usually occurs within 3 to 4 years.

The disease is due to an inherited metabolic abnormality. The babies cannot produce an enzyme (hexosaminidase A) that normally functions to break down a particular fatty substance in the body. When this enzyme is absent, the fatty substance accumulates in body cells, particularly in brain tissue.

The production of this vital enzyme is controlled by a pair of genes, one inherited from each parent. A person who has one normal gene is able to produce enough of the enzyme to prevent the occurrence of any symptoms or disability. This person with one normal and one defective gene is known as a "carrier." If only one person in a couple is a carrier, there is no danger that their children will be affected with Tay-Sachs disease. However, if both partners of a couple planning a pregnancy are carriers, then there is a 25% chance, with each pregnancy, of having a baby with two defective genes and, thus, with Tay-Sachs disease.

Anyone could be a carrier of the gene for Tay-Sachs. However, as with many other genetic disorders, certain ethnic groups have a much higher frequency of a particular gene. People at highest risk for carrying the Tay-Sachs gene are Jewish and of Eastern European descent (Ashkenazi Jews). Approximately 1 out of 30 healthy members of this Jewish group carries the gene for Tay-Sachs disease, while only 1 out of 200 members of the non-Jewish population carries it.

**Why Performed:**
The blood test is usually performed to screen for carriers among Jews of Eastern European descent, especially before such couples plan to have children. A test may also be performed on an amniotic fluid sample (see Amniocentesis, p. 208) when both parents are known to be carriers, or on a blood sample of a newborn suspected of having Tay-Sachs disease.

**Normal Values:**
Values may vary from lab to lab:
Total serum hexosaminidase: 5.0–12.9 units per liter
Hexosaminidase A: 55%–76% of total
●*Less Than Normal Values May Mean*: A complete lack of hexosaminidase A indicates Tay-Sachs disease. Decreased levels of this enzyme indicate that the person is a carrier of the Tay-Sachs gene.

**Cost:**
$160 to $180

# Testosterone

Testosterone is the major male hormone. It is produced by the testes and is responsible for the development of such secondary male sexual characteristics as beard, body hair, muscular development, and lowering of the voice.

In men, testosterone production normally begins to increase at puberty and continues to rise during adulthood, tapering off at about 40 and gradually decreasing thereafter. In women, the ovaries and adrenal glands produce small amounts of testosterone.

This test is performed on a venous blood sample (see p. 36).

### Why Performed:

To evaluate suspected problems of sexual development, to evaluate male infertility, to evaluate excess body hair and virilization in women.

### Normal Values:

Men: 300 to 1200 nanograms per deciliter (ng/dl)

Women: 30 to 95 ng/dl

Boys: less than 100 ng/dl

Girls: less than 40 ng/dl

● *Greater Than Normal Values May Mean*: Early (precocious) sexual development, testicular tumor, adrenal disease, hyperthyroidism, disease of the ovary.

● *Less Than Normal Values May Mean*: Testicular disease, pituitary disease, testicular cancer, prostate cancer, surgical removal of testes, estrogen therapy, delayed puberty, cirrhosis of the liver.

### Interfering Factors:

Sex hormones (estrogens or androgens) and some other hormones can interfere with test results.

### Cost:

$70 to $90

# Thyroid Function Tests ($T_4$, $T_3$ Uptake, FTI)

The thyroid is a butterfly-shaped gland located in the neck with one lobe on each side of the Adam's apple and a thin ridge of tissue connecting the two wings. In response to thyroid-stimulating hormone (TSH), a chemical signal from the pituitary gland in the brain, the thyroid gland produces two iodine-containing hormones, thyroxine ($T_4$) and triiodothyronine ($T_3$). These hormones regulate the metabolism of the body by increasing the rate of the reactions taking place in the body's cells.

The most common blood tests used to evaluate thyroid function are $T_4$ (thyroxine), $T_3$ *Uptake* (triiodothyronine resin uptake), and *FTI* (free thyroxine index, which is calculated by multiplying the $T_4$ value by the $T_3$ uptake value).

### Why Performed:

To evaluate a swelling or lump in the thyroid gland; symptoms of excess thyroid hormone (hyperthyroidism) such as weight loss, tremor, nervousness, rapid heart rate, diarrhea, or the sensation of always being too hot; or symptoms of too little thyroid hormone (hypothyroidism) such as weight gain, tiredness, dry skin, constipation, or the sensation of always being too cold.

Thyroid function tests may also be done to screen newborns for hypothyroidism (cretinism) or to periodically screen healthy people over the age of 35, particularly women who are prone to develop hypothyroidism. These tests may also be used to monitor the response of thyroid disease to therapy.

## Normal Values:

Values may vary from lab to lab:

$T_4$: 5–11 micrograms/deciliter

$T_3$ uptake: 25%–38%

FTI: 1.25–4.20 units (varies)

● *Greater Than Normal Values May Mean*: Hyperthyroidism, which may be due to such causes as diffuse toxic goiter (Graves' disease), toxic adenoma, toxic multinodular goiter, or excessive thyroid hormone replacement therapy.

● *Lower Than Normal Values May Mean*: Hypothyroidism (inadequate production of thyroid hormone), which may be caused by chronic (Hashimoto's) thyroiditis, thyroid atrophy, inadequate dietary intake of iodine, or medical destruction of the thyroid gland by surgery or radioactive therapy.

## Interfering Factors:

Many drugs can influence thyroid function tests, including hormones (corticosteroids, estrogens, progestins, oral contraceptives), oral anticoagulants (Coumadin), diphenylhydantoin (Dilantin), aspirin (large doses), antithyroid drugs, sulfonamides, lithium, clofibrate, and recent radioactive scanning.

## Cost:

$T_4$: $16 to $20

$T_3$ uptake: $10 to $20

FTI: $20 to $30

## Special Considerations:

★There are several other specialized tests used to evaluate thyroid function, including blood tests (see below), thyroid scan and radioactive iodine uptake tests (p. 299), thyroid ultrasound (p. 306), and thyroid biopsy (p. 359).

★*Thyroid-Stimulating Hormone (TSH):* This test measures the amount of TSH in the blood. TSH is the hormone released from the pituitary gland to cause the thyroid to secrete thyroid hormone.

★*$T_3$ by Radioimmunoassay:* This blood test measures the amount of one of the thyroid hormones. In one form of hyperthyroidism, $T_3$ is elevated but $T_4$ is normal.

★*Thyroid Antibodies and Microsomal Antibodies:* These blood tests are used to evaluate suspected autoimmune diseases such as Hashimoto's thyroiditis and Graves' disease, in which the body produces antibodies that attack its own thyroid tissue.

# Toxicology Screening (Tox Screen, Drug Screen, Coma Panel)

Drug overdose may result from an accidental or deliberate ingestion of legal or illegal drugs. A toxicology screen measures various body fluids (blood, urine, or stomach contents) for the presence and amount of potentially toxic substances. These substances usually include such drugs as pain medications (narcotics, acetaminophen), sedatives (barbiturates), tranquilizers, antidepressants, and antipsychotic medications, as well as recreational drugs like alcohol, amphetamines, and hallucinogens. A specific drug may be tested for, or a screening panel for as many as 30 different substances may be performed.

**Why Performed:**
A tox screen is usually performed in an emergency situation to evaluate such symptoms as coma, stupor, irrational behavior, hallucinations, confusion, sudden personality change, breathing difficulties, or heart irregularities which may be due to toxic substances. Most drug overdoses can be managed without measuring drug levels. A careful history, physical exam, and observation are usually sufficient. Toxicology screening, however, may be useful when the cause of the symptoms or type of overdose is not known. Depending on the type of overdose, treatment may involve a specific antidote or management strategy.

**Normal Values:**
No toxic substances detected or nontoxic levels for regularly taken medications.
●*Greater Than Normal Values May Mean*: The presence and, sometimes, amount of ingested, injected, or inhaled toxic substance are indicated. However, toxicology screens are not 100% accurate. In about 10% of tests, drugs known to have been ingested are not detected (false-negatives) and drugs not taken are detected (false-positives). For example, some nonnarcotic cough medications may be identified as narcotics. Therefore, positive results, whenever possible, should be confirmed by independent testing.

**Cost:**
$120 to $140 for blood and urine panel; individual tests vary in cost.

**Special Considerations:**
★See alcohol (p. 44) and drug monitoring (p. 69).

# Urea Nitrogen
## (Blood Urea Nitrogen, BUN)

Urea is formed in the liver, an end product of protein breakdown. It is found in the blood in the form of urea nitrogen (BUN). Most BUN is excreted into the urine by the kidney. If kidney function is impaired, or if a person is dehydrated, the BUN level will increase. Thus this test can be used as an index of kidney function.

This test is performed on a venous blood sample (see p. 36).

**Why Performed:**
When kidney disease or impairment is suspected, to monitor known kidney disease, when there is a suspected blockage in urine flow, to assess the extent of dehydration, to determine the cause of unexplained mental confusion.

**Normal Values:**
Values may vary from lab to lab:
8 to 23 milligrams per deciliter (mg/dl)
●*Greater Than Normal Values May Mean*: Kidney disease (e.g., glomerulonephritis, pyelonephritis) or prolonged urinary obstruction due to a tumor or a kidney stone. The BUN may also be increased in dehydration, starvation, fever, gastrointestinal bleeding, or other situations in which large amounts of protein are being broken down.
●*Less Than Normal Values May Mean*: Liver disease, malnutrition, excessive fluid intake.

**Interfering Factors:**
BUN levels can be elevated by drugs that can damage the kidney, including amphotericin B, cephaloridine, gentamicin, tobramycin, kanamycin, or methicillin.

**Cost:**
$5 to $20

**Special Considerations:**
★If liver disease is present, the BUN level may not be an accurate index of kidney function: even though kidney function may be good, poor liver function might produce low BUN levels.

# Uric Acid

Uric acid is a by-product from the breakdown of the body's own cells and from the metabolism of certain purine-rich foods such as liver, kidneys, and sweetbreads. Uric acid levels can build up in the blood and urine due to certain metabolic abnormalities, such as gout or kidney disease. An excess of uric acid in the blood is usually found in gout, a type of arthritis characterized by very painful swelling of the big toe and other joints. An excess of uric acid in urine can result in the formation of uric acid and calcium oxalate kidney stones.

Serum uric acid is measured on a venous blood sample (see p.36). To determine the amount of uric acid excreted in the urine, a 24-hour urine specimen is collected and analyzed (see p.39).

**Why Performed:**
Serum uric acid levels may be measured to help determine whether gout is the likely cause of an inflamed joint. They may also be used to monitor patients with leukemia, kidney failure, and those taking certain medications which increase uric acid levels. Both serum and urine acid levels are usually measured in patients with kidney stones.

**Normal Values:**
Values may vary from lab to lab:
Blood uric acid:
    Males, 4.0–8.5 milligrams/deciliter (mg/dl)
    Females, 2.7–7.3 mg/dl
Urine uric acid:
250–750 mg per 24 hours
●*Greater Than Normal Values May Mean*: Elevated serum uric acid (hyperuricemia) may be caused by either overproduction or underexcretion of uric acid. The overproduction may be due to the metabolic defect found in gout or to conditions resulting in an increased rate of destruction of body cells (leukemia, multiple myeloma, chemotherapy or radiation therapy for cancer, excess red blood cells [polycythemia vera], toxemia of pregnancy, or high fever). Underexcretion of uric acid resulting in high blood levels is found in various types of kidney disease. Increased uric acid levels in blood and urine may also be caused by many drugs, including diuretic medications (thiazides, Lasix, and ethacrynic acid), probenecid (Benemid), salicylates (aspirin), corticosteroids, and alcohol.

Elevated serum uric acid levels do not always indicate gout. Conversely, with gout uric acid is not always increased. The definitive diagnosis of gout arthritis is made by examining fluid taken from an inflamed joint (see p. 363).
●*Lower Than Normal Values May Mean*: Decreased levels of uric acid are found in some types of kidney disease. Certain medications, like allopurinol (Zyloprim), used in the treatment of gout lower uric acid in blood and urine.

**Interfering Factors:**
Drugs such as levodopa, methyldopa (Aldomet), and large doses of vitamin C may cause false-positive elevations of uric acid.

**Cost:**
$10 to $20

# Urinalysis
## (UA, Urine Test)

Several of the more important and easier to perform urine tests are grouped together and called a *routine* or *complete urinalysis*. These tests give information about the health of not only your kidneys and bladder but also nearly every organ in your body.

A routine urinalysis is usually performed in a doctor's office, clinic, or laboratory. But you can learn to perform most parts of a urinalysis at home (p. 421). A complete urinalysis consists of visual examination of the urine (color and clarity), measurement of the concentration (specific gravity) and acidity (pH), chemical tests (glucose, ketones, protein, hemoglobin, bilirubin, and urobilinogen), and an examination under a microscope. These specific parts of a urinalysis are described in detail below. The test begins with the collection of a urine specimen (see p. 38).

The chemical tests are performed with a dipstick. These "miniature laboratories" are plastic strips (about 4 inches long and ¼-inch wide) with chemically treated test pads on one end. After dipping the strip in urine, each test pad will change color if certain chemicals or substances are present in the urine. For example, the protein pad will turn various shades of green if protein

is present. The more protein, the darker the color change. The color changes are compared with a standard chart of colors to determine whether the chemicals are present and roughly in what amounts.

**Why Performed:**
A complete urinalysis is often performed as part of a routine screening exam. In addition, it is used to help evaluate a number of symptoms, including discolored urine, painful urination, abdominal or flank pain, or fever, to name a few. Since a urinalysis can give valuable information about nearly every organ system in the body, this test is often used to screen for and monitor diseases such as diabetes, kidney stones, urinary tract infections, liver disease, gallbladder disease, hypertension, and hormone disorders.

**Cost:**
$10 to $20

## Volume

The amount of urine you produce will vary depending upon the amount of fluids you drink, the loss of body fluids (by perspiration, exhaled vapor, vomiting, diarrhea, bleeding, etc.), kidney function and various hormonal influences. Urine volume can be measured by collecting all the urine excreted over a 24-hour period (see p. 39).

**Normal Values:**
On average, most adults produce between 1200 and 1500 milliliters (ml) of urine a day, with a normal range of 800 to 2000 ml (approximately 1 to 2 quarts) per day. Children normally produce somewhat less (300–1500 ml/day).

● *Greater Than Normal Values May Mean*: Excessive fluid intake (polydipsia), uncontrolled diabetes mellitus, diabetes insipidus (deficiency of antidiuretic hormone), use of diuretics (medications, caffeine, alcohol), and other kidney and hormonal disorders can produce large volumes of urine.

● *Lower Than Normal Values May Mean*: Decreased urine production (oliguria) or little or no urine excretion (anuria) can be due to decreased fluid intake, excessive fluid loss (from fever, sweating, vomiting, diarrhea), shock (severe decrease in blood pressure), toxic reactions (carbon tetrachloride poisoning, sulfonamides, transfusion reaction), or various kidney disorders. A sudden decrease in urine volume may be due to a blockage or obstruction of the urinary tract.

## Color and Clarity

Many people wonder why the color of their urine varies at different times. Some sense intuitively that changes in the color of the urine somehow reflect changes in their health—and to some degree, this is true. The color of the urine can indicate certain diseases, but it more commonly reflects changes in the concentration of the urine, various foods in the diet, or medications that color the urine. Generally the intensity of the color of urine indicates how concentrated the urine is. Darker urine owes its color to a high concentration of yellow pigment (urochrome) formed from foods and bile metabolism.

**Normal Values:**

Normal urine can vary from almost colorless to a dark yellow or amber, depending upon how concentrated it is. Reduced fluid intake or increased fluid losses (from vigorous exercise, fevers, vomiting, or diarrhea) tend to make the urine more concentrated and, therefore, darker. Usually the first urine specimen of the morning is dark and concentrated. When held up to the light and viewed, normal urine usually appears clear or slightly hazy.

**Abnormal Values:**

An unusual color in the urine can be due to changes in fluid balance, foods, medications, or various diseases. For example, a reddish or brown urine may be caused by blood, various medications, or eating blackberries or beets. Taking vitamin supplements that contain B-complex can turn your urine bright yellow. Cloudy or turbid urine can be due to pus or bacteria from a urinary tract infection, blood crystals, or residual sperm after ejaculation. Other causes of unusually colored urine are listed in the accompanying table and in sections on specific tests included in a urinalysis for blood, bilirubin, urobilinogen, red and white blood cells and so on.

---

### Causes of Changes in Color and Appearance of Urine

*Nearly Colorless*
large fluid intake
alcohol ingestion
nervousness
diuretic therapy
uncontrolled diabetes mellitus
diabetes insipidus
chronic kidney disease

*Dark or Bright Yellow*
concentrated urine (dehydration, fever, exercise, etc.)
vitamin B-complex (especially riboflavin)
yeast concentrate
food coloring
quinacrine (Atabrine, antimalarial drug)

113

### *Orange*

carotene (found in carrots and spinach)

phenazopyridine (Pyridium) (urinary anesthetic)

sulfonamides (antibiotics)

bilirubin

### *Red-Orange, Pink, or Red*

beets

blackberries

food coloring

phenolphthalein laxatives (Ex-Lax, Dorbane, Mondane, Senekot)

dioctyl calcium sulfosuccinate laxative (Doxidan)

cascara (laxative)

senna (laxative)

phenothiazine tranquilizers (Thorazine, Mellaril, Haldol)

rifampin (antibiotic)

phenazopyridine (Pyridium) (urinary anesthetic)

methyldopa (Aldomet) (antihypertensive)

phenytoin (Dilantin) (anticonvulsant)

salicylazosulfapyridine (Azulfidine) (antibiotic)

iron preparations (injectable)

pyrvinium pamoate (Povan) (antiworm medication)

aniline dyes

blood and hemoglobin

### *Green or Blue-Green*

urate crystals

methylene blue

amitriptyline (Elavil) (antidepressant)

triamterene (Dyrenium) (diuretic)

indomethacin (Indocin) (antiinflammatory)

*Pseudomonas* urinary tract infection

biliverdin

### *Brown or Brown-Black*

rhubarb

cascara (laxative)

chloroquine (Aralen) (antimalarial)

phenacetin (pain medication)

sulfonamides (antibiotic)

nitrofurantoin (antibiotic)

metronidazole (Flagyl) (antibiotic)

quinine iron preparations (injectable)

levodopa (L-dopa) (antiparkinsonism medication)

lysol poisoning

blood or hemoglobin

bilirubin

porphyrins

alkaptonuria

melanin

### *Cloudy*

crystals (urate, uric acid, carbonates, phosphates)

bacteria

pus (white blood cells)

blood (red blood cells)

mucus

prostatic fluid

sperm

### *Foamy*

bilirubin

## Odor

The odor of urine can also provide some interesting clues.

### Normal Values:

A fresh urine specimen has a slightly aromatic or "nutty" odor due to volatile acids. After standing for several hours the urine develops a pungent ammonia odor due to the decomposition of urea. Certain foods like asparagus and garlic may also produce a characteristic aroma.

### Abnormal Values:

A sweet, fruity odor to the urine is found in uncontrolled diabetes due to the excretion of ketone bodies in the urine. A foul odor may be a clue to an infection in the urinary system. If the urine of an infant smells like maple syrup, this may indicate an inherited defect in amino acid metabolism appropriately named "maple syrup urine disease." Some vitamins and several antibiotics (such as penicillin) can also produce an unusual odor in the urine.

## Specific Gravity (SG)

This test measures the ability of the kidneys to control how concentrated or dilute the urine is. Healthy kidneys should be able to adjust the amount of water excreted in urine to keep the fluids consumed and excreted in balance. When fluid intake is excessive, the kidneys should excrete a larger volume of dilute urine. When intake is limited, smaller amounts of a more concentrated urine should be excreted. The partly controlled by antidiuretic hormone, which is secreted by the pituitary gland. gland.

Specific gravity is a measure of the density of urine compared with pure water. The higher the specific gravity, the greater the amount of solid material dissolved in the urine. Specific gravity is measured by floating an instrument called a urinometer in a urine specimen, by using a refractometer, or by using a dip-and-read chemical test for specific gravity.

**Normal Values:**
The specific gravity of pure water is 1.000. The specific gravity of urine usually ranges between 1.006 and 1.030 but may go as low as 1.003 or as high as 1.035. It varies depending on the amount you eat, drink, exercise, and sweat. Normally, in the morn-

ing, after hours without any food or water, the urine will be more concentrated, with a specific gravity greater than 1.025.

●*Greater Than Normal Values May Mean*: High specific gravity (very concentrated urine) may be due to low fluid intake, high fluid losses (from sweating, vomiting, or diarrhea), excessive sugar in the urine from diabetes mellitus, excessive protein in the urine, or abnormal increases in secretion of antidiuretic hormone.

●*Lower Than Normal Values May Mean*: Low specific gravity (very dilute urine) may be due to excessive fluid intake, use of diuretic medications, severe kidney disease, or diabetes insipidus (a rare disease in which the pituitary gland in the brain fails to secrete sufficient antidiuretic hormone). People with kidney stones may be advised by their physician to drink lots of fluids throughout the day to keep their urine dilute so that kidney stones are less likely to form. In this case, frequent checking of the specific gravity can provide useful information for adjusting fluid intake.

**Special Considerations:**
★*Concentration and Dilution Tests*: If the specific gravity is abnormal on repeated measurements, additional tests, not part of a routine urinalysis, can be performed to evaluate the ability of the kidneys to properly concentrate urine. These tests are done when certain kidney, pituitary gland, or adrenal gland disorders are suspected. They are also sometimes done to evaluate unexpained edema (fluid retention and swelling).

A *concentration test* assesses the ability of the kidneys to concentrate urine when fluids are restricted. For this test you will be given a high-protein dinner with only 200 ml (less than a glass) of fluid on the night before the test. You will then fast until the following morning when you collect urine specimens at 6:00 A.M., 8:00 A.M., and 10:00 A.M., which normally should have a high specific gravity!

A *dilution test* determines the ability of your kidneys to excrete fluid after you consume a large amount of it. You will be asked to drink 1500 ml (about 5 glasses) of water within 30 minutes. A urine specimen will be collected every 30–60 minutes for the next four hours after drinking the water.

# pH

The pH is a measurement of the acidity or alkalinity of urine. It reflects the type of food you eat (certain foods are more acidic or alkaline) and the functioning of your lungs, kidneys, and metabolism.

pH is measured on a dipstick or a meter and recorded on a scale in which 1 is strongly acid, 14 is strongly alkaline and 7 is neutral.

### Normal Values:

Urine pH normally varies from 4.6 to 8.0 throughout the course of a day, with an average of 6.0, which is slightly acid.

● *Greater Than Normal Values May Mean*: An increased pH (more alkaline urine), may be found just after eating a meal. The secretion of hydrochloric acid by the stomach is balanced by a compensatory excretion of alkaline urine. A diet rich in vegetables, milk products, and citrus fruits also tends to alkalinize the urine. Certain medications such as antacids with bicarbonate, potassium citrate, and acetazolamide (Diamox) can produce alkaline urine. Increased urinary pH is also caused by prolonged vomiting, hyperventilation, aspirin overdose, and certain types of urinary tract infections and kidney disease.

In some situations an alkaline urine is desirable and encouraged as part of therapy. For example, kidney stones composed of uric acid, calcium oxalate, and crystine are less likely to form in alkaline urine. Also, certain antibiotics are more effective in killing bacteria in alkaline urine.

● *Lower Than Normal Values May Mean*: Acidic urine (pH below 6.0) is found with diets high in protein (meats and fish) or with certain foods like cranberries. Normally, during sleep you *breathe* more shallowly, the blood becomes more acid, and the kidneys compensate by excreting an acidic urine, so morning urine samples are more acidic. However, persistent acidic urine throughout the day may be a sign of severe lung disease (emphysema), uncontrolled diabetes, prolonged diarrhea, dehydration, or starvation. Certain drugs, including thiazide diuretics and large doses of vitamin C (ascorbic acid) can acidify the urine.

There are circumstances in which an acid urine is desirable. Certain types of kidney stones (calcium phosphate and calcium carbonate) are less likely to develop in acid urine. Also, acidifying the urine by drinking large amounts of cranberry juice is sometimes recommended to help prevent the growth of certain types of bacteria in the urinary tract.

### Interfering Factors:

Urine that is left standing for more than one hour without refrigeration tends to become more alkaline.

# Glucose

Urine usually contains very little glucose (sugar). However, when the blood sugar level is very high, as in diabetes mellitus, the ability of the kidneys to reabsorb the glucose is exceeded, and it spills over into the urine. The level of blood sugar at which glucose spills into the urine is known as the renal threshold and is usually between 160 and 180 mg/dl, though it may be much higher in some people. The sugar that spills into the urine carries a large volume of water with it, producing two of the classic symptoms of diabetes, excessive urination and thirst.

Sugar in the urine can be measured by two simple methods: a tablet (reducing) test such as Clinitest or the dipstick (enzymatic) test such as Clinistix, Diastix, or TesTape. You can easily learn to perform these tests at home (see p. 421).

Urine tests for glucose are usually performed along with a test for ketones (see next). They may be performed on any urine specimen, but results are best interpreted with a "double-voided" specimen. This involves urinating once and flushing it away, urinating again 30–40 minutes later, and collecting a sample. This second-voided specimen more accurately reflects current blood glucose levels and metabolic activity. But even then, the results can be misleading. Urine glucose levels may lag well behind blood levels, and many diabetics are turning to home *blood* glucose monitoring (see p. 434) as a more precise and accurate method.

**Normal Values:**
Negative (no detectable glucose).
● *Greater Than Normal Values May Mean*: Increased levels of urine glucose are scored on the dipstick test as $\frac{1}{10}$, $\frac{1}{4}$, $\frac{1}{2}$, 1, and 2 or more gram/dl (%) or in terms of milligrams per dl (100, 250, 500, 1000, 2000, or more mg/dl). Abnormal results for urine glucose should be interpreted in light of the results of tests for blood glucose (see p. 78).

The finding of glucose in the urine in small amounts is not necessarily abnormal. Following a meal rich in carbohydrates (sugars and starches), during pregnancy, or after excessive stress, most people will normally excrete a trace amount of glucose in the urine. Furthermore, some people have a low renal threshold and spill small amounts of sugar into the urine even when their blood sugar levels are normal, and they suffer no ill consequences.

In the majority of cases, however, excess glucose in the urine (glucosuria or glycosuria) is due to diabetes, a condition of inadequate insulin production from the pancreas or insensitivity to the insulin produced. Glucosuria may also occur with hyperthyroidism and adrenal gland abnormalities, liver damage, brain injury, certain types of poisoning, and certain kidney diseases which decrease the ability to reabsorb glucose from the urine. Some drugs can also cause glucose to be excreted in the urine. These include thiazide diuretics, corticosteroids, carbamazepine, ammonium chloride, large doses of nicotinic acid, lithium carbonate, and prolonged use of phenothiazine tranquilizers.

**Interfering Factors:**
Many drugs can interfere with the two tests for glucose in the urine. For example, with the Clinitest (reducing) tablets, false-positive results can be caused by ascorbic acid (vitamin C), antibiotics (cephalosporins, chloramphenicol, tetracyclines, nalidixic acid, penicillin, and sulfonamides), probenecid, methyldopa (Aldomet), aspirin (high doses), and levodopa. With the dipstick and other enzymatic tests, false results can be caused by ascorbic acid, tetracycline, levodopa (L-dopa), phenazopyridine (Pyridium), methyldopa (Aldomet), and aspirin.

## Ketones

Glucose is normally the main source of energy for body metabolism. However, if there are inadequate carbohydrates (sugars and starches) in the diet or if you have diabetes mellitus (a defect in carbohydrate metabolism), the body cannot rely upon carbohydrates for energy. Instead the body burns fat. As the fat is metabolized, by-products known as ketones or ketone bodies are produced, collect in the blood (p. 85), and are excreted in urine. These ketones can be detected with either a dipstick or tablet urine test. These tests for ketones are usually performed along with blood and urine tests for glucose.

### Normal Values:
Negative (no detectable ketones).
●*Greater Than Normal Values May Mean*: Increased amounts of ketones in the urine (ketonuria) are scored on the dipstick test as small (+ or 15 mg/dl), moderate (+ + or 40 mg/dl), and large (+ + + or greater than 80 mg/dl). Ketonuria typically occurs in diabetes. Large amounts of ketones accompanied by very high blood glucose signal a dangerous condition known as diabetic ketoacidosis, which requires immediate medical attention.

Ketones are also produced when the diet is deficient in carbohydrates. This can occur with starvation, prolonged vomiting, or low-carbohydrate diets for weight loss. Increased metabolic states such as occur with severe stress, extreme cold exposure, very strenuous exercise, prolonged fever, or pregnancy can cause a relative carbohydrate deficiency with resulting ketone production.

### Interfering Factors:
Certain drugs like phenazopyridine (Pyridium) and levodopa can cause false-positive results.

## Protein

The kidney normally filters small proteins out of the bloodstream, then reabsorbs them and puts them back into the blood. Thus, under normal conditions, no detectable amount of protein is excreted in the urine. In many kidney diseases (and a few diseases outside the kidney) this protein-saving function of the kidney is disrupted, and protein, mostly albumin, leaks into the urine. The finding of protein in the urine (proteinuria or albuminuria) is one of the most important tests for kidney disease.

There are several tests for urinary protein. A screening test is performed as part of every routine urinalysis. In this simple test a reagent strip is dipped into a fresh urine specimen. The reagent pads change color depending upon how much protein is in the urine specimen. If significant amounts of protein are found, the test is usually repeated on a first morning urine specimen. If protein is still present, more accurate measurements are then performed to determine the total amount of protein excreted in a 24-hour urine specimen.

### Normal Values:
Negative on the dipstick and less than 150 milligrams of protein per 24-hour urine specimen (mg/24 hr).
●*Greater Than Normal Values May Mean*: Increased amounts of protein in the urine (proteinuria) are scored on the dipstick test as trace, + (30 mg/dl), + + (100 mg/dl), + + + (300 mg/dl), and + + + + (over

2000 mg/dl). The most common cause of small amounts of protein in the urine is a harmless condition known as postural or orthostatic proteinuria. In this condition, found in 3%–5% of healthy young people, protein is excreted in the urine only when people are standing up; the condition is not associated with any kidney disease. If you are found to have a small amount of protein in the urine on a routine test, the test should be repeated using a urine specimen collected immediately after you get up in the morning and then after being up and walking for several hours. If you have protein in the second specimen but not the first one, then you probably have postural proteinuria, and no further testing is necessary.

Transient proteinuria may also be caused by prolonged fever, strenuous exercise, and normal pregnancy.

Persistent proteinuria can indicate kidney disorders such as glomerulonephritis, nephrosis, polycystic kidneys, renal tubular disorders, urinary tract infections, cancer of the kidneys, lupus erythematosus, venous congestion of the kidney, and diabetic or hypertensive kidney damage. In addition, proteinuria may be caused by heart failure, toxemia of pregnancy, anemia, leukemia, multiple myeloma, and certain poisonings (mercury, lead, opiates).

**Interfering Factors:**
Contamination of the urine specimen with heavy mucus, vaginal or prostatic secretions, residual semen, blood, or large amounts of white blood cells (pus) can alter test results. On certain tests for proteinuria false-positive results can occur with x-ray contrast material, tolbutamide, acetazolamide, sodium bicarbonate, para-aminosalicylic acid (PAS), and antibiotics (penicillin, sulfasoxazole, cephalosporins).

False-negatives can be due to very dilute urine, highly alkaline urine, and the presence of certain types of bacteria in the urine (urea-splitting organisms).

**Special Considerations:**
★*Bence Jones Protein*: There is a special test which detects a certain type of protein in the urine known as Bence Jones protein. This abnormal protein is found in the urine of 50% of patients with multiple myeloma, a cancer of the bone marrow. The cancer cells produce large amounts of this abnormal protein, which is then excreted in the urine. This test is usually performed when multiple myeloma is suspected from abnormal bone x-rays, unexplained bone pain, anemia, and weakness.

## Blood and Hemoglobin

Normally red blood cells and hemoglobin (the oxygen-carrying molecule in red blood cells) are not found in the urine. If the kidneys, ureter, bladder, or urethra is irritated or diseased, blood may leak into the urine. A small amount of blood may not be visible to the naked eye, but can usually be detected by placing a chemically treated dipstick in a urine specimen. The results of this chemical test are usually compared with the findings of the microscopic examination of the urine sediment (see later in this section) to see if red blood cells are present.

**Normal Values:**
Negative (no blood or hemoglobin detected).

●*Greater Than Normal Values May Mean*: The presence of blood or hemoglobin in the urine is scored on the dipstick test as + (small), + + (moderate), or + + +

(large). If red blood cells and hemoglobin are present in the urine (hematuria and hemoglobinuria), this is usually a sign of kidney injury, kidney inflammation (glomerulonephritis), a kidney or bladder tumor, a kidney or bladder stone, or an infection in the urinary tract. If only hemoglobin is present in the urine (hemoglobinuria), this suggests increased destruction of red blood cells in the bloodstream (hemolysis) due to drugs (including certain antibiotics and anticoagulants), infections (malaria), toxins (poisonous mushrooms), severe burn or crush injuries, or an allergic reaction to transfused blood.

Hemoglobin in the urine can also be caused by trauma from strenuous physical exercise (so-called march or jogger's hemoglobinuria) or by a condition known as paroxysmal nocturnal hemoglobinuria. If you have unexplained blood or hemoglobin in your urine, the test should be repeated when you have not exercised vigorously for 24–48 hours. If the abnormality persists, further tests such as urine culture (p. 131), intravenous pyelogram (p. 269), or cystoscopy (p. 322) may be necessary.

### Interfering Factors:

False-negative results may occur with the use of high doses of ascorbic acid (vitamin C) either as a dietary supplement or as a perservative used with certain antibiotics (such as tetracycline). False-positive results can occur with contamination of the urine specimen with menstrual blood. The dipstick test for hemoglobin will also show a positive result if another pigment (myoglobin) is present in the urine. Myoglobin is normally found in heart and skeletal muscle. When a muscle is severely damaged, myoglobin is released into the bloodstream and eventually excreted in the urine. Excessive amounts of myoglobin in the urine indicate muscle damage from trauma (crush injuries, heart attack), muscle diseases, or excessive exercise ("march" or "jogger's" myoglobinuria).

## Bilirubin

Bilirubin is a by-product of the breakdown of hemoglobin, the oxygen-carrying molecule in red blood cells. Normally the hemoglobin released from old or damaged red blood cells is metabolized in the liver and excreted in bile into the intestines as bilirubin. (It is the bilirubin that gives the yellow-brown color to stools).

Bilirubin is not normally found in urine. Large amounts may give the urine a dark red-orange color and result in a yellow foam if shaken. Smaller amounts are invisible but may be detected by a change in color on the bilirubin section of the dipstick test.

### Normal Values:

Negative (no detectable bilirubin).

● *Greater Than Normal Values May Mean*: Increased amounts of bilirubin in the urine (bilirubinuria) are scored on the dipstick test as + (small) + + (moderate), or + + + (large). Bilirubin in the urine is usually a sign of liver cell damage or blockage of the flow of bile from the liver or gallbladder. Damaged liver cells (hepatitis or cirrhosis) may be the result of infections, excessive alcohol use, or exposure to toxic chemicals or drugs. The flow of bile may be obstructed by gallstones, tumors, or strictures of the bile ducts. The test for urine bilirubin is a very sensitive indicator of liver disease, often appearing positive before the development of symptoms such as jaundice (a yellow discoloration of the skin due to the accumulation of bilirubin). The results of the urine test for bilirubin should be considered along with the blood tests for bilirubin (see p. 52) and urine urobilinogen (discussed next).

### Interfering Factors:

The urine specimen should be tested within one hour of collection, since the bilirubin decomposes rapidly at room temperature and on exposure to light. Large amounts of ingested vitamin C can give a false-negative result. False-positives can be caused by aspirin, phenazopyridine (Pyridium), and phenothiazine (tranquilizers) such as chlorpromazine (Thorazine).

## Urobilinogen

Bilirubin, a by-product of the breakdown of red blood cells by the liver, is excreted in bile into the intestine. There the bilirubin is further broken down by intestinal bacteria into a yellow pigment called urobilinogen. Normally, the bulk of urobilinogen is excreted in the stool, while only trace amounts are absorbed and excreted in the urine. Tests for urobilinogen, when compared with other tests, can help determine whether jaundice (yellow skin due to increased bilirubin) is caused by liver cell disease, obstruction of the bile ducts, or increased destruction of red blood cells.

The test is performed either on a random urine specimen with a dip-and-read reagent strip or on a 2-hour urine specimen. Since the excretion of urobilinogen normally peaks in the afternoon, the 2-hour urine specimens are collected between 1 and 3 P.M. or 2 and 4 P.M.

### Normal Values:

On the dipstick test the color should read yellow-green to yellow, indicating very low amounts of urobilinogen. Normal values for the 2-hour test are 0.1–1.1 Ehrlich units per 2-hour specimen for women and 0.3–2.1 Ehrlich units per 2-hour specimen for men.

- *Greater Than Normal Values May Mean*: Increased amounts of urobilinogen in the urine are scored on the dipstick test as 2, 4, 8, or 12 Ehrlich units/dl. Increased urobilinogen can indicate increased destruction of red blood cells (hemolytic anemia) or liver damage. The liver damage may be caused by cirrhosis or hepatitis (an inflammation of liver cells due to infection, alcohol excess, toxic chemicals or drugs).
- *Lower Than Normal Values May Mean*: Gallstones, inflammation, or tumors can block the flow of bile into the intestines. Since no bilirubin then reaches the intestinal bacteria, no urobilinogen is produced. Decreased urobilinogen also occurs when intestinal bacteria are killed by treatment with certain antibiotics.

### Interfering Factors:

Since the urobilinogen quickly degrades, this test should be performed within 30–60 minutes of specimen collection. False-positive results can be caused by any of the following medications: acetazolamide (Diamox), sodium bicarbonate, aspirin, phenazopyridine (Pyridium), procaine, sulfonamides (e.g., Gantrisin), para-aminosalicylic acid (PAS), and phenothiazine tranquilizers (e.g., Thorazine). False-negative results can be produced by ingestion of large amounts of vitamin C or ammonium chloride.

## Microscopic Analysis

In this part of a urinalysis a few drops of the urine specimen are viewed under a microscope. This can provide important information about the kidneys and the rest of the urinary tract. It may also help explain other abnormalities noted from the chemical tests of the urine.

The urine specimen is spun rapidly in a centrifuge for about five minutes, causing the solid materials to settle to the bottom. This sediment is then placed on a slide and examined by microscope. The types of material that may be found include cells, casts, crystals, bacteria, and miscellaneous substances.

## Cells

Three types of cells are sometimes seen in the urine: red blood cells (RBCs), white blood cells (WBCs), and epithelial cells. Under high magnification, the types and numbers of cells in a standard area called a high-power field (HPF) are counted.

**Normal Values:**
> 0–3 red blood cells per high-power field (RBC/HPF)
> 0–5 white blood cells per high-power field (WBC/HPF)
> few epithelial cells per high-power field
> ● *Greater Than Normal Values May Mean*:

*Red blood cells* in the urine (hematuria) may arise from anywhere in the urinary tract. They may result from kidney or bladder trauma, kidney stones, infections or inflammation in the urinary tract (glomerulonephritis, pyelonephritis, cystitis, prostatitis, or urethritis), tumors in the kidney or bladder, bleeding disorders, or kidney damage from hypertension. Reactions to certain drugs such as salicylates (aspirin), anticoagulants (coumarin), antibiotics (sulfonamides, methicillin), and phenylbutazone can also cause red blood cells in

the urine. Sometimes the blood is due to contamination with menstrual blood. Vigorous exercise may cause the release of red blood cells into the urine, but this is regarded as a harmless finding—if the urine is reexamined after several days without strenuous exercise, the red blood cells should not be present.

*White blood cells* or pus in the urine (pyuria) suggests bladder infection (cystitis), kidney infection (pyelonephritis), urethritis, or glomerulonephritis. Certain drugs such as methicillin, ampicillin, kanamycin, allopurinol, and aspirin can also produce white blood cells in the urine. When such cells are present, a urine culture (p. 131) may be performed to detect the presence of bacteria.

*Epithelial cells* are the specialized cells that cover body surfaces, including the kidney tubules, bladder, and urethra. These cells are continually aging, shedding, and being replaced; thus a few epithelial cells are normally found in the urine. Large number of certain types of epithelial cells, however, may indicate inflammation or degeneration of the kidney tubules.

## Casts

Casts are cylindrical plugs of protein gel and cellular debris which form in abnormal kidney tubules and are then flushed out with the flow of urine. There are several types of casts: red blood cell casts, white blood cell casts, epithelial casts, hyaline casts, granular casts, and waxy or fatty casts. Each type suggests different kinds of kidney disease.

**Normal Values:**
Normally no casts are found in the urine except occasionally for a few hyaline casts.

•*Greater Than Normal Values May Mean*: *Red blood cell casts* suggest acute inflammation or poor blood supply to the kidneys as in acute glomerulonephritis, sickle-cell disease, and subacute bacterial endocarditis.

*White blood cell casts* are usually found in acute glomerulonephritis or pyelonephritis, nephrotic syndrome, and bacterial infections.

*Epithelial cell casts* suggest renal tubular damage, eclampsia, nephrosis, and heavy metal poisoning.

*Hyaline casts* occur when the diseased kidney allows protein to leak from the bloodstream into the kidney tubules. This can occur with inflammation or trauma such as fever, strenuous exercise, shock, and heart failure.

*Granular casts* form in inflamed and diseased kidneys and with chronic lead poisoning.

*Waxy and fatty casts* are found in chronic renal disease.

## Crystals

An examination of the urine sediment can reveal some rather striking—and often beautiful—crystal formations. Each different type of crystal has a distinctive shape and color.

### Normal Values:
A few crystals such as urates, uric acid, and calcium oxalate may be normally found in the urine.

•*Greater Than Normal Values May Mean*: Excessive amounts of crystals or the presence of certain types of crystals may give a clue to the cause of kidney stones (p. 85) or metabolic abnormalities. Certain drugs such as sulfonamides and ascorbic acid (vitamin C) may cause increased levels of crystals to form.

## Bacteria

Bacteria can sometimes be seen in the microscopic examination of urine sediment.

### Normal Values:
No bacteria present.

•*Greater Than Normal Values May Mean*: Bacteria in the urine suggest an infection in the kidney, bladder, or urethra. This can be supported by finding white blood cells in the urine and confirmed by finding significant bacterial growth on urine cultures (p. 131). However, bacteria in the urine may also be due to contamination during urine collection or storage.

## Miscellaneous

The urine sediment may also contain various other substances, including mucous strands, hair, yeast, parasites (such as *Trichomonas vaginalis* or schistosomal ova), and sperm.

# Vitamin B₁₂ (Cyanocobalamin)

Vitamin $B_{12}$ is a water-soluble vitamin necessary for the formation of red blood cells, DNA synthesis, and growth. It is the one vitamin that plants cannot synthesize; it is derived almost entirely from meat, shellfish, milk products, and eggs. Even yeast, which is an excellent source of the other B vitamins, does not contain $B_{12}$ (except for yeasts specially grown on a medium rich in $B_{12}$). Thus vegetarians who do not eat milk or eggs should take vitamin $B_{12}$ supplements or $B_{12}$-enriched nutritional yeast. People who are not strict vegetarians are unlikely to develop $B_{12}$ deficiencies unless they have malabsorption syndromes.

Blood folate levels (p. 75) are usually tested at the same time as $B_{12}$ because the diagnosis of certain types of anemia requires measurements of both folate and $B_{12}$.

You will be asked to fast for 10–12 hours before the blood sample is collected.

### Why Performed:
To help in the diagnosis of megaloblastic anemia which is characterized by the larger than normal red blood cells; to help diagnose certain disorders of the nervous system, suspected vitamin $B_{12}$ deficiency, or suspected malabsorption syndromes.

### Normal Values:
Values may vary from lab to lab:

200–1100 picograms per milliliter (pg/ml)

● *Greater Than Normal Values May Mean*: Excessive dietary $B_{12}$ intake, liver disease, some leukemias, polycythemia vera.

● *Less Than Normal Values May Mean*: Pernicious anemia (see p. 63), inadequate dietary $B_{12}$ intake, disorders of intestinal absorption, hyperthyroidism, pregnancy. Decreased values are also sometimes seen if part or all of the stomach has been surgically removed.

### Interfering Factors:
Failure to observe pretest fast, previous administration of $B_{12}$, previous administration of radionuclides used in nuclear medicine tests.

### Cost:
$20 to $40. If radioactive $B_{12}$ is used, this test may cost $100 to $200.

# 2 Testing for Infection

**N**o one lives alone. We share our body with trillions of microscopic house guests—bacteria, protozoa, viruses, and fungi. Hundreds of different species peaceably inhabit every square inch of our skin. Microorganisms are everywhere: in the spray from a sneeze, in the water we drink, in the food we eat. If all the microbes that live in an average adult body were put together, they would fill a coffee cup. Those that live outside the intestine would fill a thimble.

The presence of these "bugs" does not mean that we have a disease. Our body's customary lodgers, our normal *flora*, can actually help keep us healthy. A few of these hardworking microbes produce some of the vitamins we need. Others bolster our immune system. Still others keep less friendly invaders away. Without these friendly visitors we would be in big trouble, for hostile organisms would almost certainly take their place. Many women, for example, get vaginal infections after taking antibiotics that kill their normal flora.

We only get into trouble when there is a deficiency in our immune system, a break in our body's natural defenses (e.g., a wound), if we are exposed to a particularly aggressive disease-producing organism (pathogen), or if our normal flora wander into forbidden territory—as when bacteria from the rectal or vaginal area find their way into the bladder. The result is an infection. This can be something as common as a cold or sore throat, or something as serious as an infection of the heart or brain.

There are several ways to test for infection: We can do blood tests that look for antibodies produced to fight infecting organisms. We can do skin tests that can give us information about our body's immune response to current or previous infections. We can stain a sample of body fluid and examine it under a microscope. Or we can attempt to "culture" or grow the organism in a special medium in the laboratory.

Microscopic exams and cultures are done not only to determine whether an infection is present but to help identify the responsible microbe. Symptoms of infection may include fever and chills, rashes, swelling, a puslike discharge, or increasing tenderness in the affected area. A swab or fluid sample from the suspect area is collected and sent to the laboratory for examination. Some types of culture specimen can be collected at home (see Home Throat

Cultures, p. 438). Some cultures can be grown at home as well (see Self-Testing for Urinary Tract Infection, p. 428).

The great majority of cultures are done to test for bacteria. Cultures for viruses and fungi are done much less frequently.

The areas most commonly tested are the throat, urethra, vagina, and rectum. Blood, urine, sputum, stool, and fluids from wounds and sores can also be examined.

Specimens collected during a spinal tap, joint tap, abdominal tap, pleural tap, and from various tissue biopsies are also frequently tested for infection.

There are two ways to test for bacteria: the specimen can be examined directly under a microscope or it can be placed in a nutritive medium, allowed to grow and multiply, and then examined.

# Microscopic Examination and Cultures

MICROSCOPIC EXAMINATION: samples to be examined by microscope are placed on a slide and allowed to dry, are *fixed* by passing the slide through a flame or dipping or spraying it with a liquid, and are then *stained* with one or more dyes before being examined.

The most frequently used stain is called the *Gram stain*, a mixture of crystal violet and iodine dyes. Organisms that stain purple are called *gram-positive*. Those that stain pale pink are called *gram-negative*. The advantage of a Gram stain is that it can give preliminary results within minutes so that treatment can be started without waiting for the culture, which may take 2–10 days. When tuberculosis is suspected, another kind of stain, an *acid-fast stain*, may be used.

Bacteria are identified on microscopic exam by their shape and their response to the stains used to prepare specimens. The two most most common shapes for bacteria are rod-shaped (*bacillus*, plural: *bacilli*) and round (*coccus*, plural: *cocci*). The report from a microscopic examination of a sample usually consists of a description of the color and shape of any bacteria seen, e.g., "gram-negative rods" or "gram-positive cocci."

CULTURES: A culture is a test in which a sample from your body (e.g., blood, urine, pus) is introduced into a gelatinous nutrient medium under conditions in which the suspected organism or organisms will grow and spread. Different media, environments, and temperatures are used when different bacteria are suspected. Most bacteria require oxygen to grow (*aerobic* bacteria). Others (*anaerobic* bacteria) can only grow in an oxygen-free environment.

It usually takes 2–10 days for culture reports to be available. Preliminary reports may be provided in some cases. Culture reports for tuberculosis may take as long as 6 weeks.

If no bacterial growth occurs, the test is reported as "negative." The presence of certain bacteria may be normal in certain cultures—e.g., *Escherichia coli* are normally found in the stool. If abnormal bacteria are detected, the test is reported as "positive."

When bacterial colonies do grow on a culture, they can be identified in two ways: by the distinctive shape and color of the colonies they form, or by making slides of specimens from the colonies and examining them by microscope as described previously.

Test results are sometimes inconclusive. This may be due to an inadequate specimen, overgrowth of the culture medium with normal bacteria, or improper specimen collection or handling. The results of a bacterial culture will be negative if the infection is produced by a virus.

### Antibiotic Sensitivity Testing

Small doses of various antibiotics are sometimes placed on the culture medium to help determine which one will be most effective against the disease-producing organism. If an antibiotic limits the growth of an organism, that organism is said to be *sensitive* to the antibiotic. If growth is not affected, the organism is said to be *resistant* to the antibiotic. This test can be extremely useful in choosing the best treatment: The drugs that inhibit or stop bacterial growth in the culture medium are usually the most effective in the body as well.

In general, specimens for culture should be collected before starting antibiotic therapy, as antibiotics can alter bacterial growth and make it difficult to interpret test results.

A typical lab report might look like this:

Gram stain: Gram-negative rods
Organism: *E. coli*

Colony count: Greater than 100,000 colonies per cc
Sensitivities:
Ampicillin, R (resistant)
Sulfa, I (intermediate)
Nitrofurantoin, S (sensitive)

# Blood Cultures

An infection in the bloodstream (*bacteremia* or *septicemia*) is always a serious matter: Blood-borne bacteria can easily spread to any part of the body. Such infections are most frequently seen in persons with decreased immunity. This may be due to age (infants and the very elderly), disease (cancers and immune diseases), or drugs (steroids or cancer chemotherapy).

### Why Performed:

This test is done in suspected bacterial infections of the bloodstream. The chief symptoms of such an infection are usually chills and fever. It is also performed in suspected infections of the heart valves (endocarditis).

### Preparation:

Tell your doctor if you are taking or have recently taken antibiotics.

### Procedure:

The sample or samples for this test are collected at your bedside or in a doctor's office or clinic by a physician, nurse, or blood-drawing technician (phlebotomist). The sample is usually taken from a vein in the bend of your arm, just opposite your elbow. Because blood samples are easily contaminated with bacteria from the skin, the person collecting the samples will perform a thorough cleansing procedure before inserting the needle—an iodine wash followed by an alcohol wash. To increase the chances of identifying the infecting organism two or three samples are usually taken from different sites. Additional samples may be taken over the next day or two.

### How Does It Feel?
You may feel a brief pain as the needle is inserted into your vein. This should feel no different from any other blood drawing.

### Risks:
There is a slight risk of bruising and bleeding at the puncture site. This risk can be reduced by applying firm pressure for 3– 5 minutes after the sample is taken.

### Results:
No bacteria are normally found in the bloodstream, but some organisms can temporarily invade the blood during the early stages of infections of the kidneys, throat, or other parts of the body. This can be a mild, transitory finding and may not indicate serious infection. Persistent high levels of bacteria in the blood usually indicate a serious blood-borne bacterial infection.

It usually takes 1–3 days for blood cultures to detect most common organisms. However, some organisms require 7–10 days to show up on culture.

About 5% of blood cultures are contaminated with normal skin bacteria (usually *Staphylococcus epidermidis*). Samples drawn from catheters and intravenous needles are also frequently contaminated. However, these samples are occasionally useful in determining the organisms responsible for blood infections caused by catheters.

### Cost:
Costs will vary depending on the type and number of organisms isolated and whether antibiotic sensitivity testing is required. Most blood cultures cost between $25 and $80.

# Sputum Cultures

A wide variety of infections can occur within the lungs (*pneumonia*) or in the airways leading to the lungs (*bronchitis*). A sputum culture is used to identify the bacteria that may be causing such infections.

### Why Performed:
This test is done in suspected infections of the lungs or airways, especially if a chest x-ray suggests infection. Symptoms may include difficulty in breathing, pain with breathing, or a cough that produces bloody or greenish-brown sputum. This test is also used to help diagnose tuberculosis.

### Preparation:
Tell your doctor if you are taking or have recently taken antibiotics. You should drink as much fluid as possible: this keeps the membranes in your respiratory tract moist and will help you cough up the needed sample.

### Procedure:
You will be asked to cough deeply and to spit any sputum you are able to bring up into a sterile cup. Sputum is not the same as saliva: Saliva is a clear, watery liquid produced in the mouth. Sputum is a thick, cloudy secretion produced in the lungs and in the airways leading to the lungs. Sometimes a doctor, nurse, or physical therapist will help you produce a sample by tapping

on your chest to loosen the sputum. Occasionally someone who has trouble coughing up sputum may be asked to inhale an aerosol mist to help bring up a sample.

Sometimes a sample is obtained during *bronchoscopy* (see p. 315). On rare occasions a soft, lubricated catheter is inserted through a nostril and down the throat to collect the needed specimen (*tracheal aspiration*). In a few extremely rare cases the sample may be obtained by inserting a needle through the neck into the trachea (*transtracheal aspiration* or *tracheal tap*).

### How Does It Feel?

If you inhale an aerosol mist, you may feel a deep, uncontrollable urge to cough. If tracheal suctioning is used, you may experience deep coughing as the catheter passes through the back of your throat, and may find it hard to breathe for the few seconds the catheter is in place.

### Risks:

In the rare cases in which tracheal suctioning is necessary, patients with severe asthma or bronchitis may experience breathing difficulties. A tracheal tap may result in the accidental injection of air into the tissues of the neck.

### Results:

Sputum that has passed through the mouth is inevitably contaminated with bacteria that normally live there—these include some types of *Streptococcus*, diptheroids, *Staphylococcus*, and *Hemophilius*. Disease-producing organisms found in sputum include *Streptococcus pneumoniae* (pneumococci), *Klebsiella pneumoniae*, and *Mycobacterium tuberculosis* (TB). Results are usually available within a few days, but cultures for TB may take as long as six weeks.

### Cost:

Costs will vary depending on the type and number of organisms isolated and whether sensitivity testing is required. Most sputum cultures cost between $25 and $80.

# Stool Cultures

As many as 50 different kinds of bacteria may *normally* be present in the intestine of a healthy person—more than are found in any other part of the body. Either the presence of an abnormal organism or the overabundance of a normal one can produce infection.

### Why Performed:

This test is done in suspected intestinal infections. Symptoms may include prolonged, unexplained diarrhea, bloody diarrhea, increased quantities of gas, lower abdominal cramping, or fever. This test may also be performed on people (especially food handlers) who, though free of symptoms, may have an infectious organism in their stool and may be spreading it to others. Such people are called *carriers*.

### Preparation:

Unless instructed differently by your doctor, you should, if possible, avoid the following for two weeks before the sample is collected: antacids, antidiarrheal drugs, antiparasite drugs, antibiotics, enemas, laxatives, and x-ray exams in which you are asked to swallow barium contrast materials. All these substances can interfere with test results.

**Procedure:**

The sample for this test may be obtained either at home or at the hospital. If you are in the hospital, your nurse will help you collect the sample. If you are at home, you will be given one or more stool collection kits (one for each day on which you are to collect a specimen). Each kit contains a number of applicator sticks and two sterile vials containing different preservatives.

Collect the specimens as follows:

1. Pass stool (but no urine) into a dry container.
2. Using one of the applicator sticks, place a lump of stool about the size of a nickel in each of the two vials. Using the applicator stick, break up the sample and stir the mixture until a uniform consistency is reached.
3. Replace the screw-on caps and label each vial with your name, your doctor's name, and the date the specimen was collected. Use one kit for each day's collection. Unless otherwise directed, collect specimens only once a day.

Either solid or liquid stool can be collected. If collecting liquid stool, it may be easier to line the container with newspaper to help absorb excess liquid. Sealed vials may be delivered or mailed (in the special mailing tube provided) to your doctor's office or directly to a laboratory. Wash your hands well after collecting the specimen to avoid spreading bacteria.

A specimen may also be collected by your doctor using a cotton swab inserted into the rectum during an exam.

**Risks:**

The only risk is that of exposing others to infectious organisms in the stool sample.

**Results:**

Some of the more common infectious organisms and the diseases they produce are *Shigella* (dysentery, shigellosis), *Salmonella* (typhoid fever, enterocolitis), *Campylobacter fetus* (gastroenteritis), and *Vibrio cholerae* (cholera).

**Cost:**

Cost will vary depending on the type and number of organisms isolated and whether sensitivity testing is required. Most stool cultures cost between $25 and $80.

**Special Considerations:**

★*Ova and Parasite Test*—The term *parasite* is used to refer to a number of infective organisms that are neither bacteria nor viruses. These most commonly infect the intestines (though the parasitic organism *Trichomonas* is a frequent cause of vaginal infection, see p. 177), and include pinworms (see p. 447), roundworms, tapeworms, amoebas, *Giardia*, and others. These parasites and their eggs can frequently be seen by microscopic examination of a stool sample.

Parasitic disease of the intestine is particularly common in travelers who have recently visited tropical countries or other places where parasites are common and in homosexual men. When such infection is suspected, an ova and parasites test is often ordered, usually as part of a stool exam.

# Throat Cultures

Many organisms can produce a sore throat, but infections with group A beta-hemolytic streptococci (group A strep) are of special concern because they can spread to the kidneys (producing glomerulonephritis) or to the heart valves (producing rheumatic heart disease). The purpose of nearly all throat cultures is to detect infections caused by group A streptococci or gonorrhea.

### Why Performed:

This test is done in cases of sore throat that are accompanied by fever, enlarged tonsils with white spots (pus), and swollen lymph nodes ("swollen glands"), or when certain infections (e.g., gonorrhea) are suspected elsewhere in the body.

Some doctors may choose to treat a throat infection with antibiotics on the basis of symptoms alone, without doing a culture. If one family member is experiencing recurrent sore throats, other family members may be cultured to determine whether they have mild, symptomless strep infections. Such people (called carriers) may be transmitting the infection.

### Preparation:

Tell your doctor if you are taking or have recently taken antibiotics.

### Procedure:

The sample for this test is usually collected in a doctor's office or clinic, but can be collected at home (p. 438). You will be asked to open your mouth as wide as possible. The person taking the sample will examine your throat and may press your tongue down with a depressor. He or she will then swab each side of the back of your throat with a long, cotton-tipped swab. Only one sample is taken for suspected strep infections. If other bacteria are suspected, two samples may be collected.

### How Does It Feel?

You may feel a brief impulse to gag when the swab touches the back of your throat.

### Risks:

There are no known risks of this procedure.

### Results:

Several different kinds of bacteria are normally found in the throat—including a few organisms capable of causing disease. Increased numbers of these bacteria may mean that disease is present. Some of the bacteria causing throat infections, and the conditions they cause, are *Streptococcus pyogenes* (strep throat, scarlet fever), *Neisseria gonorrhoeae* (gonorrhea), *Corynebacterium diphtheriae* (diphtheria), and *Bordetella pertussis* (whooping cough).

### Cost:

Cost will vary depending on the type and number of organisms isolated and whether sensitivity testing is required. Most throat cultures cost between $15 and $30.

# Urine Cultures

Bladder infections and other urinary tract infections are much more common in females. This is because the female urethra is substantially shorter than that of males, making it easier for bacteria to work their way into the normally sterile urine in the bladder. The female urethra is also much closer to the anus, the source of the bacteria that cause most urinary tract infections.

A urinalysis (p. 112) is usually performed at the same time this test is done. Antibiotic sensitivity testing and counts of the number of bacteria present can usually help determine appropriate therapy.

### Why Performed:

This test is done in suspected infections of the bladder, kidney, or other parts of the urinary tract. Symptoms may include pain or burning on urination, frequent urination, urgency before urinating, blood in the urine, foul-smelling urine, or pain in the abdomen or lower back. This test is also done when such abnormalities as an increased number of white cells (which suggests infection) are detected on a routine urinalysis. The test is also sometimes used to check for possible infection in patients with catheters in their bladders.

**Preparation:**

Tell your doctor if you are taking or have recently taken antibiotics.

**Procedure:**

You will be instructed in how to cleanse your genital area, excrete a small amount of urine, then collect a "midstream" sample in a sterile container (see Collecting a Urine Specimen, p. 38). The sample must be cultured quickly, as bacteria can multiply rapidly. If the sample cannot be cultured at once, it should be refrigerated.

**Risks:**

There is no known risk of this procedure.

**Results:**

The urine in the bladder is normally sterile, but bacteria are normally found in the urethra (the tube leading from the bladder to the outside of the body). These bacteria often get into urine samples. It is usually possible to distinguish between bacteria from the urethra and a true bladder infection by determining the number of organisms in a given quantity of urine (colony count).

A colony count of 100,000 or more per cubic millimeter of urine indicates an infection of the urinary tract. Colony counts of 100 to 100,000 could be due either to infection or to contamination by bacteria from the urethra. A repeat test may be needed. Colony counts of 100 or less are assumed to be due to contamination.

This test may not detect some mild infections or infections caused by organisms which do not grow in routine cultures.

**Cost:**

Cost will vary depending on the type and number of organisms isolated and whether sensitivity testing is required. Most urine cultures cost between $25 and $80.

# Skin and Wound Cultures

Any cut, scratch, wound, or other break in the skin or other tissues provides a hospitable site for bacterial growth. Prompt treatment of wound infections can prevent their spread to other parts of the body and can help minimize scarring.

**Why Performed:**

This test is done to determine whether a sore, wound, injury, surgical incision, or burn is infected. Typical symptoms include pain, redness, tenderness, warmth, and the presence of pus.

**Preparation:**

Tell your doctor if you are taking or have recently taken antibiotics.

**Procedure:**

The person collecting the specimen will insert a sterile, cotton-tipped swab into the suspect area and may also squeeze out a small sample of pus or other fluid. Specimens may be gathered from the ear canal, eye, wounds, a sore on the skin, or from other areas. If an anaerobic culture is to be done, a sample of fluid may be drawn up into a syringe to keep from exposing the specimen to air.

### How Does It Feel?

If the wound is sore or tender, you may feel some pain when the specimen is collected.

### Risks:

There is a very slight risk that the infection may be spread by the examiner's efforts to collect a sample.

### Results:

Some of the bacteria that most commonly produce wound infections are those normally found on skin, especially staphylococci and streptococci.

### Cost:

Cost may vary depending on the type and number of organisms isolated and whether sensitivity testing is required. Most skin and wound cultures cost between $25 and $80.

## Viral Cultures

With the exception of cultures for herpes, (p. 143), viral cultures are rarely done. This is because the equipment required is extremely complex and expensive and because these cultures take so long to complete that the results are rarely useful in planning treatment. Most viral cultures are performed in government or university laboratories.

# Other Tests for Infection

## Tuberculin Skin Tests
## (Purified Protein Derivative, PPD; Old Tuberculin, OT; Tine Test)

A tuberculin skin test helps determine whether you were ever infected by the bacteria that cause tuberculosis. A small amount of purified protein derivative (PPD) is extracted from dead TB bacteria and injected into your skin. If you were infected with TB or vaccinated against TB at any time in the past, your immune system will produce swelling at the injection site 1–2 days after the injection.

### Why Performed:

This is a screening test for tuberculosis infection. It may be performed every few years on children and young adults on a routine basis. TB skin tests are also recommended for those at high risk, such as people who have contact with an individual known to have tuberculosis, people living in communities or migrating from areas (like southeast Asia) where the prevalence of tuberculosis is known to be high, health care personnel exposed to tuberculosis, and people with signs or symptoms of tuberculosis such as a persistent cough, night sweats, weight loss, or an abnormal chest x-ray suggesting tuberculosis.

### Preparation:

Tell your doctor if
> You have ever had a positive skin test for tuberculosis in the past
> You have ever had tuberculosis
> You have ever been vaccinated against tuberculosis (known as BCG vaccine)
> You have recently been vaccinated for measles, mumps, rubella, or polio
> You are taking any medications, particularly steroids (cortisone) or immunosuppressive drugs

### Procedure:

This test is performed in a doctor's office or hospital by a physician, nurse, or technician. The injection is usually made in the skin on the underside of your forearm. The area will be first cleansed with alcohol and allowed to dry. The test material is injected into the skin with either a small syringe or an instrument with several tiny prongs. A circle may be drawn around the injection site with a pen. The test takes 2–3 minutes.

The test is read 48–72 hours later. You may be asked to return to have the test interpreted, or you may be instructed on how to read the test yourself (see later).

### How Does It Feel?

You may feel a brief, stinging sensation as the substance is injected. Since the needle is so thin and the injection is made only in the skin, the sensation is usually less painful than other injections.

If you have a positive reaction, it may itch. It is important that you not scratch the test site, as this may produce inflammation that will interfere with reading the test. If necessary cover the test site with a bandage to prevent scratching.

If you have a strongly positive reaction, it may be painful. Cold compresses may help.

### Risks:

If you have or have had active TB or BCG vaccination, there is a slight risk of a severe allergic reaction to the injection. The reaction may produce considerable swelling, loss of skin, and pain at the injection site, but can usually be treated successfully.

There is no chance of getting an active TB infection from this test because no living TB organisms are injected.

### Results:

If you ever had a previous tuberculosis infection or were vaccinated against tuberculosis, your immune system will recognize the injected TB extract and will react by producing redness, swelling, and perhaps blistering at the injection site. The reaction is interpreted 48 to 72 hours after the injection.

The amount of swelling and hardness (induration), not redness, is the key to reading the skin test. Rub your finger firmly over the injection site. A raised, hard area larger than 10 millimeters across (slightly less than a half inch), indicates a positive test. A swelling of 5–9 millimeters is a borderline or doubtful result and may have to be repeated. Less than 5 millimeters of swelling or none at all (no matter how much redness is present) indicates a negative reaction. If you have any swelling at the injection site or are unsure about reading the test yourself, check with a health professional within the 48- to 72-hour time period.

A positive TB skin test does not mean you have active infectious tuberculosis. The test cannot distinguish between active infections and previous infections which are dormant, or infection with a harmless organism related to tuberculosis (atypical mycobacteria). Further tests, including a chest x-ray and, in some cases, a sputum culture (p. 128), may be necessary.

For most people, a positive TB skin test will always remain positive, so repeat tests are unnecessary.

### Cost:
$10 to $15

### Special Considerations:

★ *Other Skin Tests:* There are other skin tests to detect current or previous infection with different organisms, such as histoplasmosis and coccidioidomycosis ("Valley Fever"). Skin tests may also be performed to test the immune system in people with severe, recurring or unusual infections or cancer in which a defect in immune function is suspected. With these tests small samples of several common infectious agents such as yeast, mumps, staphylococci, or streptococci are injected into the skin. If the immune system is working properly, the body will recognize these common agents and produce a small skin eruption. Failure to react may indicate a deficiency in the immune system.

★ *Scabies Test*—Scabies is a tiny mite which burrows into the skin causing tiny red bumps and extreme itching which is frequently worse at night. This condition is diagnosed by opening one or more of the bumps with a needle or scalpel and smearing the contents on a slide. The slide is then viewed under a microscope to look for the mite, eggs, or droppings.

★ *Tests for Fungus*—Certain skin, oral, and vaginal infections can be caused by fungi. Athlete's foot, thrush, ringworm, "jock itch," and vaginal yeast infections (p. 177) are all fungal infections. These conditions can sometimes be diagnosed from the history and symptoms alone, but if the diagnosis is in doubt, fungal scrapings should be done.

The scraping is placed on a slide along with a few drops of potassium hydroxide (KOH). This serves to dissolve the skin but leaves the fungus cells intact. Blood tests for fungal infections can also be done.

# Infectious Disease Antibody Tests

When there is an infection in any part of your body, your immune system produces antibodies against the infecting organism. Some of these specific antibodies can be measured. This can help your doctor determine whether you have had an infection caused by a specific organism.

Antibody levels (titers) are frequently repeated to help determine whether your antibody level is falling or rising. These results may suggest that the infection is currently active.

Below are descriptions of the more commonly done infectious disease antibody tests.

## AIDS Antibody Test
### (HTLV-III)

Acquired Immune Deficiency Syndrome (AIDS) is a lethal disease in which the immune system is damaged making the body unable to defend itself against certain infections and cancers. The probable cause of AIDS has been identified as a virus, known as human T-cell lymphotropic virus type III (HTLV-III). When infected with the virus the body produces antibodies that can now be detected by a blood test. The AIDS virus is thought to be spread primarily by intimate sexual contact, sharing needles, or blood transfusions.

**Why Performed:**
The test is designed to screen for the presence of antibodies to HTLV-III which indicates past or present infection with the virus. The test does not diagnose AIDS or

AIDS Related Condition (ARC). It is primarily used to screen potential donors of blood, plasma, sperm, body organs, or other tissues for the presence of antibodies to the AIDS virus. People with positive antibody tests should not be donors.

**Normal Values:**
Values may vary from lab to lab:

Negative (no significant levels of AIDS antibodies detected)

●*Greater Than Normal Values May Mean*: A positive test indicates the likely presence of antibodies to HTLV-III and suggests a current or past infection with the virus. A positive test does not indicate immunity to the disease and does not diagnose AIDS. Positive tests are usually repeated and may be confirmed with another type of test (e.g., Western blot test). The significance of a positive antibody test is not fully known. Current evidence suggests that only 10%–15% of infected people go on to develop AIDS; the majority of people with positive tests remain infected but without symptoms.

The test is not 100% accurate. When performed on large numbers of people who are at low risk for being exposed to the virus, many of the positive test results are actually false positives and these people have not been infected by the virus.

People with positive test results should consult their physicians or the local public health authorities for current information and advice.

**Cost:**
Usually performed for free at designated AIDS testing centers or at blood banks.

# Cold Agglutinins

Cold agglutinins are a type of antibody that increases markedly in the blood of people infected with a variety of microorganisms, most notably mycoplasma. This microorganism commonly causes a type of pneumonia occurring mainly in young adults. The name, cold agglutinins, derives from the observation that these antibodies tend to cause red blood cells to clump together (agglutinate) at lower temperatures.

**Why Performed:**
This test is most often used to evaluate a suspected mycoplasma-caused pneumonia. It is also sometimes used to aid in the diagnosis of certain viral diseases and some cancers.

**Normal Values:**
Values may vary from lab to lab:
An antibody level (titer) of less than 1:16 is generally normal although higher levels may be normal in older people.
● *Greater Than Normal Values May Mean*: High or increasing titers of cold agglutinins suggest a mycoplasma infection but may also be due to viral diseases or certain cancers.

**Cost:**
$15 to $25

# Hepatitis Virus Tests

Hepatitis (inflammation of the liver) can be caused by alcohol, drugs, other toxins, or one of several types of virus infections. The body responds to virus infections by producing specific antibodies to fight the infection. Blood tests to diagnose viral hepatitis detect either these specific antibodies or parts of the virus particle itself (antigens). These tests can help identify the three types of viral hepatitis which differ in cause, severity, prevention, and treatment.

*Hepatitis A*, formerly called infectious hepatitis, is caused by a virus which is shed in feces. Therefore, it is usually spread by contaminated water or food or close contact with an infected person. Symptoms usually develop 2 to 6 weeks after exposure, the disease is usually mild, and recovery complete. Hepatitis A can sometimes be prevented by an injection of gamma globulin. A blood test (*hepatitis A virus antibody* or *anti-HAV*) measures whether the body has formed antibodies in response to the presence of hepatitis A virus.

*Hepatitis B*, also known as serum hepatitis, is most often acquired by contact with hepatitis virus-infected blood from transfusions, contaminated needles or medical instruments, or sexual contact. Symptoms develop from 6 to 26 weeks after exposure, may persist and lead to severe chronic liver disease. A blood test for *hepatitis B surface antigen (HBsAg)*, which was formerly known as hepatitis-associated antigen or Australian antigen, is usually positive during a hepatitis B infection. In about 10% of people infected, the HBsAg may remain permanently in the blood. Even though such people may have no symptoms, they are carriers and may transmit the infection to others.

*Non-A, non-B hepatitis* is a less well understood type of hepatitis which usually develops after blood transfusions. There are no currently available tests for this type of hepatitis though some may soon be available. It is usually said to exist when the blood tests for the other types of hepatitis are negative.

**Why Performed:**
The test for HBsAg is often used to evaluate findings suggestive of hepatitis such as persistent flulike symptoms, fatigue, loss of appetite, abdominal pain, nausea and vomiting, enlarged liver, dark-colored urine, yellow skin (jaundice), and abnormal liver function tests (pp. 52, 45, 101). The HBsAg may also be used to screen people at high risk of contracting or transmitting hepatitis B such as food handlers, medical personnel, and blood donors. Two additional tests, *hepatitis B surface antibody* (*HBsAb*) and *hepatitis B core antibody* (*HBcAb*), may also be performed to detect previous exposure and immunity to hepatitis B in people at high risk (doctors, dentists, nurses, drug abusers, and male homosexuals). If the test for immunity is negative, then immunization with a vaccine for hepatitis B is often recommended.

**Normal Values:**
Negative for the presence of viral hepatitis antigens or antibodies.
 • *Greater Than Normal Values May Mean*: A positive hepatitis A antibody test implies current or past hepatitis A infection.

A positive HBsAg implies current or past hepatitis B infection. A person with HBsAg-positive blood should not donate blood. A positive hepatitis B surface antibody or hepatitis B core antibody suggests past hepatitis B infection with current immunity.

Negative anti-HAV and HBsAg tests suggest non-A, non-B hepatitis or some other cause for symptoms.

**Cost:**
$20 to $30 for each test.

# Mononucleosis Tests
## (Mono Test, Mono Spot Test, Heterophil Test)

Mononucleosis is a common viral disease which can produce a variety of signs and symptoms—including sore throat, swollen lymph nodes, profound fatigue, headache, and abdominal pain. It has been called "the kissing disease" because of the way it is sometimes transmitted, especially among high school and college students. This disease is produced by the Epstein-Barr virus, and the test detects the presence of anti-Epstein-Barr antibodies.

There are two general types of test for mono:

Spot tests are performed on a microscope slide by mixing a drop of blood with test reagents. Results of spot tests are read as either positive or negative.

The heterophil test measures the concentration of antibodies in the blood. Results may be reported either as positive or negative or as a ratio or titer, e.g., 1:56 or 1:112.

**Why Performed:**
To help diagnose suspected cases of mononucleosis.

**Normal Values:**
Values may vary from lab to lab:
 Negative or titer of less than 1:112
 • *Greater Than Normal Values May Mean*: The spot test is a screening not a definitive test. If the results of the spot test are positive, the heterophil test may be performed, as some conditions other than mono can produce a positive spot test. A heterophil

test result of positive or a titer of more than 1:224 suggests mononucleosis. If the test is done in the first week of the illness, the result may be negative even though the person really has mono, since the antibodies may take some time to develop. Thus if an early test is negative and symptoms persist, the test should be repeated.

### Interfering Factors:
People addicted to narcotics may have high levels of antibodies to Epstein-Barr virus even though they do not have mononucleosis.

### Cost:
$8 to $25

# Rubella Tests

Rubella (German measles) is a mild, self-limited viral disease in children, but can produce serious problems in pregnant women—birth defects, spontaneous abortion, and stillbirths. The earlier the infection occurs in a woman's pregnancy, the greater the risks to the fetus. It is important for every woman to be tested before becoming pregnant to make sure she has antibodies to rubella—and is thus not susceptible to infection during pregnancy. If a newly pregnant mother discovers that she has no antibodies to rubella, she should avoid sick children who may have measles. This test may be repeated if she becomes ill.

### Why Performed:
To determine whether a prospective mother or newly pregnant woman is susceptible to rubella. It is also recommended to screen for health workers who come in contact with pregnant women.

### Normal Values:
Values may vary from lab to lab:
Titers of 1:16 or more indicate immunity to rubella.
●*Less Than Normal Values May Mean*: A titer of 1:8 or less indicates lack of immunity to rubella infection. Rubella immunization is usually recommended.

### Cost:
$8 to $25

# Toxoplasmosis Tests

Toxoplasmosis is a disease caused by a parasite commonly carried by domestic cats, sheep, and many other animals. Cats usually show no symptoms of this disease, but can pass it to humans via their feces. (Toxoplasmosis is sometimes called cat-box disease.) Symptoms can include muscle and nerve damage, swollen lymph nodes, eye infections, and damaged heart muscle.

The most serious complications of toxoplasmosis result when a pregnant woman passes the disease to her unborn baby. This can result in birth defects, stillbirth, or abortion. At birth the affected child may be smaller than expected and may show signs of brain damage, damage to the eyes, and other organ damage. This test looks for antibodies to the toxoplasmosis parasite in a blood sample.

**Why Performed:**

As part of routine screening for pregnant women, or when toxoplasmosis is suspected—especially in an infant or young child.

**Normal Values:**

Values may vary from lab to lab:
    Antitoxoplasmosis titer of 1:128 or less.

● *Greater Than Normal Values May Mean*: Titers of 1:256 or more are considered positive. Titers greater than 1:1000 indicate active disease. A sudden rise in titer suggests toxoplasmosis.

**Cost:**

$25 to $50

# Sexually Transmitted Disease Tests

## Gonorrhea Tests

Gonorrhea is the most common sexually transmitted disease. It is popularly known as "the clap." Health workers frequently speak of it as "GC," short for *gonococci*, the bacteria that cause the disease.

Early diagnosis of suspected gonorrhea infections is very important: Gonorrhea can almost always be cured with antibiotics, but if left untreated can be serious. Since women infected with this disease often have no symptoms, they may not realize they have the disease until complications develop. The most serious complication is severe pelvic infection.

This test is done to determine whether a person has gonorrhea. A sample of vaginal and cervical secretions or penile discharge is taken. Part of the sample is examined under a microscope. Another part is spread on a special gonorrhea culture plate. If infection of the anus, throat, or eyes is suspected, samples may be taken from these areas as well.

**Why Performed:**

*In women*—Gonorrhea infections of the vagina sometimes produce a thick yellow or greenish-yellow discharge, but there is frequently no discharge at all—about 98% of women with gonorrhea have no noticeable symptoms. As a result, many cases of gonorrhea in women go untreated. This can result in passing the infection to sexual partners and the spread of the infection to a woman's fallopian tubes, ovaries, and abdominal cavity. This is called pelvic inflammatory disease (PID).

PID can produce fever and abdominal pain. The scarring resulting from PID can block the passage of the unfertilized egg to the uterus, resulting in inability to have children. Widespread gonorrhea can also affect the skin, the joints, and the bloodstream and in extreme cases can cause death.

This test should be done when a woman develops a vaginal infection or has sexual contact with a partner who may have gonorrhea. Since gonorrhea can be a "silent disease" in women and can have serious consequences, women who have multiple sexual partners, some of whom might have this disease, may wish to have the test performed periodically even if symptoms are not present.

*In pregnant women*—Gonorrhea can cause serious infections in newborn babies and was once a frequent cause of blindness in infants. Preventive eyedrops are now used routinely in all hospital deliveries. Pregnant women should have a gonorrhea culture performed early in pregnancy. Repeat cultures should be done if there is any reason to suspect she might have been exposed to gonorrhea.

*In men*—When a man has gonorrhea there is usually a yellow or greenish-yellow discharge from the tip of the penis. Burning on urination is often present. But about 10% of men with gonorrhea have no noticeable symptoms.

A culture should be done any time a man notices a discharge from the penis. It should also be done after a man has had intercourse with a sexual partner who may have had gonorrhea.

Both men and women who have gonorrhea should have another culture about two weeks after treatment to be sure that the infection has been cured.

**Preparation:**

*Women*—Do not douche for 24 hours before the test.

*Men*—Do not urinate for 1 hour before the test.

**Procedure:**

The sample for this test is collected in a doctor's office, clinic, or hospital by a physician or other health professional.

*Women*—You will be asked to remove all your clothes below the waist and to lie on your back on an examining table with your feet up in stirrups, as with a normal pelvic exam.

The examiner will insert an instrument (vaginal speculum) into the vagina. The speculum will be lubricated only with warm water, since other lubricants can interfere with the test.

The examiner will then insert a sterile, dry cotton swab into the opening (os) of the cervix. He or she will then rotate the swab, leave the swab in place for several seconds, and then withdraw it. The speculum will then be removed.

Sometimes the tube through which the urine leaves your body (urethra) is also cultured. If this is to be done, the examiner will cleanse the genital region, will gently massage or "milk" the urethra, and will then introduce a cotton swab or sterile wire loop into the urethra to collect a sample.

*Men*—A thin cotton-tipped swab will be inserted into the urethra to collect a sample of the discharge. You may be asked to "milk" a sample of the discharge from your penis onto a miscroscope slide or onto a cotton applicator

*Both men and women*—If your anus is to be cultured, the examiner will introduce a sterile cotton swab into your anus, leave it in place for a few seconds, then remove it. If an infection of the throat is suspected, the examiner will ask you to sit or stand with your head back and mouth open. A tongue blade may be used to hold your tongue down. He or she will then rub a sterile cotton-tipped swab over the sides of the back of your throat.

A screening blood test for syphilis (p. ■■■) is often performed when gonorrhea is suspected.

The collection of samples usually takes 5–10 minutes.

## How Does It Feel?

*Women*—This test is normally no more uncomfortable than a regular pelvic exam. If you have an inflammation of the vaginal area, the insertion of the speculum and the collection of the sample may be slightly painful.

The more you are able to relax, the easier and more comfortable the test will be. You can help by taking deep, slow breaths and relaxing your lower abdominal muscles as much as possible. In rare cases you may notice a small amount of vaginal bleeding after the test.

*Men*—You may experience a brief stinging sensation when the cotton-tipped swab is inserted into your urethra. Any discomfort should last only a few seconds.

## Risks:

There are no known risks of this test.

## Results:

A portion of the specimen is sometimes smeared on a microscope slide and stained with Gram's stain. Organisms that stain purple are called *gram-positive*. Those that stain pale pink are called *gram-negative*. The presence of gram-negative pairs of small, round bacteria *(diplococci)* suggest gonorrhea. The results of a Gram stain are usually available within an hour. A Gram stain is

sometimes done so that treatment can be started without waiting for the culture, which may take 2–5 days.

There are normally no gonorrhea bacteria (*Neisseria Gonorrhoeae*) in the cervix, urethra, anus, throat, or eyes. A positive culture means that you have a gonorrhea infection.

If you have symptoms characteristic of gonorrhea and/or have been exposed to a sexual partner with the disease, you will probably be treated with antibiotics immediately after the test is done. Your sexual partner should also be treated.

If you receive an antibiotic you will probably be advised to have a repeat culture 3–7 days after completing treatment to be sure that the infection has been cured. It is especially important that you have this repeat test.

If you do have gonorrhea, it is important that you refrain from sexual contact until the disease is treated and cured. You should also inform all recent sexual partners of the last several months that you have gonorrhea, and advise them to seek medical care.

If test results are negative, the symptoms may have been caused by another organism, probably chlamydia. This condition is called nonspecific urethritis (NSU) and is also treated with antibiotics.

A small percentage of people will turn out to have gonorrhea even though their test results are negative, so if symptoms persist after a negative test or treatment, see your doctor for possible repeat testing.

## Cost:

This test usually costs about $20 to $30, but is available free at many public health clinics. Call your local health department for information.

**Special Considerations:**

★*Telling Your Partner(s)*—In most states doctors are required by law to report the names and addresses of any patient diagnosed with gonorrhea. In some states doctors are also required to ask you for the names and addresses of recent sexual partners. You are not required to provide this information. You may simply say that you will tell your partner or partners yourself. If you do supply the names of your partners, they will be contacted confidentially by the public health department and advised to have a test for gonorrhea.

Telling a sexual partner you have gonorrhea can be one of life's less pleasant tasks. Nonetheless, it is something you should do as soon as possible, to prevent serious complications for your partner and to stop the possible spread of the disease.

★*Penicillin-Resistant Gonorrhea*—Some strains of gonorrhea are not sensitive to penicillin, but are sensitive to other drugs. This is one reason it's important to be retested 3–7 days after treatment. If the infection is still present, you will be treated with a different antibiotic—one that kills penicillin-resistant strains.

# Herpes Tests

There are two types of herpes simplex virus (HSV). HSV type 1 usually causes oral cold sores and fever blisters. HSV type 2 usually causes sores on and around the penis and vagina. It is usually, but not always, spread by sexual contact. (A different virus causes a disease called shingles or herpes zoster.)

Genital herpes is characterized by an initial attack of genital sores followed by a lifelong latent period, sometimes punctuated by recurrent active outbreaks. In this test, scrapings from a suspect sore are examined under a microscope and/or cultured to determine whether it is caused by herpes.

**Why Performed:**

The symptoms of herpes infection include one or more clusters of small, tender blisters on or around the genitals. The sores are usually preceded by a characteristic itching, burning, or tingling.

A person's first episode of herpes ordinarily occurs between 2 and 20 days after exposure to a sexual partner with an active herpes sore. This initial episode is usually the most severe. It may be accompanied by fever, swollen lymph nodes in the groin or other sores or rashes and may last for 2–3 weeks. Subsequent attacks are almost always less severe: they usually last 4–10 days and may occur frequently, infrequently, or not at all.

A diagnosis is usually made on the basis of history and symptoms. If there has been known exposure to a sexual partner with herpes and the signs and symptoms are characteristic of herpes, testing is probably not needed. However, if it is not clear from your history and symptoms whether you have herpes, these tests may provide the answer.

A vaginal herpes infection can be transferred from mother to baby as the newborn child passes through the birth canal. To prevent this, any pregnant woman who has ever had herpes should have regular herpes cultures during the last part of her pregnancy. If active herpes is present at the time of birth, a cesarean delivery may be done to protect the baby.

Because of a suspected link between herpes and cervical cancer, women with recurrent herpes should have a Pap test every 6–12 months.

**Preparation:**
No special preparation is needed.

**Procedure:**
There are two tests for herpes:

*Tzanck Test*—The sore (lesion) is scraped with a scalpel and the scrapings are spread on a slide and stained. Your doctor then examines the slide under a microscope, looking for giant cells and inclusion bodies which are characteristic of a herpes infection.

*Herpes Virus Culture*—Scrapings and/or fluid from the sores are collected on a cotton swab and sent to a laboratory equipped to perform viral cultures.

**How Does It Feel?**
You may find it painful when the sores are scraped or rubbed in order to collect the specimen.

**Risks:**
There are no known risks of this test.

**Results:**
*Tzanck Test*—The results of this test are available immediately, since the doctor does it right in the office. If no giant cells or inclusion bodies are found, the test is negative. There is a high rate of false-negative results (the test is negative despite the fact that you really do have herpes).

*Herpes Virus Culture*—Results of this test usually take 7–10 days. The culture is considerably more accurate than the Tzanck smear, but may also produce false-negative results if not done when the lesions are fresh and active. If no herpes is found in the culture, the test is negative. If the virus does appear in the culture, the test is positive.

■

If you suspect that you may have herpes or another sexually transmitted disease, you should avoid sexual contact until it is diagnosed.

Besides being one of the most common sexually transmitted diseases, genital herpes is one of the most feared, because there is as yet no known cure. But except for the possibility that a new mother may pass the infection on to her baby, genital herpes is an infection with no serious complications. And the physical manifestations are at worst a minor annoyance.

Sixty percent of us have some immunity to herpes viruses and are therefore extremely unlikely to get the disease. While there is no cure for herpes, people with active outbreaks may find some relief with some recent medications. Fortunately, it appears that the disease is only contagious when active genital sores are present.

**Cost:**
Cultures: $50 to $90
Microscopic exam of skin scrapings: $10 to $25

# Syphilis Tests
## (VDRL, RPR, FTA-ABS)

Syphilis is an infection caused by the bacterium *Treponema pallidum*. It is almost always transmitted through sexual contact, although pregnant women can also transfer the infection to their babies.

Syphilis has several stages. *Primary sy-*

*philis* is characterized by a sore on the penis, vagina, anus, mouth, or any other area that may have come in contact with an infected lesion. This sore, known as a *chancre* (pronounced "shanker"), is usually painless, with a hardened, red rim. The sore usually occurs within 3 weeks of initial contact, although it may not appear for several months. Even without treatment the sore heals spontaneously in 2–6 weeks. Often the sore is not noticed, particularly in women, where the lesion may be inside the vagina.

*Secondary syphilis* occurs 1 week to 6 months after the chancre heals. A rash appears on the skin, often on the palms of the hands and soles of the feet. Again, if untreated the rash heals and no further symptoms may appear until 10–20 years later, when *tertiary syphilis* begins. This stage of the disease can cause severe heart disease, brain damage, spinal cord damage, blindness, and even death.

More than a dozen lab tests are available to diagnose syphilis. The most common screening test is the *VDRL* (Venereal Disease Research Laboratory) or the *RPR* (rapid plasma reagin). These two blood tests detect an antibodylike substance in the blood which forms when a syphilis infection is present. Both tests are inexpensive and easy to perform. However, as many as 25% of people with early syphilis will *not* be detected on these screening tests. And many other conditions can produce a false-positive test.

The *FTA-ABS* (fluorescent treponemal antibody absorption) test is a more sensitive and more specific blood test for detecting syphilis. It is usually used to confirm the presence of syphilis when the VDRL or RPR is positive. But even the FTA-ABS may not always reveal syphilis until 3 or more weeks after the disease begins.

When sores are present, fluid from the sores can be examined with a miscroscope against a dark field. This *dark-field examination* may reveal the characteristic spiral-shaped organisms that cause syphilis.

## Why Performed:

Since syphilis can be present without symptoms, a VDRL or equivalent blood test is often performed as a screening test. This test is required in many states before marriage and during early pregnancy. In addition, if you have multiple sexual partners, you should have this test performed at least every 5–10 years, perhaps as often as every 1–2 years. Having multiple partners, of course, increases your risk of getting syphilis.

A VDRL test should also be performed on anyone with an undiagnosed genital sore, another sexually transmitted disease (such as gonorrhea), or a history of contact with a partner who may have syphilis. If these tests are negative (i.e., if they show no evidence of syphilis), the VDRL test should be repeated in several weeks to be sure an early infection was not missed.

## Preparation:

Tell your doctor if you are taking any medications, especially antibiotics.

It is sometimes recommended that you not drink any alcohol for 24 hours before the VDRL test, since alcohol can cause a false-negative result.

## Procedure:

For the blood tests, a small sample of blood will be drawn from a vein, usually in your arm. The dark-field exam is available in only a few clinics. In this test, a small scraping is taken from a genital sore and viewed under a special microscope.

**Risks:**

There are no risks with these tests.

**Results:**

The preliminary results of these tests may be available within a few hours or may take several days. If syphilis is suspected, you should refrain from sexual activity until the results are known.

In a person who does not have syphilis the results of the VDRL or RPR test will be "negative" or "nonreactive." If the VDRL or RPR result is "reactive," the strength of the reaction will be estimated in terms of titers. A titer of 1:64 is strongly reactive, whereas titers of 1:8 or 1:4 are weakly reactive. A reactive VDRL or RPR suggests that a syphilis infection is present. However, conditions other than syphilis can produce a positive reaction. These conditions include malaria, leprosy, infectious mononucleosis, infectious hepatitis, systemic lupus erythematosus (SLE), rheumatoid arthritis, pregnancy, and even old age. Therefore, if the VDRL or RPR is reactive, the more specific FTA-ABS test will be performed to confirm the diagnosis of syphilis.

The presence of corkscrew-shaped organisms on the dark-field exam also indicates syphilis.

Most states require physicians and laboratories to report all cases of syphilis to the local health department. If you test positive for syphilis, you will probably be contacted by a health department representative to be sure that you have been treated properly and that any recent sexual contacts are notified and tested.

Syphilis is treated with antibiotics, usually penicillin. However, follow-up tests after treatment are essential. In successfully treated syphilis the VDRL will gradually return to nonreactive or to a very low, stable reactive level (e.g., 1:4). A sudden rise in the VDRL might indicate reinfection. The FTA-ABS, however, tends to remain positive for many years or for life even after successful treatment.

**Special Considerations:**

★The VDRL and FTA tests are usually performed on a blood sample, but may be done on a sample of cerebrospinal fluid obtained by a lumbar tap (p. 367) to diagnose the spread of late syphilis to the nervous system.

**Cost:**

VDRL or RPR: $3 to $6
FTA-ABS: $15 to $30
Dark-field microscopic exam: $20 to $30

★*Chlamydia trachomatis* is now the most common sexually transmitted disease in the United States. It can infect the eye, the urethra, and the pelvic organs in women (pelvic inflammatory disease) which may result in scarring of the fallopian tubes, infertility, and other complications. While the infection may be announced by a pus-like discharge from the penis or vagina, burning on urination, or pain, many chlamydial infections occur without any symptoms. Therefore, screening tests for silent infections may be recommended for sexually active men and women, especially those with multiple sexual partners or a history of other sexually transmitted infections.

Testing for chlamydia used to be difficult, requiring tissue culture tests available at only a few laboratories. Several newer tests allow for easier, quicker (within hours), and cheaper ($10 to $20) screening. A fluid specimen from the urethra or cervix is painlessly collected on a swab.

Unfortunately, these newer tests are not 100% accurate. False negative results may occur in 10%–15% of tests and false positive results are found in 3%–5% of cases. Treatment usually consists of a course of antibiotics (tetracyline or erythromycin).

# 3 Testing for Heart Disease

**E**very day your heart pumps 2000 gallons of blood through 70,000 miles of blood vessels. In this way the cells in your body are supplied with oxygen and vital nutrients, carbon dioxide and other waste products are removed, and a variety of chemical messengers (hormones) are carried throughout the body. The heart usually performs this monumental task without much fuss or complaint. But, for many people, there comes a time when it can no longer meet the body's needs.

Nearly one in four Americans have some form of cardiovascular disease. Each year more than one and a half million Americans suffer heart attacks. Half a million of them die. Heart disease is responsible for nearly as many deaths as cancer, accidents, pneumonia, influenza, and all other causes combined.

The key to diagnosing heart disease is still a careful history (description of symptoms) and physical examination. But there are now scores of tests to detect and measure the severity of the many forms of heart disease.

Tests for heart disease are commonly divided into two categories: *noninvasive* and *invasive*. Except for drawing blood samples, noninvasive tests do not involve entering the body, do not alter the events being observed, and involve little or no risk. This category includes such tests as the measurement of cholesterol, electrocardiograms (ECG), nuclear scanning of the heart, and ultrasound examination of the heart.

Invasive tests, such as cardiac catheterization, involve entering the body, usually with a thin tube (catheter) threaded through a blood vessel and into the heart. These invasive tests involve considerably greater risk but may offer the only means of obtaining critical diagnostic information.

Most of the tests used to evaluate the cardiovascular system are described in this chapter. A few are described elsewhere: home blood pressure monitoring (p. 413), arterial blood gases (p. 50), carotid arteriography (p. 237), and venogram (p. 283).

# Cholesterol and Triglyceride
## (Blood Lipids)

Elevated blood cholesterol levels are a major risk factor for heart disease. Cholesterol is a fatty substance (lipid) found in nearly every body tissue. It is an essential building block of cell membranes, bile acids, and sex hormones. Part of the cholesterol is derived from the diet. Some is produced in the body.

High blood cholesterol levels are associated with the development of coronary artery disease, a condition in which the arteries that supply blood to the heart are narrowed or blocked. The arteries normally have a smooth inner lining, but cholesterol deposits (known as *plaques*) can form in the artery walls, partially or totally blocking the blood flow. Studies show that cholesterol plaques form more commonly in people with high blood cholesterol levels.

Since fatty substances do not dissolve in water, cholesterol can be transported through the bloodstream only when attached to proteins in complexes called *lipoproteins*. There are several different types of lipoproteins, each with a different size, density, and composition. The different forms in which cholesterol exists in the body appear to be very important.

LDL (low-density lipoprotein) cholesterol seems to be the "bad" type of cholesterol. This is the cholesterol that forms deposits in the artery walls. HDL (high-density lipoprotein) cholesterol is the "good" cholesterol. It may help to protect people from coronary heart disease by acting as a scavenger by removing excess cholesterol from the artery walls. This means that high levels of HDL cholesterol and low levels of LDL cholesterol are both desirable goals in the effort to prevent heart disease.

These new findings about the different forms of cholesterol have led to separate tests to measure not only total cholesterol levels but also the levels of the HDL (and sometimes the LDL) cholesterol portions.

Another fatty substance (lipid) in the body is *triglyceride*, which acts as a major form of stored energy. Triglyceride levels are often measured along with cholesterol to screen for risk of heart disease. This is probably not necessary, since elevated triglyceride levels, in the absence of increased cholesterol, do not appear to be a risk factor for coronary heart disease.

**When Performed:**
The test is often done if you have other risk factors for heart disease such as high blood pressure, smoking, diabetes, family history of early heart disease, symptoms that suggest possible heart disease, or signs that suggest high cholesterol such as yellow fatty deposits in the skin (xanthomatosis). It is also often done as a screening test for generally healthy people to determine whether their cholesterol level is within safe limits.

How often to have your cholesterol level checked is a matter of debate. If your level is low, checking once or twice every 10 years is probably sufficient. If your cholesterol level is high, more frequent monitoring may be indicated.

Your triglyceride level does not usually have to be measured unless you have elevated cholesterol levels, a history of coronary heart disease developing at an early age in your family, signs like fatty deposits in the skin (xanthomatosis), or inflammation of the pancreas (a condition sometimes associated with very high triglyceride levels).

The tests for both cholesterol and triglycerides are performed on blood samples drawn from a vein. Cholesterol levels can be measured without having to fast. If the triglyceride level is being measured, the blood sample should be collected after a 12- to 14-hour fast (except for water), as triglyceride levels are elevated by food and alcohol.

**Normal Values:**

Most laboratories list "normal" cholesterol levels as approximately 150–280 milligrams per 100 milliliters (mg/dl or mg%) with the upper limit of "normal" extending to 330 mg/dl in people older than 50 or 60. Triglyceride levels below 200 mg/dl are also considered normal.

These "normal" values can be misleading because they represent *average*, not necessarily *ideal* or *healthy* levels. The higher levels of cholesterol, even though still within the "normal" range, are associated with increased risk of heart disease. For example, a middle-aged man with a total cholesterol level of 250 mg/dl is nearly twice as likely to develop coronary artery disease as a man with a level of 200 mg/dl. Therefore, many experts now consider levels below 200 mg/dl as a healthier goal.

●*Greater Than Normal Values May Mean*: High total cholesterol levels, low HDL cholesterol levels, or high ratios of total cholesterol to HDL correlate with increased risk of developing coronary heart disease (see table).

The total cholesterol and HDL cholesterol levels can be considered separately, or a ratio of total cholesterol to HDL can be calculated. Sometimes the increased risk from a moderately elevated total cholesterol level can be counteracted by an increased HDL cholesterol level—and therefore a lower total cholesterol to HDL ratio.

The finding of an elevated total cholesterol level is particularly significant in younger people, since the narrowing of the coronary arteries develops gradually over many years.

In spite of the association between elevated cholesterol and heart disease, it is interesting to note that the majority of people who suffer heart attacks do *not* have greatly elevated cholesterol levels. Clearly,

## Cholesterol and Risk of Coronary Heart Disease

| Risk | Total Cholesterol | HDL Cholesterol | | Total Cholesterol to HDL Ratio | |
|------|-------------------|-----|-------|-----|-------|
| | | Men | Women | Men | Women |
| Very low risk (½ average risk) | 150 | 65 | 75 | 3.4 | 3.3 |
| Low risk | 200 | 55 | 65 | 4.0 | 3.8 |
| Average risk | 225 | 45 | 55 | 5.0 | 4.5 |
| Moderate risk (2 × average risk) | 260 | 25 | 40 | 9.5 | 7.0 |
| High risk (3+ × average risk) | >300 | <25 | <40 | >23 | >11 |

other factors must be involved in determining those who get heart disease and those who don't. Nevertheless, the risk of heart disease with elevated total cholesterol levels (or low HDL cholesterol levels) is magnified if you have other risk factors such as cigarette smoking or high blood pressure.

Elevated triglyceride levels, in the absence of increased cholesterol levels, do not appear to be a risk factor for heart disease. Therefore, in most instances the discovery of moderately high levels of triglycerides usually requires no action. However, if the triglyceride level is markedly elevated (greater than 1000 mg/dl), there is an increased risk of developing pancreatic disease.

Elevated blood lipids may be a clue to other disorders besides heart disease. For example, increased cholesterol or triglyceride levels are found with low thyroid hormone production (hypothyroidism), obstruction of the flow of bile, pancreatitis, kidney disease (nephrotic syndrome), poorly controlled diabetes, and pregnancy. In addition, recent consumption of alcohol or food may increase triglycerides.

●*Lower Than Normal Values May Mean*: Low levels of HDL cholesterol may be a strong factor in increasing one's risk of heart disease. Low total cholesterol levels, on the other hand, are associated with low rates of heart disease.

However, some recent research suggests that low total cholesterol levels (less than 180 mg/dl) may be associated with slightly *increased* risk of colon cancer and stroke. This association is still open to question and is the subject of ongoing investigation. If true, this might suggest that an optimal cholesterol level is between 180 and 200 mg/dl rather than "the lower the better." Unusually low cholesterol levels are found in severe liver disease (cirrhosis and hepatitis) and malnutrition due to malabsorption or inadequate diet.

### Interfering Factors:
Elevated or falsely elevated cholesterol levels can be caused by epilepsy medications (phenytoin), thiazide diuretics, vitamins A and D, cortisone, male hormones, tranquilizers, epinephrine, and oral contraceptives. Lowered or falsely lowered cholesterol levels may be due to certain antibiotics (tetracycline, neomycin), aspirin, high doses of niacin (vitamin $B_3$), certain female hormones, and certain drugs designed to lower cholesterol.

### Cost:
Cholesterol: $10 to $15
HDL cholesterol: $25 to $30
Triglycerides: $15 to $20

### Special Considerations:
★A number of lifestyle changes appear to have a favorable effect on blood cholesterol levels. Decreasing saturated (animal) fats and cholesterol in the diet and increasing fiber and complex carbohydrates can decrease cholesterol levels by 10% to 20%. Weight loss also decreases blood cholesterol. HDL cholesterol (the "good" cholesterol) can be increased somewhat by vigorous physical exercise, stopping smoking, and correcting obesity. Moderate consumption of alcohol (up to 3 drinks per day) can also increase HDL cholesterol, but the benefits of alcohol consumption must be balanced against the increased risk of alcoholism, cirrhosis, cancer, and traffic accidents.

# Heart Attack Enzymes
## (Cardiac Enzyme Studies: Creatine Phosphokinase, CPK; Serum Glutamic Oxaloacetic Transaminase, SGOT; Lactic Dehydrogenase, LDH)

Testing a blood sample for increased levels of three enzymes (CPK, SGOT, and LDH) can be useful in confirming a heart attack. Low levels of these enzymes are normally found in your bloodstream. However, if your heart muscle is injured (as in a heart attack), these enzymes leak out of damaged heart muscle cells, and blood levels become elevated.

These enzymes are also found in other parts of the body besides heart muscle. When these other tissues are damaged, increased blood enzyme levels can also result. Therefore, cardiac enzyme studies must always be interpreted in light of your symptoms, physical examination, and electrocardiogram (ECG). Blood samples for these cardiac enzyme tests are usually drawn every 12–24 hours for several days after a suspected heart attack to look for the characteristic rise and fall in the enzyme levels.

*Creatine Phosphokinase (CPK or CK)* is found mainly in heart muscle, the liver, skeletal muscle (such as in the arms and legs), and the brain. CPK can be separated into different subunits (known as CPK isoenzymes or "bands") to help determine whether the CPK comes from heart muscle or some other damaged tissue.

*Serum Glutamic Oxaloacetic Transaminase (SGOT)* has recently been renamed aspartate aminotransferase (AST). This enzyme is found in heart and liver and to a much lesser extent in other tissues (see p. 101). This test is the least accurate of the cardiac enzymes in indicating disease specifically due to heart muscle injury.

*Lactic Dehydrogenase (LDH)* is found in many body tissues including heart, liver, kidney, skeletal muscle, brain, and lungs. LDH, like CPK, may be divided into different subfractions or isoenzymes ($LDH_1$ through $LDH_5$) to determine which damaged tissues produced the elevations in blood LDH.

**When Performed:**
Cardiac enzyme studies are usually performed when a heart attack is suspected (due to abnormal electrocardiogram, chest pain, shortness of breath, nausea, sweating, etc.). Repeated or "serial" enzyme tests are performed to look for sequential increases in enzyme levels that can indicate a heart attack or extension of heart muscle damage. Because each of these enzymes is found in other organs besides the heart, these tests can also be useful in detecting or monitoring the progress of other diseases of the liver, muscle, or blood.

**Normal Values:**
The normal values and units for these tests vary considerably in different laboratories. Some examples are given here but check with your lab or doctor for specific values:

Total CPK:
> 55–170 international units per liter (IU/l) (males)
> 30–135 IU/l (females)

CPK isoenzymes:
> $CPK_1$ (BB) (brain) 0 IU/l (0% total CPK)
> $CPK_2$ (MB) (heart) 0–7 IU/l (less than 4%–6% of total CPK)

CPK$_3$ (MM) (skeletal muscle) 5–
70 IU/l (greater than 94%–96%
total CPK)
SGOT (AST):
5–40 IU/liter
Total LDH:
80–120 IU/liter
LDH isoenzymes:
LDH$_1$ 17%–27% of total LDH
LDH$_2$ 27%–37% of total LDH
LDH$_3$ 18%–25% of total LDH
LDH$_4$ 3%–8% of total LDH
LDH$_5$ 0%–5% of total LDH

● *Greater Than Normal Values May Mean*: Cardiac enzymes must always be interpreted in light of symptoms, history, physical examination, and findings on electrocardiogram. Also, these tests are often repeated over several days for comparison.

*CPK*: The blood levels of CPK typically increase within 2–6 hours after a heart attack, reach peak concentrations within 18–24 hours, and fall to normal levels within 3 days. Therefore, CPK is the earliest enzyme indicator of a heart attack. However, since an elevated total CPK may be due to other causes (vigorous exercise, intramuscular injections, crush injuries to muscles, muscular dystrophy, muscle inflammation, etc.), the more specific CPK isoenzymes should be examined. The CPK$_1$ (BB) isoenzyme or band comes mainly from brain tissue. CPK$_2$ (MB) is derived from damaged heart muscle, and CPK$_3$ (MM) comes mostly from skeletal muscle. Therefore, if the total CPK is elevated in a person who has collapsed while jogging or in a person who has received an intramuscular injection, the CPK might be from skeletal, not heart muscle. However, if CPK$_2$ (MB) from heart muscle is greater than 5% of the total CPK or greater than 10 IU/liter, heart muscle damage is indicated. This cardiac damage may be due to a heart attack, inflammation

of the heart muscle (myocarditis), or recent heart surgery. If CPK levels continue to rise after 2–3 days, this may suggest that the heart attack is progressing and more heart muscle is being damaged.

*SGOT (AST)*: After a heart attack SGOT levels begin to rise within 6–10 hours, peak at 12–48 hours, and return to normal within 5 days. The degree of elevation of SGOT roughly indicates the amount and extent of heart muscle damage. However, elevations of SGOT can also occur with liver disease (hepatitis and cirrhosis), muscular dystrophy, blood clots in the lungs (pulmonary emboli), pancreatitis, certain types of anemia, and certain infections (like infectious mononucleosis). Since elevated SGOT levels occur with so many other diseases, this test is not considered a specific test for heart attacks, even though SGOT levels are increased in 95% of heart attacks.

*LDH*: Following a heart attack, blood levels of LDH begin to rise within 24–72 hours, peak at 2–5 days, and remain elevated for as long as 14 days. Therefore, LDH may be useful in diagnosing a heart attack that occurred several days earlier. Increased LDH, however, can also be due to liver disease, certain anemias and leukemias, cancer, and pulmonary emboli. The LDH isoenzymes can help identify the source of the LDH. LDH$_2$ is normally greater than LDH$_1$. However, if the ratio is reversed ("flipped LDH ratio"), so that LDH$_1$ is greater than LDH$_2$, this is evidence that a heart attack has occurred.

**Cost:**
CPK: $15 to $20 (CPK isoenzymes, $30
to $50)
SGOT (AST): $15 to $20
LDH: $15 to $20 (LDH isoenzymes, $30
to $50)

# Electrocardiogram
## (ECG, EKG)

An electrocardiogram is a graphic recording of the electrical activity generated by your heart. The electrocardiogram is often referred to as an ECG or EKG (an abbreviation derived from the German word *electrokardiogramma*). The electrical signals produced by your heart are detected by small metal discs (electrodes) which are attached to your skin on various parts of your body. The detected electrical activity is recorded as a characteristic series of wavy lines on graph paper.

### Why Performed:

While an ECG measures only about 50 beats (your heart beats about 100,000 times each day), this small sample can give important information about the rhythm of the heart and the size and position of the heart chambers. It can also sometimes detect inflammation or damage to the heart muscle as well as abnormalities in the minerals that control the electrical activity of the heart.

There is considerable controversy over whether an electrocardiogram is useful in people who do not have symptoms of heart disease. You probably do not need a "routine" ECG unless you have symptoms suggesting heart disease (unexplained chest pain, shortness of breath, dizziness, faintness, or palpitations), or you have several risk factors for heart disease (high blood pressure, elevated blood cholesterol levels, cigarette smoking, diabetes, or a family history of heart attack below the age of 60).

Electrocardiograms are most often performed to evaluate unexplained chest pain when a heart attack is suspected. But not every chest pain requires an ECG. Electrocardiograms are also used to monitor the effectiveness and side effects of certain drugs which may affect the heart and to check the function of artificial pacemakers (devices inserted into the heart to maintain a normal heart rhythm).

### Preparation:

Tell your doctor if you are taking any medications. Certain medications can influence the interpretation of the ECG.

There is no need to restrict food or fluids before the test. All jewelry should be removed from your neck and wrists. You will also need to remove your clothing above the waist and expose your forearms and lower legs (stockings will have to be taken off). You may be asked to put on a dressing gown for the test.

### Procedure:

An electrocardiogram is usually performed by a technician and then interpreted ("read") by a physician. It can be performed in a clinic, doctor's office, laboratory, or at your bedside with a portable machine.

You will be asked to lie on a bed or table. Certain areas on your arms, legs, and chest will be cleaned to remove skin oils and sweat. If the chest area is particularly hairy, it may be necessary to shave small areas to attach the electrode discs. A special ECG paste or small pads soaked in alcohol are placed on the skin to improve electrical conduction.

Next a metal disc (known as an electrode or "lead") is attached to the skin on each arm and leg with thick rubber straps or adhesive. A fifth electrode is attached to the chest by a small rubber suction cup. This "chest lead" is repositioned at six different locations on your chest during the test to measure the electrical activity from different directions. In a standard "12-lead" ECG, 12 different "views" of the electrical activity of the heart can be created by recording from different pairs of electrodes. The electrical activity is converted by the ECG machine into wavy lines on moving graph paper ("a tracing").

It is important not to move or talk during the recording because muscular activity can cause inaccurate results ("artifacts") on the tracing. Relax, lie still, and breathe normally unless specifically asked to hold your breath.

The procedure takes 5–10 minutes. Sometimes a longer period of recording ("a rhythm strip") is done to look at your heart's rhythm over a minute or longer. After the procedure the electrode paste is wiped off.

### How Does It Feel?

An ECG is a painless procedure. The electrodes and conducting paste may feel cold when first applied.

### Risks:

There is no risk associated with an ECG. The electrodes only detect electrical impulses produced by your heart. No electricity passes through your body and, therefore, there is no possibility of receiving an electric shock.

### Results:

The wavy lines of the ECG tracing show a characteristic pattern of electrical impulses as your heart beats. The different parts of the heartbeat are called the P wave, the QRS complex, the ST segment, and the T wave. Deviations from normal patterns may indicate various types of heart disease. However, "abnormal" ECG patterns may also be due to errors in recording or errors in interpretation (mistaking normal variations for abnormalities). Conversely, a

"normal" ECG can occur even in the presence of heart disease. Therefore, the ECG should always be interpreted in light of symptoms, history, physical examination, and, if necessary, other test results.

*Disorders of Rhythm*: Various irregular rhythms, known as *arrhythmias*, may be detected on an ECG. Excessively rapid heart rates are called *tachycardia*, while slow rates are called *bradycardia*. Other disorders of rhythm such as *fibrillation* or *flutter* may be noted along with disorders of nerve conduction such as heart block or conduction delays.

*Coronary Artery Disease and Heart Attacks*: If the coronary arteries supplying blood to the heart muscle are blocked, the muscle tissue may suffer from a lack of oxygen (*ischemia*) or may even die (*infarction*). This damage to the heart muscle may show up on the electrocardiogram. However, the ECG in a person having a heart attack may initially appear normal or unchanged. Therefore, the ECG may be repeated over several days (serial ECGs) to look for characteristic signs of heart muscle damage. Other tests, including blood tests for cardiac enzymes (p. 151), may also be needed to diagnose a heart attack. Sometimes borderline abnormalities such as "nonspecific ST-T wave changes" are noted. These findings are of questionable significance.

*Heart Enlargement*: The ECG may reveal enlargement (hypertrophy) of the various chambers of the heart due to heart failure, excessive strain, disease of the heart valves, or congenital heart diseases.

*Inflammation of the Heart*: Certain changes on the ECG may indicate an inflammation of the heart muscle (*myocarditis*) or the sac that surrounds the heart (*pericarditis*).

*Mineral Changes*: Proper contraction of the heart depends upon normal levels of minerals such as calcium and potassium in the blood. Excessive or deficient amounts of these electrolytes result in characteristic abnormalities in the ECG.

**Cost:**
$20 to $50, including interpretation by a physician.

**Special Considerations:**
★An electrocardiogram taken at rest may fail to reveal certain abnormalities of the heart. Therefore, additional tests including *exercise* or *stress electrocardiograms* have been developed to show the response of the heart to an increased demand to pump blood (discussed next).

★*Ambulatory (Holter) monitoring* records the activity of your heart over 24–48 hours rather than just the few seconds that are recorded on an ECG (see p. 158).

★A *vectorcardiogram* is a more complex form of ECG which creates a three-dimensional view of the electrical activity of the heart. It is sometimes used to clarify borderline or abnormal electrocardiograms.

# Exercise Electrocardiogram
## (Stress Test, Cardiac Stress Test, Treadmill Test, Exercise Test, Exercise Tolerance Test)

An exercise or stress electrocardiogram (ECG) evaluates the heart's response to the stress of physical exercise. The electrical activity of the heart, blood pressure, and heart rate are monitored while you walk on a motor-driven treadmill or pedal a stationary bicycle. During exercise the heart's need for oxygen increases. If the coronary arteries which carry oxygenated blood to the heart muscle are blocked or narrowed, the heart may not get enough oxygen during exercise. The oxygen-deprived heart may produce abnormalities in the ECG. Since these abnormalities often don't appear on a ECG taken at rest, the exercise test is more sensitive in detecting coronary heart disease.

**Why Performed:**
An exercise stress test is most often performed to determine the cause of unexplained chest pain when coronary heart disease is suspected. In patients with known heart disease an exercise test may be useful in determining the severity of the disease and the present exercise capacity in order to help plan treatment and rehabilitation. Stress tests are often performed following a heart attack or heart surgery to determine the capacity of the heart for exercise or work. On the basis of this information advice can be given on an appropriate initial exercise program as well as daily activities.

An exercise test may also be used to look for abnormal heart rhythms when symptoms such as dizziness, fainting, or palpitations occur during exercise or activity.

The use of a stress ECG to test people without symptoms of heart disease is quite controversial. Some experts recommend that anyone over the age of 35 who has been generally inactive should have a stress test to look for "silent" heart disease before starting an exercise program. Others, including ourselves, disagree. Because heart disease is relatively rare in younger people without symptoms, the stress tests can frequently be inaccurate and is often misleading. Many of these people will have falsely abnormal (false-positive) tests and may be subjected to needless anxiety and further testing.

If, however, you are over the age of 40, have been sedentary for many years, and have other risk factors for heart disease (high blood pressure, cigarette smoking, elevated cholesterol levels, and a family history of heart attacks at young ages), then a stress ECG might be helpful before undertaking a strenuous exercise program.

**Preparation:**

Tell your doctor if you are taking any medications.

Before the test you may be asked to sign a consent form. Use this as an opportunity to discuss with your doctor any concerns you have about the need for the test, how it is performed, or the risks.

You should not eat, smoke, drink alcohol or caffeinated beverages for 2–3 hours before the test. Continue taking all regularly prescribed medications unless your doctor directs otherwise. Your doctor may ask you to taper off certain heart medications a few days before the test. Wear comfortable shoes and loose, lightweight shorts or slacks. Men are usually barechested during the test, while women often wear a bra, short-sleeved blouse or dressing gown.

**Procedure:**

An exercise test is usually performed in an office, clinic, or special hospital lab by a technician or physician. If the test is done by a technician, a physician should be available in the testing area.

To prepare your skin for the placement of the ECG electrodes, several areas on your chest will be shaved (if necessary), cleaned with alcohol, and gently rubbed or scratched to remove dead skin and excess oils. Several small metal discs (electrodes) will be attached to your chest with adhesive. A gel or paste will be placed between the electrode and your skin to improve conduction of the electrical impulses. The electrodes are then connected with long wires to an ECG machine, which will record the electrical activity of your heart as a series of wavy lines on moving graph paper. Your chest may be loosely wrapped with an elastic band to keep the electrodes from falling off during exercise. A blood pressure cuff will be wrapped snugly around your upper arm so that your blood pressure can be checked every few minutes during the test.

You will be shown how to step on and off the slowly moving treadmill. Place both hands on the railing in front of you to help maintain your balance, but don't try to support your weight on this bar. It is important not to grip the bar tightly, since this can interfere with the recording and interpretation of the test.

At first the treadmill will move slowly in a level or slightly inclined position. As the test progresses, the speed and/or steepness of the treadmill will be increased so that you will be walking faster and faster "uphill."

If a stationary bicycle is used, you will sit on the bicycle, and the seat and handlebars will be adjusted so that you can pedal comfortably. Use the handlebars to maintain balance, not to support your weight. You will be asked to pedal fast enough to maintain a certain speed. The resistance will then be gradually increased, making it harder to pedal.

In both the treadmill and the bicycle tests your ECG, heart rate, and blood pressure will be recorded during the exercise. The work load is gradually increased until you reach your maximum or "target" heart rate or until you experience fatigue, extreme shortness of breath, or chest pain. The test may be stopped if you develop abnormalities on the ECG or blood pressure measurements.

When the exercise phase is completed you will be asked to lie down and rest. Your ECG and blood pressure will be checked for about 5 to 10 minutes during this recovery period. The electrodes are then removed from your chest, and you may resume your normal activities. You should not take a hot bath for at least one hour, since hot water after vigorous exercise can make you feel dizzy and faint. The entire test usually takes 15–30 minutes.

## How Does It Feel?

The room may feel cool at first, but you will warm up rapidly when you begin to exercise. The preparation of the electrode sites on your chest may produce a burning or stinging sensation. The blood pressure cuff on your arm will be inflated every few minutes, producing a squeezing sensation. You may also feel slightly off-balance when your blood pressure is being taken, since you may have to take your hand off the support railing.

During the exercise you may experience leg cramps or soreness, fatigue, breathlessness, lightheadedness, dry mouth, perspiration, and perhaps some chest discomfort. Mention these sensations as you notice them to the technician or doctor.

*Patient Comments*: "I felt nervous before the test. I wasn't sure how far I could go. But once I started exercising I felt much more relaxed."

"I tried to remember this was a test of my heart, not a competitive athletic contest."

## Risks:

There is no possibility of electric shock during the test, since the electrodes only detect the electrical impulses produced by your heart. Exercise testing is generally safe. In a large study involving 73 medical centers and 170,000 exercise tests, death occurred in less than 1 in 10,000 patients. Sometimes transient episodes of irregular heart rhythms may develop, but they can usually be quickly corrected. Though the risks are minimal, emergency equipment and a physician trained in resuscitation should be available in the testing area.

## Results:

Your doctor may be able to discuss with you the preliminary results immediately after the test, though a complete interpretation may take several days. Chest pain during exercise, abnormalities in the heart rhythm or ECG tracing (particularly in the so-called ST segment), or a fall in blood pressure (blood pressure normally rises during exercise) may indicate heart disease.

Unfortunately, this test is frequently inaccurate, inconclusive or subject to varying interpretations. Many people (20%–30%) who have normal stress tests still have significant heart disease (false-negatives). On the other hand, 20%–50% of people who have "positive" or abnormal exercise tests, have essentially normal coronary arteries (false-positives). Further tests such as thallium scanning (p. 167) or coronary arteriography (p. 162) are often necessary to confirm the presence and extent of heart disease.

## Cost:

$100 to $250

# Ambulatory Electrocardiogram
## (Holter Monitoring)

Ambulatory electrocardiography, commonly known as Holter monitoring after its originator, provides a continuous record of the electrical activity of the heart over a 24- or 48-hour period. Certain abnormalities of heart rhythm may occur intermittently, sometimes only once or twice a day. A standard ECG (p. 153) monitors only 40–50 heartbeats and can easily miss these episodic irregularities. Ambulatory monitoring can record more than 100,000 heartbeats over 24 hours and is, therefore, more likely to detect transient abnormalities.

Another advantage of ambulatory (which means walking and moving about) ECG monitoring is that the heart can be observed during normal daily activities. Many heart irregularities show up only with such activities as exercise, eating, sexual activity, emotional stress, going to the bathroom, or even sleeping. A continuous 24-hour recording is much more likely to detect abnormalities associated with such activities.

## Why Performed:

An ambulatory ECG is often used to look for transient irregularities of your heartbeat (*arrhythmias*). Symptoms such as dizziness, fainting, unexplained chest pain or shortness of breath, or the sensation of pounding or skipped heartbeats (*palpitations*) may be due to episodes of irregular heartbeat. Ambulatory monitoring is also used to look for abnormalities in people with known heart disease—for instance, following a heart attack, before and after discharge from the hospital. Monitoring may also be helpful in checking the effectiveness of therapy (drugs or pacemakers) to regulate the heart rhythm.

## Preparation:

Tell your doctor if you are taking any medications, or you are allergic to adhesive tape.

Shower or bathe just before your test, since you will not be able to do so during the ECG recording period. Wear a loose-fitting blouse or shirt. Avoid wearing jewelry or metallic clothing, which will interfere with the recording. Women should wear no bra or a bra without underwiring. You should wear a watch and a strong leather or plastic belt to hold the recorder.

## Procedure:

For this test you will wear a portable, lightweight (less than 2 pounds), battery-operated instrument which looks like a small tape recorder. This monitor is connected to several electrodes taped to your chest which detect the electrical impulses from your heart. The impulses are recorded on magnetic tape and later analyzed.

You will be fitted with the monitor and electrodes by a technician in a doctor's office, ECG laboratory, or hospital room. Several areas on your chest will be shaved, if necessary, and then cleaned with alcohol and rubbed gently to remove dead skin and excess oils. A small amount of electrode paste or gel will be applied to these areas to improve conduction. Several electrodes (small metal discs surrounded by adhesive) will then be attached to your chest.

Thin wires connect the electrodes to the portable recording instrument, which is worn on a belt at your waist or on a shoulder strap. You may be briefly hooked up to a standard ECG machine to make sure that the electrodes are working properly.

You should then go about your normal daily activities while wearing the monitor. You will be given a log to record the exact times when you exercise, climb stairs, eat, urinate, have a bowel movement, engage in sexual activity, smoke cigarettes, sleep, get emotionally upset, take medications, or perform other activities. You should also carefully record in the log the exact time and duration of any symptoms such as dizziness, fainting or near-fainting, chest pain, or palpitations. For example, you might note: "12:30 P.M. ate lunch. 1:00 P.M. argument with boss/chest tightness for several minutes." Some recording instruments have an "events" button you should press when you experience any symptoms. This will mark the exact time of these symptoms on the tape. The accuracy and usefulness of this test depend upon your careful and detailed recording of the times, activities, and symptoms.

You will not be able to bathe (except for a careful sponge bath) or do anything else that might get the recorder or electrodes wet during the recording period. A flashing monitor light on the recorder means that one of the electrodes or lead wires may be loose. Press on the center of each electrode disc to see if you can restore the contact.

Try to sleep on your back, with the recorder carefully positioned at your side so that the electrodes are not pulled off. If one of the electrodes does come off, notify your doctor or technician. Signals from electronic equipment in your environment can sometimes interfere with the recording, so during the recorded period try to avoid magnets, metal detectors, high-voltage areas, garage door openers, remote control TV, CB radios, microwave ovens, and electric blankets.

At the end of the specified recording period (usually 24 hours) you will return to the technician to have the recorder and electrodes removed, or you will be instructed on how to remove the electrodes yourself.

### How Does It Feel?

You may feel a burning or stinging sensation when your chest is rubbed to prepare the electrode sites. The electrode sites may itch slightly during the recording, and the skin on your chest may be slightly irritated when the electrodes are removed. The recording unit only weighs a pound or two, so carrying it should not be particularly uncomfortable.

### Risks:

There is no risk associated with this test. The electrodes only detect the electrical impulses produced by your heart. No electricity is put into your body, and there is no possibility of receiving an electric shock.

### What Do the Results Mean?

The magnetic tape will be analyzed using a high-speed electronic scanner and then reviewed by a specially trained physician. The results should be available within several days. The majority of people will show an occasional irregularity in their heart rhythm. The importance of these irregularities (arrhythmias) depends upon the type, frequency, duration, and association with the symptoms. Irregular rhythms occurring at the same time you are having symptoms such as dizziness or chest pain suggest that the heart abnormalities may be causing the symptoms.

Electrical abnormalities such as "ST-T wave changes" suggest that the heart muscle is not getting enough oxygen due to narrowing of the arteries feeding the heart.

The finding of abnormal beats such as "PVCs" (premature ventricular contractions) after a heart attack suggests that the heart rhythms should be monitored more closely after discharge from the hospital.

Ambulatory ECG monitoring also provides valuable information on how effectively drugs or pacemakers are controlling the heart rhythm.

The results of an ambulatory ECG must always be interpreted in light of history, symptoms, and other tests.

**Cost:**
$150 to $250

**Special Considerations:**

★Another type of monitor is used to evaluate patients with symptoms that occur very infrequently. A person wears the monitor for 5 to 7 days but turns it on only if symptoms develop.

★A new monitoring system allows immediate transfer of the ECG signals to your doctor over the telephone. With this method of monitoring, your doctor can recommend immediate action if an abnormality is present.

# Echocardiogram
## (Cardiac Echo)

In this test sound waves are used to evaluate the size, shape, and motion of the heart. Ultrahigh-frequency sound waves well beyond the range of human hearing are directed into your chest. Some of the sound waves are reflected off the various structures of the heart. These echoes are converted into images of your heart which can be viewed on a TV screen. Echocardiography, one type of diagnostic ultrasound (see p. 303), is a safe, painless, quick, and

relatively low-cost way to evaluate the internal structures and function of the heart.

There are two types of echocardiogram. A time-motion or M-mode echocardiogram is a chart display showing the motion of the heart structures toward and away from the transmitter on the chest. The real time, two-dimensional, or B-mode echocardiogram presents an actual cross-sectional picture of the heart in motion. Most often both types of echocardiogram are performed.

**Why Performed:**
An echocardiogram is most often performed to evaluate abnormal heart sounds (murmurs or clicks), an enlarged heart, unexplained chest pains, shortness of breath, palpitations, or strokes (which may be due to blood clots from the heart). Echocardiograms are also sometimes useful in following the progress of patients with artificial heart valves.

**Preparation:**
No restriction of food or fluids is necessary before the test. You will be asked to remove all clothing and jewelry from the waist up and put on a hospital gown.

**Procedure:**
An echocardiogram is usually performed in a special laboratory in a hospital, office, or clinic, but it can sometimes be done at your hospital bed. The test is performed by a specially trained ultrasound technician or physician. You will be asked to lie on your back on a bed or table. Small metal discs (electrodes) will be taped to your arms and legs to record your ECG during the test. Next a small amount of oil or gel is rubbed on the left side of your chest to help improve the transmission of sound waves. A small instrument (transducer) which looks like a microphone is pressed firmly against

your chest and moved slowly back and forth. This instrument transmits sound waves into the chest and picks up the echoes as they are reflected back. These echoes are transmitted to a TV screen to form an image of your heart and recorded for later viewing and evaluation. The room is usually darkened to brighten the details on the screen. At times you will be asked to hold very still, breathe in and out very slowly, hold your breath, or lie on your left side. After the test is completed, usually in 15–45 minutes, the gel is wiped off your chest.

### How Does It Feel?

An echocardiogram is a painless procedure. The gel may feel a bit cold and slippery when rubbed on your chest. The transducer head is pressed firmly against your chest but is usually not uncomfortable. You won't be able to hear the sounds waves since they are above the range of human hearing.

*Patient Comments*: "I had a quite enjoyable time. It didn't hurt at all. A few times I was able to look at the TV screen. It was fascinating to see an image of my own heart! The technology is remarkable!"

### Risks:

There are no known risks associated with echocardiography. No x-rays or electrical current is put into your body during this test.

### Results:

If the test is performed by a technician, you will have to wait several days to hear about results, until the images have been reviewed by a doctor. If the test is performed by a doctor, the preliminary results may be available immediately.

The size of the heart chambers and thickness of the muscular walls will be measured. The four heart valves (aortic, mitral, tricuspid, and pulmonary) will be checked for excessive narrowness (stenosis), failure to close properly (insufficiency), or abnormal collections of bacteria on the heart valves (endocarditis). The chambers of the heart should be free of any tumors, and there should not be an excessive amount of fluid in the sac surrounding the heart (pericardial effusion). Abnormal movement of the heart muscle walls may indicate areas of muscle not receiving adequate blood supply due to narrowing of the coronary arteries.

### Cost:

$200 to $300

### Special Considerations:

★There are two other tests which can be used to record the sounds and vibrations produced by the heart. A *phonocardiogram* provides a visual record of the sounds made as the blood flows through the heart. This test can clarify and document the heart sounds and murmurs that your doctor may hear by listening with a stethoscope over your heart. An *apexcardiogram* is a graphic recording of the movement of the chest wall caused by the heart's pumping action. The vibrations produced in the carotid artery and jugular veins in the neck can also be recorded to evaluate heart failure and disease of the heart valves.

# Cardiac Catheterization and Coronary Angiography
## (Cardiac Cath, Heart Catheterization, Coronary Arteriography)

This test is used to determine the severity and location of blocked arteries supplying the heart, the degree of impairment of heart function due to disease of the heart valves, and the ability of the heart to effectively pump blood throughout the body. The test is accomplished by inserting a thin, hollow, flexible tube (catheter) into a vein or artery in an arm or leg. The catheter is then gently threaded along this artery or vein until it reaches the heart. Once it reaches the proper position a number of measurements and tests can be performed: the blood pressure in the various chambers of the heart can be measured, samples of blood can be taken, and a contrast material (dye) can be injected. Because the blood in the heart and vessels is not ordinarily apparent on x-ray, the contrast material (dye) is injected into the blood, and as the dye flows through the chambers and blood vessels of the heart, it makes them visible.

The most common form of cardiac catheterization is known as coronary angiography or arteriography. In this test, the contrast material is injected directly into the coronary arteries (the blood vessels that feed the heart muscle). Narrowing or blockage of these vital blood vessels by fatty deposits can be seen on the pictures taken as the dye flows through the arteries.

**Why Performed:**

Since cardiac catheterization involves some risk, it is recommended only after such noninvasive tests as electrocardiogram (p. 151), exercise stress tests (p. 155), echocardiogram (p. 160), or nuclear medicine tests (pp. 167–173) suggest the presence of significant heart disease or fail to explain persistent symptoms.

Cardiac catheterization is usually performed when a person's ability to carry out daily activities is significantly limited by cardiac symptoms such as chest pain or shortness of breath. This test can clarify the extent and type of disease, whether it involves narrowed coronary arteries, poorly functioning heart muscle, damaged heart valves, or congenital heart defects. It is a necessary test to determine whether surgery is needed to try to correct these problems. Cardiac catheterization is also sometimes used to evaluate the results of heart surgery, particularly if symptoms persist or reoccur after replacement of heart valves or coronary artery bypass surgery.

**Preparation:**

Tell your doctor if

You have allergies to any medications, anesthetics, or iodine contrast dyes used in previous x-ray tests

You are taking any medications

You have had bleeding problems

You might be pregnant

You will be asked to sign a consent form before the test. Use this opportunity to discuss with your doctor any concerns you have about the need for the test, how it is performed, or the risks.

If you are not already a patient in the hospital, you will probably be admitted the day before the test, although some doctors can arrange to admit and discharge patients on the same day. You will have a physical examination, some blood tests, chest x-ray, electrocardiogram, and possibly other non-invasive heart tests. If you are taking any medications, ask your doctor whether you should continue to take them.

You will be asked not to eat or drink anything for about six hours before the test. About one hour before the procedure you may be given a sedative medication to help you relax. It will not put you to sleep, since it is important that you be awake to follow instructions during the test. Before the test, remove any necklaces or bracelets and remove nail polish from fingernails and toenails; this permits better observation of the blood circulation in your fingers and toes. Certain areas on your arms and groin will be shaved to prepare possible sites for the catheter insertion. Be sure to empty your bladder completely just before the test.

### Procedure:

You will be transported to the cardiac catheterization laboratory ("cath lab") and transferred onto a flat table under a large x-ray machine. All around the room you will see various types of sophisticated monitoring equipment. The test is performed by a specially trained physician and one or two assistants. The doctor will wear sterile gloves, gown, and sometimes a mask.

Several small electrodes will be applied to your legs and arms. These will be connected to an ECG machine to continuously record the electrical activity of your heart during the test. A small needle or tube may be inserted into a vein in one of your arms to give you fluids or medications.

The site for your catheter insertion may be a vein or artery at the crease of your elbow or a blood vessel in your groin. The selected area is cleansed with an antiseptic solution. You will then be draped with sterile towels except for an opening over the insertion site. The preparation up to this point may take 30 minutes or more.

Next a small amount of a local anesthetic is injected to numb the skin over the insertion site. The blood vessel is then punctured by a special needle or exposed by making a small incision in the skin (cutdown). The catheter is then slipped through a tiny slit in the blood vessel. The catheter is slowly advanced through the blood vessel while the doctor watches its progress on the x-ray screen. The lights are usually dimmed in the room to make it easier to see the x-ray screen. You may be asked to hold your breath or move slightly to help the passage of the catheter. The catheter tip is moved into various positions in the heart's blood vessels and chambers. Pressures are recorded and blood samples may be withdrawn through the catheter.

A small amount of contrast material may be injected through the catheter into your heart chamber or one of the coronary arteries. Movie pictures are taken of the dye as it moves through your heart. The table may be tilted in different directions or a movable x-ray machine repositioned to obtain different views of your heart. You may be asked to cough (this helps clear the contrast material out of your heart) or breathe deeply and hold it (this can help clarify the image). You should try to lie as still as possible, since motion can distort the x-ray pictures. If you ask the doctor, you may be able to watch the TV monitor so you can see the images of your own heart and coronary arteries.

Depending upon the type of test being performed, at certain times you may be asked to dissolve a nitroglycerin tablet under your tongue to dilate the blood vessels or may be given an injection of a medication (ergonovine maleate) which causes the coronary arteries to constrict. To help measure the flow of oxygen in the circu-

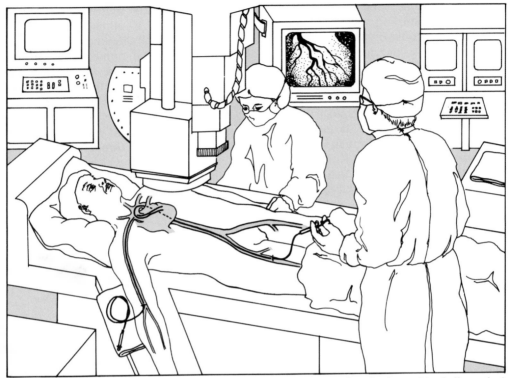

**Catheterization and Coronary Angiography.** *During cardiac catheterization a thin, hollow tube is inserted into a blood vessel in the arm or groin, and a dye is injected while x-ray pictures of the heart are taken.*

lation, you may also be asked to breathe into a special mouthpiece.

After all the necessary pictures and measurements have been taken, the catheter will be removed. If the catheter insertion site is in the arm, a few stitches will be put in to close the skin. If the insertion site is in the groin, firm pressure will be put over the area for about 10 minutes to stop the bleeding. Then a special pressure dressing may be placed over the area, sometimes including a small sandbag which will stay in place for several hours.

The entire procedure usually takes 1–2 hours but may take longer if additional tests are required. The length of the test is not an indication of the seriousness of your condition.

After the test you will be taken to your room, where a nurse will periodically monitor your vital signs (heart rate, blood pressure, and temperature) and check for signs of bleeding at the insertion site. The pulses, color, and temperature of the arm or leg in which the catheter was inserted will also be periodically checked.

The contrast material that was injected may make you pass more urine than usual, so you should replace these fluids by drinking plenty of liquids for several hours. You will be asked to lie in bed with your arm or leg extended for 4–6 hours. After that you can move about freely but should avoid any strenuous activity for at least 1−2 days or as otherwise advised. Depending upon the results of the test and whether any complications develop, you may be sent home either after being observed for 6 hours or on the next day. If any stitches were placed in your arm, they will be removed in 5−7 days.

## How Does It Feel?

When the local anesthetic is injected to numb your skin over the catheter insertion site you will feel a sharp sting. When the catheter is inserted you will feel either nothing or a brief, sharp pain. The movement of the catheter through your blood vessel may produce a periodic pressure sensation but is not usually considered painful. Patients commonly experience some "skipped" heartbeats for a few seconds when the catheter touches the walls of the heart.

If a contrast material is injected you may feel a flushed sensation, ranging from mild warmth to searing heat, spread through your body. This will last about 20−30 seconds. You may also experience some nausea, lightheadedness, chest pain, irregular heartbeat, the urge to cough, a headache, mild itching or hives from the contrast material. If this occurs, let your doctor know. Some people also report a brief metallic or salty taste from the contrast material.

During the procedure you will hear a loud, sharp clacking sound from the automatic x-ray film changer and a whining noise from the movie camera.

For many the most uncomfortable aspect of the test is having to lie still for an hour or more on the hard table. You may feel some stiffness or cramping. Ask for cushions or pillows and try to get as comfortable as possible at the start of the procedure.

If you experience chest pain, extreme shortness of breath, dizziness, trouble speaking or swallowing, or paralysis in any part of the body after the test, notify your doctor or nurse. You can expect some soreness, redness, and bruising at the insertion site. But if you feel extreme coldness, pain, numbness, or whiteness in your arm or leg, report this to your doctor or nurse immediately. These signs could indicate a blockage of blood flow.

*Patient Comments*: "It was very exciting. All the hustle and bustle, surrounded by fancy machines. It was fascinating to see my own heart on the x-ray screen. At one point I felt a warm flush. It kept getting hotter and hotter. First in the heart area and then spreading all over. Finally it eased up and faded."

## Risks:

Cardiac catheterization provides extremely important information about your heart, but it does involve significant risks. As with any test, the possible benefits of the test have to be weighed against the risks. You should thoroughly discuss the risks in your case with your doctor.

In the past few years cardiac catheterization has become a much safer procedure. Each year over 1 million cardiac catheterizations are done in the United States alone. Serious complications are rare and are more likely to occur in sicker, older patients or at medical centers that do fewer catheterizations. The chance of a serious complication such as a heart attack is less than 1 in 100 and the risk of death is usually less than 1 in 1000.

Less serious complications include some pain, swelling and tenderness at the catheter insertion site or an irritation of the vein by the catheter (thrombophlebitis). These can usually be treated with warm compresses. Some people experience an allergic reaction to the contrast material with hives and itching and, rarely, shortness of breath, fever, and shock. These allergic reactions can usually be controlled with medications. The contrast material that is excreted in the urine can on rare occasion cause kidney damage.

A serious, though still rare complication can occur if the catheter tip dislodges a blood clot or some debris from the inside wall of the artery. This clot or debris can travel through the bloodstream until it lodges in a smaller artery, blocking the blood flow. If this occurs in an artery supplying the heart, it can cause a heart attack. If it occurs in an artery feeding the brain, it can produce a stroke, with possible loss of speech, sensation, or movement. It can also occur at the catheter insertion site, causing a blockage of blood flow to the arm or leg and requiring surgery to restore the blood circulation.

Rarely the procedure can produce a persistent abnormal heart rhythm. This can cause a heart attack, but more commonly corrects itself or becomes normal after treatment with medications.

Cardiac catheterization does involve some radiation exposure, which varies considerably depending upon how difficult it is to position the catheter and how long the procedure lasts. Compared with other x-ray tests, the radiation exposure for cardiac catheterization is medium for total body exposure and medium for exposure to the reproductive organs. Discuss the possibility of gonadal shielding with your doctor. Since a developing fetus is very sensitive to radiation, this test is not usually recommended for pregnant women.

**Results:**
Your doctor may be able to discuss with you some of the preliminary findings im-

mediately after the test, though complete analysis of the x-rays and measurements may take several days.

Cardiac catheterization, depending upon the type of study performed, can provide information about the size and position of the heart chambers, the function of the heart valves, the ability of the muscular heart walls to contract, and the degree of obstruction of the coronary arteries.

If the coronary arteries which supply the heart muscle are injected with dye, movie pictures, known as a cineangiogram or "cine," show the interior outline of the arteries. This may reveal a complete blockage (obstruction) or narrowing (stenosis) of the three main arteries or branches by the fatty cholesterol deposits of atherosclerosis. Generally a narrowing greater than 70% is considered highly significant, depending upon the location of the blockage. Depending upon the findings, surgical bypass of the blockage or transcutaneous coronary angioplasty (see later) may be recommended in one or more areas.

During catheterization the ability of the muscular walls of the heart to contract can be studied. Damage to the heart muscle and areas of heart muscle not receiving adequate blood supply may be seen on so-called "wall-motion" studies.

The valves of the heart can also be studied by measuring the pressures in the different chambers of the heart and by injecting dye into the chambers. The presence and degree of stenosis (narrowing of the opening) or incompetence (failure to completely close or leaky valves) can be evaluated. Catheterization can also provide information to help decide whether a damaged valve should be replaced with an artificial valve.

Catheterization may also reveal heart defects present since birth (congenital heart disease), such as a hole in a wall (septum) separating the chambers of the heart. These septal defects can cause "shunting" of the blood, in which blood bypasses the lungs and fails to pick up oxygen or in which oxygenated blood fails to be pumped out into the tissues where it is needed. The information collected during catheterization may suggest the need for surgical repair of these defects.

### Cost:
$2000 to $3000 (including hospital charges)

### Special Considerations:
★*His Bundle Electrocardiography:* A normal heartbeat is initiated by an electrical discharge in a special area of the heart. This electrical impulse is transmitted to the rest of the heart muscle through a conduction system. Parts of this conduction pathway may be damaged (for example, by a heart attack), causing slowed or abnormal heart rhythms. While some evidence of a conduction abnormality may appear on a routine ECG, special measurements of these electrical impulses can be made during cardiac catheterization. The impulses are recorded as they move through a part of the conduction system known as the His bundle.

★*Transcutaneous Coronary Artery Angioplasty:* Cardiac catheterization can now also be used to treat some blockages of the coronary arteries. A special catheter containing a balloon is inserted and threaded into a narrowed segment of a coronary artery. The balloon is then inflated, stretching the narrowed opening of the artery and improving the blood flow to the heart muscle. In another experimental technique, emergency treatment for a heart attack is provided by advancing a catheter into a coronary artery which has been suddenly blocked by a blood clot. A small amount of an enzyme (streptokinase) is injected through the catheter to dissolve the blood clot and restore blood flow through the artery.

★*Pulmonary Artery Catheterization:* In very ill patients it is possible to monitor the function of the heart and fluid balance in the body by inserting a special "Swan-Ganz" catheter. This catheter is threaded through a vein in the arm, neck, or groin. A small balloon attached to the tip of the catheter is inflated and carried through the bloodstream to various positions in the heart. Pressures in the various chambers of the heart are then measured. The catheter is usually left in place for several days.

# Thallium Scan
## (Thallium Myocardial Imaging, "Cold Spot" Imaging, Myocardial Perfusion Imaging, Thallium Scintigraphy)

Narrowing of the arteries that supply the heart muscle is known as coronary artery disease. If blood flow through one of these narrowed arteries is suddenly completely blocked, a heart attack occurs and the heart muscle supplied by the occluded artery dies (myocardial infarction).

Thallium scans are performed to determine the amount of blood reaching the heart muscle as well as to determine the location and size of the area of injured muscle after a heart attack.

Blood flow to the heart muscle can be measured either by injecting a contrast material directly into the arteries supplying the heart (coronary arteriography, p. 162) or,

167

as in this test, by using small amounts of a radioactive tracer material (thallium). The thallium is injected into a vein in the arm. A special camera then measures the amount of radioactivity that reaches the heart muscle. The parts of the heart muscle that are receiving adequate blood supply will pick up the tracer. Areas with poor blood supply and damaged cells will not pick up the radioactive material and, therefore, appear as dark areas ("cold spots") on the scan. Thallium scans may be done at rest or after vigorous exercise.

### Why Performed:

This test is frequently done to evaluate persistent unexplained chest pain. It may also be performed to clarify abnormalities found on exercise stress tests (p. 155). As many as 20% of people with an abnormal exercise ECG have normal blood flow to the heart muscle on thallium imaging. This type of noninvasive testing is also useful after coronary artery bypass surgery to determine whether the grafted vessels are working properly.

Thallium imaging may also be used when coronary arteriography reveals borderline narrowed blood vessels. If the thallium scan demonstrates that the narrowed vessels are supplying the heart muscle with sufficient blood, there may be no need for coronary bypass surgery.

### Preparation:

Tell your doctor if
> You have allergies to any medications or anesthetics
> You are taking any medications
> You might be pregnant

Before the test you will be asked to sign a consent form. Use this opportunity to discuss with your doctor any concerns you have about the need for the test, how it is performed, or the risks.

You should not eat or drink anything for at least 3 hours before the test. If you are having an exercise thallium scan, you should also avoid alcohol, tobacco, caffeinated beverages, and unprescribed medications for at least 24 hours before the test. Ask your doctor whether you should continue taking any prescribed medications. You will be exercising vigorously during the test, so wear comfortable shoes and loose shorts or pants. Men are usually barechested during the test. Women usually wear a bra, gown, or loose blouse. You should remove all jewelry before the test.

### Procedure:

The test is usually performed in a specially equipped room in a hospital radiology or nuclear medicine department. An overnight stay in the hospital is usually not necessary. The test is done by a physician and technician trained in cardiovascular nuclear medicine.

*Resting Imaging:* A tourniquet will be placed around your upper arm to help locate the vein at the bend of your arm. The area will be cleansed and a tiny amount of the radioactive thallium injected into the vein. You will then be asked to lie on your back on a table with a very large scintillation camera above your chest. This camera measures the radioactivity emitted by the thallium; it does not expose your body to any radiation. Each scan takes 5–10 minutes. You should lie very still during each scan. Several scans will be taken with you lying in different positions. The entire test takes 30–40 minutes, after which you can resume your normal activities.

*Exercise Imaging:* In the exercise or stress thallium test you will be asked to exercise on a treadmill or stationary bicycle before the thallium is injected. Before the exercise, electrodes will be attached to your chest, arms, and legs as in a standard electrocardiogram (ECG). To prepare you for the electrodes, the skin on your chest is first shaved (if necessary), scrubbed, and mildly abraded before the electrodes are secured. An intravenous line (IV) will be placed in a vein in your arm for the thallium injection. A blood pressure cuff will be placed on your other arm.

You will then be asked to walk on the moving treadmill, slowly at first, then with gradually increasing speed. You can use the railing in front of you for balance, but don't lean on it. You will be asked to exercise until you experience symptoms of chest pain, extreme fatigue, dizziness, or breathlessness, or until your blood pressure or ECG indicates you have reached your maximal exercise tolerance.

The thallium will then be injected, and you will be asked to continue to exercise 30 to 60 seconds longer. You will then lie down on a table with the large scintillation camera above you.

Three to five minutes after the injection, the scanning begins. During each scan you should lie completely still. Each scan takes 5–10 minutes. Between scans you will be asked to change position for other views. The entire test takes 60–90 minutes.

Additional ("redistribution") scans will be ordered after you rest for 2–4 hours. No further exercise will be necessary, and you may resume normal diet and activities after the redistribution scans. As there will be a long wait for this final scan, you may wish to bring something to read or other material for quiet activity.

## How Does It Feel?

The scanning procedure itself is painless. You may feel a brief stinging or burning sensation when the needle is inserted into the vein in your arm. When your skin is prepared for the ECG electrodes, you may feel some slight burning and itching. Lying completely still on the table during the scans may be somewhat uncomfortable. If you are having the scan after exercising, you may notice chest pain, breathlessness, lightheadedness, fatigue, and aching in your leg muscles during the exercise. Report these sensations to the examiner as they occur. If the symptoms are extreme, you will be asked to stop or slow down.

## Risks:

Thallium scans are generally quite safe. The amount of radiation exposure is approximately equivalent to one chest x-ray. Even though the radiation dose is very small, the test is not recommended during pregnancy or breast-feeding except in an emergency.

The risk from the exercise portion depends on the condition of your heart and general level of health. There is a minimal risk of developing irregularities in the heart rhythm or having a heart attack during the test. The risk of death in an exercise test is about 1 in 10,000. You should discuss the particular risks in your case with your doctor.

## Results:

The results of the test should be available a day or two after the test, sometimes sooner. Areas of heart muscle with inadequate blood supply or damaged cells appear as dark "cold spots" on the images. It is not possible with thallium scanning to determine whether the "cold spot" is due to new or old damage to the heart muscle. However, the thallium scans are sensitive enough to detect about 90% of significant coronary heart disease.

## Cost:

Resting imaging: $150 to $300
Exercise imaging: $300 to $500

# Infarct Imaging
## ("Hot Spot" Myocardial Imaging or Scintigraphy, Infarct-Avid Imaging)

If the blood flow through one of the arteries feeding the heart is blocked, a heart attack occurs and the heart muscle supplied by the occluded artery dies (myocardial infarction). To confirm the presence or absence of a heart attack, an infarct scan can be performed. In this test a small amount of radioactive material (technetium pyrophosphate) is injected into a vein in the arm. This radioactive tracer travels through the bloodstream to the heart, where it becomes bound to injured heart muscle. A special scintillation camera detects the radioactivity and creates a picture which shows areas of injured heart muscle as bright "hot spots." These images show not only the presence of a heart attack but also the size and location of the damage.

### Why Performed:
Most of the time the diagnosis of heart attack can be made based on characteristic symptoms (chest pain, shortness of breath, sweating, etc.), abnormalities on ECG (p. 153), and the measurement of cardiac enzymes released into the bloodstream by damaged heart muscle (p. 151). However, when the diagnosis is unclear, an infarct scan is sometimes used. This type of nuclear scan is not accurate until about 12 to 72 hours after the heart attack, so it cannot be used immediately after a suspected heart attack. However, infarct scans can be performed several days after the onset of symptoms to see whether a heart attack has occurred.

The test is also useful in evaluating patients after coronary bypass surgery, since during the postoperative period the ECG and heart muscle enzyme tests may not accurately indicate a heart attack.

### Preparation:
Tell your doctor if
> You have allergies to any medications or anesthetics
> You are taking any medications
> You might be pregnant

You do not need to restrict foods or fluids before the test. Remove all jewelry and metal objects from the chest area before the test.

### Procedure:
This test is performed in a specially equipped room in a hospital nuclear medicine or radiology department. Hospitalization is not necessarily required unless the test shows evidence of a recent heart attack. The test is done by a physician and a technician trained in cardiovascular nuclear medicine.

A tourniquet is placed around your upper arm to help locate the vein at the bend of your arm. The area is cleansed and a small amount of radioactive technetium pyrophosphate is injected. You will have to wait for 2–3 hours while the radioactive material circulates through your blood and is picked up by the heart muscle.

You will then lie on your back on a table with a very large camera positioned above your chest. This scintillation camera detects the radioactivity from the injected tracer. The camera itself does not put any radiation into your body.

You will have to hold very still for about 10 minutes while each scan is being made. Several scans will be made with you lying in different positions. Between the scans you will be free to move or talk. The test takes 30–60 minutes, not including the 2–3 hour wait. You may wish to bring something to read or some other material for quiet activity to occupy your time while waiting.

### How Does It Feel?
You may feel a brief stinging sensation when the needle is inserted in your arm. The scan itself is painless, but lying on the table and holding still for each scan may be slightly uncomfortable. Be sure to get as comfortable as you can before each scan; ask for a pillow, blankets, or a mattress pad for the table.

### Risks:
There is very little risk associated with this type of nuclear scan. Most of the radioactive substance is eliminated from your body within a few days, and the radiation dose is small (approximately 110 millirads, or the equivalent of five chest x-rays). Even though the radiation dose is low, the test is not recommended during pregnancy or breast-feeding unless it is an emergency.

### Results:
The results are usually available the same day the test is performed. Normally the radioactive tracer is picked up by the ribs and the breastbone but not by the heart muscle. A "hot spot" (bright area) on the scan indicates the accumulation of the tracer in an injured area of the heart. In most patients with an acute heart attack, the hot spots won't show up until 12 hours after the onset of chest pain. The "hot spots" are most visible between 48 and 72 hours after an attack and disappear after one week. Therefore the timing of the test is critical in interpreting the results.

This type of test accurately detects about 90% of heart muscle damage due to a heart attack. However, in about 15% of cases the scan produces a false-positive, incorrectly indicating an area of heart muscle damage. In addition to a heart attack, there are other causes of "hot spots" or a "positive" scan. These include severe angina (decreased blood flow to heart muscle), inflammation or trauma of the heart muscle, and tumors of the heart. Therefore, the results must be carefully correlated with other tests.

### Cost:
$200 to $300

# Cardiac Blood Pool Imaging
## (First-Pass and Gated Equilibrium Scanning)

Several new nuclear medicine tests have been developed to evaluate the ability of the heart muscle to contract normally and pump blood effectively throughout the body. A small amount of a radioactive material (technetium-labeled albumin or red blood cells) is injected into the bloodstream through a vein in the arm. A special camera linked to a high-speed computer detects the radioactively labeled blood as it makes its initial pass through the heart ("first-pass imaging"). The camera then creates multiple images as the walls of the heart contract to expel the labeled blood. This new, noninvasive test carries little or no risk and can sometimes be used instead of the riskier cardiac catheterization.

### Why Performed:
These tests are most often ordered to evaluate the failure of the heart to pump blood adequately (congestive heart failure), in-

adequate blood supply to the heart muscle (coronary artery disease), and heart and vessels abnormalities present at birth (congenital heart disease). They are sometimes performed to evaluate chest pain or shortness of breath when the cause is unclear from previous studies.

### Preparation:

Tell your doctor if

> You have allergies to any medications or anesthetics
>
> You are taking any medications
>
> You might be pregnant

There is no need to restrict food or fluids before this test. Remove all jewelry before the test. If an exercise portion is planned for the test, wear comfortable shoes and loose-fitting clothing and ask your doctor about special preparations.

### Procedure:

The test is done in a specially equipped room in a hospital radiology or nuclear medicine department. An overnight stay in the hospital is usually not necessary. The test is done by a physician and a technician trained in cardiovascular nuclear medicine.

Electrodes for the electrocardiogram (ECG) are attached to your chest. You will lie on your back on a table with a large scintillation camera above your chest. A tourniquet is placed around your upper arm to help locate the vein in the bend of your arm. A tiny amount of radioactive material is injected into the vein. The camera follows the course of the material as it circulates through your heart. The camera itself does not expose your body to any radiation.

You will be asked to assume several different positions while scans are taken. During the 5 minutes it takes for each scan you should remain silent and motionless.

Depending upon the type of test, you may be given a nitroglcerin tablet under your tongue or you may be asked to exercise during the test. The test takes from 10 to 60 minutes or more, depending on which studies are performed. After the test you may resume normal activities.

### How Does It Feel?

Except for a brief, sharp pain when the needle is inserted into the vein in your arm, the procedure is painless. You may find it slightly uncomfortable to lie motionless during each scan. Try to make yourself as comfortable as possible before the scan starts. Don't hesitate to ask for a blanket, pillow, or mattress pad for the table.

### Risks:

There is very little risk associated with cardiac blood pool scans. Most of the radioactive material is eliminated from your body within a few days, and the total radiation dose is very small (approximately equivalent to one chest x-ray). Even though the radiation risk is minimal, pregnant or breast-feeding women usually should not have these tests except in an emergency.

### Results:

The test results are usually available a day or two after the test is done. The distribution of the radioactively labeled blood is viewed as it circulates through the chambers of the heart and great vessels. The amount of blood pumped out of the left ventricle during a contraction, the "ejection fraction," is normally between 55% and 65%. If the muscular wall of the ventricle is damaged, the ejection fraction will be reduced, reflecting the poor ability of the heart to pump the blood.

The motion of the walls of the heart is also examined. Immobile or poorly moving areas may reflect dead or blood-starved (ischemic) heart muscle or may be due to an abnormal ballooning-out of the wall (aneurysm). This test may also reveal leaky heart valves or holes between the heart chambers.

**Cost:**
$300 to $500

# Pericardial Tap (Pericardiocentesis)

The pericardium is a double-layered sac surrounding the heart. Normally there is a very small amount of fluid in this sac to lubricate the heart and reduce friction when the heart expands and contracts. In certain diseases an excess of fluid (effusion) collects within the pericardium.

In this test a needle is inserted through the chest wall and into the sac. Fluid is removed and examined in the laboratory to help determine the cause of the pericardial effusion. This procedure may also be performed therapeutically to remove fluid compressing the heart or to treat pericardial tumors with anticancer drugs.

**Why Performed:**
Sometimes fluid can collect very rapidly in the pericardium, putting pressure on the heart and interfering with the pumping of blood (pericardial tamponade). This can result from trauma, like a gunshot or stab wound to the chest, or from a massive heart attack with rupture of the heart muscle. An emergency pericardial tap to quickly remove the accumulated fluid can be lifesaving.

A pericardial tap can also be done on a nonemergency basis to determine the reason for an excess collection of fluid around the heart. The presence of this fluid is usually suggested by characteristic abnormalities on physical examination, chest x-ray, electrocardiogram, and echocardiogram.

**Preparation:**
Tell your doctor if
> You have allergies to any medications or anesthetics
> You are taking any medications, particularly anticoagulants
> You have had bleeding problems

Unless the procedure is being performed on an emergency basis, you will be asked to sign a consent form. Use this as an opportunity to discuss with your doctor any concerns you have about the need for the test, how it is performed, and the risks.

There is no need to restrict food or fluids before the test. Some blood tests, including checks for anemia and blood clotting problems, are usually performed before the procedure.

**Procedure:**
A pericardial tap is usually performed in your hospital room or in a cardiac procedure room by a doctor (usually a cardiologist or heart surgeon). An IV will be placed in a vein in your arm and electrodes taped on your arms and legs to monitor your ECG during the test. You may also be given a mild sedative to help you relax before the procedure. You will be leaning back at a 45-degree angle on the bed or table. First your chest will be shaved (if necessary), cleansed with an antiseptic solution, and covered with sterile drapes.

A small amount of local anesthetic will be injected to numb the skin and deeper tissues. Then a long (4"–5"), thin needle will be carefully inserted just below your breastbone. Sometimes an alternative site between your ribs on the left side over your heart is selected. The needle is slowly advanced into the pericardial sac and fluid is withdrawn and sent to the laboratory. At different times during the procedure you may be asked to hold your breath. After all the fluid is removed the needle is withdrawn and pressure is applied to the needle site for several minutes to stop any bleeding. The procedure takes about 10–20 minutes. After the test you will have a chest x-ray to check for damage to the lungs. You will be closely observed for several hours, with frequent checks of blood pressure, heart rate, and breathing rate.

### How Does It Feel?

You will feel a brief, stinging pain when the local anesthetic is injected. When the needle is inserted into the pericardial sac you will probably feel a sensation of pressure. You may also notice some irregular or "skipped" heartbeats during the test. However, if you feel a severe chest pain or shortness of breath during or after the procedure, notify your doctor immediately.

### Risks:

A pericardial tap can be a hazardous procedure, although few serious or life-threatening complications occur when performed by an experienced doctor. It is possible for the needle to puncture the heart or one of its blood vessels. In rare instances the needle may also puncture the lung, liver, or stomach. These complications may require surgery to repair.

If the needle touches the heart, an irregular heartbeat (arrhythmia) may be triggered, but the irregularity usually stops when the needle is removed. There is also a slight chance of developing or spreading an infection when the needle is inserted. This can usually be treated with antibiotics.

### Results:

The excess fluid removed during the tap will be sent to the laboratory for analysis. Some of the results will be available within hours, while others may take days or weeks. The results may reveal infection (viral, bacterial, tubercular, fungal), inflammation, cancer, uremia (inability of the kidneys to adequately excrete waste products), or rupture of the wall of the heart.

### Cost:

$100 to $200

### Special Considerations:

★*Pericardial Biopsy:* To diagnose some diseases of the pericardium it is necessary to remove a small sample of tissue (biopsy) from the pericardial sac. This is a surgical procedure performed in an operating room. A small incision is made in the chest wall, and a small specimen of pericardial tissue is removed and examined under a microscope.

# 4

# Tests for Women

## Vaginal Self-Examination

Using a hand-held mirror, a light and a small instrument known as a speculum, it is possible for women to examine their external genitals, vagina, and cervix (the part of the uterus or womb that extends into the vagina). This exam allows a woman to better understand her own body, to know what is normal for her, and to identify problems early which might need medical assistance.

Vaginal self-examination is a supplement to, not substitute for, regular complete pelvic exams and Pap smears (see p. 179) by a physician or nurse practitioner. A good way to learn more about the self-examination techniques described here is to review them with your health care provider or with a self-help group at a women's health center.

### Why Performed:
The main usefulness of vaginal self-examination is to increase a woman's awareness and knowledge of her own body. It may also be helpful as an initial self-screening of vaginal sores, irritations, or discharge. You can also look for an IUD string if you cannot locate it by feeling, or check the location of the cervix to better understand the proper placement of a diaphragm. Vaginal self-examination may also be used to note changes in cervical mucus as part of fertility awareness for birth control or achieving pregnancy (see p. 195).

Vaginal self-examination with a speculum is not advised during or just after pregnancy, after recent gynecological surgery, or just after an abortion, since there is a slightly increased chance of complications, mostly infection, at those times.

### Equipment:
- Flashlight or gooseneck lamp.
- A hand-held mirror, preferably with a long handle.
- A vaginal speculum: This is a small instrument with two duck-bill blades which open to allow you to view the vaginal walls and neck of the uterus (cervix). A speculum may be made of metal, which is more expensive ($10–$12), or clear plastic, which is less expensive ($2–$3),

more readily available, and warmer. If your doctor or nurse uses a disposable plastic speculum, ask to keep yours after your next exam. Or you can buy a speculum from a medical supply store, some pharmacies, some community and women's clinics, or by mail from the Self-Care Catalog, Box 999, Pt. Reyes, CA 94956. Both plastic models (about $4) and stainless steel models (about $14) are available.

Specula come in small, medium, or large sizes. Most women can comfortably use a medium size. If you have ever been told that you have a deep or hard-to-find cervix, you should consider trying a large size. Ask your health care provider which size he or she would recommend for you.

### Procedure:

Sit with your knees bent and feet well apart, and lean backward slightly. You should choose a firm surface (floor, bed, or couch) and support your back with pillows. Hold the hand mirror in front of your vagina and start by identifying the major structures: the labia majora and minora (the outer and inner fleshy lips of the vulva), the clitoris (the bump of erectile tissue covered by a hood found at the upper intersection of the labia), the urethral opening (the hole through which urine flows, which is often difficult to see), the vaginal opening, and the anus.

If you are using a metal speculum, warm it by running it under warm (not hot) water. Lubricate your speculum with a water-soluble jelly (K-Y Jelly) or plain, warm water to make insertion smoother and easier. Hold the speculum at the base of the blades, with the blades closed and the handle pointing to one side. Make a conscious effort to relax your vagina and abdominal muscles. Using the fingers of

your other hand, spread the vaginal lips apart and gently glide the closed blades of the speculum into the vaginal opening, aiming for the small of your back. If inserting the speculum is painful, stop and try again. When you have inserted it as far as the base of the blades, turn the speculum so that the handle is facing upward, and gently open the blades.

Now shine the flashlight into the mirror and reflect the light into your vagina, which the speculum has stretched open. Readjust the light, mirror, and speculum until you can see well into the vagina. You should be able to see the reddish-pink walls of the vagina, which have slight folds or ridges known as rugae.

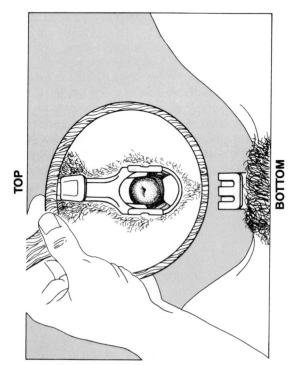

**Vaginal Self-Exam.** *A view of the cervix as seen in the mirror during vaginal self-examination.*

At the end of the vagina you may also be able to see the cervix, which appears as a rounded donut about the size of a quarter with a hole or slit in the center (the cervical os). The cervix is often difficult to locate. You might try moving the speculum in or out a little or slightly to the right or left, until the cervix pops into view. Don't be discouraged if you can't see the cervix on the first try. Take the speculum out and try locating your cervix first by reaching your finger into the vagina before reinserting the speculum. You may want to get help from a friend, self-help group or health worker. It gets easier with practice.

Once you do locate the cervix lock the speculum in its open position. Spend a few moments examining the cervix and the vaginal walls. When you are finished, unlock the speculum but keep the blades slightly open to avoid pinching the vaginal walls and slowly withdraw it. Wash your speculum with warm soapy water.

**Results:**

Redness and itching of the labia and vaginal area suggest a vaginal infection, abrasion (often from sexual activity without sufficient lubrication), or chemical irritation (often from feminine hygiene sprays, contraceptive jellies or foam, or douches). Painful blisters or small ulcerated sores may indicate a possible herpes infection. Painless ulcerated sores (chancres) may indicate syphilis. Lumps beneath the skin in the vaginal lips suggest a cyst or, if tender, an infection (abscess). Roughened, raised, whitish spots on the skin may be warts. It is wise to discuss any of these findings with a health worker.

Each woman will have a characteristic vaginal discharge which is usual for her in terms of its amount, color, odor, and consistency. A normal discharge is usually clear to cloudy-white, smells slightly acidic (like vinegar), may be thick or thin, and changes slightly throughout the menstrual cycle. If you notice a change in your normal discharge, such as an increased amount, foul smell, or associated itching or burning, this is usually a sign of a vaginal infection. Consult your health worker for further evaluation.

The cervix may normally have a small reddened area or bluish lump (cyst). The opening (os) of the cervix may be round and closed (usually in women who haven't had a child) or more open and slitlike (in women who have had a vaginal birth). If there is redness around the cervical opening it may be either normal or a sign of an infection (cervicitis). You may note a discharge from the os which varies at different times in your menstrual cycle. If you have an IUD you should see the string coming out of the cervical opening. Again, it is a good idea to review these findings, or any significant changes, with your health worker.

# Test for Vaginitis (Wet Mount)

Vaginitis means simply an inflammation of the vagina and vulva. Even though it is often due to infection, it may or may not be sexually transmitted.

Vaginitis is usually accompanied by itching, pain, and a vaginal discharge. Most women will experience at least one episode of vaginitis at some time in their lives.

In this test, your health worker performs a pelvic examination, and takes a sample of vaginal discharge. This sample is examined for fungus (yeast), parasite (*Tri-*

chomonas) and bacterial (*Hemophilus* or *Gardnerella*) infections.

### Why Performed:

This test is done when a woman experiences unusual vaginal irritation, itching, burning, rash, odor, swelling, or excessive discharge that lasts more than a few days or is very uncomfortable. It may also be done when a vaginal discharge is detected during a routine pelvic exam.

### Preparation:

Do not douche for 24 hours before this test.

### Procedure:

The sample for this test is collected in a doctor's office, clinic, or hospital by a physician, nurse, nurse practitioner, or other health worker.

You will be asked to remove all your clothes below the waist, and to lie on your back on an examining table with your legs up in stirrups.

The examiner will insert a speculum into your vagina. The speculum will be lubricated only with warm water, since other lubricants can interfere with the test.

The examiner will then insert a sterile, moist cotton swab into your vagina, take a sample of the discharge, remove the swab, and then remove the speculum.

Sometimes a sample is also taken from the urethra, the tube through which the urine leaves the body. If this is to be done, the examiner will insert a second moist cotton swab into the urethral opening.

The collection of the specimen usually takes less than 5 minutes.

Two slides are prepared—one with a few drops of salt (saline) solution, the other with a few drops of potassium hydroxide solution. The slides are usually examined under a microscope in your clinician's office immediately after the sample is taken.

### How Does It Feel?

This test is normally no more uncomfortable than a regular pelvic exam. The more you are able to relax, the more comfortable the test will be. You can help by taking deep, slow breaths and relaxing your lower abdominal muscles as much as possible.

If you have an inflammation of the vaginal area, the insertion of the speculum and collection of the sample may be somewhat painful.

In rare cases there may be a small amount of bleeding after this test.

### Risks:

There are no risks involved with this test.

### Results:

Results are usually available within 5–10 minutes. Test results will indicate whether an infection is present. It is possible to have a vaginal inflammation without an infection. If this is the case, it may be due to chemical irritation (e.g., from bubble bath or vaginal spray), mechanical abrasion, or atrophic vaginitis due to lack of estrogen.

The most common vaginal infections and the characteristic symptoms of each are as follows:

- *Yeast infection* (moniliasis, candidiasis, caused by *Candida albicans*): white, cheesy discharge, often with severe itching, vaginal inflammation or rash, painful intercourse. Microscopic exam may show branching yeast filaments.
- *Trichomoniasis* ("trich," caused by a single celled protozoan parasite, *Trichomonas vaginalis*): yellowish, frothy, foul-smelling discharge, often with vaginal inflammation, pain on urination or intercourse, lower abdominal pain. Single-celled moving organism may be seen on microscopic exam.
- *Nonspecific vaginitis* (caused by the bacterium *Gardnerella vaginalis*, also called

*Hemophilus vaginalis*): heavy, white, fishy-smelling discharge, sometimes with vaginal rash or painful intercourse. Bacteria or "clue" cells may be seen on microscopic exam.

The symptoms of these three infections can be quite similar, but different treatments are indicated for each. This test can almost always determine which one or combination of the three organisms is responsible. Sometimes the test suggests that the infection may be due to gonorrhea. If so, a gonorrhea culture (p. 140) will be taken.

### Cost:

This test is most frequently done as part of a doctor's visit, and there is usually no extra charge.

### Special Considerations:

★*Treating the Male Partner in Trichomonal and Bacterial Infections*—Trichomonal organisms can be passed by sexual contract, and men can have a low-grade infection without symptoms. If a woman's regular sexual partner has such an infection, she will very likely be reinfected by him after she receives treatment. (This is sometimes called a "ping-pong infection.") In such cases it is necessary for the male sexual partners of women with trichomonal infection to receive treatment as well. It may also be necessary to treat the male partner when a woman has a recurring bacterial infection of the vagina.

# Pap Smear

In this test a doctor or nurse practitioner takes a sample of cells from the vagina and cervix (the entrance to the uterus). The sample is sent to a laboratory, where a technician examines the cells under a microscope.

The Papanicolaou (Pap) smear is used primarily to screen for cervical cancer. It is one of the most frequently performed medical tests; approximately 25 million Pap tests are done per year in the United States.

### Why Performed:

How often you should have a Pap smear is a matter of debate. The American Cancer Society (ACS) suggests that women between 20 and 40 who are not in a high-risk category and who have had two previous normal Pap smears should have this test every three years. The ACS recommends that women over 40, those in a high-risk category, and those who have had a recent positive Pap smear should have a Pap smear more frequently—either yearly or as advised by their doctor. The American College of Obstetrics and Gynecology still recommends a yearly Pap smear for all women.

High risk of cervical cancer seems to be associated with the following:

Personal history of cervical or uterine cancer
Previous abnormal Pap test
Early age of first sexual intercourse
Multiple sexual partners
History of genital herpes infection or genital warts
Women whose mothers took DES (diethylstilbestrol) during pregnancy

The risk of cervical cancer is also higher in women who smoke or take birth control pills and lower in those who use condoms or diaphragms for birth control.

If you are concerned about one or more of these risk factors, you may wish to discuss with your doctor whether you are in a high-risk group and should thus have a Pap test more frequently.

If your uterus and cervix have been removed for a cancerous condition, you should discuss appropriate screening with your doctor. If they have been removed for a noncancerous condition, a Pap smear every three years is probably sufficient.

In addition to testing for cancer, the Pap test is occasionally used to detect inflammation of the cervix, to evaluate response to therapy for conditions of the cervix, and to detect infection.

**Preparation:**

Tell your doctor if
    You have ever had an abnormal Pap smear
    You are taking any of the medications listed at the end of this discussion
    You are using birth control pills
    You might be pregnant

Ideally, this test should not be done during your menstrual period. The presence of blood cells may interfere with test results. However, if you are experiencing abnormal vaginal bleeding, it may help determine the cause of the bleeding.

Avoid douching, vaginal medications, tampon use, and tub bathing for 24 hours before this test. Some physicians suggest that you refrain from vaginal intercourse for 24 hours before the test.

For your own comfort, empty your bladder just before the test.

**Procedure:**

The sample is obtained by a physician or nurse practitioner during an examination of your pelvic organs. You will be asked to remove all clothing below the waist and to lie on your back on an examining table with your feet raised and supported by stirrups.

A vaginal speculum (a small instrument with two duck-bill blades which hold the vagina open for examination) is inserted. No lubricant (other than warm water) is used, because it might get into the Pap smear specimen. The examiner then reaches into the vagina with a swab or spatula (sometimes both swab and spatula are used) and takes several samples of cells and fluid.

Two or three samples are usually taken as follows:

1. A cotton swab is inserted into the opening (os) of the cervix and/or
2. A spatula is scraped gently against the cervix and/or
3. A swab or spatula is rubbed against the wall of the vagina just below the cervix

The samples are spread on a microscope slide, sprayed with or dipped in a fixative, and sent to a lab. Taking a Pap specimen usually takes 2–3 minutes. It is usually done as the first part of the pelvic exam.

At the lab, your cell sample is stained with a special dye, then examined under a microscope by a physician specialist (pathologist) or a trained technician (cytologist).

**How Does It Feel?**

You may feel some discomfort when the speculum is inserted. You may notice a slight feeling of pressure when the sample is being taken. There may be a small amount of bleeding after the test.

**Risks:**

There is little or no risk associated with this test.

**Results:**

Results are usually available in 1–2 weeks. Dr. George Papanicolaou, for whom the Pap smear is named, established five diagnostic classifications for Pap results. Classes I and II mean "negative for cancer." Classes IV and V mean "it looks like it could be cancer." Class III covers anything that does not fit easily into any of the other classes. In some laboratories Class III is used to mean "I don't really know." Other laboratories use Class III to mean "atypical cells, but not cancer cells, are present."

More recently, another method of classifying Pap smears has come into widespread use. This system divides Pap smears into three main categories: *benign* (noncancerous), *precancerous* (showing abnormal cell changes called cervical interstitial neoplasia, CIN), and *malignant* (possibly cancerous).

If you receive an abnormal Pap smear (Class III in the old system or precancerous, CIN, in the new system), it does not necessarily mean that you have cancer. It *does* mean that you should have another Pap

---

## Other Terms Sometimes Used in Pap Test Reports

| Term | Meaning |
|---|---|
| Negative | No abnormal cells. |
| Inconclusive | Sample is inadequate. Repeat sample is needed. |
| Atypical | Some cells appear abnormal but not precancerous. Repeat test is needed. |
| Suspicious | Some abnormal cells that may or may not be cancerous. Discuss with your physician. |
| Positive | Cells appear cancerous. Discuss with your physician. |
| Inflammatory | No cancer cells seen, but signs of inflammation are present. If symptoms appear, discuss possible treatment with your physician. |
| Hemorrhagic | Blood cells are present in sample. This could be due to menstruation or to slight bleeding produced by the spatula when the sample was taken, but could also be due to disease condition. If not sure of the cause, consult with your physician. |
| Trichomonas | A minor vaginal infection is present. If vaginal discharge, itching, or other symptoms of infection are bothersome, consult with your clinician. |
| Estrogen level | Some Pap tests show signs of low estrogen levels. This may or may not be reported. Low estrogen levels occur with age, breast-feeding, onset of menopause, and after surgical removal of the ovaries. |
| Endocervical cells | This indicates that some of the cells are of the type that normally come from inside the cervix. An adequate sample of these cells is necessary for an accurate Pap result. |

smear. If a vaginal infection is present, it should be treated before the second Pap smear is done.

If the repeat Pap is also abnormal, or if your first Pap result shows Class IV or V or malignant cells, further tests will be needed—probably a colposcopy and a cervical biopsy—to determine a final diagnosis.

Pap smears do not diagnose cervical cancer; they only screen for it. Even when a Pap report says that cancer cells were seen, there is about a 20% chance that you do not have cancer. On the other hand, about 10% of cancers are not detected by this test. The great majority of abnormal Paps are due to premalignant changes, which can be dealt with by early treatment.

A normal Pap smear is not a guarantee that there is no cancer anywhere in the genital tract. Although it occasionally detects cancerous cells from the lining of the uterus (endometrium), a Pap smear is not an accurate screening test for endometrial or ovarian cancer.

Some medications (see listing below) can alter Pap smear results. The most important of these are hormones and chemotherapeutic agents used to treat cancers.

## Drugs That May Affect Pap Smears

Bleomycin (Blenoxane)—used in cancer chemotherapy

Busulfan (Myleran)—used to treat some leukemias

Chlorambucil (Leukeran)—used to treat leukemias, lymphomas, and Hodgkin's disease

Colchicine (Colbenemid)—used to treat chronic, gouty arthritis

Cyclophosphamide (Cytoxan)—used to treat lymphomas, leukemias, multiple myelomas, and other malignancies

Doxorubicin (Adriamycin)—used to treat leukemias, lymphomas, and other malignancies

Estrogen (Premarin, many other brands)—used to eliminate or modify postmenopausal symptoms, to prevent osteoporosis, in breast and prostate cancer, in birth control pills

5-Fluorouracil (Adrucil)—used to treat cancers of the colon, rectum, breast, stomach, and pancreas

6-Mercaptopurine (Purinethol)—used to treat leukemia

Methotrexate—used in the treatment of some cancers and in some very severe cases of psoriasis which do not respond to other therapies

Mithramycin (Mithracin)—used to treat tumors of the testes and some other cancers

Periwinkle—an herbal remedy

Podophyllin—used to treat venereal warts and other skin tumors

Progestins (progesterone)—a hormone used in birth control pills and in postmenopausal hormone therapy

Silver nitrate—used to prevent infections in the eyes of newborn infants

Thiotepa—used to treat certain cancers

Source: William A. Nahhas: The Pap smear. *Diagnosis*, Vol. 1, No. 3, pp. 60–68, July/August 1979.

**Cost:**
A doctor's visit to have the sample collected usually costs about $25 to $40. The Pap smear itself usually costs about $10 to $15.

### Frequency of Pap Smear Results

| Result | Frequency |
| --- | --- |
| Normal | 90 in 100 |
| Inflammatory | 1 in 20 |
| Mild CIN | 1 in 30 |
| Severe CIN | 1 in 500 |
| Malignant | 1 in 1000 |

Source: Stewart, Felecia, et al.: *My Body, My Health: The Concerned Woman's Guide to Gynecology.* New York: Wiley Medical Publications, 1979, p. 400.

# Colposcopy and Cervical Biopsy

A colposcope is a diagnostic instrument used to obtain a magnified view of the surface cells of the vagina and cervix (opening to the uterus). Since the image is magnified 10 to 40 times normal size, abnormalities can be seen which are often missed by the naked eye. If abnormal areas are spotted, small tissue samples (biopsies) can be collected for laboratory examination to diagnose possibly cancerous or precancerous conditions.

**Why Performed:**
Colposcopy is often the first test done if you have an abnormal Pap smear (see preceding test) or a lesion on your vaginal lips (vulva), vagina, or cervix. Colposcopy and biopsy can help determine whether a cancer is present. Colposcopy may be performed every 6 to 12 months to monitor precancerous abnormalities (dysplasia) or to look for recurrent abnormalities after treatment. It may also be used to evaluate unexplained pain or bleeding during intercourse. Some gynecologists recommend colposcopy for women whose mothers took diethylstilbestrol (DES) during pregnancy, since these women are at increased risk for vaginal and cervical cancer. Colposcopy is quick, painless, and can often eliminate the need for more extensive procedures such as cone biopsy of the cervix (see later).

**Preparation:**
Tell your doctor if
   You are taking any medications
   You have had any bleeding problems
   You are having menstrual bleeding
   You think you might be pregnant

No special preparation is necessary. For your comfort, empty your bladder before the exam. Douching before the exam is not recommended, as it may disrupt the surface cells and cause a false-negative result. Colposcopy cannot be done satisfactorily during your menstrual period, so discuss with your doctor the best time to schedule the exam.

**Procedure:**
Colposcopy can be done as part of a regular pelvic exam in a gynecologist's office. You will be asked to lie on your back on the table with your feet up in the stirrups. As with a routine pelvic exam, a speculum will be inserted into your vagina and slightly opened, making your cervix visible. Your cervix will be swabbed with a chemical solution (acetic acid) to highlight abnormal areas. The colposcope will then be positioned at the entrance of your vagina and

your doctor will look through the eyepieces at a magnified view of the surface of the vagina and cervix. Photographs may be taken.

Samples of suspicious areas will be removed using a small biopsy forceps. Usually several biopsy samples are collected and sent to the laboratory to be examined under a microscope, to look for cancerous changes in the cells. In addition, the inside canal of the cervix may be scraped gently with a tiny spoon-shaped instrument (curet) to obtain tissue samples from that difficult-to-view area. Colposcopy and biopsy usually take 10 to 15 minutes to perform.

If a biopsy is performed, there may be a small amount of bleeding, which often stops by itself or may be stopped by direct pressure, chemical cautery, or electrocautery. If necessary a pad or tampon may be used. Leave the tampon in place for 8 to 24 hours or as advised. If a biopsy was performed, avoid sexual intercourse, douching, or using additional tampons for one week (or as advised) to allow your cervix to heal.

### How Does It Feel?

Colposcopy is essentially a painless procedure. The colposcope itself never touches you. Insertion of the vaginal speculum can be slightly uncomfortable if it is not properly warmed and gently placed. The cervix does not contain many pain-sensing nerves, so during a biopsy you may feel only a brief pinching sensation followed by mild cramping. Some vaginal bleeding and a slight discharge are normal after a biopsy for up to one week. However, if heavy bleeding (more than a menstrual period), fever, pelvic pain, or a foul-smelling vaginal discharge occurs, notify your doctor.

### Risks:

Colposcopy itself poses no risk. A biopsy may rarely lead to prolonged vaginal bleeding or a pelvic infection, which will require further treatment.

### Results:

The surface of the cervix and vagina will be examined for abnormal patterns in the blood vessels or whitish patches suggestive of cancer or precancerous lesions. Areas of inflammation, erosion, and atrophy may also be noted.

The laboratory results from biopsies will take several days. The tissue will be examined under a microscope for cancer cells or precancerous changes (dysplasia or carcinoma in situ). The results from the biopsies, Pap smears, and colposcopic exam are compared. If the results are inconsistent or inconclusive, repeat testing or a cervical cone biopsy may be necessary.

### Cost:

Colposcopy: $50 to $100
Colposcopy and cervical biopsy: $100 to $150

### Special Considerations:

★*Cone Biopsy:* If the colposcopic exam or cervical biopsy does not reveal the cause of an abnormal Pap smear or if it shows cervical cancer or precancerous lesions, a more extensive biopsy procedure may be indicated. A cone biopsy (cervical conization) is performed in an operating room under a general anesthetic (see p. 465). A small cone of tissue is removed from the cervix and examined under a microscope for cancerous changes in the cells. In many cases, the cone biopsy serves as the treatment as well, since all the diseased tissue may be removed during the biopsy. The possible complications of a cone biopsy—including extensive bleeding, infection, and problems with later pregnancies—and the alternatives to cone biopsy should be discussed with your doctor if this procedure is recommended.

# Endometrial Biopsy
## (Dilation and Curettage, D & C; Vabra Aspiration)

The uterus is lined by a layer of tissue called the endometrium which changes throughout the menstrual cycle. In this test a small sample of this uterine lining is removed and examined under a microscope.

A more extensive version of the endometrial biopsy is called a dilation and curettage (D & C). In this procedure, instead of just removing a small sample, the doctor removes as much of the uterine lining as possible.

**Why Performed:**
An endometrial biopsy is most frequently done to determine the cause of a change in menstrual bleeding pattern—most commonly heavy or prolonged bleeding, irregular bleeding, or bleeding in women who have already gone through menopause.

This test is also sometimes performed on women who have been unable to become pregnant. In such cases a specimen is taken 3–5 days before a normal menstrual period is expected. Results will usually show whether the uterine lining is properly prepared to receive a fertilized egg.

It can also be used as a screening test for endometrial cancer before starting estrogen therapy. This is recommended for all postmenopausal women receiving estrogen therapy, but especially for those at higher risk of developing uterine cancer—women who are obese, are diabetic, or have never had children are at increased risk. The test may also be repeated a year or two after starting hormone therapy in high-risk women.

A D & C may be used for both diagnosis and treatment of irregular menstrual bleeding. It is also sometimes performed to remove any tissue from the fetus or placenta after an abortion or miscarriage.

**Preparation:**
Tell your doctor if
    You are allergic to any medications or anesthetics
    You are taking any medications
    You have had bleeding problems
    You might be pregnant

You will be asked to sign a consent form authorizing this procedure. Use this opportunity to discuss with your doctor any concerns you may have about the need for the test, the risks of the test, or how and when it will be performed.

If a general anesthetic will be used, you should take nothing by mouth for at least 10 hours before this test.

**Procedure:**
If the test will require hospitalization, you will be admitted the night before. Routine blood and urine studies will usually be done. In most cases you will be able to return home the day after the test.

Endometrial biopsy is usually performed by a gynecologist or a family practitioner. It is usually done without anesthetic, although local anesthesia is sometimes used. (A general anesthetic is sometimes used if a D & C is planned.)

You will be asked to lie on your back with your feet in stirrups. The doctor will perform a pelvic examination, insert a speculum into the vagina, and hold the cervix with an instrument called a tenaculum. The sample is then collected through a small, hollow plastic tube (cannula) which is passed through the opening in the cervix and into the uterus. The cannula is connected to a suction apparatus. Only a small amount of uterine lining is removed.

Dilation and curettage usually require general or spinal anesthesia. The procedure is usually performed in a hospital operating room. The cervical opening is made gradually wider using a series of dilators of increasing size. A small spoon-shaped instrument (curette) is then passed through the cervix and into the uterus. The top layer of the inner lining of the uterus is carefully scraped off and removed. The samples of uterine lining are then sent to a laboratory for examination.

These tests usually take 10–30 minutes. Afterward you will be observed for 2–4 hours. If no complications develop, you will be allowed to return home.

You should plan to rest and to refrain from heavy lifting for the next 24 hours. Do not douche or engage in sexual intercourse for three days after this test or as advised.

You may be asked to take your temperature daily for three days after this test. Notify your doctor if you notice a fever. You should use a tampon or menstrual pad and should notify your doctor if you experience heavy bleeding—more than one tampon or menstrual pad per hour.

### How Does It Feel?

The instruments may feel cold. If no anesthetic is used, you will probably feel some cramping as the instrument is inserted into your uterus and some additional cramping when the sample is collected. Women who have had this test usually describe the cramping as mild to moderate.

If general anesthesia is used, you will probably receive a sedative injection about an hour before you are taken to the operating room. The injection will make you feel very sleepy and relaxed. During the procedure itself you will feel nothing since you will be asleep.

After you wake up you will feel drowsy for several hours. For a day or two after the procedure you may notice some tiredness and some general aches and pains (the aftereffects of the anesthetic) and a mild sore throat (the result of the endotracheal tube). Throat lozenges and warm salt-water gargling may help with the sore throat.

### Risks:

The risks of this procedure include perforation of the uterus or tearing of the cervix (both extremely rare) and prolonged bleeding after the test. There is also a small chance of infection.

If done in the early stages of pregnancy, this procedure can produce abortion. If there is any chance you might be pregnant, a pregnancy test will usually be done before the procedure.

If general anesthesia is used, there is a small but significant risk of death from complications of anesthesia (see p. 465).

You should discuss the risks in your particular situation with your doctor.

### Results:

Results are usually available in about one week.

Abnormal vaginal bleeding may be due to polyps, endometrial cancer, or other causes. This test will usually determine the cause of such bleeding.

In addition to its use in diagnosis, a D & C is sometimes used to treat certain types of abnormal vaginal bleeding.

If done to investigate infertility, this test can usually determine whether the uterine lining is being properly stimulated by the hormones estrogen and progesterone to allow implantation of a fertilized egg.

### Cost:
Endometrial biopsy: $60 to $80
D & C: $300 to $500

### Special Considerations:
★*Vabra Aspiration*: In this procedure a suction device is inserted into the uterus, and a sample of endometrial tissue is withdrawn for analysis. This can be done as an office procedure and usually does not require anesthesia. You may feel some cramping as the instrument is inserted and as the sample is removed.

# Breast Self-Examination

Breast cancer is the leading cause of cancer death in American women, with over 37,000 deaths per year. It is estimated that nearly 1 in 11 women will develop breast cancer at some time in her life. Unfortunately, the causes of breast cancer are not known, so it is not clear how it can be prevented. However, it can often be treated successfully if detected early, before the cancer spreads.

Over 90% of all breast cancers are first discovered by women themselves, often by accident. Breast self-examination (BSE) is a simple technique that helps women get to know their breasts so that they can notice changes which may indicate early breast cancer.

Several studies suggest that women who practice BSE are more likely to discover breast cancers when chances of cure are significantly higher. In fact, one study estimated that regular breast self-examination might reduce breast cancer deaths by nearly one quarter. It's simple, quick and convenient, and may save your life.

BSE is not a substitute for regular breast examinations by a nurse or doctor and x-ray examinations (mammography, see p. 189). However, professional exams on a yearly basis are not enough. Only by doing regular BSE can you develop a sense of what is normal for your breasts. Then if you notice a change you can seek further professional help.

### Why Performed:
Breast cancer can occur at any age, though it is more common in women over 40. Monthly breast self-examination is recommended for women starting in their teens and continuing throughout their lives. Though breast cancer is very rare in men, occasional BSE by men may be helpful in detecting early, more curable cancers.

### Procedure:
The best time to examine your breasts is usually a week after the start of your menstrual period. At this time your breasts are likely to be less swollen and easier to examine. If your menses are irregular or have stopped due to menopause or a hysterectomy, just pick one day that is easy to remember each month. Many women choose the first day of the month. Others choose a day that has the same number as their birthday. The important thing is to do BSE once a month, every month.

BSE consists of three parts:

1. *Breast exam in the bath or shower.* While sitting or standing, place one arm over your head and lightly soap your breast on that side. Then using the flat surface of your fingers (not the fingertips), gently

move your hand over your breast, feeling carefully for any lumps or thickening.

2. *Observing your breasts in a mirror.* Stand in front of a mirror with good lighting. View your breasts carefully, first with your hands at your sides, then with hands raised high above your head, and finally with your hands pushing firmly on your hips to contract the chest muscles. Compare the right and left breasts in each maneuver, noting any flattening or bulging on one side but not the other, any puckering or dimpling of the skin, or any distortions of the nipples. Squeeze each nipple gently between the thumb and index finger, and look for a discharge.

3. *Breast exam lying down.* Lie down and place a small pillow or folded towel under your right shoulder and place your right arm above your head. This distributes the breast tissue more evenly on the chest, making it easier to examine. Using the flat portion of the first three or four fingers of your left hand, begin to feel the right breast by pressing firmly on a spot. Then move your whole hand slowly in small circular motions so that the breast tissue slides back and forth under your fingers. You must press firmly to feel all the breast tissue between your skin and chest wall. Focus your full attention on your fingers as you begin to systematically examine your entire breast.

One way to ensure you cover the whole breast is to imagine your breast is the face of a clock. Starting at the top of the outer edge of your breast at 12 o'clock, move slowly to 1 o'clock and so on around the breast back to 12. Then move an inch toward the nipple and circle the breast again, and another inch—and so on, until reaching the nipple. Slide your fingers from one area to another without picking up your hand. Don't forget to feel under the nipple and in the armpit. You can use any pattern you like, but be sure not to skip any areas

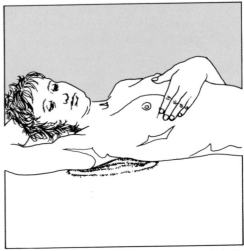

**Breast Self-Exam.** *With one arm extended all areas of the breast are carefully examined for lumps with the fingers of the opposite hand.*

and pay special attention to the area between the nipple and the armpit, the most common location of tumors. Then move the pillow to the left and repeat the procedure using the right hand to examine the left breast.

The next time you have your breasts examined by a health professional, ask to have your BSE technique observed and, if necessary, corrected. Some health professionals have rubber breast models which contain examples of what breast lumps may feel like. Immediately after you have been checked by a health professional is a good time to go home and repeat the BSE technique, and do it every day for a month or so until you can form a clear mental picture of what is normal for you. Some women even draw a picture of their breasts to help remember any areas which are different or difficult to examine. Don't be discouraged. It takes some practice.

## Results:

Every woman's breasts are different. That's why it is so important to know your own breasts so that you can report changes. One of your breasts is likely to be larger than the other. This is normal. You may also notice that your breasts change throughout the menstrual cycle. You'll often notice increased swelling and tenderness before your menses start.

If you notice new wrinkling or dimpling of the skin, retraction of the nipple, or puckering of the breast on one side, report this to your health professional. If you see a red scaling rash or sore on your nipple, have this checked as well.

As you are examining your breasts you may find a crescent of firm tissue in the lower curve of the breast below the nipple. This is normal. If you find a lump, don't panic. Remember, 8 out of 10 lumps are not cancer. A lump is most often either a small cyst or a fibroadenoma, which is noncancerous. Still, any new lump should be checked without delay by a health professional. Don't expect a lump to be the size of an egg; most often lumps are pea-sized. You may notice certain areas that feel grainy, stringy, or thickened. Have these areas checked by a health professional. Most often they are normal, but you should become intimately familiar with these areas so that you can notice any change.

If you notice a nipple discharge, note the color and consistency. A clear or milky discharge may be due to nursing, breast stimulation, hormones, or many other causes. A bloody discharge may be a benign growth or breast cancer. Discuss any discharge with a health professional.

If an abnormality is found, your doctor may recommend observation, with reexamination in several weeks, a mammogram (p. 189), or a breast biopsy or aspiration (p. 193).

## Special Considerations:

★A new type of home screening device known as a Breast Cancer Screening Indicator (BCSI) has recently been developed. It consists of two round pads which you wear inside your bra for 15 minutes once a month. The pads contain chemical heat sensors which change color depending upon the temperature of the underlying breast tissue. "Hot" spots may indicate a growing tumor or other breast disease which will need further evaluation. The product will be marketed by Faberge and sold for approximately $10 for two sets of pads. The pads are not reusable. Studies are currently under way to determine the accuracy and usefulness of this breast cancer screening approach.

# Mammogram

A mammogram is an x-ray picture of the breasts (mammary glands) used to evaluate breast symptoms or to search for early signs of breast cancer. Cancer of the breast is the most common cancer in women. Nearly 1 in 11 women will develop breast cancer during her lifetime. Many of the more than 37,000 women who die each year from breast cancer in the United States alone could have been saved if the cancer had been detected earlier.

Early detection of breast cancer is best accomplished by a combination of monthly breast self-examination (see p. 187), periodic physical examination by a trained professional, and mammography. More than one third of small cancers can be seen on a mammogram before they can be felt by the patient or a doctor. These early or "minimal" cancers can be cured 95% of the time, so early detection of breast cancer is critical.

There are two basic types of mammography: *Film-screen mammography* and *xeromammography.* Film-screen mammography detects the x-rays transmitted through the breast on a fluorescent screen and records the image on an x-ray film. In xeromammography the x-rays are recorded on an electrostatically charged x-ray plate and then transferred onto a special paper as a blue-on-white photographic print. The lower-radiation-dose film-screen mammograms are more commonly used.

**Why Performed:**

If you have symptoms of breast disease such as a lump, nipple discharge, new retraction of the nipple, dimpling of the skin on one area of the breast, or persistent breast pain, a mammogram may be helpful in determining the cause of the symptoms.

However, there is some controversy and honest disagreement on when and how often women *without symptoms* should have screening mammograms to look for early breast cancer.

The American Cancer Society now recommends a single baseline mammogram for women between the ages of 35–40, screening yearly or every two years for ages 40–49, and then every year for women over the age of 50.

The National Cancer Institute has stated that high-risk women "may consider mammography as an annual procedure." High-risk women include all women over the age of 50, women over 40 with a history of premenopausal breast cancer in the family (mother, sister, or grandmother), or women over 35 who have already developed cancer in one breast.

The American College of Radiology now recommends mammograms every 1–2 years for women over the age of 40.

Another approach recommends screening mammograms on a yearly basis primarily for those women at increased risk for breast cancer or with large or lumpy breasts which are difficult to evaluate by self-exam or professional physical examination. Factors increasing the risk of breast cancer include previous history of breast cancer, family history of breast cancer in mother or sister, and no history of childbearing or a first child after the age of 35.

We suggest you discuss with your doctor when and how often to have a mammogram.

**Preparation:**

Tell your doctor if you might be pregnant or are breast-feeding.

You will have to undress from the waist up and wear a gown for this x-ray exam. On the day of the exam do not use any deodorant, perfume, powders, or ointments under your arm or on your breasts. Residue from these substances on your skin can obscure the mammograms.

Before the exam remove any jewelry from your neck.

**Procedure:**

Mammograms are done in an x-ray department of a hospital, clinic, or doctor's office. The films are made by a radiology technician and interpreted by a radiologist.

After undressing from the waist up, you will be asked to take a sitting, standing, or lying position for the x-rays, depending upon the type of equipment used. One breast at a time is examined. Your breast will rest on a flat surface which contains the x-ray plate, and a device called a compressor will be pressed firmly against your breast to help flatten out the breast tissue. You may be asked to lift your arm or use your hand to hold your other breast out of the way. For a few seconds while the picture is being taken, you will be asked to hold your breath. Usually two pictures are made of each breast—one from the top and one from the side. Then the procedure is repeated for the other breast.

The exam itself usually takes about 10–15 minutes. You may be asked to wait a few minutes while the films are developed and checked to see if they are satisfactory or if repeat films are needed.

## How Does It Feel?

At first it may feel cold when you place your breast on the x-ray table or plate. When the compression device is pressed against your breast this is usually moderately uncomfortable.

*Patient Comments*:

"The mammogram only hurt a bit when my breasts were pressed against the tray. I was slightly embarrassed sitting there with my breasts exposed, but the technician was understanding and tried to respect my privacy."

## Risks:

Several years ago there was great concern about the risks of developing cancer from the radiation of mammography itself. However, the newer x-ray techniques have dramatically reduced the radiation exposure. The risk of developing breast cancer from mammography remains theoretical and, at worst, is exceedingly low. For example, it has been estimated that the risk of dying from a mammogram appears to be no greater than that of traveling in a car for 300 miles or riding a bicycle for 10 miles. For most women the risk of dying from an undetected breast cancer is far greater. Therefore, we feel that the benefits of routine mammography far outweigh the unproven risks.

Because a fetus is more sensitive to radiation exposure, routine mammography should be avoided if you are pregnant. However, if you have breast abnormalities that must be checked, single views can be performed with abdominal shielding by lead apron. Also mammography is usually not performed in breast-feeding women since the breasts are engorged and the x-rays are more difficult to interpret.

## Results:

Your mammograms will be read by a radiologist. It requires special training and a great deal of experience to accurately interpret the subtleties of mammography. If the reading is questionable, or suggests a cancer, sometimes it is helpful to get a second opinion. Many radiologists will automatically request another opinion from a colleague.

The mammogram will be examined carefully for masses, calcifications, or distortion of the normal breast architecture. A well-outlined, discrete spot on a mammogram suggests a benign (noncancerous) lesion such as a cyst. An irregular, poorly outlined, dense area with fine calcium deposits (microcalcifications) suggests a cancer.

A mammogram usually reveals about 90%–95% of all breast cancers. However, that means between 5% and 10% of cancers could be missed. Therefore, mammography should be combined with a careful physical examination of the breasts as well as monthly breast self-examination. Even if the mammogram is "normal," suspicious breast lumps should be aspirated or biopsied (see p. 193) for a definite diagnosis.

Some mammograms are very difficult to interpret. This is particularly true in younger women with dense, glandular breasts.

**Cost:**

$80 to $160 (may be less in specially designed breast screening centers). Although many health insurance programs do not cover screening tests, most will pay for mammography if specifically ordered by your physician to "rule out" breast cancer.

**Special Considerations:**

★Mammography is the most accurate clinical test for breast cancer. Other techniques are under investigation but do not currently offer the accuracy necessary for routine breast cancer screening. *Thermography* involves measuring the heat given off by different areas of the breast. A cancer usually gives off more heat than normal breast tissue due to the increased metabolic activity and blood supply. *Ultrasound* (see next test) creates images of the breast tissue from sound waves directed into the breast. This technique is sometimes helpful in determining whether a breast lump is a fluid-filled cyst or a solid tumor. *Transillumination* or *diaphanography* is an experimental technique which shines a bright light through the breast tissue to detect abnormalities.

# Breast Ultrasound

In this test a small instrument (transducer) which emits high-frequency sound waves is passed back and forth over the breasts. A microphone on the transducer picks up the sound waves as they are reflected back from the tissues within the breasts. This information is processed by a computer, and an image of the inside of the breasts and the adjacent structures is displayed on a TV screen.

**Why Performed:**

This test is most frequently done to help determine whether a breast lump is cancerous. It is also used to aid in the diagnosis of other diseases of the breast.

Lumps that increase and decrease in size over the course of your menstrual period are more likely to be noncancerous. They are usually due to cystic breast disease. Cystic lumps are also more likely to be painful, especially just before menstruation.

Cancerous lumps are more likely to remain unchanged during menstruation. They tend to be nontender and are more likely to occur in the upper, outer portion of the breast.

This test is often especially effective in evaluating small lumps and lumps close to the chest wall and in examining the denser breast tissue of younger women.

This test is not considered as accurate as mammography (see preceding test) and is therefore not recommended as a screening test. It is used as an adjunct to mammography.

**Preparation:**

You will be asked to undress from the waist up and to put on a hospital gown. Remove all jewelry from your neck.

**Procedure:**

A small ultrasound transducer will be passed back and forth over your breasts. You may be asked to lie on your stomach with your breasts immersed in a warm water bath, or a water-filled chamber may be lowered over your breasts while further scans are done. The procedure varies at different hospitals and clinics. Ask your doctor how the test will be performed at the facility where you will have the test.

## How Does It Feel?

You should feel no discomfort. If you are asked to immerse your breasts in a water bath, you may find the water somewhat cool.

## Risks:

There is no known risk of this test.

## Results:

This test can usually distinguish between a solid lump (tumor) and a fluid-filled (cystic) lump. It cannot usually distinguish a benign tumor from a cancerous tumor; breast biopsy (see next test) may be needed to do this.

## Cost:

$80 to $100

# Breast Biopsy and Aspiration

In a breast biopsy a small sample of breast tissue is removed and examined under a microscope for signs of cancer. There are two kinds of breast biopsy: *open biopsy*, a surgical procedure in which an incision is made and the entire lump or slice of it is removed, and *needle biopsy*, in which a core of tissue is removed from the lump by a needle inserted through the skin.

In *needle aspiration* a needle is inserted into a lump or cyst to remove any fluid that may be present.

## Why Performed:

This test may be indicated if a lump in your breast is discovered. Most lumps are first detected by a woman herself.

Some lumpiness of the breasts is normal. Fibrocystic breasts have many soft, fluid-filled lumpy areas which tend to enlarge and become tender just before menstruation and to shrink or disappear when your period is finished.

Needle aspiration is sometimes used to determine whether a lump is filled with fluid (such a lump is called a *cyst*). If it is, aspiration will frequently make it disappear completely. If little or no fluid is obtained by aspiration, a biopsy may be recommended.

Breast biopsy is most frequently done to determine whether a breast lump is due to cancer. Lumps produced by cancers are often painless, nontender, harder and more irregular in shape and are not affected by the menstrual cycle. Other suspicious signs include persistently inflamed areas of the breast and a bloody discharge from the nipple. For more information on breast lumps see breast self-examination, p. 187.

Breast biopsies are sometimes performed when a suspicious area is seen on a mammogram (see p. 189). Even if a mammogram is normal, a biopsy is usually necessary to rule out cancer if a lump or other symptoms are present.

## Preparation:

Tell your doctor if

You have allergies to any drugs or anesthetics

You are taking any medications

You have had bleeding problems

You might be pregnant

You will be asked to sign a consent form authorizing this procedure. Use this opportunity to discuss with your doctor any concerns you may have about the need for the test, the risks of the test, or how it will be performed. In some open biopsies, some women may choose to have a mastectomy performed at once if the lump turns out to be cancer. A full, frank discussion of all possibilities well in advance of the test is most desirable.

*Needle Aspiration*: No special preparation is needed.

*Biopsy*: If your biopsy will be performed with local anesthetic, no special preparation is needed.

If general anesthesia is used, you should not eat or drink anything for 8–12 hours before the test. If your stomach is empty there is less risk of vomiting and complications. Pretest blood and urine studies and a chest x-ray may be required. You will be asked to take nothing by mouth beginning at midnight on the night before the test is to be done. If you are taking medications, ask your doctor whether to continue them.

**Procedure:**

*Needle Aspiration*: The sample is usually collected by a physician in a doctor's office. You will be asked to remove all clothing above the waist and to lie on a padded examining table.

The area over the lump is cleaned with an antiseptic solution. Local anesthetic is sometimes used. Your doctor steadies the lump between two fingers, inserts the needle, removes any fluid that may be present, and then checks to see whether the lump has disappeared. The needle is removed and a bandage is applied.

This procedure takes less than 5 minutes.

*Needle Biopsy*: This is usually done by a physician in the doctor's office. You will be asked to remove all clothing above the waist and to sit or lie with your hands at your sides. Your doctor will cleanse the biopsy site, inject a local anesthetic, and then insert a needle through the skin and into the tissue to be biopsied. The needle is then withdrawn and the sample is placed in a specimen bottle and sent to the laboratory. Pressure is applied to the biopsy site to help stop the bleeding, and a bandage is applied.

This procedure takes 5–10 minutes.

*Open Biopsy*: This test is usually done under general anesthesia (see p. 465) in an operating room by a surgeon, an anesthesiologist, and one or more assistants. A sedative medication is usually given by injection about an hour before the procedure begins. An intravenous (IV) line will be placed in a vein, usually in your arm.

During the procedure you will be given a mixture of anesthetic gases and oxygen through a hollow endotracheal tube, which is inserted through your mouth into the airway (trachea) which leads to your lungs.

After you are anesthetized, the surgeon makes an incision with a scalpel and carefully dissects the surrounding tissue away until the lump is revealed. The surgeon may then remove either the entire lump (excision biopsy or "lumpectomy") or just a part of it (incision biopsy).

The size, location, and appearance of the lump will determine which procedure will be used. Be sure to discuss all possibilities—including the possibility of mastectomy if the lump turns out to be cancer—with your surgeon in advance. The wound is then closed with stitches, and a bandage is applied.

This procedure usually takes 30–45 minutes. After the biopsy is completed, you will be taken to the recovery room and observed until you are fully awake and your gag reflex has recovered. You can then return to your hospital room.

You can resume your regular diet at once, and by the next day you can begin normal acitivities. You may choose to wear a bra or not after this test, whichever makes you more comfortable.

### How Does It Feel?

With a needle aspiration done under local anesthesia you will feel only a small sting when the anesthetic is injected. If anesthesia is not used, you will feel a sharp, brief sting when the aspiration needle is inserted.

In the needle biopsy, you will feel a small sting from the needle used to introduce the local anesthetic, and may feel some pressure when the biopsy needle is inserted.

After an incision biopsy you may notice a temporary bruising of the skin around the incision.

You may experience aching and tenderness at the biopsy site for about 2 days (needle biopsy) to one week (open biopsy). If the pain persists or is accompanied by redness, discharge, or fever, notify your doctor.

### Risks:

There is a very slight chance of infection. This can usually be treated with antibiotics. If a general anesthetic is used, there is a small but significant risk of death from complications of anesthesia (see p. 465).

A needle aspiration or biopsy usually leaves no scar. An open biopsy will leave a small scar. The scar almost always fades and becomes less noticeable in 6–12 months after the operation.

### Results:

In needle aspiration, the fluid may be withdawn from a cyst, causing the lump to immediately disappear. Occasionally the fluid in the cyst may reaccumulate and the lump will return.

If a frozen section is performed (see p. 344), the results will be available within an hour. Otherwise, the results of the biopsy will be available within 2–3 days.

About 80% of all breast lumps are not cancerous. The most common benign (noncancerous) findings are normal breast tissue, fibrocystic lumps, and fibroadenoma. The most common breast cancer is adenocarcinoma. If cancer is found you will need to discuss treatment alternatives with your doctor.

In a needle biopsy, there is a slight chance that a cancer may be missed. Also, the specimen is occasionally found to be inadequate and the procedure must be repeated.

### Cost:

Needle aspiration: $50 to $75
Needle biopsy: $70 to $100
Open biopsy: $400 to $800

### Special Considerations:

★*Estrogen and Progesterone Receptor Assays*: Some breast cancers are responsive to treatment with hormone manipulation (e.g., removal of ovaries, pituitary or adrenal glands, or antiestrogen drugs). To determine which tumors are more likely to respond to this type of treatment, estrogen and progesterone receptors can be measured in the biopsy specimens.

# Fertility Awareness

Fertility awareness, also known as natural family planning, involves observing your body to determine when you are likely to be fertile. This knowledge can help you avoid pregnancy, but can also help you plan intercourse to increase your chances of getting pregnant.

A woman is usually fertile for about 5 days each month around the middle of her menstrual cycle. At this time, an egg is released from an ovary (ovulation), and if it is not fertilized by a sperm, the menstrual period will normally start 14 days later. The key is determining exactly when the egg will be released.

There are four basic methods for detecting ovulation:

*Rhythm or Calendar Method*: With this method you predict the time of ovulation based on a record of your previous menstrual cycles. An estimate is made on which days you are likely to be fertile.

*Basal Body Temperature (BBT) Method*: The lowest temperature that a healthy person typically achieves during the day is known as the basal body temperature (BBT). In most women, due to the natural cyclic changes in female hormones, basal body temperature falls slightly just before ovulation and then rises just after ovulation. By carefully measuring your BBT every morning before getting out of bed and recording it on a chart, you may be able to estimate the time of ovulation.

*Mucus Method*: The amount, texture, and appearance of the mucus found in the vagina changes throughout the menstrual cycle. Before ovulation the mucus is scant, thick, cloudy, and slightly sticky, whereas just before and during ovulation the mucus produced by the cervix (the opening to the uterus) becomes abundant, elastic and stretchy (see later), slippery, thin, and clear. By observing and recording the character of the mucus over several cycles, you can more accurately predict when ovulation occurs. The systematic observation of cervical mucus is sometimes known as the Billings Method.

*Combined (Symptothermal) Method*: In this approach you measure basal body temperature, assess cervical mucus, and also observe for other signs of ovulation such as breast tenderness, abdominal pain, and changes in mood around the time of ovulation.

## Why Performed:

Fertility awareness can be used as a form of birth control or as a means to increase the chances of becoming pregnant. Some couples use these methods as a form of natural birth control because of religious or personal beliefs. Others prefer it because they feel it has fewer side effects than drugs, surgery, or mechanical devices. Still others like the increased awareness and knowledge about how the female reproductive cycle functions.

Fertility awareness when used for birth control is not without problems. It's not very effective if you have irregular menstrual cycles or inconsistent basal body temperature charts. It also requires considerable effort to learn the method as well as three or more months of diligent observation and record keeping before it can be used for birth control. Fertility awareness for birth control also requires that you either abstain from vaginal intercourse or use some other method of birth control during the fertile days. And, as with other methods of birth control, even when the method is practiced carefully, unwanted pregnancies can occur (see discussion later on the effectiveness of birth control methods).

## Equipment:

Basal body temperature is measured by a special type of thermometer (basal body temperature or ovulation thermometer), which has more gradations (tenths of degrees) to allow more precise measurements than an ordinary thermometer. These thermometers are available in most pharmacies or family planning clinics for about $3–$7 and often come with calendar charts and directions. Basal body temperature thermometers are also available by mail for about $8 from the Self-Care Catalog, Box 999, Pt. Reyes, CA 94956.

An electronic thermometer linked to a minicomputer has recently been developed. It records your daily temperature, compares it with your basal body temperature pattern and then flashes a green light when the "safe," nonfertile period has been reached. It sells for about $100 and is also available from the Self-Care Catalog.

## Procedure:

*Basal Body Temperature (BBT) Method*: Take your temperature using a special ovulation thermometer every morning for several months and record the temperature on a chart or graph (see sample chart p.198). The temperature may be taken orally or rectally, but be sure to use the same site each day. Always take your temperature just after awakening and before smoking, eating, drinking, or beginning any activity. Leave the thermometer in place for a full 5 minutes. Shake down the thermometer after each use. Don't wait until the next morning to shake it down. Even the activity of shaking can alter your basal temperature.

*Mucus Method*: Each day insert one finger into the vagina and note the amount of mucus, its color, and thickness or thinness. In addition, you should test the "stretchiness" of the mucus (technically known as *spinnbarkeit*) by stretching a drop of the mucus between your index finger and thumb. Note how long a strand of mucus you can make before it breaks, and record this along with the other observations on your calendar.

*Combined (Symptothermal) Method*: In addition to recording your BBT and cervical mucus observations, each day note the presence of red or brown vaginal spotting, pain in the lower abdomen, breast tenderness, swelling or fullness of the va-

ginal lips (vulva), abdominal bloating, and increased sexual interest.

## Results:

In general, it is possible to become pregnant for a period of 5 days each month. This includes 2 days before ovulation, since sperm can survive in the female reproductive tract for at least 48 hours. The fertile period also includes 2 days after ovulation during which the egg can be fertilized.

*Basal Body Temperature (BBT)*: Your basal body temperature usually drops 0.4 degree or more below your normal temperature a day or so before ovulation and then rises 0.4 degree or more above your baseline temperature and stays elevated until just before your menstrual period begins. Since the classic rise in your BBT doesn't occur until *after* ovulation, if you have intercourse just before or during ovulation, you may become pregnant. If you do not wish to become pregnant, you should avoid intercourse (or use a back-up form of birth control) from the end of the menstrual period until three days after ovulation. You can assume your fertile days are over only when your temperature has risen and remained elevated for three full days. Temperatures on these three days should be consistently higher than on any of the previous days in that cycle.

Unfortunately, many women do not show this classic temperature pattern, making prediction of ovulation much more difficult. You should keep BBT temperature charts for at least three monthly cycles to determine your typical pattern before using this as a birth control method. Many factors can influence the accuracy of the charts. Illness (especially with fever), drug use (aspirin, alcohol, birth control pills), sleeplessness, emotional upset, travel, and stress can all upset the BBT pattern.

The effectiveness of any birth control

## Basal Temperature Guide and Mucus Chart

*Dates of this cycle* September 20 *through* October 21     *Number of days in this cycle* 32

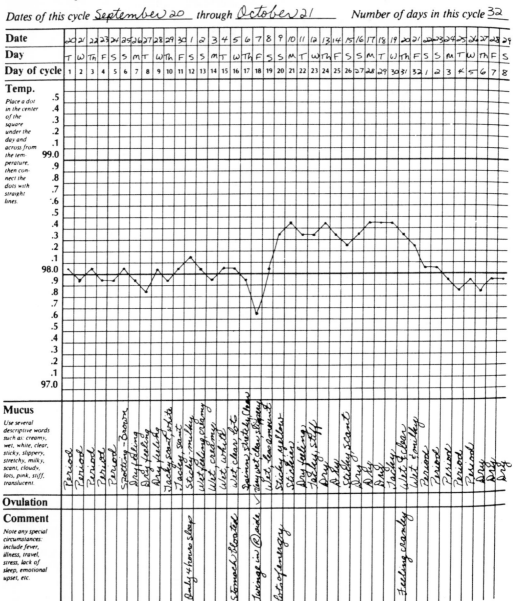

# Basal Temperature Guide and Mucus Chart

*Dates of this cycle* _____ *through* _____ *Number of days in this cycle* ____

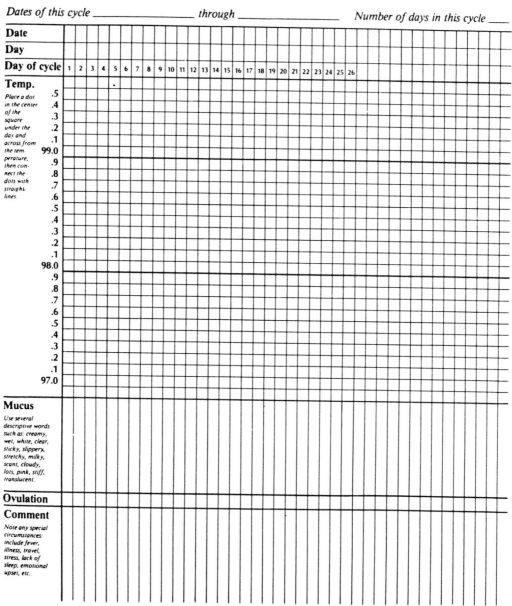

| Date | | | | | | | | | | | | | | | | | | | | | | | | | | |
|---|---|---|---|---|---|---|---|---|---|---|---|---|---|---|---|---|---|---|---|---|---|---|---|---|---|---|
| **Day** | | | | | | | | | | | | | | | | | | | | | | | | | | |
| **Day of cycle** | 1 | 2 | 3 | 4 | 5 | 6 | 7 | 8 | 9 | 10 | 11 | 12 | 13 | 14 | 15 | 16 | 17 | 18 | 19 | 20 | 21 | 22 | 23 | 24 | 25 | 26 |

**Temp.**

*Place a dot in the center of the square under the day and across from the temperature, then connect the dots with straight lines.*

.5
.4
.3
.2
.1
99.0
.9
.8
.7
.6
.5
.4
.3
.2
.1
98.0
.9
.8
.7
.6
.5
.4
.3
.2
.1
97.0

**Mucus**

*Use several descriptive words such as: creamy, wet, white, clear, sticky, slippery, stretchy, milky, scant, cloudy, lots, pink, stiff, translucent.*

**Ovulation**

**Comment**

*Note any special circumstances: include fever, illness, travel, stress, lack of sleep, emotional upset, etc.*

method is usually expressed as the percentage of women who do not get pregnant during one year of use of the given method. When BBT is used as the sole method of birth control it has been shown to be 80%–93% effective. If vaginal intercourse occurs only after the temperature pattern clearly indicates that the fertile days are over, the effectiveness is 93%–99%. For comparison, the effectiveness of the rhythm or calendar method is about 70%.

*Mucus Method*: Before ovulation cervical mucus tends to be very scant, cloudy, whitish to yellow, and slightly sticky. Just before ovulation the mucus tends to become abundant, clear, slippery, and stretchy, resembling raw egg white. At the time of ovulation your cervical mucus will usually stretch more than an inch, sometimes several inches, between your fingers. For birth control, avoid vaginal intercourse or use another birth control method as soon as you notice a thinning and stretchiness of your vaginal mucus until a full three days after the peak ovulatory mucus changes are noted. The safest days for unprotected intercourse are from the fourth day after these mucus changes through the menstrual period. Therefore, for added safety you may wish to use an alternative form of birth control from the end of the menstrual period until three days after the cervical mucus changes.

Some women do not follow this typical pattern of cervical mucus change. As with basal body temperatures, you should record at least three or four cycles to establish a pattern before using this as a method of birth control. Vaginal lubrication, spermicides (jelly, foam, or cream), douching, vaginal infections with discharge, and semen can interfere with the proper interpretation of cervical mucus. When cervical mucus observation is used as the sole means of birth control, it is usually about 80% ef-

fective. However, in one study when intercourse was avoided until three days after a clear indication of ovulation, the effectiveness approached 99%.

*Symptothermal Method*: Many women experience symptoms such as spotting, breast tenderness, vulvar fullness, abdominal bloating, sharp twinges of lower abdominal pain, and increased libido around the time of ovulation. The abdominal pain, known as *mittelschmerz* ("midcycle pain"), is a sharp one in the right or left side of the lower abdomen, felt as the egg is released from the ovary. When these symptoms are combined with BBT and cervical mucus observation to determine ovulation, the effectiveness of birth control is nearly 99%, provided no unprotected intercourse occurs until several days after ovulation, but drops to 80%–93% if intercourse occurs both before and after ovulation.

Remember, sperm can survive inside the female reproductive tract for 48 hours or longer. Therefore, if you have unprotected intercourse a day or two before ovulation and only abstain after you notice your temperature drop or your cervical mucus change, it may be too late to prevent pregnancy.

If you are trying to get pregnant, fertility awareness can help. A characteristic drop and then rise in BBT or the cervical mucus changes provide indirect evidence that ovulation is occurring (see Fertility Testing, p. 201). Couples wanting pregnancy should have intercourse every day or every other day from the 9th day after the start of the menstrual period until three days after the BBT elevation or peak cervical mucus changes to maximize the opportunities for fertilization.

### Special Considerations:

★We strongly recommend that if you plan to use these methods for birth control, you receive more complete instruction and demonstration from a trained instructor. For more information, see the books listed in the appendix (p. 474), contact your doctor, nurse practitioner, family planning clinic, or write to The Couple to Couple League, P.O. Box 11084, Cincinnati, Ohio 42511, or Natural Family Planning Federation of America, 1221 Massachusetts Ave., NW, Washington, D.C. 20005.

★Cervical mucus can also be tested for the presence of glucose (sugar), which increases at the time of ovulation. A sample of cervical mucus is collected on a fingertip and then touched to a strip of yellow TesTape (available without prescription from most pharmacies). The tape turns dark blue at the time of ovulation and lighter shades of blue and green before ovulation. Cervical mucus will also, at the time of ovulation, develop a branching pattern like a fern when examined under a low-power microscope. Again, these methods alone are not considered reliable but may be used in combination with the others.

★Several new products are being developed to improve the ease and accuracy of fertility awareness. One instrument measures the viscosity of the cervical mucus. Another device, an impedometer, measures the electrical conductivity of the vagina, which changes at the time of ovulation. OvuSTICK (by Monoclonal Antibodies, Inc.) is a new test designed to detect hormone changes in the urine which signal ovulation.

# Fertility Testing

About one in five couples have difficulty conceiving. Problems with the male or female reproductive systems, or both, may be the cause. The most common causes of female infertility include incorrect timing of intercourse, blocked fallopian tubes, vaginal or cervical disorders, hormone imbalances, problems of the ovaries, emotional factors, drugs, and radiation exposure. Tests can be performed to determine which of the factors, if any, is involved.

**Why Performed:**
These tests are normally performed only after a couple have been having unprotected intercourse for at least 12 months without conceiving. If the woman is over 30, the evaluation may be performed after 6 months instead.

**Procedure:**
Before these tests are done you will be asked to give a complete medical history and will have a complete physical exam, including a pelvic exam.
● *First Phase*
*Semen Analysis* (p. 221)—Determines the number, structure, and movement of sperm.

*Postcoital Test*—This test is done a day or two before a woman's expected day of ovulation. The couple has intercourse the day of the exam. No lubricants should be used, and the woman should not douche. Immediately afterward the woman goes to a clinic or doctor's office for a pelvic examination. A sample of the cervical mucus is taken and examined under the microscope.

The number and movement of the sperm in the cervical mucus are examined. A certain number (10 or more per high-power field) of active sperm cells should be seen. If sperm cells have not reached the cervix, you and your partner may wish to discuss appropriate sexual techniques and positions with your doctor. If the sperm are present but not active, it may indicate a problem in the cervical environment.

The mucus itself is also examined. At ovulation, cervical mucus is normally abundant, watery, elastic, and clear. When spread on a glass slide, it dries in a fern pattern. When you are not ovulating the mucus is scant, sticky, and cloudy and does not dry in a fern pattern.

*Blood Tests*—May reveal a hormone imbalance, infection, or other problem. These may include a complete blood count (p. 61), test for syphilis (p. 144), blood type and Rh factor (p. 53), thyroid function tests (p. 108), progesterone, (p. 94), prolactin (p. 95), FSH (p. 76), and LH (p. 88).

*Basal Body Temperature* (p. 195)—Can help determine if a normal ovulatory cycle is present.

● *Second Phase*

*Hysterosalpingogram* (below)—Can help determine if the uterus and fallopian tubes are healthy and whether the fallopian tubes are blocked.

*Endometrial Biopsy* (p. 185)—Can determine if the lining of the uterus is responding appropriately to hormones.

● *Third Phase*

*Laparoscopy* (p. 325)—Used to check for scar tissue around the tubes and ovaries and for endometriosis, abnormal growths of uterine tissue in the abdominal cavity.

*Hysteroscopy*—Used to look inside the uterus to examine the uterine lining.

# Hysterosalpingogram

This test is most frequently done when a woman has questions about her ability to have children. Infections of the pelvic or-

gans can produce severe scarring of the fallopian tubes. This scarring can close both tubes, thus blocking the normal path by which the female egg passes into the uterus. If this happens, fertilization cannot occur.

In this test a dye which shows up on x-ray is injected through the cervix into the uterus, and up into the fallopian tubes. X-rays are then taken. The x-rays usually show any abnormality that might block the egg's passage into the uterus. They also show any abnormalities on the inside of the uterus which might prevent implantation of the fertilized egg.

**Why Performed:**

This procedure is one of a number of tests performed to evaluate infertility in women. It is also sometimes done to investigate suspected problems of the lining of the uterus, to determine the cause of repeated miscarriages or of excessively painful menstruation. It is sometimes performed before surgery, to give the surgeon a good idea of the anatomy of the region, or after surgery to evaluate the result.

**Preparation:**

Tell your doctor if

You have allergies to x-ray contrast material or to any medications

You are taking any medications

You might be pregnant

You may be asked to fast for several hours before the test; check with your doctor for specific instructions. You may be offered a mild sedative such as diazepam (Valium) to help you relax.

You may be asked to sign a consent form authorizing this procedure. Use this opportunity to discuss with your doctor any concerns you may have about the need for the test, the risks of the test, or how and when it will be performed.

You will be asked to remove all clothing below the waist and to put on a hospital gown. For your own comfort you should empty your bladder just before the test begins.

**Procedure:**

This test is done in a hospital x-ray department by a radiologist or gynecologist and an assistant. You will be asked to lie on your back with your legs up in stirrups in the same position as that taken for the pelvic exam. A lower abdominal x-ray is taken.

A vaginal speculum is inserted and an instrument called a tenaculum is attached to hold the cervix in place. The cervix is then cleaned, and a cannula (hollow tube) is inserted into the cervix. The x-ray contrast material (dye) is then injected through the cannula. If the fallopian tubes are normal, the contrast material will flow through them and spill into the abdominal cavity. If they are blocked by scar tissue, the contrast medium does not pass through.

The abdomen is viewed on a TV screen (fluoroscope) while the contrast medium is injected and x-rays are taken. If side views are needed, the table may be tilted, or you may be asked to change position. Another x-ray of the pelvis may be taken 24 hours later.

This test usually takes 15–30 minutes. There is no medical reason to abstain from intercourse after the test is finished.

**How Does It Feel?**

You will probably feel a cramping sensation similar to menstrual cramps. The amount and duration of discomfort vary with the condition of the fallopian tubes, the kind of contrast material used, and the pressure under which the contrast material is injected. Contrast material injected at high pressure into a blocked tube can produce severe pain which last several hours. Water-soluble contrast material may produce a short burst of pain as it spills into the abdominal cavity.

After the test some of the residual contrast material may leak out of the vagina. You may also notice a bloody vaginal discharge for several days after the test. If the discharge is very heavy (more than one tampon or menstrual pad per hour) or continues for more than 3–4 days, or if you develop a fever or extreme abdominal pain, you should notify your doctor.

*Patient Comments:* "The table was hard and cold and the position was embarrassing and uncomfortable. There was minimal pain during the test—just a brief, sharp cramping. It was fascinating to be able to watch the whole thing on the TV monitor. Afterward I could feel fluid moving around in my abdomen. I had some cramping and passed some blood for four days after the test."

**Risks:**

There is some risk (less than 1 in 100) of a pelvic infection following this test. The risk may be higher in women with a history of previous pelvic infections. If infection does occur, it can usually be managed by antibiotics.

There is some risk of damage to the uterus or fallopian tubes when the dye is injected under pressure.

When an oil-based contrast medium (such as Lipiodol) is used, there is a very slight risk of the oil getting into the bloodstream (oil emboli); this can result in a pulmonary embolism (a blockage of blood flow to a section of the lung), a very serious side effect. Adhesions (scar tissue connecting abdominal organs) can also result from the oil-based substance. Adhesions may occur with water-based contrast material as well, but these are much less common. For these reasons water-based contrast media are usually used. (Oil-based contrast materials are occasionally used because they produce less muscular spasm, and they generally produce a better-quality picture.)

There is always some concern about the effects of exposure to any radiation, including the low-level radiation of diagnostic x-rays. Extremely high levels of radiation have been shown to cause various diseases and birth defects. However, if this test is really necessary, the radiation risk is generally very low compared with the potential benefits of the test.

Compared with other x-rays, the radiation exposure from this test is low for the total body but high for the female reproductive organs. Because a developing fetus is very sensitive to radiation, this test should not be done on pregnant women. (For more on x-ray risks, see p. 227.)

The specific risks in your particular situation should be discussed with your physician.

### Results:
Your doctor will usually be able to discuss preliminary results with you immediately after the test. If contrast material reaches the abdominal cavity, this indicates that the tubes are not completely blocked. If an abnormality is found, other tests such as laparoscopy (see p. 323) may be needed to determine appropriate treatment.

### Cost:
$100 to $150

### Special Considerations:
★Most infertility specialists recommend that this test be performed in the first 10 days of the menstrual cycle. This is to avoid the possibility of doing the test on a woman who is pregnant. Doing the test within this period also reduces the risk of backflow and implantation of endometrial tissue into the abdominal cavity (endometriosis).

★Some studies suggest that having a hysterosalpingogram may actually increase a woman's chance of getting pregnant. This may be because the injection of dye dislodges mucous plugs, straightens the tubes, breaks through filmy adhesions, stimulates cervical mucus production, stimulates the action of the tubes, or suppresses infections.

# Culdocentesis

This procedure is used to check for free fluid in a woman's lower abdominal cavity (*cul-de-sac*).

### Why Performed:
This test is used to evaluate pain in a woman's lower abdomen and pelvic region, particularly when a ruptured tubal pregnancy (ectopic pregnancy) or ovarian cyst is suspected.

### Procedure:
This test is done by a physician and an assistant. You will be asked to walk or sit up for a short time before the test begins; this will encourage the drainage of fluids into the lower abdomen. You will then be asked to lie down on your back with your knees or heels resting in stirrups.

A pelvic exam will be done. The physician will then grasp the cervix with an instrument (tenaculum), lift it slightly, and insert a long, thin needle through the vaginal wall below the uterus. If fluid is found in the space behind the uterus (cul-de-sac), a sample is drawn up into the syringe. If no fluid is found, a second or third attempt may be made at a slightly different angle.

### How Does It Feel?

Many women experience an uncomfortable pulling sensation when the cervix is grasped. The insertion of the needle may cause a brief, sharp pain. Most physicians perform this procedure without anesthesia, since injecting local anesthesia may interfere with the results and may be as painful as the test itself. A sedative is sometimes given before the test.

### Risks:

There is a slight risk of inadvertently puncturing a mass, a cyst, an ectopic pregnancy, or a pregnancy in a retroverted uterus. The best safeguard against this occurrence is a careful pelvic exam before the test. If a hard, immobile mass is felt in the cul-de-sac on pelvic examination, this test should not be done.

### Results:

In about half of all culdocenteses (taps), no fluid is found. This is called a dry tap. However, a dry tap does not mean that fluid is not present. Further tests such as pelvic ultrasound (p. 307) or laparoscopy (p. 323) may be needed to make a diagnosis.

This test is used to diagnose ectopic pregnancy or tubal infections. It can also help detect ruptured ovarian cysts and ovarian cancer. If fresh blood is found, emergency surgery may be needed. If an infection is present, a culture of the fluid can suggest the appropriate treatment.

### Cost:

$50 to $100

# Fetal Ultrasound
## (Obstetric Ultrasound, B-Scan, Obstetric Sonogram)

In this test a small instrument (transducer) which emits high-frequency sound waves is passed back and forth across the abdomen a number of times. The transducer picks up the sound waves reflected from the developing baby inside the uterus. This information is processed by a computer, and an image of the baby and the uterus will be displayed on a TV screen.

### Why Performed:

This test is used to determine how old the fetus is (gestational age), to demonstrate the presence of fetal heartbeat, and to detect faster- or slower-than-normal fetal growth. It is also used to locate and evaluate the placenta (a large, flat organ to which the baby's umbilical cord is attached), to check for twins or other multiple pregnancies, and to evaluate some types of suspected birth defects.

The test can be used to confirm pregnancy, to check for ectopic pregnancy (a fetus implanted in the abdominal cavity or fallopian tubes instead of the uterus), and to detect fetal death. In addition, this test is sometimes used after childbirth to check for infection or for pieces of the placenta that were not expelled.

There is considerable disagreement among physicians about when this test should be done. It is our opinion that this test is indicated only if there is increased risk of a problem. We agree with a National Institutes of Health consensus panel, which concluded that this test should not be done routinely on all pregnant women. Panel members felt that roughly one third of pregnant women are at sufficient risk of problems of pregnancy that this test would be recommended. Such problems include a history of problem pregnancy, multiple pregnancy, decreased fetal heart rate or fetal movements, or amniocentesis test results suggesting a birth defect or fetal distress.

### Preparation:

As a full bladder is usually required, you will be asked to drink several glasses of water (about 32 ounces) about an hour before the test. You will be asked not to urinate until the test is finished. A full bladder pushes the bowel up out of the pelvic area, makes it easier to identify the surrounding structures, and ensures better transmission of the sound waves.

You will be asked to undress and to put on a hospital gown.

### Procedure:

This test is performed by a specially trained physician (radiologist or obstetrician) or an ultrasound technician. It is done in an ultrasound room in a hospital or doctor's office.

You will be asked to lie on your back on a padded examining table. The techni-

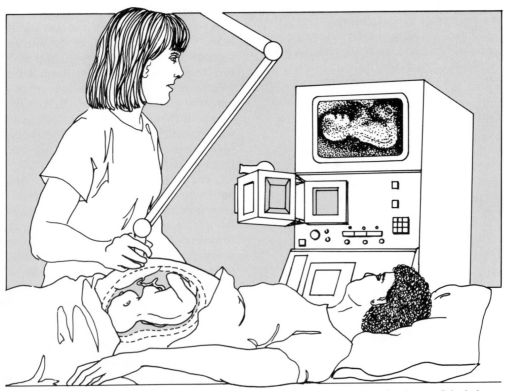

**Fetal Ultrasound.** *Sound waves are directed into the uterus, creating a "sound" picture of the baby.*

cian will apply a gel or oil to your abdomen to improve transmission of the sound waves.

The examiner will then move a transducer up and down over your abdomen a number of times and then repeat the process in a side-to-side direction. Scans at other angles may also be done. If your baby's head is deep inside your pelvis, you may be asked to lie with your head down and feet raised while additional scans are done.

The reflected sound waves will be converted to an image on a TV screen. You will probably be able to watch your baby's image. Photos of the TV image will be taken to create a permanent record.

After the test the gel will be wiped off and you will be able to return home (or to your hospital room) immediately. The test usually takes 20 minutes, but may take longer if additional scans are needed. You can urinate as soon as the test is finished.

## How Does It Feel?

The gel may be cold when it is first applied. You will hear or feel nothing at all from the sound waves. You will feel a light pressure from the transducer as it passes over your abdomen.

You will probably be aware of an uncomfortable feeling of pressure in your bladder and an urge to urinate.

If you are asked to assume the head-lowered, legs-raised position, you may find it slightly difficult to take a full breath, since your baby's weight may push upward against your lungs.

## Risks:

Many doctors consider this test to be completely harmless, and while the available evidence suggests that this may be the case, there is no absolute proof of its total safety. As with all newly introduced technologies, there is some chance that long-term effects could be discovered at a future date.

The studies that have been done show no increased risk of birth defects among babies who received ultrasound before birth. This is true even for Doppler ultrasound or Doptone (see Special Considerations), which exposes your baby to many hundreds of times the exposure used in a regular ultrasound scan.

## Results:

The radiologist may be able to provide a preliminary report during and immediately after the test. Full results should be available the next day.

*Fetal (gestational) age*—The fetal age can usually be determined to within 1 week if the exam is done before the 20th week of pregnancy, to within 1 to 2 weeks if the exam is done between the 20th and 30th weeks of pregnancy, and to within 3 to 3½ weeks if it is done after the 30th week of pregnancy.

*Confirming pregnancy*—This test can confirm pregnancy by 4–6 weeks after fertilization.

*Checking fetal growth*—This is done by comparing the size of the baby's head, limbs, and body with standard tables.

*Checking the shape and function of fetal organs*—The shape and function of your baby's bowel, heart, and bladder can be checked. The baby's breathing movements may also be seen after 30 weeks of fetal age.

*Checking the placenta*—The normal shape and development of the placenta can be checked.

*Multiple pregnancies*—The presence of twins or other multiple pregnancies can usually be determined by about the 8th week of pregnancy.

*Fetal sex*—The sex of the fetus can sometimes, but not always, be determined by about the 30th week of pregnancy. Determination of sex by this test depends on the position of the baby in the uterus.

*Birth defects*—Many, but not all, major birth defects can be detected by this test.

*Other findings*—Pelvic masses, ectopic pregnancies, and fetal death can also be detected by this test, but normal results of this test do not guarantee a normal baby.

## Cost:

$100 to $200

## Special Considerations:

★Ultrasound is done by some obstetricians in their offices. Whereas radiologists are required to have special training in ultrasound, this is not always required of obstetricians. Although some obstetricians haven taken special training and are very proficient in doing and reading these scans, others may not be.

If you feel that you may need an ultrasound examination and are considering having it performed in your obstetrician's office, make sure that your doctor has had special training in ultrasound. In addition, you should ask that a complete, not a partial, ultrasound exam be done and that a complete record of the exam, including a photograph and all interpretations of the findings, be made part of your permanent medical record.

★If your doctor suggests an ultrasound but you are not convinced that it is really needed, you should obtain a second opinion from a radiologist or an obstetrician with special training in ultrasound.

★*Doppler Ultrasound (Doptone)*—This is a limited ultrasound exam done at 10–11 weeks of fetal age by some obstetricians to be sure the fetal heart is beating. This exam is usually much less expensive than a complete ultrasound exam, but it provides less information (only whether a heartbeat is present) and exposes your baby to a quantity of ultrasound many hundreds of times that of a normal ultrasound scan. In addition, the test is performed at a period during which the baby's organs are especially vulnerable to damage. (Regular ultrasound scans are usually done later in pregnancy.)

Thus, if you are concerned about protecting your baby from the seemingly remote possibility of ultrasound-produced damage, the best precaution would seem to be avoiding Doppler ultrasound.

# Amniocentesis

All expectant parents hope for a normal healthy baby, but 3%–5% of newborns have a significant birth defect. For some couples the risk of a genetic defect is even higher. Over the past 10–15 years a technique called amniocentesis has been developed to help these high-risk couples by detecting certain genetic abnormalities before the fetus is born.

In this test a needle is inserted through the pregnant mother's abdomen into the uterus (womb). Within the uterus, the fetus floats in a fluid-filled sac (amniotic sac), and a small amount of the fluid can be withdrawn. This amniotic fluid contains cells shed by the developing fetus as well as chemical by-products which can give important clues to fetal health.

There are two major uses of amniocentesis. It may be performed early in pregnancy to detect birth defects or later in pregnancy when a problem is suspected. Unfortunately not all birth defects can be detected by amniocentesis. In fact, many of the most common birth defects such as congenital heart disease, cleft lip and palate, and certain types of mental retardation cannot be diagnosed by this test. However, amniocentesis can detect chromosomal disorders such as Down's syndrome (mongolism); other structural defects such as spina bifida ("open spine" or incomplete development of the spinal cord) and anencephaly (incomplete development of the brain); as well as over 100 very rare inherited metabolic disorders.

Since the genetic disorders that can be detected are generally severely disabling and incurable, abortion is usually offered. If you would not consider having an abortion no matter what the results, then the test is probably inappropriate.

In addition to its use in genetic screening early in pregnancy, amniocentesis can be used later in pregnancy to help in the management of a problem pregnancy. For example, amniocentesis may help determine if a distressed fetus is mature enough to survive an early birth or if a fetus is at risk because of an Rh incompatiblity with the mother's blood (see. p. 53).

### Why Performed:

*Amniocentesis to Detect Birth Defects:* For the average couple without known risk factors, the probability of a serious birth defect that can be diagnosed by amniocentesis is very low. Because there is a risk from the procedure itself, as well as considerable expense, amniocentesis is reserved for couples at higher risk for genetic disorders. If you answer yes to any of the following questions about risk factors, amniocentesis may be indicated:

● Will you (the mother) be age 35 or older when the baby is due?
   YES_____NO_____
   The risk of having a baby with a chromosomal abnormality such as Down's

syndrome (mongolism) increases significantly in women 35 or older.

● Have you or the baby's father ever had a previous infant born with a chromosomal abnormality (e.g., Down's syndrome) or abnormal development of the spinal cord or brain (e.g., neural tube defects such as spina bifida) or other serious birth defect?
   YES_____NO_____

● Have you or the baby's father ever been told that you have an unusual chromosomal arrangement (translocation)?
   YES_____NO_____

● Have you and the baby's father ever been told that you are *both* carriers of the same gene for an inherited disorder such as Tay Sachs disease, sickle-cell disease, or thalassemia (Mediterranean anemia)?
   YES_____NO_____

● Do you have a family history of a known sex-linked disorder, such as hemophilia or Duchenne muscular dystrophy, that is related to the sex chromosomes?
   YES_____NO_____
   These so-called sex-linked abnormalities can be carried by women and passed onto their sons.

● Have you, or a previous spouse of this baby's father, had three or more spontaneous miscarriages?
   YES_____NO_____
   In some cases an unusual chromosomal arrangement may be responsible for the miscarriages. Therefore, chromosomal studies may be performed on the parents.

*Amniocentesis for Problem Pregnancies:* Amniocentesis may be recommended for a woman in whom a premature delivery is anticipated. The maturity of the fetus, particularly of its lungs, can be measured to determine the likelihood that the fetus can survive. Also, if there is early rupture of the membranes ("bag of waters"), amniocentesis can be used to determine the presence of an infection. A series of amniocenteses may also be performed during the last half of pregnancy in an Rh-negative mother carrying an Rh-positive fetus. This helps the physician determine whether the blood type incompatibility is affecting the health of the baby and whether early delivery is recommended.

### Preparation:

There is no need to restrict food or fluids before this test. You may be asked to empty your bladder just before the test. Occasionally you may be asked to get down on your hands and knees and bounce up and down to stir up some of the fetal cells in the amniotic fluid for better sampling. Before the procedure you will be asked to sign a consent form. Use this opportunity to discuss the need for the test, risks, and how it is performed.

### Procedure:

Amniocentesis is performed by a physician (usually an obstetrician, radiologist, or geneticist) and an assistant in an office or ultrasound department of a hospital. An overnight stay in the hospital is not required.

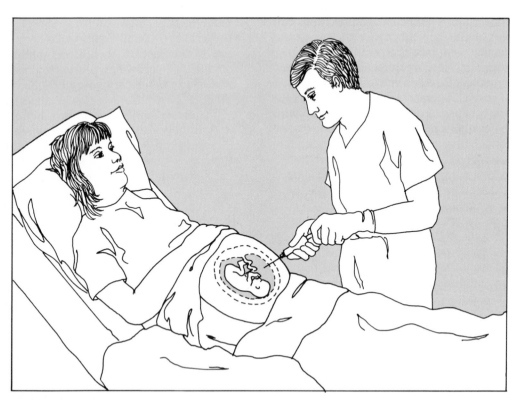

**Amniocentesis.** *During amniocentesis a needle is inserted into the uterus, and a small sample of the fluid surrounding the fetus is withdrawn.*

If the test is being performed to detect birth defects, it is done between the 14th and 18th week of pregnancy (counted from the last menstrual period). By that time there is ample amniotic fluid to sample. If the test is being performed to check fetal maturity, infection, or Rh incompatibility, it is done later in pregnancy, usually in the third trimester.

First an ultrasound examination (see p. 205) is performed by sending high-frequency sound waves through the abdomen. These sound waves bounce back to create a picture of the uterus, fetus, and placenta on a screen. This examination checks the approximate fetal age and allows the doctor to select the safest position to insert the needle to avoid injuring the fetus or placenta.

For the amniocentesis you will lie on your back with your upper body slightly elevated to relax the abdominal muscles. Your lower abdomen is cleansed with an antiseptic solution and covered with sterile drapes. A small amount of local anesthetic may be injected into the skin. Then a very thin needle approximately 4 inches long is gently inserted through the skin in the lower abdomen and into the uterus. A small amount of fluid (1–2 tablespoons) is withdrawn into the syringe, and the needle is removed. Pressure is placed over the puncture site for a minute or so to stop any bleeding.

The amniotic sac contains about 250 milliliters of fluid at the time the procedure is done, so that removing 20–30 ml or so is not significant and is quickly replaced. The fluid that has been removed is transferred to test tubes and sent to the laboratory for analysis. The procedure itself usually takes 15–20 minutes, but allow some additional time for arrival and recovery. After the test you should not exert yourself for about an hour, but after that you can resume normal activities unless otherwise advised.

## How Does It Feel?

If an anesthetic is injected, you will feel a sharp stinging or burning sensation for a few seconds. During the insertion of the needle into the amniotic sac you will feel a sharp pain lasting a few seconds, similar to having your blood drawn. When the fluid is withdrawn some women describe a mild "pulling" sensation or pressure in the lower abdomen. You will be more comfortable if you breathe slowly and let your abdominal muscles remain soft and relaxed during the procedure.

After the procedure, you may experience some mild lower abdominal cramping. However, if you notice significant abdominal pain or cramping, chills, fever, dizziness, or a leakage of fluid or blood from the vagina or puncture site, notify your doctor immediately.

## Risks:

While amniocentesis is generally a very safe procedure, there is a slight chance of triggering a spontaneous abortion (miscarriage). There is also a slight possibility of introducing an infection or injuring the fetus. Every attempt is made to insert the needle in a safe location, and the fetus usually floats away from the needle tip. Usually the risk of having an abnormal baby greatly outweighs the risk of the procedure when it is performed in high-risk pregnancies.

## Results:

When amniocentesis is done to look for birth defects in early pregnancy, it usually takes 3 to 6 weeks for the laboratory analysis to be completed. The fetal cells normally found in the amniotic fluid are grown ("cultured") and the fluid is tested for various chemicals. Less than 3% of amniocentesis procedures have to be repeated because of insufficient fluid, failure of the cells to grow in culture, or borderline results.

Fortunately, in over 95% of cases the results of such testing show no abnormalities and the parents can proceed with the pregnancy without undue anxiety. However, since only a few disorders can be tested for, *a normal amniocentesis does not guarantee a normal child.*

The cells of the fetus are carefully analyzed (see Chromosomal Analysis, p. 60) to look for the proper number and arrangement of chromosomes. Chromosomes are packages of hereditary material (genes) which determine overall development. Normally, there are exactly 46 chromosomes in each cell. The most common problem found on amniocentesis is Down's syndrome (mongolism), in which there is an extra number-21 chromosome, resulting in 47 rather than 46 chromosomes. Other chromosome problems can also be detected. Occasionally, chromosome abnormalities are found for which the significance or consequences are not known. Overall, chromosomal studies are over 99% accurate.

Amniocentesis can also indicate the sex of the fetus. For some suspected inherited disorders that are carried by the sex chromosomes, such as hemophilia, this is critical information. In most instances, however, you can choose whether or not you wish to be told the sex of the fetus before birth.

Sometimes a different type of abnormality is detected. For example, abnormal levels of a chemical called alpha-fetoprotein (p. 46) in the amniotic fluid suggests a serious disorder in the development of the nervous system (neural tube defects such as spina bifida or anencephaly). Other biochemical tests may reveal any of over 100 inherited metabolic disorders. The accuracy of these biochemical tests varies with the disorder studied.

If a serious abnormality is detected, it most often represents a severe, often fatal, physical handicap or mental retardation. Such abnormal results pose a difficult and emotionally charged decision for the parents: whether to abort the pregnancy or to make plans to have a seriously handicapped child. The decision is obviously the parents', but discussion with a physician or genetic counselor can be of considerable help in informing parents of the risks and options. It is also wise to carefully consider, before the amniocentesis is performed, what choice you would make. If abortion of a seriously defective fetus is not considered a possible choice, amniocentesis should not be performed in the first place.

Analysis of amniotic fluid performed later in pregnancy can also provide clues as to the maturity of the fetus and likelihood of survival should a premature delivery be necessary. Chemicals such as lecithin and sphingomyelin are measured, and the ratio of these chemicals (L/S ratio) is a fair predictor of lung maturity. These results are combined with other chemical tests to estimate fetal maturity.

The finding of large amounts of bilirubin, a pigment from the destruction of red blood cells, may indicate hemolytic disease of the newborn from Rh incompatibility. In this case, an early delivery of the baby or transfusion while the baby is in the uterus may be indicated.

The amniotic fluid may also be examined for evidence of infection if the membranes rupture early. An early delivery is usually performed if an infection is present.

**Cost:**

Amniocentesis for birth defects: $600–$900 (includes procedure, laboratory analysis, and genetic counseling)

Amniocentesis for problem pregnancies: $125–$200

**Special Considerations:**

★*Chorionic Villi Biopsy (CVB):* This is a new technique which may replace amniocentesis in screening for genetic disease. In this test, the doctor inserts a thin hollow tube (catheter) through the vagina and cervix into the uterus. Small tissue samples are taken by suction of the chorion, a layer of tissue surrounding the amniotic sac and the fetus. This tissue contains cells which have a genetic composition similar to that of the fetus. This test can be performed earlier in pregnancy (at 8–9 weeks) than amniocentesis and provides results within 1–2 days rather than the 3 to 6 weeks required for amniocentesis results. The safety of this procedure is currently being investigated.

★*Fetoscopy:* This is a new experimental technique which allows direct visualization of the fetus. A long, thin fiberoptic tube is inserted directly through a small incision in the abdomen into the uterus. The fetus can be viewed and fetal blood samples can be drawn to diagnose certain hereditary anemias such as thalassemia as well as hemophilia. Fetoscopy carries a higher risk of miscarriage (3%–5%) than amniocentesis and is available in only a few medical centers.

# Electronic Fetal Monitoring
## (EFM) (External and Internal Fetal Monitoring, Nonstress and Stress Test, Oxytocin Challenge Test)

In this test a record is made of an unborn baby's heartbeat and the contractions of the mother's uterus. This test is used to evaluate your baby's well-being during labor and to detect early signs of potential problems. It is also used to monitor your baby during the nonstress test and the oxytocin challenge test (see Special Considerations below).

Abnormal readings may indicate that some treatment is needed to help the baby. Sometimes a change in the mother's position or extra oxygen can relieve the problem. Occasionally forceps are needed to help deliver the baby. In extreme cases, a cesarean section may be indicated.

**Why Performed:**

The use of electronic fetal monitoring during high-risk pregnancies (e.g., when the mother has diabetes or high blood pressure or when the baby is being born prematurely) is now widely accepted. However, although EFM is now used routinely for all women in labor in many hospitals, its value for low-risk mothers is not universally accepted. Some researchers feel that it decreases the quality of the birthing experience because it limits the mother's freedom of movement, discourages physical examination by the clinician, and restricts the mother's physical contact with friends and family.

Critics charge that for normal births, electronic fetal monitoring is an expensive and unnecessary technologic intrusion into the birth process, and that EFM allows the hospital to increase fees and to decrease the amount of individual staff attention each mother receives. Some have expressed concern that once the machines have been purchased by the hospital, there is considerable economic pressure to use them whenever possible.

There is considerable evidence that careful physical exams can do just as well for healthy mothers of healthy babies. The National Center for Health Services has concluded that there is no scientific evidence that continuous electronic fetal monitoring prevents brain damage or otherwise improves infant health, except in problem pregnancies.

Many proponents of fetal monitoring, on the other hand, feel that all labors should be monitored by this test because complications can arise even with a seemingly healthy mother and baby. They argue that even though regular, careful physical exams may be just as good as the electronic monitoring, such careful and time-consuming individual care is not always possible on a busy and understaffed delivery floor. Many obstetricians are enthusiastic about the use of continuous monitoring.

This is a test about which it is especially important to have a full and open discussion with your clinician—ideally well before the time you are due to actually deliver your baby. You may wish to draft a written agreement which can be reviewed in advance by any physicians who might end up supervising your delivery if your own obstetrician is not available.

Some alternatives to discuss:
- No monitoring unless physical exam detects a possible problem.
- Your physician will run an initial EFM strip for 15 or 30 minutes when you are first admitted to the maternity department. If all is well, the monitoring will be discontinued and you will be checked by stethoscope and physical examination alone. If any problem arises during the test strip or later, you agree to continuous monitoring throughout the rest of your labor.
- Continuous monitoring will be done throughout labor.

**Preparation:**
No special preparation is needed.

**Procedure:**
There are two kinds of EFM: external and internal. In external monitoring, two belts are placed around your abdomen. In internal monitoring, a small device is attached to your baby's scalp.

*External EFM*—The two belts hold two small instruments in place. One instrument uses ultrasound to detect your baby's heart rate. The other measures the changes in pressure produced when your uterus contracts. A jelly or spray may be used to provide good contact for the instruments.

You will be asked to lie still and to remain mostly on your back. From time to time the position of the heart rate monitor may have to be changed as the result of your baby's movements.

External fetal monitoring can be done at any time, including early labor before your cervix is dilated and your membranes rupture.

*Internal monitoring*—In internal EFM, the baby's heart rate is measured through a tiny electrode which is placed through the mother's vagina and attached to the baby's scalp. A soft plastic tube (catheter) is also inserted through the vagina. A device connected to this tube measures labor contractions. A belt will be placed around your upper leg to keep the internal monitor in place.

The internal method can be used only after your cervix has started to dilate and your amniotic sac ("water bag") has broken. If your water bag has not broken, your doctor will have to deliberately rupture it to install the monitoring unit.

Internal EFM is much less susceptible to disturbances caused by the mother's movements than external EFM. It also allows the mother more freedom of movement.

Sometimes a combination of internal and external monitoring is used: The baby's heart rate is measured by a scalp electrode and the mother's contractions with an external belt.

With both methods, the measurements are recorded by a small machine which traces them on a long strip of paper, showing the baby's heart rate and the mother's contractions in graphic form.

### How Does It Feel?

Fetal monitoring is confining. The mother has to lie in bed and cannot move around much—and it may be quite difficult to hold still while you're in labor. The belts holding the external monitors in place may be

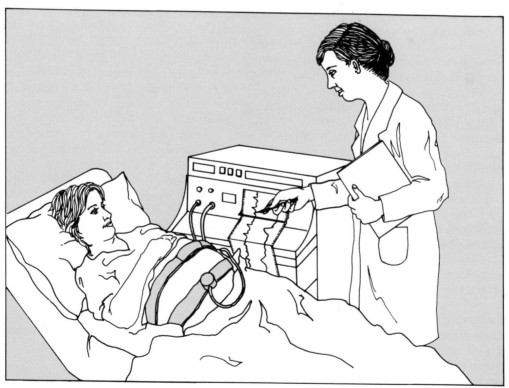

**Electronic Fetal Monitoring.** *The belts placed around the abdomen during external electronic fetal monitoring record the patterns of contraction of the uterus and the baby's heartbeat.*

slightly uncomfortable, as may the belt around your upper leg in internal monitoring.

Having the internal monitor inserted may be mildly uncomfortable.

Some mothers experience fetal monitoring as an unnecessary intrusion into a natural process. Others, particularly high-risk mothers, including those who have had trouble with earlier pregnancies, consider it very reassuring.

**Risks:**
Studies show that women who have fetal monitoring are more likely to have cesarean sections, but this may be because women with problem pregnancies are more likely to be monitored.

External fetal monitoring may be inaccurate. It can sometimes pick up artifacts—noises such as the mother's heartbeat or her stomach rumbling—which can distort the signals coming from the baby.

Fetal monitoring cannot predict every type of problem. It does not detect birth defects. Very rarely, as the result of technical problems, the monitor will indicate that a baby is normal when it is really in distress.

This test exposes both fetus and mother to a large dose of ultrasound. While there is to date no evidence that ultrasound is harmful, the long-term effects have not been fully studied.

There is a slight risk of infection in your baby as a result of improper placement of the scalp monitor.

**Results:**
This test measures the timing and strength of your uterine contractions and the response of your baby's heart to these contractions.

Some variability in heart rate is normal in healthy babies, but if your baby's heart rate decreases in response to uterine contractions, it may mean that it is in trouble. Your clinician will be watching for dips in fetal heart rate during or immediately after a uterine contraction.

There are three kinds of dips: early decelerations, late decelerations, and variable decelerations.

*Early deceleration* is caused by pressure on the baby's head. Healthy babies usually tolerate early decelerations well. The heart rate rarely falls below 100. Early decelerations are not, in general, considered very dangerous.

*Late deceleration* means that your baby's heart is slowing down at about the peak of the uterine contraction, then returning to normal between contractions. In late deceleration the rate may fall as low as 60. Repeated late deceleration patterns are often interpreted as a sign of problems in the baby's blood supply from the placenta. But there can be other causes, too; the mother's blood pressure may be low, for instance. If late deceleration pattern continues, a cesarean may need to be performed.

*Variable decelerations* show a pattern that is inconsistent from contraction to contraction. They are usually caused by compression of the umbilical cord. Repositioning the mother—either on her hands and knees or on her left side—may take the pressure off the cord. Oxygen may also be given to lessen the stress on the baby.

**Cost:**
When this test is performed as part of the labor process in the maternity department of a hospital, there is usually no additional charge. If it is done before labor begins, it usually costs $30 to $90.

**Special Considerations:**
★*Fetal Scalp Blood Sampling*—The existence of fetal distress can sometimes be

confirmed by taking a blood sample from a vein in the baby's scalp. If the blood is too acidic, it usually indicates fetal distress.

★*Nonstress Test*—This test uses electronic fetal monitoring to check your baby's well-being before labor begins. An external monitoring belt is applied. Then you (and sometimes a nurse) watch carefully for any movements by your baby. When movements are noticed, they are marked on the recording of your baby's heart rate. The results show how your baby responds to its own movements.

★*Stress Test (Oxytocin Challenge Test)*— This test is also done before labor begins. Two external monitoring belts are applied to measure your baby's heart rate and your uterine contractions. You are then given a small dose of the drug oxytocin through an intravenous (IV) needle to make your uterus contract. The baby's response to uterine contractions is then observed.

On very rare occasions, this test may result in premature labor.

★*Self-Monitoring of Fetal Movements*— Every mother is aware of her baby's movements inside her—including the fetal "kick." Several studies have shown that mothers can accurately monitor the number of these movements to check for possible problems.

This test can be performed daily for the last 12 weeks of pregnancy. Your obstetrician may give you instructions on how to count and record fetal movements. In one method, the mother simply begins looking for fetal movements first thing in the morning. She makes a mental note each time she feels her baby move until she has felt 10 different movements. She then records the time at which the tenth movement was felt. Two or three distinct kicks in a row should be counted as two or three separate movements.

If 10 movements have not been felt after 12 hours of monitoring, the mother should consult her clinician at once or should come to the clinic or hospital for further evaluation. A nonstress test (see preceding section) will probably be done.

Fewer movements may mean that the baby is beginning to have trouble. But fewer than 10 movements may occasionally occur in healthy babies as well.

# 5 Tests for Men

## Testicular Self-Examination

Even though cancer of the testicle is relatively rare, it is one of the most common cancers in men under the age of 35. The cause is unknown. Most testicular cancers are first discovered by men themselves as a lump or enlargement of the testicle. When testicular cancer is found early and treated promptly, chances for cure are excellent (90%–95%). Since testicular cancer often develops without symptoms, learning how to examine your testes may save your life.

The two testicles, or testes, are located in the scrotum, the flesh-covered sac that hangs between the legs at the base of the penis. The testicles are the male reproductive organs. They produce sperm and the male hormone testosterone (see p. 108). The testes develop within the abdomen of the male fetus and normally descend into the scrotal sac before or shortly after birth. Each testicle is approximately the size and shape of a small egg. At the back of each

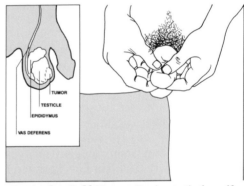

**Testicular Self-Exam.** *During testicular self-examination the leg is extended to one side, and the surface of each testicle is carefully felt. Insert shows the structures inside the scrotal sac.*

testicle is the epididymis, a coiled tube which collects and stores sperm (see illustration).

### Why Performed:
Since testicular cancer often develops without symptoms, testicular self-examination (TSE) should be performed once a month by every man between the ages of 15 and 40. After the age of 40 testicular cancer is so rare that monthly self-examination is not necessary.

**Procedure:**

Testicular self-examination is painless and takes only a minute. It is best performed after a bath or shower when the scrotal muscles are warm and relaxed. Stand and place your right leg on an elevated surface about chair height. Then gently feel the scrotal sac until you locate the right testicle. Roll the testicle gently, but firmly, between the thumb and fingers of both hands carefully exploring the surface. Repeat, lifting your left leg and examining your left testicle.

**Results:**

Each testicle should feel firm but not hard, and the surface should be very smooth, without any lumps or bumps. You may be able to feel the spongy, tubelike structure known as the epididymis on the top and down the back side of each testicle. You may find that one of the testicles (usually the left one) hangs slightly lower than the other, and one testicle may be slightly larger. This is perfectly normal. It is important for each man to become familiar with what is normal for him. If you have any questions about what is normal, ask your doctor.

If you find a small, hard lump like a pea on the surface of the testicle or you find an enlarged testicle, consult a doctor immediately. Do not delay or wait for the lump to go away. It may be a cancer.

If you cannot find one or both testicles, consult your doctor. The testicles may not have descended properly at birth.

If you feel a soft collection of thin tubes (often referred to as a "bag of worms" or "spaghetti") above the testicle, this may be a varicocele, which is a collection of dilated veins in the scrotum. Have this checked by your doctor.

If you notice the rapid onset of pain or swelling in the scrotum, you should consult a doctor immediately. These symptoms are rarely caused by testicular cancer, but may represent an infection (epididymitis) or blockage of blood flow to the testicle (torsion), which requires prompt attention.

**Special Considerations:**

★Testicular cancer is nearly 35 times more likely to occur when the testes have not properly descended into the scrotal sac or when they descend after age 6. Parents should check their children or have them checked by a doctor to be sure the testes have descended.

★Most testicular lumps are cancerous and require immediate treatment. Usually the testicle is removed surgically. In some cases, the lymph nodes may also be removed and chemotherapy or radiation therapy administered. An artificial testicle may be inserted into the scrotum so the man looks and feels normal. More importantly, virility and fertility are *not* affected, since one testicle is adequate for maintaining sexual and reproductive function.

# Self-Test for Erection Problems (Nocturnal Penile Tumescence (NPT) Stamp Test)

The inability of a man to achieve and maintain an erection is a common problem. The causes can be organic (due to a physical condition), psychologic, or a combination of both. Physical factors that can contribute to erection problems include various medications, alcohol, diabetes, arteriosclerosis, endocrine disorders, prostate disease, or spinal cord injuries. Estimates vary, but nearly half of all erection problems are now thought to be due primarily to psychologic causes.

At first it may seem unusual to suggest a home diagnostic test for erection problems (sometimes referred to as impotence). You either have erections or you don't. But the purpose of this test is to help distinguish between physical and psychologic erection problems, a matter of some importance since the approaches to treatment are quite different.

The test is based on the finding that men with psychologic erection difficulties usually still have normal erections during sleep but are often unaware of this. These sleep erections are technically referred to as nocturnal penile tumescence (NPT) and occur during certain stages of sleep known as rapid eye movement or REM sleep. By placing a ring of stamps around the penis and checking to see if the perforations are torn in the morning, it is possible to tell if an erection has occurred during the night.

## Why Performed:

Occasional erection problems are considered normal. If you can ever achieve and maintain a full erection, including during masturbation, then the physiologic mechanisms are intact and this test is unnecessary. However, if you are unable to maintain an erection at all, then the NPT stamp test may be useful in helping to determine if the cause is physical or psychologic.

## Equipment:

You will need a strip of four to six stamps for each of three nights. You can use any kind of stamps, but if you wish you can obtain official test stamps, each with NPT printed on it, from Dr. John Barry at The Oregon Health Sciences University (3181 S.W. Sam Jackson Park Road, Portland, Oregon 97201). The cost is one dollar for a sheet of NPT stamps, and the check should be made payable to "ARF Urology Gift Account." If you use postage stamps, try a strip of the one-cent variety to save money.

## Preparation:

Obtain your stamps. Do not drink alcohol or take sleep or sedative medications for at least two days before the test. These drugs can interfere with REM sleep, which is when nocturnal erections occur.

## Procedure:

Wear brief-type undershorts with a fly. Bring your penis through the fly; this leaves most of the pubic hair against the body. Wrap a strip of four to six stamps snugly around the shaft of the penis, forming an overlapping ring. Wet the overlapping stamp to seal the ring. After the stamp has dried, carefully replace your penis inside the shorts and wear the shorts to sleep. The undershorts help protect the stamps from accidentally falling off. Upon awakening, check the stamp ring to see if it has been broken along the perforations. If the tearing of the stamps awakens you, check whether you have an erection and check the degree of rigidity of the erection. Repeat the test for a total of three nights.

## Results:

If all of the perforations between any two stamps in the ring are broken on any one of the three nights, you probably had an erection. This evidence suggests that the physiologic mechanisms are functioning normally and that the erection problem is probably due to psychologic causes. If the stamp ring is unbroken on all of the three

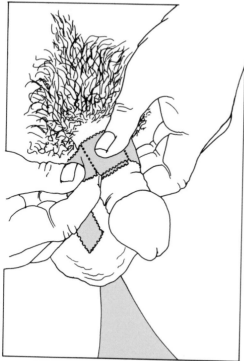

**Self-Test for Erection Problems (Stamp Test).** *A ring of stamps is wrapped around the base of the penis.*

vide valuable clues in the diagnosis and successful treatment of erection problems.

Many times physical and psychologic erection problems overlap and interact. For example, a slight degree of physiologic dysfunction can be magnified by anxiety over sexual performance. This is one reason we recommend sexual counseling in addition to this self-diagnostic test.

### Special Considerations:

★If the idea of using a ring of stamps is somehow not acceptable to you, a Velcro band is available to document nocturnal erections. This Dacomed Snap-Gauge is expensive ($25), but is reusable. They are available from Dacomed Corporation, 1701 East 179th St., Minneapolis, Minnesota 55420.

★More elaborate nocturnal penile tumescence monitoring devices with strain-gauge recorders are available. This will provide information on the number and duration of erections during sleep. However, it is quite expensive, often requiring an overnight stay in a hospital or sleep laboratory.

nights, this suggests that the erection problem is due to medications or a physical condition. In either case, you should seek the counsel of a professional who is sensitive to and informed about sexual problems.

The NPT stamp test is not foolproof. The stamps may separate due to rubbing on the shorts or rolling over in bed. If you have any doubts, repeat the test. Also, the stamp ring only measures the circumference of the penis and doesn't necessarily guarantee that the erection was fully firm, nor does it document the duration or number of erections. Further evaluation may be necessary, but the NPT stamp test can pro-

# Semen Analysis (Sperm Count, Male Fertility Test)

In about one third of all couples who have been unable to have children, male infertility is the major factor. This test is usually one of the first performed to evaluate suspected infertility in men. A sample of your semen (the thick, white, sperm-containing fluid produced by the male sexual glands) is obtained and analyzed. The evaluation of female infertility is described elsewhere (p. 201).

## Why Performed:

If you have been unable to conceive a child after a year of trying, this test may be useful in determining whether a problem in sperm production could be a cause.

This test is also used after a vasectomy to be certain that there are no sperm in the semen.

## Preparation:

Some doctors will ask that you refrain from any sexual activity, including masturbation, for 2 to 5 days before this test. Others advise that you refrain for about the same time as your usual interval between sexual activity. This period of abstinence helps ensure the buildup of a sizable sperm sample and helps standardize test results. You should not abstain from sex for a long period before this test, as prolonged abstinence can result in less-active sperm. Ask your doctor or lab for specific instructions. Also some doctors recommend abstaining from alcoholic beverages for at least 24 hours before the test.

## Procedure:

You will be asked to supply a semen sample. You should discuss the method of sample collection with your physician. You can masturbate into a sterile container in the doctor's office, clinic, or laboratory—not the most romantic setting by any means. If you live nearby and so prefer, you may be able to arrange to obtain the sample at home by masturbation, coitus interruptus, or intercourse using a special condom. Rubber condoms should not be used—the lubricants and powder with which they are packed may kill sperm. Use the plastic condom provided by your lab or physician.

After the sample has been collected, tie a knot in the condom, place it in a closed container, and take it to the laboratory within an hour. The sample should be examined as soon as possible, within two hours at the very latest. Be sure to protect the sample from sunlight and from intense heat or cold. Do not refrigerate.

Since there may be marked variations from sample to sample, several specimens may be examined over several weeks or months to look for a consistent pattern of abnormality.

## How Does It Feel?

The collection of the semen specimen does present a potentially embarrassing situation and a religious dilemma for some men. If you are uncomfortable about it, you should discuss it openly with your doctor or clergy.

## Results:

The semen specimen is analyzed in the laboratory in terms of the volume of fluid, number and structure of sperm, and movement of the sperm. The thickness of the fluid, acidity and sugar (fructose) content is also assessed. The results are usually available by the next day.

*Volume:* Normal semen volume varies from 1.5 to 5.0 milliliters per ejaculate. Abstaining from ejaculation usually increases the volume.

*Number:* Normal sperm count varies from 20 to 150 million sperm per milliliter. Men with very low counts or very high counts are less fertile. However, even men with sperm counts below 1 million have fathered children. It only takes one viable sperm to fertilize an egg. The finding of sperm in the semen after vasectomy should raise doubt as to the success of the sterilization procedure, and another form of birth control should be used.

*Shape (morphology):* At least 60% of the sperm should have normal shape and structure.

*Movement (motility):* At least 60% of the sperm should show normal forward movement indicating the potential to be able to "swim" to meet the egg.

The acidity (pH) of the semen as well as the presence of white blood cells (which suggests an infection) may also influence fertility. Many drugs, including alcohol, tobacco, marijuana, cimetidine (Tagamet), male and female hormones, and many of the drugs used to treat cancer, can impair male fertility. An estimated two million men were exposed to the drug diethylstilbestrol (DES) before birth; this drug was widely prescribed to prevent miscarriages in pregnant women in the 1950s. DES sons have high infertility rates.

Radiation exposure as well as certain pesticides and industrial toxins may also decrease fertility. Exposure of the testicles to heat can lower sperm counts. Thus men who are trying to conceive a child should avoid prolonged hot baths or saunas. Blockage of the tubes that conduct the sperm may occur from growth abnormalities or infection and results in reduced or absent sperm in the semen.

If a low sperm count or abnormal semen is found, further testing may be indicated. This might include measurement of hormones such as testosterone (p. 108), luteinizing hormone (LH, p. 88), follicle-stimulating hormone (FSH, p. 76), and prolactin (p. 95). Testicular biopsy (p. 225) is also performed in some cases to evaluate male infertility.

Another type of semen analysis, the postcoital test (p. 201), is commonly used to test how the sperm behave in the vaginal environment.

There are yet many unknowns in the field of male infertility. Even the results from all of these tests often fail to explain the cause of infertility.

**Cost:**
$25 to $50

# Prostate Biopsy

The prostate gland lies in the area behind the penis and in front of the rectum. The prostate surrounds the urethra at the neck of the bladder and secretes seminal fluid, the liquid portion of the ejaculate.

In this procedure a sample of prostate tissue is removed and examined under a microscope. This test is most frequently done to determine whether cancer of the prostate is present. Among men over 50, cancer of the prostate is second to lung cancer as the most common cause of cancer death.

This test is also sometimes done to help diagnose benign enlargement of the prostate gland (benign prostate hypertrophy or BPH).

Most prostate biopsies are performed in one of three ways:

By needle through the perineum (the area between the base of the penis and the rectum)

By needle through the wall of the rectum

By cystoscopy (see p. 322)

**Why Performed:**
This test is most frequently used when a finger (digital) rectal exam reveals an abnormal prostate, most frequently a lump or an enlarged prostate. The finding of increased amounts of alkaline phosphatase

(p. 45) in the blood may suggest the presence of a prostate cancer for which a biopsy should be done.

**Preparation:**
Tell your doctor if
You have allergies to any anesthetic
You have had bleeding problems
You are taking any medications

If the biopsy will be done through the perineum, no special preparation is necessary. If it will be done through the rectum, you will be asked to take a cleansing enema and will be instructed how to do it.

**Procedure:**
This test is done by a surgeon, usually a urologist. It is frequently performed in a doctor's office or clinic or in a hospital special procedures room or operating room. You may or may not need to be admitted to the hospital. Discuss this with your doctor.

An antibiotic may be administered shortly before the test is done to reduce the risk of infection afterward. You may be given a mild sedative, either by mouth or by injection, shortly before the test begins.

*Needle Biopsy via Perineum*—This test is performed in a hospital operating room. You will be asked to lie on one side or on your back with your knees up. The skin of the perineum (the area between the base of the penis and the rectum) will be cleansed. A local anesthetic will be injected. Occasionally general anesthesia is used (see p. 465).

A small incision (less than an inch) may be made in the perineum. Your doctor locates the prostate by placing one finger into your rectum, then inserts the needle into the prostate.

The doctor turns the needle gently, quickly withdraws it, and reinserts it into another part of the prostate. Tissue may be taken from several areas. The biopsy needle is then withdrawn, and pressure is applied to stop the bleeding. This test usually takes about 15–30 minutes.

*Needle Biopsy via Rectum*—This procedure is done by a urologist and is usually performed in a doctor's office or clinic procedures room. It is usually done without anesthetic. Different physicians have their patients assume different positions for this test—either kneeling, lying on your side, or lying on your back with your legs supported by stirrups.

The surgeon attaches a curved needle guide to his or her finger, then inserts the finger into the rectum. When the needle guide is properly placed, the biopsy needle is pushed along the guide, through the wall of the rectum, and into the prostate. The needle is rotated gently and then withdrawn. Sometimes the biopsy is done through a small scope placed in your rectum. The biopsy usually takes 15–30 minutes.

You will be asked to avoid strenuous activities for the rest of the day. There is no need to limit sexual activity. You may notice some blood in your urine for 2–3 days after the test and may also notice a small amount of rectal bleeding. This is normal. If you experience persistent bleeding, pain or fever, or if you are unable to urinate for 24 hours, notify your doctor.

**How Does It Feel?**
*Perineal Biopsy*—You may feel a slight sting as the local anesthetic is injected, and a dull pressure as the biopsy needle is inserted. You may experience some mild discomfort at the biopsy site for 1–2 days after the test.

*Rectal Biopsy*—You may experience a brief, sharp pain as the biopsy needle is inserted. You may experience some mild discomfort at the biopsy site for 1–2 days after the test.

## Risks:

This is generally a low-risk procedure. There are some possible complications, but they are not frequent and can almost always be easily treated. There is no risk of causing erection problems or infertility.

Possible complications include bleeding into the urethra or bladder, resulting in a hematoma (bleeding into an enclosed inner space), infection, inability to urinate, or excessive frequency of urination. There is also a slight risk of allergic reaction to the anesthetic or to other drugs used in the procedure. You should discuss the risks in your particular case with your doctor.

## Results:

Results are usually available in about 3 days. The cells in the tissue sample will be examined under a microscope by a pathologist. The results may show normal tissue, signs of inflammation, benign prostate hypertrophy (noncancerous prostate enlargement), or prostate cancer.

Benign prostate hypertrophy (BPH), the gradual noncancerous enlargement of the prostate gland, often begins at about age 40 and is a very common finding in older men.

If prostate cancer is present, further tests will be required to determine the extent to which the tumor has spread before some combination of the available therapies (surgery, radiation, and/or hormones) is suggested.

## Cost:

$100 to $600 (depends on procedure)

# Testicular Biopsy

The testicle (testis) is one of a pair of egg-shaped glands which hang in the scrotum, just beneath the base of the penis. The testicles are the male reproduction organs. They produce sperm and male hormones.

In this test a small sample of tissue is taken from one or both testicles and examined under a microscope to evaluate fertility.

## Why Performed:

If a semen analysis (p. 221) indicates abnormal sperm, hormone tests (testosterone, p. 108; follicle-stimulating hormone, FSH, p. 76; luteinizing hormone, LH, p. 88; and/or prolactin, p. 95) may help you and your doctors determine the cause of the abnormalities. If these tests do not provide the needed information, testicular biopsy may on rare occasion be done.

Testicular biopsy is not usually used to detect cancer of the testes. When this diagnosis is suspected, a surgical procedure is used.

## Preparation:

If this biopsy is done under local anesthesia, no special preparation is needed. If it is done under general anesthesia, a sedative medication is usually given by injection about an hour before the procedure begins. An intravenous line (IV) will be placed in a vein, usually in your arm. For more about general anesthesia, see p. 465.

## Procedure:

This test is done by a surgeon or a urologist in a doctor's office, a special procedures room, or a hospital operating room.

The skin over the testicle will be

cleansed with an antiseptic solution and the area around it covered with sterile towels. Your doctor will wear sterile gloves. It is very important that you do not touch this sterile area.

A local anesthetic will be injected into the skin of the scrotum to numb (anesthetize) the area. A small incision (about one-half inch long) is then made through the skin, and a tiny piece of testicular tissue is snipped off with small scissors. A single stitch is used to close the incision in the testicle. Another stitch is used to close the skin incision. (Absorbable sutures are used so the stitches do not need to be removed.) The procedure is usually repeated on the other testicle. The area is then bandaged.

The biopsy usually takes 15–20 minutes. You will be asked to wear an athletic supporter for several days after the procedure. This helps support the testicles while the incisions heal. You will probably be advised to refrain from sexual activity for a week or two after the biopsy. You should avoid bathing the area for several days.

### How Does It Feel?

You will feel a brief sting when the local anesthetic is injected. Other than that, the procedure itself should be painless.

The scrotum and testicle may be somewhat sore for 3–4 days after the test. Some black and blue areas may appear. Notify your doctor if you experience severe pain or fever after the test.

### Risks:

There is a slight risk of prolonged bleeding or infection from this procedure. There is no risk of erection problems or infertility as a result of this test. If general anesthesia is used, there is a small but significant risk of death from complications of anesthesia (see Anesthesia, p. 465).

### Results:

Results are usually available in 2–4 days. The biopsied tissue is examined by a pathologist for any abnormalities in sperm production or maturation. If sperm development appears normal yet semen analysis shows reduced or absent sperm, a blockage of the tube (vas deferens) that conducts the sperm from the testes to the urethra is suspected. Such a blockage can sometimes be repaired by surgery.

### Cost:

$100 to $300

# 6                                      X-Rays

**X**-rays are a form of electromagnetic radiation, like light or radio waves. X-rays can penetrate most matter—including the human body. Thus they can be used to take pictures of structures inside your body.

If you place your arm in an x-ray beam, some of the x-rays are absorbed by the tissues of your arm and some pass through. If the x-rays that pass through strike a plate of photographic film, an x-ray image of your arm results. The denser tissues, like bone, appear on the film as white, the less dense tissues, such as muscles, various shades of gray, and the empty space surrounding the arm, solid black.

Sometimes a substance that shows up on x-rays is injected into the body to highlight certain structures. Such substances are called *contrast materials, contrast media,* or *dyes.*

## How Are X-Rays Measured?

Physicists often measure x-rays in units called *roentgens* (pronounced RENT-genz), named for Wilhelm Roentgen, who discovered x-rays in 1895. But x-rays that pass through your body without being absorbed have no harmful effect. Thus for medical purposes we are mainly concerned with the *absorbed* x-ray dose. The unit of absorbed x-ray dose is the *rad*. (Absorbed x-ray doses are also sometimes expressed in units called *rems*. For medical x-rays, rads and rems have the same value, and the terms can be used interchangeably.)

Since a rad is a fairly large amount of radiation, a smaller unit, the *millirad*, is usually used to measure the radiation dose of x-rays. (The prefix *milli* means one thousandth. Thus 1 rad equals 1000 millirads.)

## How X-Rays Can Harm

X-rays can damage the human body in three ways:

1. They can damage individual cells. High radiation levels can kill cells, but the harm caused by lower doses is usually rapidly repaired. Rarely, this injury or damage to the cell can convert it to a cancer cell. Such injuries are called *somatic effects.*

2. There can be injury to the developing fetus, which can result in either malformations (i.e., birth defects), or death. Such damages are called *developmental effects.*

3. There can be injuries to the sperm or egg cells in the testes or ovaries. This damage can be passed on to future gen-

erations. Some of these injuries can result in birth defects in the individual's future offspring. These injuries are called *gonadal* or *genetic effects*.

In all the foregoing cases, the harmful effects of x-rays may not be evident for some time (many months to many years) after the x-ray exposure.

### X-Ray Risks in Perspective

Most experts believe that every x-ray exposure carries some risk. However, the risks of most x-rays are frequently as small or smaller than other risks many of us choose to take every day. For instance, the risk of getting cancer as the result of having a chest x-ray (a relatively low-dose procedure of 20–25 millirads) has been estimated as about the same as that of getting cancer from smoking two cigarettes or inhaling fumes during a 70-mile drive on a freeway. The risk from relatively high-risk procedures may be 10–20 times as great.

Those who receive the highest x-ray exposures are those who undergo repeated high-dose procedures. But these are almost invariably patients with serious medical problems who have the most to gain from the information x-rays can provide.

Further, medical x-rays are not our only source of exposure to x-rays. The average whole-body radiation dose received from natural sources (background radiation) is about 84 millirads per year. The average dose of x-rays received per year from medical x-rays is 78 millirads. Therefore, the average person receives about the same amount of radiation exposure from natural sources as from medical sources.

Your risk from x-ray exposure depends on your age (children are more sensitive to x-ray damage), the specific area of the body being x-rayed (such organs as ovaries, testes, thyroid, and bone marrow are more sensitive than others) and the amount of radiation you've received in the past.

The amount of radiation you will receive depends on the type of examination (some x-ray procedures deliver hundreds of times more radiation than others) and how often the examination is repeated (your cumulative radiation dose goes up each time an x-ray is done).

We have provided a rough estimate of the relative amount of total body radiation and reproductive organ radiation for each of the major x-ray examinations (see table, p. 230).

### Pregnant Women and Children—at Highest Risk

Developing fetuses and young children are more sensitive to x-ray damage than adults. Because of this, pregnant women should not receive any x-rays, especially lower abdominal, lower back, and hip x-rays, unless they are required for a life-threatening condition. Women who might possibly be pregnant should also avoid x-rays. X-rays of children should not be taken unless they are absolutely necessary.

### Is This X-Ray Really Needed?

There is probably more misunderstanding between health professionals and laypeople about x-rays than about any other tests currently performed. Many people are understandably concerned about the radiation dose they will receive and the damage it might do. But all too often these concerns lead people to forget what is in most cases an even *more* important question: *Is this x-ray really necessary?*

It's your doctor's job to describe the alternatives available to you and to estimate the most likely outcome of each. *Not* having an x-ray is always an alternative that should be seriously considered. The risk of not having the x-ray should then be compared with the risk of having it.

## Unnecessary X-Rays

It is our opinion that if an x-ray is really needed and is carefully performed on recently inspected equipment, the benefits are almost always worth the risks. But we are alarmed at how many unnecessary x-rays are done every day. X-rays are ordered to protect doctors from lawsuits. They are ordered as substitutes for a more time-consuming history and physical examination. They are ordered to satisfy doctors' curiosity, or because of real or imagined patient demand. They are done because it is hospital routine. They are taken when adequate x-rays already exist elsewhere.

In addition, x-rays are all too frequently ordered, taken, and interpreted by health workers without special training in radiology or by those who are not up-to-date on the latest x-ray procedures. And doctors who make a profit when they order an x-ray are more likely to order x-rays than those who do not.

## Inspection of X-Ray Machines

In addition to the problem of unnecessary x-rays, the consumer faces the problem of quality control on x-ray equipment. While the x-ray machines in all accredited hospitals must be inspected regularly, inspection of such equipment in nonhospital settings (e.g., clinics and doctor's offices) is often minimal or nonexistent.

Quality-control procedures need not be difficult or expensive: In one FDA trial program, cards containing small radiation measurement devices were mailed to dentists' offices with instructions to expose the card just as they would a patient. The exposed cards were then mailed back for analysis. The dentists received reports by mail, with the "high-dose" clinics getting consultative visits from a state inspector. As a result of the feedback provided by this study, the average patient's radiation exposure from dental x-rays was cut by 40%.

If your doctor or clinic doesn't currently have an inspection program, you may wish to let them know about a service provided by the University of Wisconsin Medical School. This service, Radiation Monitoring by Mail, is currently used by over 1000 medical facilities. The university sends each subscribing facility a number of tiny radiation-absorbing crystals. The health professional sets his or her machine to a specified radiation dose, exposes the crystal, and returns it. The university then sends back a report giving the true dose received. The service can measure radiation doses for mammography, chest x-ray, or virtually any other x-ray procedure.

Radiation Monitoring by Mail is available to clinics, hospitals, and individual practitioners. For more information contact Radiation Monitoring by Mail, Department of Medical Physics, Room 1530, Medical Sciences Center, University of Wisconsin School of Medicine, Madison, Wisconsin 53706, (608) 262-6320.

## Guidelines for Avoiding Unnecessary X-Rays

Sit down with your doctor and ask him or her to explain, in detail, why the suggested x-ray is needed. Here are some of the questions to raise:

- Is this x-ray really necessary?
- How will the results help in my diagnosis or treatment?
- How will positive or negative findings change the treatment of my condition?
- What would happen if no x-ray were taken?
- Could some or all of the needed infor-

## Comparative Radiation Exposures
## for Various X-Ray Examinations

| | Total Body Exposure (Somatic Dose) | Reproductive Organ Exposure (Gonadal/Genetic Dose)* | |
| --- | --- | --- | --- |
| | | Male | Female |
| Abdominal x-rays | Medium | Low-medium† | Medium-high |
| Arteriogram (abdominal/renal) | High | Medium† | High |
| Arteriogram (cerebral/carotid/ vertebral) | Medium | Low | Low |
| Arteriogram (lung) | Medium | Medium | Medium |
| Arthrogram | Low | Low | Low |
| Barium enema | High | Medium-high | High |
| Bronchography | Low | Low | Low |
| Cardiac catheterization | Medium | Medium | Medium |
| Chest x-ray | Low | Low | Low |
| CT scan—head | Low | Low | Low |
| CT scan—body | Medium-high | Medium-high† | Medium-high |
| Cystourethrogram | Medium | High | High |
| Dental x-rays | Low | Low | Low |
| Extremity x-rays (skeletal bone | Low | Low | Low |
| films) hip and thigh | Low | Medium | Medium |
| Gallbladder x-rays (oral cholecystogram) | Medium | Low | Low |
| Intravenous cholangiogram (with tomograms) | High | Medium | Medium |
| Percutaneous transhepatic cholangiogram | Medium | Low | Low |
| Hysterosalpingogram | Low | — | High |
| Intravenous pyelogram (IVP) | High | Medium† | High |
| Lymphangiogram | High | Medium-high† | High |
| Mammogram | Low | — | Low |
| Myelogram | Medium | Medium | Medium-high |
| Retrograde ureteropyelogram | High | High | High |
| Skull x-rays | Low | Low | Low |

**(Chart continued on next page)**

| (Continuation of chart) | Total Body Exposure (Somatic Dose) | Reproductive Organ Exposure (Gonadal/Genetic Dose)* | |
|---|---|---|---|
| | | Male | Female |
| Spine x-Rays | | | |
|    Cervical | Low | Low | Low |
|    Thoracic | Medium | Medium | Medium |
|    Lumbosacral | High | Medium† | High |
| Upper gastrointestinal series | Medium | Medium | Medium |
| Venogram | Medium | Medium† | Medium-High |

*Radiation exposure to the reproductive organs is most significant to children and people in the reproductive ages.

†With gonadal shielding.

mation be obtained by a more detailed history or physical examination, from a previously taken x-ray, or by some other low-risk diagnostic tests?

### Questions to Ask Yourself

The following are some questions you may not be comfortable asking your doctor, but should certainly ask yourself—and perhaps discuss with a family member or friend as well:

- Am I putting pressure on my doctor to order this test?
- Could my doctor be suggesting this x-ray because he or she thinks it would help prevent a lawsuit?
- Will my doctor make a profit on this x-ray?

If after considering all these questions, you still are not convinced that the test is needed, but your doctor still feels it is necessary, seek a second opinion, preferably from a radiologist (a physician who specializes in the use of x-rays).

### Questions to Ask If You Decide to Have the X-Ray

- What radiation-sensitive organs will be in the x-ray beam, and is it possible to use shielding (a lead apron or other shielding device) to protect them? (Such organs as ovaries, testes, thyroid, and bone marrow are more sensitive to radiation than other parts of the body.)
- Is the radiologic technician certified by the American Registry of Radiology Technologists?

### Communication Problems

You may find it difficult to get some doctors and dentists to take the time and trouble to deal with your concerns about x-rays. If you are like most people, you probably feel a bit uneasy even raising such questions with busy health professionals.

We encourage you to share your concerns with your doctor: doing so will inevitably work to your benefit. Don't be afraid of insulting your doctor by asking for information. Ten years ago it was rare for patients to ask such questions. Today's doctors hear them all the time.

Research shows that an attitude of confidence, relaxation, and trust promotes healing. It is just as important a part of your doctor's duties to deal with your concerns and to keep you fully informed as it is to help you make decisions about diagnosis and treatment. You should assume—and if necessary, demand—that your concerns be taken seriously.

### Doctors Feel Frustrated, Too

It's also important for you to understand some of your doctor's concerns about x-rays. Many physicians and dentists feel that their patients have been unduly alarmed by scare headlines about x-ray exposure.

Respect your doctor's concerns, but stick to your guns. Be assertive, not aggressive. If you find that after several attempts you cannot get your doctor to take your concerns seriously, or if you find that he or she can not give you clear, understandable answers to your questions, find another doctor.

### Reactions to Contrast Media

Because x-rays can distinguish only between structures of *different* density, and because many of the structures to be studied have roughly the *same* density, it is sometimes necessary to use *contrast materials* (contrast agents, contrast media, dyes) to obtain more detailed x-rays. Contrast materials can be injected (into a vein or an artery), swallowed, inhaled, or suffused into a hollow space or organ.

The risks of contrast material are mainly associated with injection. The death rate resulting from the intravenous injection of contrast material is approximately 1 in 40,000. It is important to distinguish the common minor side effects of such injections from rarer but potentially more serious allergic or neurologic reactions.

*Side effects* occur in roughly half of all persons receiving injected contrast material. Symptoms include a feeling of warmth, a mild flushing, tingling sensations, a slight giddiness, a metallic taste in the mouth, nausea, and rarely vomiting. These are mild, temporary, self-limited and not life-threatening. No treatment is necessary.

*Allergic or neurologic reactions* are rare and can almost always be successfully treated. Symptoms may include hives, widespread itching, irregular heartbeat, rapid pulse, very slow pulse, or clouding of consciousness.

If you have had a previous allergic or neurologic reaction to contrast material, you may be at a higher risk of having one again. However, studies show that some people who believe that they have had an allergic reaction to contrast material actually had an anxiety reaction to the procedure. Other possible risk factors include allergies to iodine, hay fever, hives, or eczema.

If you are at increased risk of an allergic reaction, yet the procedure is really necessary, you may be treated for several days before the test with steroid and antihistamine medications to minimize the risk of reaction.

### A Healthy Caution

In summary, we recommend that you exercise a healthy caution when your health professional suggests that an x-ray may be needed. Ask questions to assure yourself that the test really is necessary. But remember too that the overall risk from most x-rays is very low. And don't forget to consider the substantial benefits of x-rays when the information they can provide really is needed.

# Abdominal X-Ray
## (KUB, Flat Plate, Abdominal Scout Film)

In this test one or more x-rays are taken, allowing your doctor to examine some of your abdominal organs, such as the large and small intestine, stomach, spleen, and diaphragm (the sheet of muscle just under the lungs). If used mainly to examine the kidneys, ureters, and bladder, this x-ray is often referred to as a KUB.

### Why Performed:
The abdominal x-ray is frequently done as an early step in evaluating suspected problems of the urinary system (such as a kidney stone) or the gastrointestinal system (such as a blockage or perforation of the intestine). This test can help evaluate undiagnosed abdominal or flank pain, or persistent unexplained nausea and vomiting. It can also be used to locate foreign objects that have been swallowed.

### Preparation:
Tell your doctor if
> You might be pregnant
> You have an IUD
> You have had previous x-ray exams using barium contrast media or have taken bismuth-containing medications like Peptobismol within the past 4 days. Barium and bismuth can show up on the x-ray films and interfere with test results

No restrictions of food or fluid or other advance preparation is usually necessary. Before the test begins, remove any clothing, jewelry, or other objects between the neck and the hips.

### Procedure:
This procedure is performed by an x-ray technician in a doctor's office or a hospital radiology department.

You will be asked to lie on your back on an x-ray table. The x-ray machine will be positioned over your abdomen. You will be asked to hold your breath while the x-rays are being taken. Be sure to lie very still to avoid blurring the x-rays.

In many cases only a single x-ray is taken, but sometimes a three-way abdominal series is done. This series includes one film standing, one film lying on your back, and one lying on your side.

The procedure usually takes about 5–10 minutes. You will be asked to wait (usually about 5 minutes) until the x-rays are developed so that repeat films can be taken if necessary.

### How Does It Feel?
You will feel no discomfort from the x-ray itself, but the x-ray table may feel hard and the room may be chilly. If the x-ray is being taken because of abdominal pain, you may find the required movements and positions somewhat uncomfortable.

### Risks:
There is always some concern about the effects of exposure to any radiation, including the low-level radiation of diagnostic x-rays. Extremely high levels of radiation have been shown to cause various diseases and birth defects. However, if this test is really necessary, the radiation risk is generally very low compared with the potential benefits of the test.

Compared with other x-rays, the radiation exposure from this test is medium for total body exposure, low to medium for the male reproductive organs, and medium to high for the female reproductive organs. Because a developing fetus is very sensitive to radiation, this test is not usually recommended for pregnant women. The ovaries cannot be shielded during this exam, as they lie too close to the organs to be x-rayed. Men should have lead shields placed over their testes. (For more on x-ray risks, see p. 227.)

**Results:**

In an emergency the results of an abdominal x-ray can be available within minutes. Otherwise results may take a day.

The position, shape, and size of your kidneys may be determined from these x-rays. The ureters (the tubes that carry urine from the kidneys to the bladder) are not normally visible in this type of x-ray. If they do appear, it may mean that they contain kidney stones.

Some types of gallstones may also show up on the x-ray. Dilated bowel or abnormal gas patterns may suggest an intestinal blockage. The appearance of free air inside the abdominal cavity may be due to perforation of the stomach or intestines. Gas, feces, fluid (ascites), or foreign bodies in the intestine may also be seen.

**Cost:**

Single film: about $35 to $60
Three-way: about $70 to $100

# Arteriogram—General
## (Angiogram)

The arteries can't normally be seen in standard x-rays, so in this test a contrast material is injected into one or more arteries so that they can be visualized. The contrast material is usually injected through a long, thin, flexible tube (catheter) which is inserted and threaded through an artery to the site to be x-rayed.

Standard arteriography can be used to evaluate arteries in the arms, legs, chest, and abdomen. There are also special arteriographic procedures for the arteries in the heart (p. 162), lung (p. 241), and brain (p. 237).

**Why Performed:**

Arteriography is used to evaluate suspected abnormalities of blood flow to an area. This can be due to rupture of blood vessels, outpouchings of blood vessels (aneurysms), birth defects in the arteries, blood clots, and other causes of blocked blood flow.

**Preparation:**

Tell your doctor if

You have ever had an allergic reaction to x-ray contrast material or any other iodine-containing compound

You have allergies to any medication, pollen, or other substance

You are taking any medications

You have had bleeding problems

You might be pregnant

You will be asked to sign a consent form authorizing this procedure. Use this opportunity to discuss with your doctor any concerns you may have about the need for the test, the risks of the test, or how and when it will be performed.

Routine blood tests will be performed before this test. You will be asked to abstain from all food for 6–10 hours before the test. You may or may not be asked to abstain from fluids as well. Ask your doctor for specific instructions.

You may receive a sedative and/or pain pill about an hour before the procedure to help you relax.

You will be asked to put on a hospital

gown. Remove all dentures, jewelry, or other objects that might appear on the x-ray. As the procedure may be a long one, it's a good idea to empty your bladder just before the test begins.

You will be observed for several hours after the test, so you may want to bring something to read or material for some other quiet activity to occupy yourself during this period.

If you are having this test as an outpatient, you should arrange to have someone take you home 4–8 hours after the procedure; check with your doctor in advance to learn when you will be able to leave the hospital.

**Procedure:**

This test is done in a hospital x-ray department by a radiologist and one or more x-ray technicians. You will be asked to lie on your back on an x-ray table in the middle of a room filled with x-ray machines and various other electronic equipment. A fluoroscopy unit—a long, round column-like device containing an x-ray tube—will be directly above you. This device will move up and down from time to time during the procedure. It will be connected to a TV monitor nearby. ECG leads may be taped to your arms and legs to monitor the electrical activity of your heart during the procedure.

The part of your body to be examined may be secured with sandbags, straps, or tape to keep it from moving during the test. An intravenous (IV) needle may be placed on the back of your hand or on the inside of your elbow; this gives your doctor a way to administer drugs or provide additional fluids as needed.

The site at which the catheter will be inserted will be shaved, cleansed, and surrounded with sterile drapes. The femoral artery in your groin is usually used, but sometimes an artery in your arm is used instead, depending on the location of the area to be examined.

The radiologist will inject a small amount of local anesthetic at the catheter insertion site. Once the area is numb, a tiny incision is made through the skin. An arterial needle is used to enter the artery; then a thin, sterile tube (catheter) is introduced through the needle and into the artery and threaded to the section of your body to be examined. The catheter location is verified by x-ray.

Once the catheter tip is properly placed, the contrast material will be injected through the catheter. A rapid series of x-rays will be taken, developed immediately, and reviewed. Depending on the findings, more contrast material may be injected and more x-rays taken.

The catheter will be kept open by flushing with a saline solution containing heparin, an anticoagulant which keeps the blood around the catheter from clotting. Your pulse, blood pressure, and breathing rate are usually monitored during the procedure.

After the study is completed the catheter will be withdrawn and pressure will be applied to the insertion site for 10–15 minutes to stop any bleeding. The puncture site will then be checked and a tight bandage applied.

An arteriogram usually takes between 1 and 3 hours, depending on the part of the body examined and the number of x-rays required. After the test is finished you should remain quietly in bed for 4 to 6 hours, unless otherwise advised. Pain medication will be provided if needed. A nurse will check your pulse and blood pressure during this time.

You will be given instructions about the care of the leg or arm into which the catheter was inserted. Discuss these aftercare measures thoroughly with your doctor.

If your arm was used as the insertion site, you should not allow anyone to draw blood or take your blood pressure from the affected arm for several days—until the incision site has completely healed. During the first 24 hours the affected leg or arm should be kept from bending at the puncture site.

### How Does It Feel?

The injection of local anesthetic may sting briefly. Some people experience a brief, sharp pain when the catheter is inserted into the artery. Some also feel a pressure within the artery as the catheter is advanced. Let your doctor know if you are uncomfortable; this discomfort may be relieved by additional injections of anesthetic.

When the contrast material is injected, you will probably feel a burning sensation in the area being studied. Ask your doctor to tell you in advance where and when you will feel the heat. For some people, the sensation of heat can be quite extreme; for others it is relatively mild. This sensation lasts only a few seconds.

You may also experience a brief headache, flushing of the face, and a salty or metallic taste in your mouth. These sensations will also pass quickly. A few patients experience some nausea and vomiting, but this is very rare.

Most patients become somewhat uncomfortable because of the long time they must spend lying on a hard table. You may be more comfortable if you ask for pads or a blanket before the procedure begins.

You may experience some pain and swelling at the injection site for a day or two after the procedure. Signs that an artery may be blocked include pain or a loss of temperature, color, pulse, or sensation in the arm or leg into which the catheter is inserted. Be sure to inform the doctor immediately if you notice any such symptoms either during or after the procedure.

### Risks:

This procedure does involve some risk, so you should thoroughly understand the need for the test before proceeding. There are a number of possible complications, and although the risk of any one major problem is extremely small, they can add up to a significant risk.

There is the possibility of a reaction to the iodine contrast material. This can range from itching, hives, and wheezing to very rare cases of severe reactions which can result in death. Most problems can be controlled by medication. Be sure to tell your doctor if you have had any sensitivity or allergy to iodine-containing substances or if you have allergies of any kind (e.g., hay fever, eczema, hives, food allergies).

There is also some risk that the catheter may damage an artery or knock loose a piece of clotted blood or a piece of an artery wall. Such a dislodged object can block blood flow and create damage to the brain (stroke) or to other vital organs. This complication occurs in fewer than 5 in 1000 patients. There is a slight risk of bleeding, blockage of blood flow, or infection at the catheter insertion site.

There is always some concern about the effects of exposure to any radiation, including the low-level radiation of diagnostic x-rays. Extremely high levels of radiation have been shown to cause various diseases and birth defects. However, if this test is really necessary, the radiation risk is generally very low compared with the potential benefits of the test.

Radiation exposure from this test depends on the area examined. Because a developing fetus is very sensitive to radiation, this test is not usually recommended for pregnant women. (For more on x-ray risks, see p. 227.)

*Patient Comments*:

"It was scary being surrounded by all that equipment, and the injection made me feel hot all over, but after they put the catheter in, I enjoyed watching myself on the TV monitor. It's important to have your doctor explain everything in advance—that made me much less anxious."

## Results:

Your doctor may be able to discuss preliminary results immediately after the test. A full report is usually available within 1–2 days.

Contrast material will flow quickly and evenly through normal arteries. Contrast material that leaks out of the blood vessels may indicate internal bleeding. The arteriogram may reveal an outpouching of a blood vessel (aneurysm). Narrowed arteries may suggest a disease of the blood vessels such as cholesterol deposits, inherited disorders, spasm, or other conditions. A complete blockage of a vessel may indicate a blood clot.

Displacement of blood vessels may be due to tumors or internal bleeding. An abnormal network of new arteries may indicate a tumor. Understanding a tumor's blood supply is useful in planning appropriate treatment.

## Cost:

$1000 to $2000

## Special Considerations:

★*Digital Subtraction Angiography (DSA)* —This new test, now available at only a few medical centers, is quickly revolutionizing the practice of angiography and arteriography. Instead of introducing a long catheter through an artery in your leg and into the arteries to be examined, your doctor injects the contrast material through a catheter placed in a vein in your arm or leg.

Computers make DSA possible. The x-ray machine takes two pictures, and the computer then "subtracts" one picture from the other. The resulting image shows only the arteries to be studied.

This technique substantially reduces the risk of stroke or damage to the artery. However, this method may not produce as much information as regular arteriography. Some people who undergo DSA may need to have a standard arteriogram as well.

As a small percentage of people having DSA feel nauseous, it's a good idea not to eat for 2–3 hours before the test.

The exam usually takes 30 minutes to an hour. After the test you will be asked to wait in a recovery room for 30 minutes to an hour to be sure that you have not experienced a reaction to the contrast material.

# Arteriogram— Cerebral/Carotid/ Vertebral
## (Cerebral Angiogram, Carotid Angiogram)

In this test a contrast material, which makes blood vessels stand out in x-rays, is injected into one or both carotid and/or vertebral arteries in your neck. X-rays are then taken to study the flow of blood through the brain. The contrast medium is introduced through a long, narrow, flexible tube (catheter) which is inserted into an artery, usually in your leg.

## Why Performed:

This test is used to evaluate such symptoms as frequent severe headaches, memory loss, slurred speech, dizziness, blurred or double vision, weakness or numbness, and loss of coordination or balance. It is frequently performed to get more exact information after an abnormality has been detected either by a CT scan of the head (see p. 256) or a brain scan (see p. 289). It is most commonly used in confirmed or suspected cases of stroke, tumor, bulging of the artery walls (aneurysm), clot (thrombosis), narrowing or blockage (occlusion) of the arteries, and to evaluate the arteries of the head and neck before or after corrective surgery.

## Preparation:

Tell your doctor if

You are taking any medications

You have ever had an allergic reaction to x-ray contrast material or any other iodine-containing substance

You have ever had an allergic reaction to any medication, pollen, or other substance

You have had bleeding problems

You might be pregnant

You will be asked to sign a consent form authorizing this procedure. Use this opportunity to discuss with your doctor any concerns you may have about the need for the test, the risks of the test, or how it will be performed.

You should arrange to have someone drive you home 7–9 hours after the procedure; check with your doctor to see when you will be able to leave the hospital. You will undergo routine blood tests and a complete examination of your nervous system

(neurologic exam) before the procedure is performed.

You will be asked to abstain from all food for 4–8 hours before the test. You may or may not be asked to abstain from fluids as well; ask your physician for instructions. Before the test, remove all dentures, hairpins, necklaces, earrings, or other objects which might appear on the x-ray. Your hair should be unbraided. You will be asked to put on a hospital gown.

You may receive a sedative and/or pain pill before or during the procedure to help you relax. In rare cases an extremely nervous adult patient and children who are unable to cooperate may be given a general anesthetic.

As the procedure is a lengthy one, it's a good idea to empty your bladder just before the test begins.

## Procedure:

This procedure is performed by a radiologist and one or more x-ray technicians in the x-ray department of a hospital.

You will be asked to lie on your back on a hard x-ray table in the middle of a room filled with x-ray machines and various other electronic equipment. You will be lying directly beneath a long, round columnlike fluoroscope, which is connected to a TV monitor. This device will move up and down from time to time during the procedure.

Your head will be positioned and then immobilized with a strap, tape, or sandbags. ECG leads may be taped to your arms and legs to monitor the electrical activity of your heart during the procedure. The injection site usually overlying an artery in the groin will be shaved and cleansed with an iodine solution. A local anesthetic will be injected.

You will be asked to lie still with your

arms at your side. A needle will be inserted into the femoral artery in your groin. A long flexible tube (catheter) will be inserted through the needle and threaded up through the main vessels of the abdomen and chest until it is properly placed in one of the arteries of the neck. Proper placement will be verified by x-ray pictures displayed on the monitor.

If the femoral artery cannot be used, the test may be done by injecting the contrast medium directly into the arteries of the neck. If the injection site is the neck, you will be asked to extend your head back with your chin pointing up.

The contrast medium (dye) is injected and a series of x-rays is taken. Be sure to keep very still while x-rays are being taken to avoid blurring the x-ray image.

The x-ray technician may apply pressure to the artery on one side of your neck while dye is injected into the artery on the other side. This can demonstrate whether the artery through which the dye is flowing is capable of supplying blood to the entire head.

The x-rays are developed and reviewed immediately. Depending on the findings, more contrast medium may be injected and more x-rays taken. The catheter may be kept open by flushing it periodically with saline solution containing heparin, which keeps the blood within the catheter from clotting. Your pulse, blood pressure, and breathing rate are usually monitored during the procedure.

After the study is completed, the needle or catheter will be withdrawn, and pressure will be applied to the insertion site for 10–15 minutes to stop any bleeding. The puncture site will then be checked and a tight bandage applied.

This test usually takes 1–3 hours depending on how long it takes to place the catheter and how many x-rays are taken.

The leg into which the catheter was inserted should be kept straight and checked regularly for 12 hours after the procedure. If you have the test as an outpatient, you will be sent home after about 6 hours. You should try to keep your leg as straight as possible and you should remain in bed for the rest of the day. You will be given instructions for home care, and pain medication will be provided if needed. If you remain in the hospital, you will be asked to lie still in bed and will be checked regularly for 12–24 hours after the test.

You can help relieve any discomfort in the 24 hours after the test by applying an ice pack intermittently to the injection site. After the initial 24-hour period, occasional warm soaks can help relieve pain and aid healing of the injection site.

### How Does It Feel?

If you find the table hard or feel cold, you may wish to request a blanket, pad, or pillow.

You will feel a brief sting as the local anesthetic is injected. The anesthetic numbs the skin, but not the artery. You will feel a brief, sharp pain as the catheter is first inserted into the artery and may experience a feeling of pressure in the artery as the catheter is advanced. Let your doctor know what you are feeling; this discomfort may be relieved by additional injections of local anesthetic.

When the dye is injected you will feel a burning sensation in your face and head and may experience a brief headache or feel flushed on the side of your face that was injected. A few people experience nausea. These symptoms should last only briefly. If the exam goes on long enough for the local anesthetic to wear off, you may experience pain at the catheter insertion site.

You may notice some tenderness and

bruising at the injection site after the test. If you notice facial weakness, visual disturbance, or slurred speech, or if your leg becomes cool, pale, or numb during or following the procedure, notify your doctor.

### Risks:

This procedure does involve a small but meaningful risk, so be sure you thoroughly understand the necessity for the test before proceeding. There are a number of possible complications, and although the risk of any one major problem is extremely small, they can add up to a significant risk.

There is the possibility of a reaction to the contrast medium. This can range from itching, hives, and wheezing to very rare cases of severe reaction which can result in death. Most problems can be controlled by medication. Be sure to tell your doctor if you have had any sensitivity or allergy to iodine-containing substances or if you have allergies of any kind (e.g., hay fever, eczema, hives, food allergies).

There is also some risk that the catheter may damage an artery or knock loose a piece of an artery wall. Such a dislodged object can block blood flow and create damage to the brain (stroke). This happens in fewer than 1 in 100 patients.

Perforation of the artery wall is rare but possible. Clotting or bleeding at the puncture site can result in a partial blockage of blood to the affected leg.

There is always some concern about the effects of exposure to any radiation, including the low-level radiation of diagnostic x-rays. Extremely high levels of radiation have been shown to cause various diseases and birth defects. However, if this test is really necessary, the radiation risk is generally very low compared with the potential benefits of the test.

Compared with other x-rays, the radiation exposure from this test is medium for total body exposure and low for exposure to the reproductive organs. Because a developing fetus is very sensitive to radiation, this test is not usually recommended for pregnant women. (For more on x-ray risks see p. 227).

Be sure to discuss the particular risks in your case with your doctor.

### Results:

The radiologist may be able to discuss preliminary results immediately after the test. Full results should be ready in 1–2 days.

Any contrast material that flows out of the blood vessels may indicate internal bleeding. Narrowed arteries may suggest disease of the blood vessels such as cholesterol deposits, inherited disorders, spasm, or other conditions. Displacement of the vessels may be due to tumors or bleeding within the skull. Abnormal growth or formation of arteries may indicate a tumor, aneurysm, or arterial-venous (AV) malformation.

### Cost:

$1000 to $1500

### Special Considerations:

★*Four-Vessel Study*—In this test the catheter is positioned up to four different times, so that contrast material can flow into each of the four arteries supplying the head and neck: the right and left carotid arteries and the right and left vertebral arteries.

★*Arch Study*—In this test the catheter is withdrawn from the neck and contrast material is injected into the aorta, the large artery between the carotids and the heart. This allows your doctor to see the arteries as they branch off the aorta within the chest.

★*Digital Subtraction Angiography (DSA)*—see p. 237.

# Arteriogram—Lung
## (Pulmonary Arteriography, Pulmonary Angiography)

This test permits evaluation of the blood vessels within the lungs. A contrast medium is injected into the arteries leading to the lungs so that x-ray pictures of these vessels can be taken.

### Why Performed:

This test is used to diagnose suspected blood clots and other blockages of blood flow in the lung. Such a blockage is called a *pulmonary embolism.* Symptoms that suggest a possible pulmonary embolism include sudden onset of chest pain accompanied by shortness of breath and rapid heartbeat. When pulmonary embolism is suspected, a chest x-ray and lung scan are usually done before this test. If a lung scan (see p. 295) shows abnormal findings, a pulmonary arteriogram may be performed.

### Preparation:

Tell your doctor if
    You might be pregnant
    You are taking any medication
    You have ever had an allergic reaction to x-ray contrast material or other iodine-containing substance
    You have ever had an allergic reaction to any medication, food, pollen, or other substance

You will be asked to fast for approximately 8 hours and to abstain from water for 1 hour before the test. You will be asked to put on a hospital gown and to remove all jewelry or other objects that might appear on the x-rays.

You will be asked to sign a consent form authorizing this procedure. Use this opportunity to discuss with your doctor any concerns you may have about the need for the test, the risks of the test, or how and when it will be performed.

### Procedure:

This test is done in a hospital x-ray department by a radiologist and one or two x-ray technicians. It is rarely done as an outpatient procedure.

You will be asked to lie on your back on a hard x-ray table in the middle of a room full of electronic and x-ray equipment. You will be lying beneath a long, round, columnlike fluoroscope, which is connected to a TV monitor. This device will move up and down during the procedure. ECG leads will be attached to your arms and legs to monitor your heart during the procedure.

The injection site is usually a vein in the groin or at the elbow. The site is shaved if necessary, cleansed with an iodine solution, and a local anesthetic is injected. A small incision is made in the skin, and a long, thin, flexible tube (catheter) is inserted through the skin and into the underlying artery.

The catheter is then threaded along the chosen vessel, through the heart, and into the pulmonary artery, which leads to the lungs. The movement of the catheter is checked on the TV monitor.

When the catheter tip is positioned in the pulmonary artery, the contrast material will be injected. As the contrast material passes through the lungs, a rapid series of x-rays is taken. During the injection you will be asked to take a breath and hold it for several seconds. The process may be repeated on the artery leading to the other lung. If a clot is found on one side, the other side is usually not done.

After the needed x-rays have been obtained, the catheter is slowly withdrawn, and pressure is applied to the insertion site for several minutes to stop any bleeding.

The test usually takes about 1 to 1½ hours. You will be instructed on proper care for the catheter insertion site. You should remain in bed for 24 hours following the test. If you notice increasing chest pain or shortness of breath, let your nurse or doctor know immediately.

## How Does It Feel?

You may feel a brief stinging as the local anesthetic is injected, a brief sharp pain as the catheter is first inserted, and some pressure in the vein as the catheter is advanced.

When the contrast material (dye) is injected you will feel a burning sensation starting in your chest and spreading throughout your body. A few patients experience nausea. These symptoms should last only briefly. You may feel the urge to cough during the injection, but try to avoid doing so. If the exam goes on long enough for the local anesthetic to wear off, you may experience pain at the catheter insertion site.

## Risks:

This procedure does involve some risk, so you should thoroughly understand the need for the test before proceeding. There are a number of possible complications, and although the risk of any one major problem is extremely small, they can add up to a significant risk.

There is the possibility of a reaction to the iodine contrast material. This can range from itching, hives, and wheezing to very rare cases of severe reactions which can result in death. Most problems can be controlled by medication. Be sure to tell your doctor if you have had any sensitivity or allergy to iodine-containing substances or if you have allergies of any kind (e.g., hay fever, eczema, hives, food allergies).

If the catheter is introduced through the femoral vein, there is some risk that the catheter may dislodge a blood clot. Such a dislodged clot can travel to the lungs and cause a pulmonary embolism, the very condition this test is usually used to diagnose.

There is also a slight risk of bleeding, blockage of blood flow, or infection at the catheter insertion site.

There is always some concern about the effects of exposure to any radiation, including the low-level radiation of diagnostic x-rays. Extremely high levels of radiation have been shown to cause various diseases and birth defects. However, if this test is really necessary, the radiation risk is generally very low compared with the potential benefits of the test.

Compared with other x-rays, the radiation exposure from this test is medium for total body exposure and medium for exposure to the reproductive organs. Because a developing fetus is very sensitive to radiation, this test is not usually recommended for pregnant women. (For more on x-ray risks, see p. 227.)

## Results:

Results are usually available immediately after the test.

If the vessels of the lungs are normal, the contrast material will be evenly spread and will flow through without interruption. Blockages in blood flow may be caused by a blood clot in an artery supplying the lungs (pulmonary embolism), narrowed blood vessels, or displaced blood vessels due to a tumor.

## Cost:

$1000 to $1500

# Arthrogram
# (Arthrography)

In this test a fluid containing a contrast medium is injected into a joint. This allows your doctor to visualize the interior structures of the joint on x-rays.

Arthrograms can be taken of any joint in the body, but they are most commonly done on the knee and shoulder joints. Arthrography can provide much more information about a joint problem than a standard x-ray because it shows both the bones and the soft tissues of the joint—the cartilage, ligaments, and bursae (saclike structures filled with thick fluid which reduces friction in many of your body's joints).

## Why Performed:

Arthrography is usually used to evaluate an injured or arthritic joint. A typical use of this test is to evaluate persistent unexplained pain or limitation of movement in a knee or shoulder joint. It can be very useful in deciding whether a knee or shoulder injury requires surgery. The most frequent use of this test is to evaluate suspected tears in the cartilage of the knee. Arthrography can also be used to evaluate the function of artificial joints.

If your doctor needs more information to decide how to treat your knee problem, you may face a choice between having an arthrogram or arthroscopy (see p. 312). Arthroscopy is a surgical procedure in which a thin viewing tube is inserted into the joint through a small incision. There are advantages and disadvantages to each test. The choice of procedure will depend on the location of the suspected problem. Fortunately, many of the areas that are difficult to assess by arthroscopy are easy to examine by arthrography, and vice versa. The arthrogram allows your doctor to look at the entire joint space, while in arthroscopy it may be possible to adequately examine only certain areas.

Arthrography can be used to examine both the inner and outer aspects of the knee, while in arthroscopy it is usually possible to examine only one or the other. There is less risk, discomfort, and cost with an arthrogram. Arthroscopy, however, is preferred if it is very likely that surgery will be necessary, since certain surgical procedures can also be done through the arthroscope.

If arthrography does not reveal the source of the problem, should arthroscopy be done? Usually not. A "negative" result usually means that surgery is not needed. If severe symptoms continue, however, arthroscopy may be necessary at a later time.

## Preparation:

Tell your doctor if
    You might be pregnant
    You have ever had an allergic reaction
        to x-ray contrast material or any
        other iodine-containing substance

You will be asked to sign a consent form authorizing this procedure. Use this opportunity to discuss with your doctor any concerns you may have about the need for the test, the risks of the test, or how it will be performed.

There is no need to restrict food or fluids. Empty your bladder just before the test.

## Procedure:

The test is usually performed under local anesthesia by a physician (usually a radiologist) and a radiology technician. It is done in a hospital x-ray suite or in a radiologist's office and is frequently done on an outpatient basis. This test is rarely done under general anesthesia; if so, it is performed in an operating room.

You will be asked to sit or lie with the joint to be examined under a fluoroscopy tube, a long, round columnlike device connected to a TV monitor. The joint and the injection site are shaved, cleaned with an antiseptic solution, and draped with sterile towels. A local anesthetic is injected. The doctor then inserts a needle into the joint space. The needle's progress is usually checked on the TV monitor.

Once the needle is properly placed, a sample of the joint fluid is withdrawn. This is usually sent to the laboratory for analysis. The x-ray contrast material is injected into the joint space. Sometimes a small amount of air is also injected. The needle is then withdrawn. A bandage is then placed over the injection site.

Your doctor will ask you to move the joint in order to spread the contrast material through the joint space. X-rays are then taken. If your knee is being examined, you may be asked to take a few steps or to run in place. The doctor may also move or stretch the joint while further x-rays are taken or further observations are made on the TV monitor. A series of x-ray pictures will be taken with the joint in various positions.

This procedure usually takes 25–35 minutes. You will probably be advised to rest the joint for 12 hours after the test. (The contrast medium is absorbed quickly, but the air can remain for up to 24 hours.) You should avoid dancing, jogging, or other strenuous activity for 1–2 days. If swelling occurs, ice applied intermittently to the joint may help reduce it.

If the procedure was done on the knee, wrap your knee in an elastic bandage for 12–24 hours after the test.

## How Does It Feel?

The x-ray table will be hard and may be cold. You may feel a brief sting when the local anesthetic is injected.

There will be a feeling of dull pressure when the needle is inserted and a tingling warmth and fullness within the joint when the contrast material (dye) is injected. Try to relax when the needle is being inserted. If your muscles tighten, it makes the joint space smaller and more difficult to enter. The movement and repositioning of the joint may be momentarily painful.

You may experience mild pain, tenderness, and swelling in the joint after the test, and you may hear a grating or crackling sound when you move the joint. This usually lasts less than 24 hours. If you notice persistent pain, tenderness, or swelling of the joint, notify your doctor.

*Patient Comments*:

"The worst part was when the radiologist started twisting my knee back and forth. It hurt somewhat but surprised me more than anything. Afterward the joint felt soggy and noisy, like a shoe filled with water."

## Risks:

Possible complications of this procedure include infection at the site of the injection (very rare) and allergic reaction to the contrast material (see Reactions to Contrast Media, p. 232).

There is always some concern about the effects of exposure to any radiation, including the low-level radiation of diagnostic x-rays. Extremely high levels of radiation have been shown to cause various diseases and birth defects. However, if this test is really necessary, the radiation risk is generally very low compared with the potential benefits of the test.

Compared with other x-rays, the radiation exposure from this test is relatively low for total body exposure and low for exposure to the reproductive organs. Ask your doctor if lead shielding could be used to protect your reproductive organs while the x-rays are being taken. Because a developing fetus is very sensitive to radiation, this test is not usually recommended for pregnant women. (For more on x-ray risks, see p. 227.)

**Results:**

The radiologist may be able to discuss the findings with you during or immediately after the test.

*Knee*—the most common abnormal findings are tears in the wedge-shaped cartilage pad on the inside of the knee (medial meniscal tears), disorders of bone growth, cartilage disorders, torn ligaments, and disruption of the joint capsule.

*Shoulder*—the most common abnormal findings are adhesions of the joint capsule, inflammation or rupture of the tendon sheath, tears in the muscles that surround the joint, and damage resulting from dislocations of the head of the humerus (the bone of the upper arm).

**Cost:**

| | |
|---|---|
| Knee: | $130 to $180 |
| Shoulder: | $100 to $150 |
| Other: | $100 to $180 |

# Barium Enema
## (BE, BaE, Lower Gastrointestinal Series)

A barium enema is an x-ray examination of the large intestine (colon). To make the intestine visible on x-ray, liquid barium sulfate is instilled through the anus to fill the colon. The barium blocks x-rays, causing the barium-filled colon to show up as a white shadow on the x-ray film. This test is useful in detecting or confirming the presence of polyps, tumors, and inflammation of the colon (see illustration, p. 281).

There are two types of barium enema. In the "single-contrast" study the colon is filled with barium only. In the "double-contrast" or "air-contrast" study, the colon is first coated with a thin layer of barium and then filled with air. The double-contrast barium enema is more time-consuming and somewhat more uncomfortable, but offers a much more detailed view of the inner lining (mucosa) of the colon, and is more sensitive in detecting small polyps, cancers, or inflammation. The single-contrast study is often done first. If the results do not permit a diagnosis or if there is a strong suspicion of colon cancer, an air-contrast study is then performed.

**Why Performed:**

This test is often used to detect colon cancer. The first signs of a cancer might be blood in the stool (either visible or detected on a stool blood test, see p. 443), a change in bowel habits (persistent diarrhea, constipation, or narrowed, pencil-thin stool), or unexplained lower abdominal pain. However, a barium enema should be ordered only after you have had a thorough history and physical examination, usually including a proctosigmoidoscopy (see p. 335). The cause of symptoms can sometimes be determined in this way without a barium enema.

A barium enema is not generally accepted as a useful screening test for colon cancer in people without symptoms. However, this test may be recommended for some people who are at high risk in developing colon cancer due to a personal or family history of colon cancer, intestinal polyps, or ulcerative colitis.

A barium enema may also be used to document the presence and extent of inflammatory bowel disease such as ulcerative colitis or granulomatous colitis (Crohn's disease).

This test is of doubtful value in evaluating chronic constipation (a common reason for ordering this test), a brief episode of diarrhea, or abdominal pain, particularly in younger people. Also, CT scans and ultrasound are now the tests of choice for the initial evaluation of most abdominal masses. A barium enema is no longer considered necessary before routine surgical repair of hernias.

### Preparation:

Tell your doctor if
  You might be pregnant

The preparation for a barium enema involves a very thorough cleaning of your large intestine. An accurate test depends on your colon being free of stool and gas. Even a small amount of stool material can mask or be mistaken for an abnormality. If your colon is not clear, the test will have to be postponed or repeated.

Nearly every doctor and x-ray department has a slightly different ritual for bowel cleaning and preparation, so check with your doctor for details. In general, it is recommended that you start on a clear-liquid diet (no solid, high-residue foods) for 1 to 3 days before the exam. On the day before the exam you should drink very large amounts of noncarbonated clear liquids. You will also be instructed to take a combination of laxatives or cathartics, usually castor oil, magnesium citrate, or bisacodyl (Dulcolax). The day before the test you will need to take a warm-tap-water enema. On

the day of the exam you may be instructed to repeat the tap-water enemas until the return is clear of any stool particles.

If you have a lot of anal soreness or irritation after the laxatives and enemas, ask for a local anesthetic salve to numb the anal area during the exam. The salve should be applied 15–20 minutes before the exam is to start.

You will be asked to remove all your clothing and put on a special gown. You may want to bring along a robe and socks to keep warm, although some of the barium may get on them during the exam.

### Procedure:

The test is performed by a radiologist and one or two assistants in an office or hospital radiology department. Overnight hospitalization is not usually necessary.

You will be asked to lie on the x-ray table while a preliminary x-ray film is taken. While lying on your side, a well-lubricated enema tube will be inserted gently into your rectum. The barium, stored in a bag, is then allowed to flow slowly into your colon. A small balloon on the enema tip may be inflated to help you hold in the barium. Tightening your anal sphincter muscle against the tube may also help.

The doctor will observe the flow of the barium through your colon on an x-ray fluoroscope screen like a TV monitor. You will be asked to turn in different positions and the table may tilt slightly to obtain different views (sides, front, and back). The doctor may also press gently on your abdomen with his hand or plastic paddle to help move the barium through your intestines. At certain times "snapshot" x-ray pictures called "spot films" will be taken of different areas of your colon. You will be asked to hold your breath and lie completely still for a few seconds while these pictures are being taken.

The enema tube is then removed, and you will be given a bedpan or escorted to the toilet. You will be asked to expel as much of the barium as you can. One or two additional x-ray pictures (postevacuation films) will then be taken. If a double- or air-contrast study is being performed, the enema tube will be reinserted and a small amount of air will be gently instilled into your colon. A thin layer of barium will then coat the air-filled colon. This procedure gives more detailed x-ray pictures. You will then again be asked to empty your colon.

A single-contrast study usually takes 30–45 minutes, although the actual time the barium is held inside is only 10–15 minutes. A double- or air-contrast study may take up to an hour. After the exam you may resume your regular diet unless otherwise instructed. Be sure to drink plenty of liquids to replace lost fluids and help flush the remaining barium out of your colon.

### How Does It Feel?

The procedure may be somewhat uncomfortable and tiring, but fortunately it does not last very long.

Many patients report that the preparation and bowel cleaning are the most taxing part of the test. The castor oil has an unpleasant taste. The frequent bowel movements can be exhausting. And the anal area can become quite sore (warm sitz baths or local anesthetic salve can ease this discomfort.)

The test itself is also potentially embarrassing. Patients are often afraid that they won't be able to hold the barium in and that it will leak onto them or onto the table. Be assured that though these mishaps do happen, the physicians and technicians who perform this procedure are accustomed to them and will be able to help you. You can decrease your own anxiety by discussing the possibility of a spill with the technician before starting the procedure. If the technician doesn't bring up the matter, you might say: "I understand that it's sometimes difficult to hold the barium in. I'm worried about that."

As the barium first flows into your colon it may feel a bit cool. As the colon fills you may feel a full sensation, moderate cramping and an uncontrollable urge to have a bowel movement. If an air-contrast study is performed, you may feel increased cramping or gas pains from the distention of the large intestine when the air is introduced. Taking slow deep breaths through your mouth can help you relax.

The x-ray table is hard and sometimes cold. You will also hear loud snapping and banging noises from time to time as the x-ray film cassettes slide into place.

The examination as a whole can be extremely tiring, particularly in elderly or debilitated patients. You may feel tired for a day or so after the test. It may be a good idea to arrange for someone to drive you home after the test.

For 1–2 days after the test you may notice some of the residual barium (a whitish or pinkish material) in your bowel movements. If you notice rectal bleeding, severe abdominal pain, or fever notify your doctor.

*Patient Comments:*

"The preparation and laxatives were the hardest part. My rectum became very sore, and I was crampy from so much laxative, but they said it was necessary to be sure the system was cleaned out."

"I felt apprehensive and wondered if I would be able to hold the barium in. I did lose a bit. It was a little messy and embarrassing, but the technician said they see it all the time. That helped me relax."

**Risks:**

There is always some concern about the effects of exposure to any radiation, including the low-level radiation of diagnostic x-rays. Extremely high levels of radiation have been shown to cause various diseases and birth defects. However, if this test is really necessary, the radiation risk is generally very low compared with the benefits.

Compared with other x-rays, the radiation exposure of a barium enema is relatively high for total body exposure, medium to high for the male reproductive organs, and high for the female reproductive organs. Shielding of the gonads from radiation during the exam is difficult, since the shielding might block areas that need to be examined on the x-ray. Because a developing fetus is very sensitive to radiation, this test is not usually recommended for pregnant women.

Occasionally the barium remaining in the colon hardens, causing severe constipation (impaction). Drink large amounts of fluids and, if necessary, take an enema or mild laxative after the test.

A more serious, though exceedingly rare, complication is perforation of the bowel. Under the pressure from the barium or air, a weakened section of the colon may rupture, allowing the intestinal contents to spill into the abdominal cavity. This may occur in patients with a weakened bowel wall from severe colitis. Surgical repair and antibiotics are often required. Rupture of the colon occurs in less than 1 in 5000 examinations.

**Results:**

The radiologist will make observations during the fluoroscopic examination and will record some of the findings on x-ray films. Preliminary results may be discussed with you immediately after the exam or on the following day.

Sections of the colon that fail to fill with barium ("filling defects") suggest a possible cancer. Further examination with colonoscopy and biopsy (p. 319) will be needed. Any polyps that are detected will also have to be removed or biopsied to determine if they are cancerous. Polyps are small growths on the inner wall of the colon.

A common finding is diverticulosis, in which multiple small outpouches form from the colon wall. These are not cancerous but can become inflamed (diverticulitis). Disruptions and inflammation of the inner lining of the intestine may indicate inflammatory bowel disease (either ulcerative colitis or Crohn's disease). An acute appendicitis or twisted loop of bowel may also be seen on a barium enema.

There are limits to a barium enema. Small polyps or cancers may be missed, often because remaining stool hides the lesions. Also, the lower end of the large intestine (rectosigmoid colon) is often better examined by proctosigmoidoscopy than with a barium enema.

**Cost:**

Single-contrast: $90 to $150
Double- or air-contrast: $110 to $170

**Special Considerations:**

★If an upper gastrointestinal series x-ray study is planned, it should be performed after the barium enema. The barium swallowed during an upper GI series may take several days to pass and, therefore, can interfere with the barium study of the colon.

# Bronchogram
## (Bronchography)

The full outline of the bronchial airways within the lung cannot be seen on a regular chest x-ray. In this test a contrast material which is visible on x-ray is injected into the airways of the lungs. X-rays are then taken. This provides a picture of the bronchi—the tubes that carry your breath from your throat and windpipe to the tissues of your lungs.

### Why Performed:
This test is used to investigate such conditions as bronchitis (inflammation of the airways), bronchiectasis (the production of large amounts of sputum by enlarged bronchi), hemoptysis (blood in the sputum), or fistula (an abnormal opening between the respiratory system and some other part of the body—e.g., the esophagus, stomach, or outer chest wall).

This test is now performed less frequently than it was before the development of bronchoscopy (see p. 315). It is occasionally done to guide the doctor who will be doing bronchoscopy and to provide a record of conditions found by bronchoscopy.

### Preparation:
Tell your doctor if

You might be pregnant

You have ever had an allergic reaction to x-ray contrast material, any other iodine-containing substance, or local anesthetics

You may be asked to sign a consent form authorizing this procedure. Use this opportunity to discuss with your doctor any concerns you may have about the need for the test, the risks of the test, or how and when it will be performed.

You will be asked to abstain from all food or fluid for 8–12 hours before the procedure. You may be asked to brush and floss your teeth thoroughly the night before the test and to repeat this procedure again on the morning of the test; this decreases the number of bacteria that could be introduced into the lungs during the test.

If you have a great deal of bronchial secretions, postural drainage may be arranged for one or more days preceding this test. Postural drainage is a procedure designed to help clear the airways of secretions. It is performed by lying in a head-down position, sometimes with another person tapping you vigorously on the back.

Before the test you should remove dentures, jewelry, or other objects that might show up in the x-ray. For your own comfort, empty your bladder just before the test begins.

### Procedure:
This test is performed in a hospital x-ray department by a physician and an x-ray technologist.

You will receive one or more medications 30–45 minutes before the procedure; these are to relieve anxiety, reduce coughing and gagging, and decrease secretions in the bronchi.

You will be asked to position yourself on a hard x-ray table. Your throat will be sprayed and swabbed with a topical anesthetic. Additional anesthetic will be sprayed down your throat. This will make you cough, the coughing helps to spread the anesthetic.

You will be asked to sit up or to lie in a semiupright position. A soft flexible tube (catheter) will be inserted into your nose or mouth and threaded down your throat to the place where your windpipe (trachea) branches into the bronchi which lead to your right and left lungs. (Sometimes a bronchoscope may be used. If so, it will be inserted through your mouth—see Bronchoscopy, p. 315.)

Throughout the procedure your doctor will be taking x-rays with a fluoroscopy machine and watching the resulting images of your chest on a TV monitor.

The catheter is directed into the main bronchus on the side to be studied. Contrast material is then injected. You will be asked to breathe in deeply; this will help spread the contrast material.

Try to cough as little as possible; coughing can push the catheter out of position and prolong the test. It may be helpful to pant like a dog to keep from coughing.

You may then be asked to assume various positions to further spread the contrast material (dye). The spread of the dye is watched on a fluoroscope, and individual x-ray films are taken. You will be asked to lie down while additional x-rays are taken.

Finally, you will be asked to sit up and cough as hard as you can to get rid of the contrast material. After you've coughed up as much as you can, additional films will be taken.

If both lungs are to be examined, the second may be done at a later time. This procedure is sometimes performed under a general anesthetic (see p. 465), especially when bronchoscopy is also to be done.

After the test is completed, postural drainage (in which you lie with your head lower than your feet) or other chest physical therapy may be provided to help you cough up the remaining material. Another fluid may be sprayed into your bronchi to help wash the contrast material out.

You should not have anything to eat or drink until the anesthetic has worn off, usually 2–3 hours.

## How Does It Feel?

This is a physically and emotionally trying test. It may be a good idea to have a friend or a hospital staff member with whom you are especially familiar and comfortable stay with you during the procedure for support.

The anesthetic spray may taste unpleasant and may make your tongue and throat feel swollen. When the catheter passes through the back of your throat, you may find yourself gagging and coughing.

Once the tip of the catheter has passed your throat, the procedure gets easier, but when it reaches the bottom of your windpipe, you may again have a strong urge to cough.

You may feel as though you are having trouble breathing during the procedure—don't worry, you will receive plenty of oxygen and your airway will not be blocked. The more you can relax, the easier it will be for the doctor to pass the catheter.

After the test you may have a sore throat. After the anesthetic has worn off, you may wish to use throat lozenges or a warm-salt-water gargle to relieve the discomfort.

You should plan on a full day of rest after the procedure.

You may have sore chest muscles from coughing. It is common to develop a fever after the procedure—the result of chemical irritation to the lungs. The fever will normally disappear within 48 hours. If it persists longer, notify your doctor.

## Risks:

There is an extremely small risk that the windpipe could be punctured: in rare cases this can result in the collapse of a lung. There is also a small risk of pneumonia.

This can be produced by the contrast medium itself ("chemical" pneumonia) or by bacteria introduced during the test. Such pneumonias usually heal by themselves or may require antibiotic treatment. There is a very small risk of reaction to the contrast medium.

There is always some concern about the effects of exposure to any radiation, including the low-level radiation of diagnostic x-rays. Extremely high levels of radiation have been shown to cause various diseases and birth defects. However, if the test is really necessary, the radiation risk is generally very low compared with the benefits.

Compared with other x-rays, the radiation exposure from bronchography is relatively low for total body exposure and low for exposure to the reproductive organs. Since a developing fetus is very sensitive to radiation, this test is not usually recommended for pregnant women. (For more on x-ray risks, see p. 227).

### Results:

Preliminary results may be available immediately after the test or by the next day.

The x-rays may show widening of the bronchial tubes (bronchiectasis) or blockage of the bronchial tubes by cysts, cavities, tumors, or foreign objects.

### Cost:

One side: $250 to $300
Both sides: $300 to $350

# Chest X-ray

The chest x-ray is the most frequently performed x-ray procedure. It provides a picture of the organs and structures within the chest: the lungs, blood vessels in the lungs, heart, large arteries leading in and out of the heart, and the right and left sides of the diaphragm (the thin sheet of muscle just below the lungs). A chest x-ray can provide a rough screening for disorders of these structures as well as the ribs, collarbone, breasts, and the upper part of the spine. However, more specific x-rays are usually necessary if abnormalities are detected.

### Why Performed:

Chest x-rays are often ordered when a medical history, physical exam, or the results of other medical tests suggest disease of the chest. They can be especially helpful in evaluating persistent cough, coughing up blood (hemoptysis), chest pain, difficulty in breathing, fever of unknown cause, or chest injury. They are also frequently done when active tuberculosis or lung cancer is suspected.

A chest x-ray should usually not be required as a condition of employment. However, certain workers (such as asbestos workers) are exposed to potentially damaging substances and should have periodic screening chest x-rays.

Although the chest x-ray is an excellent method of detecting a wide variety of problems, this test is sometimes overused. For instance, x-ray screening for tuberculosis was once routine. There is now general agreement that routine chest x-rays should not be done on healthy people for screening purposes. Chest x-rays should also probably not be done

As a requirement of hospital admission for persons under 40 with no evidence of lung disease

On heavy smokers without symptoms to screen for cancer (see Special Considerations)

On a daily basis for patients with uncomplicated pneumonia

On former tuberculosis patients who have fully recovered and are now without symptoms

## Preparation:

Tell your doctor if

You might be pregnant

You have had a previous chest x-ray within the past 12 months

You will be asked to remove all clothing above the waist, including your bra, and to remove any jewelry around your neck.

## Procedure:

The chest x-ray may be taken at a doctor's office, a radiologist's office, a clinic, a hospital radiology department, or your bedside in a hospital. The film will be taken by a radiologic technician and will be interpreted by a physician, usually a radiologist.

Two films are usually taken—a *PA or posterior-anterior view*, in which the x-rays pass through your chest from back (posterior) to front (anterior), and a *lateral view*, in which the x-rays pass through your body from one side to the other. Sometimes only a PA view is taken.

*PA View*—You will be positioned with your chest against a film holder and your hands on your hips, with your shoulders forward. The x-ray tube will be placed about 6 feet behind you. You will then be asked to take a deep breath and hold it while the

film is exposed. Be sure to hold your breath as directed, and remain very still while the x-ray is being taken.

*Lateral View*—You will be asked to stand with one side toward the film holder, with your arms forward or above your head to keep them out of the x-ray beam. Again you will be asked to take a deep breath and hold it while the x-ray is taken.

Additional views may be taken in special circumstances.

The test takes 5–10 minutes. You will be asked to wait while the film is developed to determine whether repeat films will be necessary.

## How Does It Feel?

There is no discomfort associated with this exam.

## Risks:

There is always some concern about the effects of exposure to any radiation, including the low-level radiation of diagnostic x-rays. Extremely high levels of radiation have been shown to cause various diseases and birth defects. However, if this test is really necessary, the radiation risk is generally very low compared with the potential benefits.

Compared with other x-rays, the radiation exposure for this test is relatively low for total body exposure and low for exposure to the reproductive organs. Because a developing fetus is very sensitive to radiation, this test is not usually recommended for pregnant women. (For more on x-ray risks, see p. 227.)

## Results:

Results should be available immediately or by the next day.

*Lungs*—A chest x-ray may reveal infection (such as pneumonia or tuberculosis) or a collapsed lung. It may also show scarring of the lung tissue, a collection of fluid around the lung (pleural effusion), or may suggest the development of emphysema (also called chronic obstructive pulmonary disease or COPD). A single spot or nodule in the lung ("coin lesion") may be due to a cyst, a benign tumor, a malformation of the blood vessels, or lung cancer. A chest x-ray is not a very sensitive test for indicating the early damage done by cigarette smoking. Even though the chest x-ray may appear normal, there can be significant airway and lung disease.

*Heart*—The size and shape of the heart and the position and shape of the large artery leading from the heart to the body (aorta) can usually be determined.

*Bones*—Fractures or other abnormalities of the ribs and the spine can sometimes be seen.

Further tests are often needed to evaluate abnormalities seen on x-ray. Some findings are not clear-cut, and different observers sometimes draw different conclusions about the same chest x-rays. Significant abnormalities can be overlooked, insignificant abnormalities can be thought to be significant, and experts frequently disagree—even with themselves—about the interpretation of chest x-rays. Therefore, when the interpretation of an x-ray is likely to make a significant difference (for example, if surgery is recommended because of the results of a chest x-ray), you should seek a second opinion.

### Cost:

$35 to $50
$60 to $80 (2 views)

### Special Considerations:

★*Screening Smokers for Lung Cancer*—Preliminary studies of screening programs show that there is little or no benefit of using chest x-rays to screen smokers who have no symptoms of lung disease. Concerned smokers should watch for the following symptoms: coughing up blood, a cough lasting more than 6 weeks, increasing shortness of breath, or significant weight loss. If any of these symptoms appear, you should have a thorough physical examination, including a chest x-ray. The most effective way to cut your risk of getting lung cancer is to reduce your exposure to inhaled tobacco smoke to the lowest possible level.

★*Nipple Markers*—Sometimes the x-ray shadows of the nipples in either men or women are difficult to distinguish from abnormal findings. If small rounded densities are seen in your first chest films, you may be asked to return for repeat films wearing nipple markers (steel or lead BBs taped to your nipples).

★*Tomogram*—This is a special x-ray procedure performed to obtain a clearly focused x-ray image of a part of the chest (or other part of the body) which is hidden by shadows in a regular x-ray or to obtain more information about a suspicious finding on a regular x-ray. In this test the x-ray tube swings back and forth above you, taking numerous films from different angles. There is a higher radiation exposure from tomography than from a regular chest x-ray.

# CT Scan—Body
## (CAT Scan of Body, Computerized Tomography of Body)

In this test a computerized axial tomography (CAT or CT) scanner is used to produce a series of cross-sectional x-ray images of a selected part of the body. A computer operates the scanner, and the resulting picture represents a slice of the body. Areas above and below the chosen slice do not appear on the image. The computer can then combine the information in several slices to create other images of the structures inside the body. These images can detect many conditions that cannot be seen in regular x-rays.

The scanner produces images by passing a pencil-thin beam of x-rays through a particular area of the body. The x-ray tube moves rapidly around the chosen slice, creating a 360-degree picture. It takes the machine only a few seconds to photograph each slice, and 10–30 slices are usually taken.

The x-ray beam is picked up by an electronic device that records the information and sends it to a computer for processing. The computer then displays the chosen slice on a TV screen. Information from several slices can be combined to create a view across the body from any angle.

Information from the scans is stored in the computer's memory and can be converted into images on a video screen at any time. Photographs of the video screen are taken to record significant findings. The information is then kept in storage on a disc or tape so that it can be examined again if necessary.

It is no overstatement to say that CT scanning has revolutionized the practice of making images of the human body. The CT scanner is the greatest advance in diagnostic imaging since the discovery of x-rays. It produces pictures with 10–20 times the detail of regular x-rays, and it can be used to make images of parts of the body that were previously difficult or impossible to obtain.

However, CT scans are more expensive than regular x-rays, and scanners are not available in all areas. And because the technique is relatively new, some doctors may be unfamiliar with all its uses.

**Why Performed:**

CT scans of the body are used to diagnose a wide variety of conditions, including the following:

- *Chest (Thorax)*—To locate suspected tumors, including Hodgkin's disease, in the space between the lungs (mediastinum); to help decide whether small lumps in the lung are cancer; to distinguish bulges (aneurysms) of the aorta (a large artery which passes down the back of the chest cavity) from tumors of the chest; and to investigate the spread of tumors into the chest from elsewhere in the body.
- *Kidney*—To confirm the presence of stones, obstructions, tumors, congenital abnormalities, infections, and other diseases of the kidneys.
- *Liver*—To diagnose tumors, abscesses, and bleeding.
- *Biliary Tract*—To evaluate jaundice (yellowing of the skin).
- *Pancreas*—To determine if there is a tumor or inflammation of the pancreas. The CT scan is replacing the use of ultrasound as the test of choice for examination of the pancreas. Although it costs more and involves radiation exposure, it can be much more accurate in many conditions. CT scans do a much better job than ultrasound in distinguishing between benign and malignant tumors of the pancreas.
- *Adrenals*—To look for tumors.
- *Spleen*—To evaluate suspected injury and other abnormalities.
- *Spine*—To investigate suspected tumors, injuries, deformities, and other problems of the backbone, discs, and spinal canal.

**Preparation:**

Tell your doctor if

You have ever had an allergic reaction to x-ray contrast material or any other iodine-containing substance

You might be pregnant

You should wear loose-fitting, comfortable clothing, with no jewelry or other objects in the area to be x-rayed. If contrast material will be used, you will be asked to abstain from food for 4 hours and from water for 1 hour before the test.

You will be asked to undress and put on a hospital gown. Be sure to remove any objects that might come into the path of the x-ray beam.

You may be asked to sign a consent form authorizing this procedure. Use this opportunity to ask any questions you may have about the need for this test or its procedure.

**Procedure:**

This test is performed in a hospital radiology department or office by a radiologist and an x-ray technician. You will be asked to lie on a table which is connected to the large CT scanner. You will be positioned so that the body part to be examined lies in the middle of the large scanner ring. The ring contains the x-ray tube and detector.

After the procedure begins, the table on which you are lying will move a small distance every few seconds—this is to position you for each new slice. The mechanism inside the scanner will move around your body and may make clicking or buzzing sounds. It is especially important that you hold completely still while the scan is being taken. Otherwise, repeat scans may be needed.

During the test you will be alone in the room. A technician will be keeping a close watch through an observation window, and you will be able to talk to him or her by a two-way intercom.

An x-ray contrast material may be used to highlight internal structures. This material may be given by mouth, by an injection, or in some cases via an enema. If contrast enhancement is to be used, a preliminary set of CT scans will be done, the contrast medium will be administered, and the CT scans will be repeated.

Afterward you will be asked to wait while the radiologist reviews the scans to be sure that they contain all the required information. Occasionally repeat or additional scans are required.

This test usually takes from 30 minutes to 1½ hours, but because delays and repeats are common, you should allow 2 hours or more.

**How Does It Feel?**

You will feel nothing from the CT scanner. If contrast material (dye) is injected, you will feel the needle going into your vein and may experience a warm, flushed sensation, and perhaps a metallic taste in your mouth as the dye is injected. This will last only a minute or two. In rare cases, some patients may experience such side effects as nausea, vomiting, and headache. If such symptoms persist after the test, notify your doctor.

If you are asked to drink a contrast material, you may find the taste unpleasant.

No aftercare is needed for a plain CT scan.

**Risks:**

If contrast material is used there is the possibility of an allergic reaction. This can range from itching, hives, and wheezing to very rare cases of severe reactions which can result in death. Most problems can be controlled by medication. Be sure to tell your doctor if you have had any sensitivity or allergy to iodine-containing substances or if you have allergies of any kind (e.g., hay fever, eczema, hives, food allergies).

There is always some concern about the effects of exposure to any radiation, including the low-level radiation of diagnostic x-rays. Extremely high levels of radiation have been shown to cause various diseases and birth defects. However, if this test is really necessary, the radiation risk is generally very low compared with the potential benefits of the test.

Compared with other x-rays, the radiation from this test is medium to high for total body exposure and medium to high for exposure of the reproductive organs depending on the area x-rayed. Discuss the possibility of shielding your reproductive organs during the test. Because a developing fetus is very sensitive to radiation, this test is not usually recommended for pregnant women. (For more on x-ray risks, see p. 227.)

**Results:**

The radiologist may be able to give you some preliminary results of the scan immediately after the test. Full results should be available in 1–2 days. The radiologist will interpret the scans and review them with your doctor, who will explain and discuss them with you. Sometimes the diagnosis is not clear-cut and further tests are needed.

The radiologist reading your CT scan will compare your findings with the normal appearance of the organ or organs examined. A diseased organ or structure may appear lighter (more dense) or darker (less dense) than usual. Or certain tissues may be displaced.

The blood vessels don't ordinarily show up in normal CT scans. These vessels, tissues with an ample supply of blood, and some tumors will stand out more readily when contrast material is given. The contrast material is also very useful in detecting bleeding inside the body.

The most common abnormalities in this test are as follows:
- *Chest*—tumors, cysts, aneurysms of the aorta, fluid in the lungs, bleeding, and other accumulations of fluid.
- *Liver*—tumors, abscesses, bleeding, cysts.
- *Biliary Tract*—dilation of the bile ducts (from blockage), gallstones.
- *Pancreas*—tumors, acute pancreatitis, chronic pancreatitis, cysts.
- *Adrenals*—tumors.
- *Spleen*—injuries.
- *Spine*—tumors, herniated discs.

**Cost:**
$400 to $800

# CT Scan—Head
# (CAT Scan—Head, Computerized Tomography—Head)

In this test a computerized axial tomography (CT or CAT) scanner is used to take a series of cross-sectional x-ray pictures of your head. A computer operates the scanner, and each resulting picture represents a slice of your head. Areas above or below the chosen slice do not appear on the image. The computer can then combine the information in several cross sections to create other images of the structures inside your head. These images can detect many conditions that cannot be seen in regular x-rays.

The scanner produces these images by passing a pencil-thin beam of x-rays through a particular area of your head. The x-ray tube moves rapidly around the chosen slice, creating a 360-degree picture. It takes only a few seconds for the machine to record each slice. In a head scan 10–15 slices are usually taken.

The x-ray beam is picked up by an electronic device that records the information and sends it to a computer for processing. The computer then displays the chosen slice on a TV screen. Information from several slices can be combined to create a view from any angle.

Information from the scans is stored in the computer's memory unit and can be converted into images on a video screen at any time. Photographs of the video screen are taken to record the findings. The information is then kept in storage in a disc or tape so that it can be examined again if necessary.

It is no overstatement to say that CT scanning has revolutionized the practice of making images of the human body. The CT scanner is the greatest advance in diagnostic imaging since the discovery of x-rays. It produces pictures with 10–20 times the detail of regular x-rays, and it can be used to make images of parts of the brain that were previously difficult or impossible to obtain.

CT scanning has proved especially useful in diagnosing problems inside the skull, including head injury. CT scans have partially or totally replaced several more painful and hazardous procedures, especially pneumoencephalography, many angiograms, and exploratory brain surgery.

However, CT scans do cost more than a regular x-ray. And because the machines required to perform the test are stagger-ingly expensive, they are not available at all medical facilities.

### Why Performed:
CT scans of the head are most often used to evaluate signs and symptoms of brain injury or disease such as unexplained paralysis, loss of sensation, visual disturbances, headache, and abnormal findings on a neurologic exam. It is usually performed to look for suspected blood clots, tumors, bleeding, infection, or to explain increased pressure within the brain. It may also be used to evaluate the effect of various types of therapy on brain tumors.

### Preparation:
Tell your doctor if
    You have ever had an allergic reaction to x-ray contrast material or any other iodine-containing substances
You might be pregnant

You may be asked to sign a consent form permitting this test. Use this opportunity to make sure that all your questions about the test are answered.

You should wear loose-fitting, comfortable clothes, with no earrings, hairpins, or other objects in the area to be x-rayed. You will be asked to remove dentures, glasses, hearing aids, and other objects that might come into the path of the x-ray beam. If contrast material will be used, you will be asked to abstain from food for 4 hours and from water for 1 hour before the test.

### Procedure:
This test is performed in a hospital radiology department by a radiologist and an x-ray technician. You will be asked to lie on a table connected to a CT scanner, a large machine with a doughnut-shaped scanner ring. Your head will be placed in

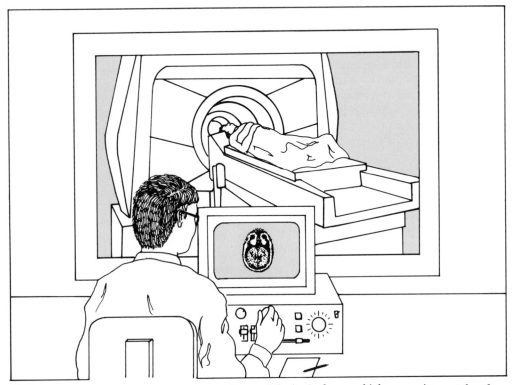

**CT Scan.** *In a CT Scan a computer creates an image of the brain from multiple x-ray pictures taken from different angles.*

a headrest in the middle of the ring. The ring contains the x-ray tube and detector. Your face will not be covered.

After the procedure begins, the table on which you are lying will move a small distance every few seconds to reposition you for each new slice. The mechanism inside the ring will move around your head and may make clicking or buzzing sounds. It is especially important that you hold completely still while the scan is being taken. Otherwise, repeat scans may be needed. During the test you will be alone in the scanner room. A technologist will be keeping a close watch on you through an observation window. You will be able to communicate with her or him via a two-way intercom.

Contrast enhancement is ordered in many CT scans of the head to highlight the internal structures. If your doctor has requested it, a contrast material will be injected into a vein in your arm, and the CT scan will be repeated.

Afterward you will be asked to wait while the radiologist reviews the scans to be sure that they contain all the required information. Occasionally repeat scans are needed.

This test usually takes about 30 minutes, but because of occasional delays and because further evaluations are sometimes necessary, you should allow an hour or more.

## How Does It Feel?

You will feel nothing from the CT scanner. No aftercare is needed for a plain CT scan. If contrast material is used, you may experience a warm, flushed sensation and perhaps a metallic taste in your mouth after it is injected. In rare cases, some patients may experience nausea, vomiting, or headache. If such symptoms persist after the test is completed, notify your doctor.

*Patient Comments:*

"When the dye was injected I felt an intense heat all over my body. Tape was used to keep my head still. When they took the tape off, it pulled my hair."

"You are left all by yourself in there while the machine is whirring around you. You feel warm all over when they inject the contrast material. It was hard to lie perfectly still. I was surprised at how big the machine was."

## Risks:

There is the possibility of a reaction to the iodine contrast material. This can range from itching, hives, and wheezing to very rare cases of severe reactions which can result in death. Most problems can be controlled by medication. Be sure to tell your doctor if you have had any sensitivity or allergy to iodine-containing substances or if you have allergies of any kind (e.g., hay fever, eczema, hives, food allergies).

There is always some concern about the effects of exposure to any radiation, including the low-level radiation of diagnostic x-rays. Extremely high levels of radiation have been shown to cause various diseases and birth defects. However, if this test is really necessary, the radiation risk is generally very low compared with the potential benefits of the test.

Compared with other x-rays, the radiation from this test is relatively low for total body exposure and low for exposure to the reproductive organs. Because a developing fetus is very sensitive to radiation, this test is not usually recommended for pregnant women. (For more on x-ray risks, see p. 227.)

## Results:

The radiologist may be able to discuss preliminary results with you immediately after the test. Full results are usually available in 1–2 days. The radiologist will analyze the scans and review them with your doctor, who will explain them and discuss them with you:

The radiologist reading your CT scan will compare your findings with the normal appearance of the skull and the brain. A diseased organ or structure may appear lighter (more dense) or darker (less dense) than usual, or certain tissues may be displaced.

The blood vessels don't ordinarily show up in CT scans done without contrast material. These vessels—as well as tissues with an ample supply of blood and some tumors—will stand out more readily when contrast material is given. The contrast material is also very useful in detecting bleeding inside the head.

The most common abnormalities found in this test are stroke, bleeding, tumors, abscesses, and excess fluid (hydrocephalus) or enlarged ventricles within the brain. (Ventricles are openings in the brain through which cerebrospinal fluid, CSF, normally flows. A blockage of normal CSF flow can result in enlarged ventricles.) Sometimes the diagnosis is not clear-cut

259

and further tests (e.g., arteriography, p. 237) are needed.

**Cost:**

$300 to $600

# Cystourethrogram
## (Retrograde Cysto-urethrography, Void-ing Cystourethrogram)

In this test a thin flexible tube (catheter) is inserted through the urethra (the channel through which urine passes from the body) and into the bladder (a hollow organ that serves as a reservoir for urine). A contrast material which is visible on x-ray is injected into the bladder through the catheter, and x-rays are taken with the contrast material in the bladder and urethra. Additional x-rays are taken with the urine flowing through the bladder and the urethra.

This test is sometimes called retrograde cystourethrography because the contrast material flows into the bladder in a direction that is the reverse of the usual direction of flow.

**Why Performed:**

This test can be useful in determining the cause of repeated urinary tract infections. It is also used to investigate suspected injuries to the bladder or urethra, to determine the cause of inability to control urinary flow (incontinence), and to detect acquired or inherited malformations of the lower urinary tract. In men this test is sometimes used to investigate suspected enlargement (hypertrophy) of the prostate, narrowing (stricture) of the urethra, and to evaluate

the status of artificial urethras. This test is sometimes performed to evaluate abnormalities first detected on an IVP (p. 269).

**Preparation:**

Tell your doctor if

You might be pregnant

You have ever had an allergic reaction to an x-ray contrast medium or any other iodine-containing substance

There is no need to restrict food or fluids before this test. You may be asked to sign a consent form authorizing this procedure. Use this as an opportunity to ask any questions you have about the need for the test, risks, or how it is performed.

You will be asked to remove your clothes and to put on a hospital gown. Be sure to empty your bladder immediately before the test begins.

**Procedure:**

This test will be performed by a radiologist or urologist and an x-ray technician in an x-ray department or urologic procedures room. It can be performed on an outpatient basis.

You will be asked to lie on your back on an x-ray table. Your genital area will be cleaned and draped with sterile towels. The doctor will insert a well-lubricated catheter through your urethra and into your bladder and will then slowly instill the contrast material through the catheter until your bladder is full. You will be asked to assume various positions while x-rays are taken.

The catheter is then removed. You will be asked to lie down on the table and urinate into a bedpan. While the contrast material flows out, additional x-rays will be taken. You may be asked to stop urinating, assume a different position, and begin again. If you are unable to urinate lying down, you may be asked to do so standing up.

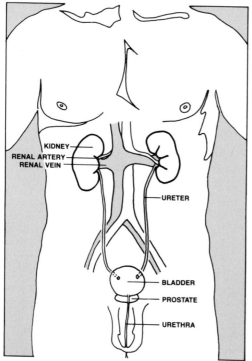

KIDNEY
RENAL ARTERY
RENAL VEIN

URETER

BLADDER

PROSTATE

URETHRA

**Urinary System.**

After the test is over, you should drink lots of fluid to help wash the contrast material out of your bladder and reduce any burning on urination.

This test usually takes 30 to 45 minutes.

### How Does It Feel?
You may feel a slight burning when the catheter is inserted. There will be a feeling of bladder fullness and an urge to urinate when the contrast medium is injected. You may feel embarrassed at having to urinate with others present. You needn't be, as the procedure is quite routine for the x-ray staff. If you find yourself feeling embarrassed, take deep, slow breaths and try to relax.

During and after the test you may feel a burning sensation on urinating, due to irritation of your urethra from the catheter. You may note blood-tinged urine for a day or two after the test. Notify your doctor if you experience chills, fever, or lower abdominal pain or if you notice persistent blood in your urine.

### Risks:
Complications are rare. Occasionally this test leads to an infection of the urinary tract. If the injections are made under too much pressure, there is some chance of damage to the bladder or urethra wall.

There is always some concern about the effects of exposure to any radiation, including the low-level radiation of diagnostic x-rays. Extremely high levels of radiation have been shown to cause various diseases and birth defects. However, if this test is really necessary, the radiation risk is generally very low compared with the potential benefits of the test.

Compared with other x-rays, the radiation from this test is medium for total body exposure and high for exposure of the reproductive organs. Because a developing fetus is very sensitive to radiation, this test is not usually recommended for pregnant women. (For more on x-ray risks, see p. 227.)

### Results:
Preliminary results should be available immediately after the test or on the next day.

In a normal bladder and urethra, the contrast material flows evenly out of the bladder through a smooth-walled urethra. Abnormal findings include stones, tumors, narrowing or outpocketing (diverticula) of the urethra or bladder, enlargement of the prostate, abnormal backward flow (reflux) of urine up into the ureters (the tubes that connect the kidneys to the bladder), or inability of the bladder to fully empty.

**Cost:**
$120 to $160

**Special Considerations:**

★*Chain Cystourethrogram*—This procedure is sometimes done on women troubled by involuntary spilling of urine (incontinence). A small amount of contrast material is injected; then a small sterile chain is introduced into the bladder through the urethra. The chain shows up on x-ray and helps show the position of the bladder and urethra. You will be asked to bear down on your abdominal muscles during this test.

★*Retrograde Urethrogram*—This test is sometimes used to examine disorders of the urethra in men. A small catheter is inserted into the tip of the penis, and a small quantity of contrast material is gently injected up the urethra. X-rays are then taken. This test can help detect the presence of lacerations, scar tissue, prostate narrowing, tumors, or malformations of the urethra.

# Dental X-Rays

Dental x-rays provide your dentist with pictures of your teeth, gums, and jaw which can be used to help diagnose and treat dental disease. Types of dental x-rays include the following:

*Bitewing*—this exposure shows the upper and lower teeth on one film. It is especially useful in detecting decay between the teeth. It also shows bone loss which can indicate severe gum disease.

*Periapical*—This is an x-ray of one entire tooth, from tip to root, with its surrounding tissues. It is used for an impacted or abscessed tooth or for investigating decay beneath an old filling, root fracture, bone defects, or the effects of gum (periodontal) disease on the bone.

*Occlusal*—This view shows the roof or floor of the mouth and is used to detect unerupted teeth, fractures of the upper or lower jaw, and to locate foreign objects.

*Panographic*—These x-rays show all the upper and lower teeth with the surrounding structures, including unerupted teeth, wisdom teeth, jawbones, and the temporomandibular joint (the place where the upper and lower jaws come together).

**Why Performed:**

The question of when dental x-rays should be done is a very controversial one. Dental x-rays can reveal many defects of the teeth and surrounding tissues which are not apparent on visual examination, but most experts agree that many dentists take too many x-rays. In 1978, the last year for which statistics are available, 82% of dental patients received x-rays.

Some of these unnecessary x-rays are due to fear of lawsuits: There is a substantial risk that a jury will find a dentist guilty of malpractice if it turns out that he or she was unaware of a condition that might have been detected by x-rays. Also, since most dentists own their own x-ray machines, there may be a strong economic incentive for dentists to order x-rays.

The American Dental Association urges dentists to use x-rays "primarily for diagnostic purposes and not routinely as part of periodic examinations." Yet one recent study showed that 95% of dentists routinely perform x-rays as part of every initial exam.

It is reasonable for your dentist to want a full set of dental x-rays as a baseline, but if you have already had such films within the past 5–10 years, repeats are probably not necessary unless there have been significant changes. Once such a baseline film exists, only bitewings (with a relatively low radiation dose) should be used for screening. Other x-rays should be taken only after an examination reveals evidence of a problem. The dentist should take a complete medical and dental history and, if possible, obtain previously taken x-rays before ordering any new films.

The National Center for Health Care Technology recommends the following guidelines for the use of bitewings in periodic screening exams:

High-risk children—posterior bitewings at intervals of up to 12 months
Low-risk children—posterior bitewings every 24 months
High-risk adults—posterior bitewings every 12 months
Low-risk adults—posterior bitewings every 36 months

A high-risk child or adult is one who is exposed to low levels of fluoride, exhibits poor daily preventive care, and has a high intake of sugars.

### Preparation:
Tell your doctor if you might be pregnant.

If a panographic x-ray is to be taken, you will be asked to remove your glasses, necklace, earrings, or other objects that might come into the x-ray beam.

### Procedure:
Before taking the x-ray, your dentist should provide you with a lead apron and collar to shield you from unnecessary radiation exposure. Ask for one if it is not provided.

For bitewing, periapical, and occlusal x-rays you will be asked to hold the cardboard carrier containing the x-ray film—sometimes in your mouth, sometimes with a finger. An x-ray machine will be positioned near your mouth. In panographic x-

rays, the film is held in a carrier outside the mouth and the x-ray tube will revolve around your jaw.

After the film and x-ray tube are in place, your dentist will step behind a protective screen. You may hear a buzzer or beeper during the time the x-ray is being taken. You should hold your head completely still during the exposure to keep from blurring the picture.

This test usually takes 5 to 10 minutes. The actual time of x-ray exposure is only a few seconds.

### How Does It Feel?
You will feel nothing at all from the x-ray. If you are asked to hold a cardboard carrier containing a piece of x-ray film in your mouth, the edges of the cardboard may feel sharp against your gums or the roof or floor of your mouth, causing minor discomfort. If it is very uncomfortable, ask to have the film repositioned.

Some people tend to gag when certain periapical films are taken. If this occurs, ask to have the film adjusted. If this doesn't improve matters, ask your dentist to spray your throat with an anesthetic. This will temporarily suppress your gag reflex.

### Risks:
There is always some concern about the effects of exposure to any radiation, including the low-level radiation of diagnostic x-rays. Extremely high levels of radiation have been shown to cause various diseases and birth defects. However, if this test is really necessary, the radiation risk is generally very low compared with the potential benefits of the test.

Compared with other x-rays, the radiation from this test is relatively low for total body exposure and low for exposure of the reproductive organs. The American Dental Association recommends the use of leaded aprons and collars on all patients to prevent unnecessary radiation exposure to the thyroid and the genitals.Because a developing fetus is very sensitive to radiation, this test is not usually recommended for pregnant women. (For more on x-ray risks, see p. 227.)

## Results:

Dental x-rays can be useful in detecting cavities between the teeth or under the gum line, decay around or under old fillings, damage to the bones supporting the teeth caused by gum (periodontal) disease, abscesses, impacted teeth (teeth whose emergence is blocked by other teeth), developmental abnormalities, dental injuries, tumors, fractures, and diseases of the bone. In addition x-rays can reveal the status of unerupted permanent teeth in children who still have their primary (baby) teeth.

Dental x-rays are also useful in evaluating and planning treatment of large or extensive cavities; in planning root canal surgery and difficult extractions; in evaluating cancer of the jaw and pain or clicking of the jaw joints; and in planning orthodontic treatment.

## Cost:

Bitewings: $5 to $10
Periapical: $6 to $12
Occlusal: $10 to $20
Panographic: $30 to $45

### Guidelines for Dental X-Rays

- Ask your dentist why the x-ray is needed.
- Don't insist that x-rays be taken if your dentist says they're not needed.
- When you change dentists, have your x-rays sent to your new dentist. This may eliminate the need to take new films.

- Keep record of dental x-rays, including type of x-ray, when taken, and where stored.
- Ask your dentist:
  —Do you use a long, open lead cylinder to decrease unnecessary exposure?
  —Do you use high-speed film?
  —Can this x-ray wait until after my pregnancy, or just after my next menstrual period?
  —Do you use an automatic timer to reduce length of exposure?

# Extremity X-Rays
## (Hand, Wrist, Arm, Foot, Knee, Ankle, Leg Films)

The purpose of this test is to obtain an x-ray picture of the bones and soft tissues of an extremity.

### Why Performed:

This test is frequently used to determine whether there has been a fracture of a bone in an extremity. It is also done to evaluate changes in the bones produced by arthritis, infection, and other bone diseases. This test is also sometimes used to locate foreign bodies (e.g., glass or metal) in wounds.

Not all injuries to the limbs require x-rays. The following guidelines will help you decide whether an injured extremity needs one or not:

- An injured extremity with visible signs of deformity should always receive an x-ray.
- An extremity with point tenderness (severe pain if pressure is applied over the injury) or severe swelling should receive an x-ray.
- A hip or thigh injury should receive an

x-ray if there is moderate to severe pain when the injured person tries to put his weight on it.

- A knee injury should be x-rayed if there is swelling, persistent pain, or inability to bend the knee.

### Preparation:

Tell your doctor if you might be pregnant.

You should remove any jewelry or other objects that might appear in the x-ray.

### Procedure:

This test is performed by a radiology technician in a hospital x-ray department or doctor's office. It is interpreted by a physician.

You will be asked to position yourself on an x-ray table with a film holder under the affected limb. Hold the limb exactly as directed by the technician.

Two or more x-rays will be taken. Sometimes x-rays of the opposite limb are taken for comparison. Sometimes it is necessary for the doctor to move or position an injured limb to produce "stress" views of the ligaments.

Sometimes x-rays need to be taken in areas other than those where obvious injury has occurred. X-rays of the lower arm or lower leg should include the full length of both bones (the radius and ulna in the arm, the tibia and fibula in the leg), as an injury at one point is frequently accompanied by another injury elsewhere. Similarly, x-rays of the thighbone (femur) should include shots of both the knee and the hip.

You will be asked to wait until the x-rays are developed to be sure that retakes are not needed.

### How Does It Feel?

You will not feel anything from the x-ray itself, though you may find some of the required positions uncomfortable. If it is necessary to apply pressure to an injured joint to obtain a "stress" view, the technician's manipulations of the injured extremity may be somewhat painful.

### Risks:

There is always some concern about the effects of exposure to any radiation, including the low-level radiation of diagnostic x-rays. Extremely high levels of radiation have been shown to cause various diseases and birth defects. However, if this test is really necessary, the radiation risk is generally very low compared with the potential benefits of the test.

Compared with other x-rays, the radiation from this test is relatively low for total body exposure. Hip and thigh films are medium and other extremity films are low in radiation exposure of the reproductive organs. Ask the physician or technician about the possibility of shielding the reproductive organs during the test. Because a developing fetus is very sensitive to radiation, this test is not usually recommended for pregnant women. (For more on x-ray risks, see p. 227.)

### Results:

Results are usually available immediately. Your doctor, a radiologist, or both will examine your x-ray for evidence of fractures, dislocations, arthritis, foreign bodies, bone infection, tumors, bone disease, and soft-tissue changes, including stretched ligaments. Sometimes the only way to determine whether an abnormality is present is to compare the suspicious area with the corresponding area on the opposite unaffected limb.

### Cost:

$35 to $80

# Gallbladder X-Rays
## (Oral Cholecystogram, OCG, Gallbladder Series)

The gallbladder is a saclike organ located under the front ribs on the right side of the abdomen. It stores bile, a yellow-green liquid produced by the liver which helps digest fats.

When you eat a fatty meal, the gallbladder contracts, pushing the bile through the bile duct and into the small intestine, where it helps digest the fat. Because fat stimulates the gallbladder, some people with gallbladder problems find that they feel better if they avoid fatty foods.

The gallbladder is not normally visible on x-rays. In this test a contrast medium is used to produce an x-ray picture of your gallbladder and bile ducts (see illustration, p. 281).

### Why Performed:
This test is used to evaluate signs and symptoms that could result from disease of the liver and/or gallbladder, such as pain in the right upper abdomen, inability to digest fatty foods, and jaundice (a condition in which the whites of the eyes and the skin take on a yellowish color). Gallbladder ultrasound (p. 304) is now commonly used instead of these x-ray examinations.

### Preparation:
Tell your doctor if
> You might be pregnant
> You have ever had an allergic reaction to x-ray contrast material or any other iodine-containing substance.
> You have had a recent barium x-ray study. (If several tests are planned, you should have this test before any barium studies, since left-over barium in your intestine can interfere with the interpretation of gallbladder x-rays.)

You will probably be asked to continue your normal diet until the day before the test. Then you should eat a high-fat meal at noon on the day before the OCG is to be done. (A high-fat meal includes plenty of eggs, butter, milk, salad oils, or fatty meats.) The fatty meal will make your gallbladder empty itself of bile. Dietary instructions vary at different institutions, so be sure to discuss the recommended preparation with your doctor.

In the late afternoon or early evening of the day before the test you should eat a fat-free meal (fruits, vegetables, bread, tea or coffee, and lean meat only). This makes the gallbladder relax and collect bile. No more food should be eaten until after the test.

Two hours after the low-fat evening meal, you will take six tablets containing the x-ray contrast material. Swallow the tablets one at a time, at five-minute intervals (to minimize nausea), swallowing one or two mouthfuls of water with each tablet. After you take the last tablet you should abstain from fluids until after the test. In some cases you may be instructed to take two tablets with each meal for one or two days before the test. Ask your doctor for specific instructions.

In the hours that follow, the contrast material will be absorbed by the small intestine, filtered out of the blood by the liver, and deposited in the gallbladder. It takes 12–14 hours from the time you take the tablets for the contrast material to reach your gallbladder.

If you should vomit up any of the tablets, notify your doctor or the hospital radiology department. The test may have to be rescheduled.

Some radiologists use the "double-dose" technique: with this method you take six tablets of contrast material the first day, and another six tablets the second day. The test is performed on the third day. If this approach is used, you will be instructed how and when to take the pills.

You may be asked to take a cleansing enema on the morning the test is to be done. If you are to take the enema at home, you will be instructed how to do it. If you are hospitalized, the nursing staff will help. The purpose of the enema is to clear the large intestine of material that might make the gallbladder x-rays hard to interpret.

Shortly before the test begins, you will be asked to remove your clothes and to put on a hospital gown.

### Procedure:

This test is performed by a radiologist and an x-ray technician. You will be asked to lie on an x-ray table and assume various positions as instructed by the doctor. X-rays will be taken. Your gallbladder may also be examined on a TV screen connected to an x-ray machine (fluoroscope).

You may then be asked to drink a high-fat formula. The presence of fat in the digestive system causes the gallbladder to contract. X-rays will be taken at 15-, 30-, and sometimes 60-minute intervals.

You will be asked to wait until the films are developed to be sure that no further studies are necessary. You can expect to be in the x-ray facility about 45 minutes. If a high-fat meal is given as part of the x-ray procedure, it may take 1–2 hours longer. A good deal of this time will be spent waiting, so you may wish to bring along something to read or material for another quiet activity. You may also wish to bring along a sweater and perhaps knee socks, as x-ray departments are sometimes a bit chilly.

Unless instructed otherwise, you can resume your normal diet as soon as the test is finished.

### How Does It Feel?

There is no pain or discomfort associated with the procedure itself. Many people experience no side effects at all from the contrast tablets. A few experience some diarrhea. (A small or moderate amount of diarrhea is a normal reaction to taking the tablets and will not interfere with test results.) Occasionally, the high-fat meal may trigger an attack of abdominal pain. Fewer still experience nausea, vomiting, cramps, and painful urination. Be sure to report any symptoms other than these to your doctor immediately.

### Risks:

There is always some concern about the effects of exposure to any radiation, including the low-level radiation of diagnostic x-rays. Extremely high levels of radiation have been shown to cause various diseases and birth defects. However, if this test is really necessary, the radiation risk is generally very low compared with the potential benefits of the test.

Compared with other x-rays, the radiation exposure from this test is as follows:

| | Total Body Dose | Reproductive Organs Male | Female |
|---|---|---|---|
| Oral cholecystogram | Medium | Low | Low |
| Intravenous cholangiogram | High | Medium | Medium |
| Percutaneous transhepatic cholangiogram | Medium | Low | Low |

Because a developing fetus is very sensitive to radiation, this test is not usually recommended for pregnant women. (For more on x-ray risks, see p. 227.)

If you have a history of severe kidney or lung damage or have ever had a hypersensitivity reaction to an x-ray contrast medium or other iodine-containing substance, you are at increased risk of injury or side effects from this test and should ask your doctor if you can substitute an ultrasound exam of your gallbladder.

**Results:**
The radiologist may be able to discuss preliminary findings with you immediately after the test. Full results should be available by the following day.

A normal gallbladder is pear-shaped with thin, smooth walls—it looks something like a balloon. The contrast material should be evenly distributed throughout the organ. All parts of the structure will be clearly outlined on the x-ray film.

The disorders most frequently detected by this test are gallstones and inflammation of the gallbladder. Tumors of the gallbladder are very rare. If your gallbladder doesn't show up clearly on x-ray, the study may need to be repeated, or an ultrasound study may be done.

**Cost:**
$80 to $120

**Special Considerations:**
★*Intravenous (IV) Cholangiogram*—This test is performed to check the bile ducts, the tubes that conduct bile from the liver to the gallbladder, and from the gallbladder to the small intestine. It is most often performed to evaluate recurring jaundice and upper abdominal pain following surgical removal of the gallbladder. This test has now been in large part replaced by gallbladder ultrasound (p. 305) and abdominal CT scan (p. 253).

A contrast material is injected into a vein in your arm and is carried via the blood to your liver, where it is excreted in the bile. The contrast-laden bile then fills the bile ducts within the liver and the common bile duct, which leads from the liver to the intestine. A series of x-ray pictures is then taken. The test lasts between 1 and 8 hours.

Except for the injection, there is nothing painful about this test, but if it goes on for many hours, it can become tiring.

This test may show a blockage of the biliary duct due to gallstones or a narrowing or blockage of the duct due to a tumor or other causes. The test costs $175 to $225.

★*Percutaneous Transhepatic Cholangiogram*—This test is sometimes performed to help your doctor determine whether jaundice is caused by a blocked bile duct or by liver disease.

You will be asked to lie on your back on the x-ray table. You will probably be given a sedative to relieve anxiety and make it easier to hold still. The skin and the liver capsule will be numbed with local anesthetic.

You will be asked to empty your lungs and to hold very still. The radiologist will watch an x-ray image on a TV screen while a needle is inserted through the skin of the upper right abdomen and into a bile duct in your liver. If a duct cannot be found after several attempts, the exam is stopped. Failure to locate a duct usually means that ducts are of normal size.

If a duct is located, a sample of bile is taken. Contrast material (dye) is then injected. You may be asked to assume several different positions to help the dye spread. The radiologist will watch the spread of the dye on the TV screen (fluoroscope). Individual x-rays will also be taken. The needle is then withdrawn and further x-rays are taken.

You will feel a small sting from the needle used to administer the anesthetic. You should feel little or no pain during the procedure, but may experience a feeling of pressure within your liver and may have a feeling of fullness as the contrast material is injected.

The table may be tilted from time to time. You will be tightly secured so there is no danger of falling.

You will need to stay in the hospital after the procedure to be sure that bleeding or bile leakage does not develop. These complications are quite rare, but if either does occur, surgery may be required to correct it.

If the injected substance passes through the liver and into the intestine, no blockage is present. If it does not, there probably is blockage. This test costs $350 to $400.

★*ERCP (Endoscopic Retrograde Cholangiopancreatogram)—see p. 342.*

# Intravenous Pyelogram (IVP, Excretory Urography)

In this test an iodine-containing contrast material which shows up on x-rays is injected into your bloodstream. This material concentrates in the kidneys, and a series of x-rays are then taken at timed intervals. The resulting films let the doctor see a series of images of the entire urinary tract—the tissue of the kidney itself, the collecting system inside the kidney, the tube running from the kidney to the bladder (ureter), and the bladder (the hollow organ that acts as a reservoir for urine). See the illustration on p. 261.

**Why Performed:**

An IVP is often performed to evaluate recurring infections of the bladder or kidney, blood in the urine (hematuria), flank pain (when a kidney stone is suspected), or changes in urination pattern or bladder function. An IVP may also be used to look for urinary tract damage following an abdominal injury. Abnormalities on blood or urine tests suggesting kidney disease may be further evaluated with an IVP.

Although an IVP is not recommended as a routine test for all people with high blood pressure, it may be helpful in those whose high blood pressure comes on suddenly, especially if blood tests suggest that kidney disease is present. An IVP may also be done if the high blood pressure is difficult to control with standard antihypertensive medications.

An IVP is frequently used to evaluate blood in the urine but should not be done if the bloody urine might be due to a known disease (such as sickle-cell anemia) or if the person runs long distances. (A condition called jogger's hematuria can result from long runs. This condition will resolve on its own if the person stops running or reduces his or her distance for a few days.)

**Preparation:**

Tell your doctor if

> You might be pregnant
>
> You have had recent abdominal surgery
>
> You have ever had an allergic reaction to x-ray contrast material or other iodine-containing substance
>
> You have ever had an allergy to any other medications

You may be asked to sign a consent form authorizing this procedure. Use this opportunity to discuss with your doctor any concerns you may have about the need for the test, the risks of the test, or how it will be performed.

You will be asked to take a laxative the afternoon before the examination. This is to remove intestinal gas and feces which could block the view on the x-rays.

You may be asked to eat only a very light dinner, or no food at all, the night before the test, and then to fast and drink no liquids until the test is completed. The required preparation can vary in different clinics and hospitals. Ask your doctor for specific instructions.

You will be left alone, lying on the x-ray table, for several 5-minute periods between x-rays, so you may wish to bring along something to read. During this time you will not be able to move unless the technician moves you. The room may be cool, so you may want to bring knee socks. If you are chilly during the test, ask for a blanket.

You will be asked to undress and to put on a hospital gown. Be sure to remove any jewelry or other objects that might come into the path of the x-ray.

## Procedure:

This test is done in a radiologist's office or in a hospital radiology department by a radiologist and an x-ray technician. It can be performed on an outpatient basis.

There are a number of possible variations on the IVP procedure, depending on the condition of the patient, the information requested, and what is found as the exam progresses.

You will be asked to urinate immediately before the procedure, so that the contrast medium will not be diluted by urine in the bladder. First you will lie on an x-ray table so that a preliminary film can be taken. This will show the radiologist the basic landmarks of your abdomen. This film will be developed and read before the next part of the test begins.

A needle will be inserted into a vein (usually on the inside of your elbow) and taped in place, for injection of the contrast material. You may wish to tell the x-ray technician which arm you would prefer to have used as the injection site.

The contrast material is then injected through the needle. It is carried by the blood to the kidneys and filtered out of the blood into the collecting system of the kidneys. As the contrast medium is distributed through the urinary tract, it can be seen on x-ray. Films are taken at regular intervals— usually at 1, 5, 10, and 15 minutes after the dye (contrast medium) is injected. Sometimes films are taken every minute for the first five minutes after a rapid infusion of the dye. It is important that you hold still while each film is taken.

These films trace the progress of the contrast medium through your urinary tract. Sometimes fluoroscopy (a special x-ray which displays a moving image on a TV screen) is also used. Sometimes special views called nephrotomograms are taken to better view the kidney tissue. These special x-rays provide an image of a cross section of the kidney.

After the 5-minute film has been taken, a compression device may be applied to your abdomen to keep the dye in the kidneys. The most common compression device is a wide belt containing two balloons that are inflated, pushing in on either side of your abdomen. These block the passage of contrast medium through the ureters. The balloons are deflated after the 10-minute film. In most cases you will then urinate and an additional film is taken to check how well your bladder has emptied.

If you have recently had abdominal surgery or have a known or suspected abdominal disorder, the compression band may not be used.

Each x-ray is developed immediately, and the radiologist sometimes decides to take additional films based on earlier x-rays. The exam usually takes about 45 minutes to one hour. After the test you should drink plenty of fluids to help wash the dye out of your system.

### How Does It Feel?

You may become hungry and thirsty as a result of not eating or drinking as instructed before the test. You might wish to bring a snack to eat or some fruit juice to drink as soon as the test is over.

You will feel a brief sting when the needle is inserted into the vein in your arm. When the dye is injected you may feel a burning sensation in your arm and warm spots or flushing throughout your body. You may also notice a salty or metallic taste in your mouth.

A few people having this test develop headaches, feel nauseous, or vomit after the injection of the dye. Fewer still experience fainting, tingling, numbness, runny nose, sneezing, or cough as a reaction to the dye. The compression belt may produce a sensation of pressure. If it should become painful, tell the technician and ask that it be readjusted.

You may feel slightly weak, nauseous, or lightheaded for a short time after the test.

*Patient Comment*:

"I felt a sharp, stinging pain as the IV was inserted, then a very subtle feeling of warmth throughout my body as the contrast medium was injected. A feeling of nausea came and went very quickly. It didn't last long. I was uncomfortable and lonely lying on the table between exposures. It seemed to take forever. The room was chilly. I was cold the whole time."

### Risks:

The radiologist or technician will ask you about any history of allergic reaction to contrast materials or other iodine-containing substances. If you do have such a history, do not proceed with the exam until you have discussed this with your doctor or radiologist.

The contrast material may produce a number of fairly minor side effects, as previously described. About 1 in 100 patients experience a minor allergic reaction (severe nausea, hives, itching). However, about 1 in 40,000 experiences a major allergic reaction: breathing difficulty, swelling of the face, profuse sweating, shock, and, in extremely sensitive people, possibly death. These side effects are quite rare and can almost always be controlled with medication. It is very important that you report any unusual feeling after the contrast material is injected—no matter how minor it may seem. This could be the key to detecting and treating an allergic reaction to the dye. Any side effects will usually occur within the first 10 minutes. Problems rarely arise once the exam is over.

There is always some concern about the effects of exposure to any radiation, including the low-level radiation of diagnostic x-rays. Extremely high levels of radiation have been shown to cause various diseases and birth defects. However, if this test is really necessary, the radiation risk is generally very low compared with the potential benefits.

Compared with other x-rays, the radiation exposure from this test is relatively high for the total body, medium for the male reproductive organs, and high for the female reproductive organs. Because a developing fetus is very sensitive to radiation, this test is not usually recommended for pregnant women. (For more on x-ray risks, see p. 227.)

Very elderly people and those with severe diabetes may be at risk of toxic damage to the kidneys resulting from injection of the contrast medium. For these persons, renal ultrasound (see p. 304), nuclear renal scans (see p. 297), and a plain abdominal x-ray may be an acceptable alternative to the IVP.

### Results:

Preliminary results are sometimes available immediately after the test. Full results are usually ready by the next day.

In reading an IVP, the radiologist follows the course of the contrast material into the kidneys, through the collecting systems of the kidney, into the ureters (the tubes leading to the bladder), to the bladder, and (in some studies) out through the urethra. The IVP may reveal kidney stones, tumors, birth defects, or other kidney diseases.

### Cost:

$120 to $170

# Lymphangiogram
## (Lymphography, Lymphangiography)

The lymphatic system consists of *lymph nodes*, which are found throughout your body, and small lymph vessels (*lymphatics*), which link the lymph nodes. The nodes (commonly called lymph glands, although they are not really glands) produce lymphocytes, a type of white blood cell which fights infection. When you have an infection your lymph nodes swell, produce white blood cells, and try to trap the organisms causing the infection. The lymph nodes also trap cancer cells and slow their spread. Thus cancers that spread (metastasize) may go first to nearby lymph nodes.

Lymph nodes and vessels aren't visible on normal x-rays. To make them visible, a contrast material must be injected into the lymphatic system. If the contrast material is injected into the foot, the lymphatics of the legs and abdomen will be outlined on x-rays. Less frequently, the dye is injected into the hands, to outline the lymph channels and nodes of the arms and upper body.

### Why Performed:

Lymphangiograms are most frequently used to investigate the possible spread of tumors, either lymphatic cancers (lymphomas) or other cancers. Lymphatic x-rays can help determine how far a cancer has spread, which is important in selecting the appropriate treatment. This test is also sometimes used to evaluate the effectiveness of cancer therapy.

Lymphatic x-rays are also used to determine the cause of unexplained swelling of an arm or leg and to check the lymphatic system for parasitic diseases such as elephantiasis.

### Preparation:

Tell your doctor if
You might be pregnant
You have any disease of the lung
You have ever had an allergic reaction to x-ray contrast material, to other iodine-containing substances, or to local anesthetic

You will be asked to sign a consent form authorizing this procedure. Use this opportunity to discuss with your doctor any concerns you may have about the need for the test, the risks of the test, or how it will be performed.

You may be asked to observe a restricted diet and to take only clear liquids for the period immediately before the test. Exact details vary in different institutions. Your nurse or doctor will give you specific instructions.

If you are having the test as an outpatient, bring someone with you to accompany you home. You may also wish to bring slippers or loose shoes to wear after the test.

There will be some long waits during the test, so you may wish to bring something to read or material for another quiet activity. Since the procedure usually involves slow injections into your feet, your hands will be free. For your own comfort, empty your bladder just before the test begins.

**Procedure:**

This test is usually performed in a radiologist's office or in the x-ray department of a clinic or hospital by a radiologist and an x-ray technician.

You may be offered a sedative to help you relax. If allergy to the contrast material is suspected, you may be given an antihistamine capsule to help prevent an allergic reaction.

You will be asked to position yourself either on a specially constructed chair or on an x-ray table. The skin of each foot will be cleaned with antiseptic. A small amount of blue dye (sometimes mixed with local anesthetic) will be injected into the webs between your toes. Within about 15 minutes, thin bluish lines, the lymph channels, will begin to appear on the skin of the top of your foot.

A local anesthetic is then injected, and a small incision is made over one of the larger blue lines (lymphatic vessels) in each foot. A tiny needle or tube (catheter) is inserted into a vessel in each foot, and a syringe filled with contrast material is connected to it. Contrast material is then automatically injected into both feet at a very slow rate. It takes about 1 to 1½ hours for all the contrast material to go in.

The injection is made very slowly to prevent damaging the delicate lymph vessels. The contrast material spreads through the lymph vessels of the leg, into the groin, and along the back of the abdominal cavity. Sometimes an x-ray tube connected to a TV screen (fluoroscope) may be used to monitor the spread of the contrast material. Sometimes the spread is checked by periodic x-rays.

When the injection is complete, the needles or catheters are removed and the incisions are stitched up and covered with sterile dressings. Since the exam takes several hours, your doctor may inject additional local anesthetic before closing the incisions with stitches. X-rays of the legs, pelvis, abdomen, and chest are then taken.

You may be instructed to consume only clear liquids until the final x-rays are taken the next day, 24 hours after the original injection. In some cases, additional x-rays are taken 48 and 72 hours after the contrast material is injected. An IVP (see p. 269) is sometimes performed at the 24-hour point.

Aftercare depends largely on the amount of pain you are experiencing. You may resume your normal activities as soon as you can comfortably do so. If your feet hurt you should relax with your feet elevated for 12–24 hours after the test. Sometimes ice packs placed intermittently on the incision sites can help reduce swelling. Keep the bandages in place for 2 days, and keep the incision sites dry.

You may experience some continued swelling of the feet after the test. This usually disappears within 7–10 days, but on occasion can last as long as a month or more.

The average procedure takes about 2½ to 3 hours, but this test can take up to 5 hours. You will need to return for additional x-rays the next day. These additional x-rays usually take 25–30 minutes and do not involve the injections of additional dye. The stitches are removed in 7–10 days.

### How Does It Feel?

You may feel a brief sting from the first needle and the blue dye, and another brief sting from the needle used to inject local anesthetic. You will not feel the small incision because of the anesthetic. You may experience a feeling of pressure when the contrast medium is injected. You may also feel some discomfort behind your knees and in your groin. You may find it difficult to remain still on the x-ray table for so long.

The incision sites may be sore for a few days after the procedure. The blue dye will discolor your urine and stool for about 48 hours and may give your skin a temporary bluish tone. Your vision, too, may take on a temporary bluish cast—things may look as though you were wearing blue-tinted glasses. These changes in your skin and vision may last as long as a week. If you notice shortness of breath, cough, fever, or persistent swelling, tenderness, or a discharge at the incision site, notify your doctor.

### Risks:

There is a slight chance that you may experience a reaction to the contrast material (see p. 232).

Infections sometimes occur at the injection site. The dye or the contrast material may cause an inflammation of the lymph vessels (lymphangitis) and fever. The inflammation can be quite painful. Damage to the lymph vessels from the test can result in swelling of the affected arm or leg.

In very rare cases a small quantity of contrast material may enter the blood and lodge in a blood vessel in the lungs, temporarily blocking blood flow to a portion of the lung. This can cause difficult breathing, chest pain, and fever. These symptoms usually disappear rapidly, but tell your doctor immediately if you notice them.

There is always some concern about the effects of exposure to any radiation, including the low-level radiation of diagnostic x-rays. Extremely high levels of radiation have been shown to cause various diseases and birth defects. However, if this test is really necessary, the radiation risk is generally very low compared with the potential benefits.

Compared with other x-rays, the radiation exposure from this test is relatively high for the total body, medium to high for the male reproductive organs, and high for the female reproductive organs. Because a developing fetus is very sensitive to radiation, this test is not usually recommended for pregnant women. (For more on x-ray risks, see p. 227.)

### Results:

Results of the test should be available by the next day.

Enlarged lymph nodes with a "foamy" appearance may indicate lymphoma (lymph cancer). Nodes or parts of nodes that fail to fill with contrast material may indicate other kinds of cancers spreading into the lymph system. Blockage of the lymph channels by tumor or infection may also be noted.

### Cost:

$400 to $750

# Myelogram

A myelogram is an x-ray study of the spinal canal, the fluid-filled space which surrounds your spinal cord. In this test a contrast material is introduced into your spinal canal and x-rays are then taken.

This test can be done at various levels of your back—if done at neck level it is called a cervical myelogram, if done in the midback it is called a thoracic myelogram, and if done in the lower back it is called a lumbar myelogram.

### Why Performed:
The myelogram can be very useful in locating and identifying problems involving the spinal cord such as slipped discs (herniated intervertebral discs), spinal cord tumors, injuries to the roots of the nerves branching off the spinal cord, and tumors in the lower part of the skull. A myelogram should be done only after a thorough neurologic exam has revealed findings such as numbness or weakness that suggest a spinal cord abnormality. A CT scan (see p. 253) is now frequently used instead of, or in addition to, this test.

### Preparation:
Tell your doctor if
> You might be pregnant
> You are taking any medications
> You have ever had an allergic reaction to x-ray contrast material, to any other iodine-containing substance, or to a local anesthetic

You may be asked to avoid all food for 4 hours preceding the test, but should drink plenty of clear liquids during this time. Instructions may vary at different institutions, so ask your doctor or radiology department for specific instructions.

### Procedure:
This test is done in a hospital x-ray department by a radiologist or neurosurgeon and an x-ray technician. You may or may not need to be admitted to the hospital. About an hour before the test you may be given an injection of a sedative or pain medication to help you relax.

The injection site—usually in the lower back, but sometimes at the base of your skull—will be shaved and cleaned with an antiseptic solution. You will be asked to lie face-down on the x-ray table with your chin extended. If a neck study is planned, you may be secured to the table with straps across your back and ankles.

A small area of skin at the chosen site may be anesthetized by injection of a local anesthetic. A longer needle will then be introduced into the spinal canal. Its position will be checked using a fluoroscope (a type of x-ray tube) connected to a TV monitor. A small sample of cerebrospinal fluid (CSF) will be removed and sent for laboratory analysis.

The x-ray contrast material will then be injected. Depending on the type of contrast material (oil-soluble or water-soluble), the needle will either be withdrawn or left in place.

Since the contrast material is heavier than the spinal fluid, it tends to be pulled downward by gravity. The technician will adjust the table so that you are sometimes head-down, sometimes feet-down, in order to move the contrast material to the area to be examined.

The radiologist will watch the spread of contrast material through the fluoroscope, and will take individual x-ray pictures. If the flow of contrast material is blocked, another injection may be made above the level of the block.

This test usually takes between 15 minutes and 1 hour. You may resume your regular diet as soon as it is over. Drink plenty of fluids after the test to help replace the CSF that was removed.

If an oil-based contrast agent is used, it is withdrawn or allowed to drip out through the needle. (If left in the body it may cause inflammation or adhesions.) You must then lie flat for 6–8 hours.

If a water-based contrast agent is used, it does not need to be removed, as it will be rapidly absorbed by your body. You must either sit up in a chair or lie with your head slightly elevated for 6–8 hours. You should not lie flat in bed for 6–8 hours. Keeping your head raised prevents the contrast material from irritating sensitive areas in your head and neck.

Your vital signs and neurologic status will be checked throughout the procedure and for several hours afterward. If you are not hospitalized, you may return home after 6 hours of observation. However, you should plan to rest for a day or two.

## How Does It Feel?

You will feel a brief sting from the small needle used to administer the local anesthetic, and a slight pressure as the longer (spinal) needle is inserted. You may feel an occasional sharp pain from the needle while it is in place. You may find the chin-extended position uncomfortable. Some people may find it difficult to swallow or to draw a full breath while in this position. In most cases this position need not be maintained for long. You may also find some of the other positions—especially those with your head lower than your body—uncomfortable. You may find it tiring to lie still on the table for an hour or more.

There is a slight chance that you will feel a brief pressure or a burning sensation as the contrast material is injected. Other common side effects include headache, flushing, nausea or vomiting, or a low-grade fever. Once the test is over, notify your doctor if you notice a feeling of extreme irritability, a severe headache, a headache that lasts more than 24 hours, or any increase of pain, weakness, or numbness in your legs.

*Patient Comments*:

"It wasn't nearly as bad as I'd feared. The shot they gave me beforehand made me very relaxed and sleepy. I felt a lot of pressure when the contrast material was injected, but there was never any pain, just a warm, burning sensation all over. I had a headache afterward—that was really the only bad thing about the test."

"When they put the needle in I felt a brief shock down my right leg—apparently they touched a nerve. It was most interesting watching the dye spread up and down my back on the TV screen. I didn't get a headache like some people do. The whole thing was not bad at all."

## Risks:

About 20% of patients will experience headache, nausea, or vomiting after the test. Seizures occur in less than 1 in 1000. Allergic reactions to the contrast material are rare. Rarely inflammation of the coverings of the brain and spinal cord (meningitis), weakness, numbness, paralysis, or inability to control bowel or bladder function develops. There is a slight risk of infection at the injection site. There is also a very small chance that the procedure will convert a preexisting incomplete blockage of the spinal canal to a complete block. If this occurs, surgery may be necessary. You should discuss the risks in your particular case with your doctor.

There is always some concern about the effects of exposure to any radiation, including the low-level radiation of diagnostic x-rays. Extremely high levels of radiation have been shown to cause various diseases and birth defects. However, if this test is really necessary, the radiation risk is generally very low compared with the potential benefits.

Compared with other x-rays, the radiation exposure from this test is medium for the total body, medium for the male reproductive organs, and medium to high for the female reproductive organs depending upon the area examined. Discuss with your doctor or radiology technician the possibility of shielding the reproductive organs during the test. Because a developing fetus is very sensitive to radiation, this test is not usually recommended for pregnant women. (For more on x-ray risks, see p. 227.)

## Results:

Results of this test are available immediately or by the next day.

Any block in the flow of dye around the spinal cord may indicate a problem. The blockage may be due to a herniated disc, a nerve root injury, an abscess, a vascular malformation, or a benign or malignant tumor (including a metastatic tumor, i.e., a tumor "seeded" from cancer elsewhere in the body).

## Cost:

$200 to $300

# Skull X-Rays

This x-ray is used to examine the bones that make up the skull, including the facial bones, nose, and sinuses.

## Why Performed:

This test is sometimes ordered to evaluate head injuries. However, the newer CT scan of the head (see p. 256), where available, has in many instances replaced skull x-rays for this purpose.

If a head injury is minor, neither x-rays nor CT scans are usually necessary. However, if any of the following signs are present, one of these tests should probably be performed:

Skull depression or facial deformity
Foreign body which can be felt through a scalp wound
Clear fluid discharge from nose or ear
Bloody discharge from ear
Bruising behind one or both ears
Black eyes on both sides
Loss of consciousness after a blow to the head
Decreasing level of consciousness
Unexplained defects of nervous system

Skull x-rays are also sometimes useful in evaluating an unusually shaped child's skull.

Special sinus x-rays may be ordered to look for a sinus infection or obstruction in cases of headache or facial pain.

## Preparation:

Tell your doctor if you might be pregnant.

No special diets or food restrictions are necessary. It is important that you remove all jewelry, eyeglasses, dentures, hearing aids, hairpins, or any other objects that might show up in the x-rays.

**Procedure:**

Skull x-rays are usually taken in a hospital radiology department or in a radiologist's office, usually by a radiology technician. The films are interpreted by a physician.

You will be asked to lie on a table or sit in a chair. Your head will be placed in various positions by the technologist. Foam pads, a headband, or sandbags may be used to make it easier to keep your head still. X-rays are usually taken from the front, back, and side. Sometimes other views are taken as well. If sinus films are needed, you will be asked to sit upright so that any fluids in your sinus cavities can be easily seen.

All films taken will normally be developed and checked before you leave the facility. If they are unsatisfactory, repeat films may be needed.

This test usually takes 10 to 20 minutes.

**How Does It Feel?**

You will not feel anything from the x-ray itself. If you have an injury of the head, you may find it uncomfortable to assume some of the required positions.

**Risks:**

There is always some concern about the effects of exposure to any radiation, including the low-level radiation of diagnostic x-rays. Extremely high levels of radiation have been shown to cause various diseases and birth defects. However, if this test is really necessary, the radiation risk is generally very low compared with the potential benefits.

Compared with other x-rays, the radiation from this test is relatively low for total body exposure and low for exposure to the reproductive organs. Because a developing fetus is very sensitive to radiation, this test is not usually recommended for pregnant women. (For more on x-ray risks, see p. 227.)

There are no notable risks other than the exposure to x-ray.

**Results:**

In viewing a skull x-ray, the radiologist is able to examine the three groups of bones that compose the skull—the vault (calvaria), the jaw (mandible), and the facial bones. The bones of the skull are so complex that views from many different angles are often necessary for adequate examination.

Skull fractures usually appear as thin translucent lines. Skull x-rays may also show erosion or decalcification of the bone, or shifts in the soft tissues inside the skull that may result from increased pressure inside the brain. Skull x-rays can also detect signs of metabolic diseases that affect the bones of the skull.

Sinus films may show evidence of infection, obstruction, bleeding, or tumors.

**Cost:**

Single film: $25 to $35
Five-film series: $90 to $125

# Spine X-Rays
## (Back Films; Vertebral Radiography; Cervical, Lumbar, or Thoracic Spine Films)

Your vertebrae are divided into five groups: 7 neck (cervical) vertebrae, 12 chest (thoracic) vertebrae, 5 lower back (lumbar) vertebrae, the sacrum (composed of 5 small, fused vertebrae), and the coccyx (composed of 4 small, fused vertebrae). The vertebrae are separated by flat pads of cartilage (intervertebral discs) which cushion the vertebrae from shock and allow movement between them.

A spine x-ray may include pictures of one or more of these divisions. The most commonly taken spine x-rays are cervical (C-spine films) and lumbosacral (LS-spine films).

### Why Performed:

Spine films are most often ordered to evaluate neck and back injuries or persistent pain, numbness, or weakness. Unfortunately, the great majority of back problems cannot be seen on regular back x-rays. This is because most back problems originate not in the spine but in the muscles, nerves, and other soft tissues of the back. The most common source of back pain—sprained or torn back muscles—never shows up on x-rays. Slipped or herniated discs, also common, can sometimes be seen on x-ray as narrowed disc spaces.

Back films were at one time used to screen healthy people for back problems. Most physicians now feel that this is not an appropriate use of x-rays. However, some employers require preemployment back x-rays to protect themselves in case of lawsuits resulting from on-the-job back injuries.

There is now general agreement among physicians that these films are of questionable value to the employer and of very little use to the person tested. If you are asked to have such an x-ray, we suggest that you discuss the matter with your prospective employers. They may be willing to settle for a thorough physical exam by a physician.

### Preparation:

Tell your doctor if you might be pregnant.

No restrictions of food or fluid are necessary. Be sure to remove any jewelry or other objects that might lie in the area being examined.

### Procedure:

This exam is performed in a hospital x-ray department or in a radiologist's office by a radiology technician. You will be asked to lie on an x-ray table and assume various positions at the direction of the technician.

If the x-ray is being taken because of a possible neck or back injury, the required positions will be modified to prevent further injury. In such situations you may be x-rayed on a stretcher.

Three to five films are usually taken. Be careful not to move when the x-ray is being taken, and hold your breath when so directed: This can help prevent the need for a repeat film.

This procedure takes about 15 minutes. If repeat films or more elaborate studies are done, it may take longer.

### How Does It Feel?

You will feel nothing from the x-ray itself. The table will be hard and may be cold. Some of the positions may be slightly uncomfortable; if they are painful, let the technician know.

### Risks:

There is always some concern about the effects of exposure to any radiation, including the low-level radiation of diagnostic x-rays. Extremely high levels of radiation have been shown to cause various diseases and birth defects. However, if this test is really necessary, the radiation risk is generally very low compared with the potential benefits.

Compared with other x-rays, the radiation from this test for total body exposure is

| Cervical | Low |
| Thoracic | Medium |
| Lumbosacral | High |

Radiation exposure to the reproductive organs is

| | Women | Men |
| --- | --- | --- |
| Cervical | Low | Low |
| Thoracic | Medium | Medium |
| Lumbosacral | High | Medium* |

*Males having this test should wear a genital shield.

Because a developing fetus is very sensitive to radiation, this test is not usually recommended for pregnant women. (For more on x-ray risks, see p. 227.)

**Results:**

Results are usually available either immediately or by the next day.

The most frequent abnormalities detected by this procedure are fractures, dislocations, deformities in the curvature of the spine, and thinning of the bone (osteoporosis).

Spine films are also used to detect and evaluate arthritis and tumors of the vertebrae and associated structures. They can also sometimes detect vertebral degeneration, bone spurs, disc problems, spinal effects of metabolic and arthritic diseases, and a number of other conditions.

If spine films indicate that abnormalities are present, further studies such as myelography (p. 275), computerized tomography (p. 253), or thermography may be necessary to determine appropriate treatment.

**Cost:**

Cervical spine: $100 to $140
Thoracic spine: $70 to $120
Lumbar spine: $70 to $150
Complete back survey: $150 to $200

# Upper Gastrointestinal (GI) Series
## (UGI, Barium Swallow, Esophagram)

Several related x-ray studies can be used to examine the upper portion of your gastrointestinal tract. In each of these you swallow a "milkshake," usually made up of barium and water. A radiologist then uses a fluoroscope connected to a TV monitor to observe the progress of the barium through your digestive tract.

If the area to be examined is the throat and esophagus, the procedure is called an *esophagram* (barium swallow). The *upper GI series* examines the esophagus, stomach, and the first part of the small intestine (duodenum). The *small bowel follow-through* is performed immediately after a UGI series to help visualize the entire 20 feet of the small intestine (duodenum, jejunum, and ileum).

**Why Performed:**

The esophagram is used to evaluate difficult swallowing and regurgitating food, which could be due to a hiatus hernia. The small bowel study is usually done to investigate symptoms like weight loss and chronic diarrhea when regional enteritis (Crohn's disease) is suspected.

Although the UGI series is one of the most frequently performed x-ray examinations, there is disagreement as to when it should be done. In some medical centers

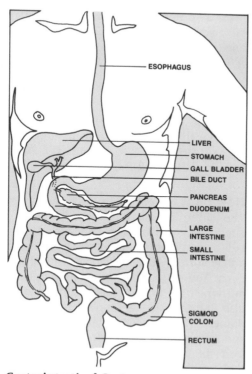

ESOPHAGUS

LIVER
STOMACH
GALL BLADDER
BILE DUCT

PANCREAS
DUODENUM

LARGE
INTESTINE

SMALL
INTESTINE

SIGMOID
COLON

RECTUM

**Gastrointestinal System.**

it is ordered for nearly every patient with problems of the upper gastrointestinal tract.

Many physicians now feel that the UGI should be used more selectively. This test is more likely to show an abnormality when performed in patients with one or more of the following:

Difficulty in swallowing
A history of an ulcer
Age greater than 50
Abdominal pain relieved by eating
Pain that occurs within an hour of eating
Heartburn (gastric reflux)
Gastrointestinal bleeding

Studies suggest that if these guidelines were followed, the use of this procedure could be substantially reduced and few abnormalities would be missed. There is general agreement that the UGI series should not be used as a routine screening test for people without symptoms.

Endoscopy, the direct viewing of the lining of the esophagus, stomach, and duodenum with an instrument, has replaced x-ray studies in some cases.

**Preparation:**
Tell your doctor if
You are taking any medications
You might be pregnant
You have ever had an allergic reaction to barium or any other x-ray contrast medium

You will be asked not to eat or drink anything for 12 hours before the examination. If you are taking any medication, ask your doctor whether you should continue it. Since smoking or chewing gum can stimulate gastric juices and slow digestion, you will be asked not to smoke or chew gum during that time. You should remove dentures and all jewelry before the test. You will be asked to undress and put on a hospital gown.

If your condition is such that your stomach cannot empty well on its own, the contents of your stomach may need to be removed through a special tube passed through your nose and down into your stomach just before the test begins.

If you are having the small bowel follow-through, there will be periods of waiting between x-rays, so you may want to bring along a book to read or material for some other quiet activity.

**Procedure:**
You will be asked to lie on your back on the x-ray table while a preliminary x-ray is taken. You may be secured to the table with a belt. The table will be tilted to bring

you to an upright position with the x-ray machine in front of you. In some cases the exam will start in the upright position and the table will later be tilted back. The technician will be sure you are comfortable during any changes in table position.

You will then be asked to swallow several mouthfuls of a thick, barium "milkshake." Throughout the procedure the radiologist will tell you when and how much to drink. You may be asked to drink 2–3 cups of the barium mixture by the end of the procedure.

The radiologist will watch the barium pass through your digestive tract on a special x-ray tube (fluoroscope) attached to a TV screen and will take individual x-ray pictures of significant findings. The table will be tilted at various angles, and you may be asked to assume various positions to help spread the barium. Your abdomen may be compressed by a belt or by the examiner's gloved hand. You may be asked to cough so that the radiologist can observe the effect on the barium flow.

If you are having a double-contrast study, you will be asked to sip the milkshake through a straw with a hole in it or to take tablets that release gas in your stomach. The air or gas helps outline the lining of the stomach and intestines in greater detail.

If the small bowel study is to be done you will then be given a thinner solution of barium to drink. The radiologist will watch as it passes along your small intestine into the lower end of the small intestine and the beginning of your large intestine (cecum). X-ray pictures will be taken every 30 minutes.

The esophagram (barium swallow) takes 10–20 minutes, the upper GI series 10–20 minutes. Both studies may be done in the same visit. The upper GI with small bowel follow-through or small bowel study takes 2–6 hours. In some cases you may be asked to return after 24 hours for an additional x-ray.

Be sure to ask if the study is finished before eating or drinking anything. You may resume your regular diet unless advised otherwise.

Some facilities may suggest that you use a laxative to prevent constipation after the test. Drinking large quantities of fluids can also help wash the barium out.

**How Does It Feel?**

The barium milkshake has a thick, chalky consistency which a few people find difficult to swallow in spite of the sweetening and flavoring—usually chocolate or strawberry. You may find it somewhat unpleasant when the table is tilted. Some people also find the pressure applied to their abdomen slightly uncomfortable.

Your stool will have a whitish color from the barium for 1 to 3 days following the procedure. If you don't notice a whitish substance in your stool within 2–3 days, or if your bowel habits undergo a marked change, let your physician know. The barium can harden and cause obstruction if it is not eliminated.

*Patient Comments:*

"I expected the barium to taste awful but it wasn't bad at all. I was a bit surprised when the table started to tilt. I was quite hungry and thirsty by the time the test was over."

**Risks:**

There is always some concern about the effects of exposure to any radiation, including the low-level radiation of diagnostic x-rays. Extremely high levels of radiation have been shown to cause various diseases and birth defects. However, if this test is really necessary, the radiation risk is generally very low compared with the potential benefits.

Compared with other x-rays, the radiation exposure from this test is medium for the total body and medium for the reproductive organs. Discuss with the radiologist or technician the possibility of reproductive-organ shielding during the test. Because a developing fetus is very sensitive to radiation, this test is not usually recommended for pregnant women. (For more on x-ray risks, see p. 227.)

The barium is not absorbed into the bloodstream, so allergic reactions are exceedingly rare. Other risks from the procedure are relatively small—mostly the chance of perforation of a weakened portion of the wall of the stomach or intestine, or a leakage of the contrast material into the abdominal cavity through a perforated ulcer. A special type of contrast material (Gastrografin) can be used if this possibility is suspected or if it is suspected that the gastrointestinal tract is obstructed. There may be some risk in using a strong laxative in the presence of an obstruction of the colon, ulcerative colitis, or some other diseases of the colon.

### Results:

Preliminary results may be available immediately or by the next day. In nearly one-half the studies, no abnormalities are found.

The esophagram may reveal a narrowing, an inflammation, or a mass obstructing the esophagus or throat or a hiatal hernia (a condition in which a portion of the stomach protrudes upward through the diaphragm). Abnormal contraction of the esophagus or reflux of digestive juices may be noted.

The UGI series may demonstrate a gastric (stomach) or duodenal (intestinal) ulcer, a tumor, or displacement of the

esophagus or stomach by a mass outside the digestive tract.

The small bowel follow-through may reveal a form of inflammatory bowel disease (Crohn's disease) or a pattern that may indicate malabsorption. Sometimes additional studies such as endoscopy (see p. 338) are necessary to clarify the findings seen on x-ray.

### Cost:

Esophagram: $90 to $120
Upper GI series: $120 to $160
Upper GI with small bowel follow-through: $160 to $200

# Venogram
## (Lower Limb Venography, Ascending Contrast Phlebography)

When a vein is blocked or becomes narrowed, the return of blood from the tissues to the heart is impaired, and you may experience pain and swelling in the affected area. Such blockages are most commonly due to a blood clot (thrombus) or to compression by a lymph node, tumor, or other source.

Veins do not normally show up on x-rays. In this test a contrast medium which can be seen on x-rays is injected into your veins. X-rays are then taken as the contrast material passes through the area to be examined.

### Why Performed:

This is the most accurate test for searching for blood clots in the deep veins of the leg (thrombophlebitis, deep vein thrombosis, or DVT). DVT typically develops quickly. The symptoms include soreness, tenderness, swelling, and redness of the lower leg, usually in the calf.

Such clots can result from surgery, prolonged bed rest, problems involving the clotting mechanism of the blood, childbirth, or injuries to a leg vein. Women taking estrogen or birth control pills are also at increased risk of blood clots.

Blood clots in the deep veins of the legs can be dangerous: Parts of the clot can break off and travel through the bloodstream, producing a blocked artery in the lung (pulmonary embolism). Accurate diagnosis and early treatment of clots in the leg veins may thus help prevent life-threatening complications.

Venography should be performed only when physical symptoms (tenderness and swelling in the legs) strongly suggest a blood clot. It should not be used for routine screening. Three less invasive tests—ultrasound (see p. 309), iodine-125 fibrinogen scan (see p. 302), and impedance plethysmography (see p. 384)—can in many cases supply the information needed to make a decision on the most appropriate therapy.

This test is also sometimes used to evaluate inherited disorders of the leg veins, to determine the cause of swollen legs, and to locate a suitable vein to be used in coronary artery bypass surgery.

### Preparation:

Tell your doctor if

You might be pregnant

You have ever had an allergic reaction to x-ray contrast material or any other iodine-containing compound

You are taking any medications (especially anticoagulants or blood thinners)

You may be asked to sign a consent form authorizing this procedure. Use this opportunity to discuss with your doctor any concerns you may have about the need for the test, the risks of the test, or how it will be performed.

You may be asked to abstain from food and to drink only clear fluids for 4 hours before the test. If this test is done on an emergency basis, no preparation is required.

### Procedure:

This test is performed in a hospital x-ray department by a radiologist and an x-ray technician.

You will be positioned upright on a tilting x-ray table and will be asked to lie in such a way that the leg to be studied doesn't bear your weight. You will be asked to relax the leg and keep it still during the x-rays.

A tourniquet will be fastened around your leg or ankle to make the veins of the foot fill with blood. A needle will then be inserted into a vein on the top of your foot. A small amount of saline solution will be injected to be sure the vein is large enough to handle the injection of contrast material. If an adequate vein can't be found in this way, a small surgical incision ("cutdown") may be made to locate a larger vein. If a cutdown is done, the area will first be numbed with a local anesthetic.

The contrast material will then be injected, and a series of x-rays will be taken of each section of the leg and lower pelvis. (The technician will need to move very quickly to accomplish this.) You will be asked to assume a number of different positions so that x-rays can be taken.

When the x-rays are completed, your leg will be elevated. Sterile saline solution will be injected into the vein to help flush out the contrast material. The needle will then be removed and a bandage will be placed on the injection site.

This test usually takes 30 to 45 minutes. You can resume your normal diet as soon as the test is over. If fever, redness, bleeding, or increased leg pain and swelling develops, let your doctor know at once.

### How Does It Feel?

The x-ray table will be hard and may be cold. You may feel a bit uneasy when the table tilts—don't worry, you will be secured either by belts or by holding onto handles on the table. You may experience a warm, burning sensation in your leg as the dye (contrast material) is injected. You may feel as if your leg is falling asleep. Some patients find this sensation quite uncomfortable. You may also notice some cramping in the leg. Your leg may be sore for a day or two afterward as a result of irritation from the dye.

### Risks:

There is a risk of an allergic reaction to the dye used in this test. If you have ever had an allergic reaction to any x-ray dye or any other iodine-containing substance, be sure to tell your doctor.

There is always some concern about the effects of exposure to any radiation, including the low-level radiation of diagnostic x-rays. Extremely high levels of radiation have been shown to cause various diseases and birth defects. However, if this test is really necessary, the radiation risk is generally very low compared with the potential benefits.

Compared with other x-rays, the radiation exposure from this test is medium for the total body, medium for the male reproductive organs, and medium to high for the female reproductive organs. Because a developing fetus is very sensitive to radiation, this test is not usually recommended for pregnant women. (For more on x-ray risks, see p. 227.)

Possible complications of the test include inflammation and damage to the leg veins. This test can even, rarely, cause DVT—the condition it is designed to detect.

### Results:

Results of this test are usually available within an hour or two.

In a person with normal leg veins, the dye spreads quickly and evenly through all the deep veins of the leg. A venogram that shows blockage of blood flow to one or more of the deep veins of the leg, abrupt termination of a vein, or increased flow through the smaller connecting (collateral) veins suggests the presence of blood clots.

If a deep vein blood clot (thrombophlebitis) is found, you will be advised to come into the hospital and observe strict bed rest with your leg elevated and receive regular doses of heparin, a blood-thinning medication.

### Cost:

$130 to $200

# 7

# Nuclear Scans

**N**uclear medicine is the branch of medicine that uses radioactive materials to diagnose and treat disease. Nuclear scanning permits the size, shape, location and, perhaps most importantly, the function of various internal organs to be evaluated in a way not possible with ordinary x-rays.

Radionuclides, sometimes known as radioactive tracers or radioisotopes, are substances that emit atomic radiation. To produce a nuclear scan a very small amount of a specific radionuclide is swallowed, injected, or inhaled. The radioactive material then distributes itself throughout the body, concentrating in the chosen target organ such as the brain, thyroid, liver, or kidney. The body is then "scanned" with a special camera which records the radiation emitted by the radionuclide and creates a picture or scan of the target organ. The nuclear medicine camera or scanner functions like a large Geiger counter. Though it looks like a large x-ray machine, it is not, and it does not expose you to any additional radiation. It only measures the radiation in the radionuclide tracer.

Some radionuclides concentrate in abnormal or diseased tissue (such as tumors). This forms "hot spots" on the scans. Other radionuclides concentrate in normal tissue and avoid abnormal areas. In these scans abnormalities appear as areas of decreased radioactive labeling ("cold spots"). The images often require considerable skill and experience to interpret. The interpretation is done by a specially trained physician who specializes in nuclear medicine.

Except for the brief needle stick required for injection of the radioactive tracer in some of these tests, nuclear scans are painless. Patients are often concerned about having radioactive materials put into their body. In most instances nuclear scans involve no more, and often less, radiation exposure than major x-ray procedures. The amount of radioactive material used is very small and most of it is eliminated from the body within a few hours to a few days. Still, because fetuses and infants are far more sensitive to radiation, nuclear scans are not usually recommended for pregnant or breast-feeding women or young children. The radiation risk from nuclear scans is generally quite small, and the central question, as with all tests, is whether the test is necessary. If it is necessary, then the benefits will greatly outweigh the risks. Nuclear scans often provide important diagnostic information at considerably less risk, discomfort, and cost than other more invasive diagnostic procedures.

In the sections that follow we describe the major scans used to evaluate bone, brain, gallbladder, liver, spleen, lung, kidney, and thyroid. The nuclear medicine tests used to evaluate the heart are described in the section Testing for Heart Disease (p. 167). A special blood test which uses radioactive materials to test for difficulty in absorbing vitamin $B_{12}$ (Schilling test) is described on p. 99.

# Bone Scan
# (Bone Scintigraphy)

In this test an image of the skeleton is made by a special scanning camera after the injection of a very small amount of radioactive substance. This radioactive material (radionuclide or radioisotope tracer) travels through the bloodstream and attaches to bone. It shows up in increased amounts ("hot spots") in areas of abnormal bone. The bone scan is more sensitive than regular x-rays in detecting the early signs of bone cancers, infection, or slight fractures.

### Why Performed:
Bone scans are frequently done to determine whether a known cancer (such as breast or prostate cancer) has spread (metastasized) to the bone. This so-called staging of the cancer helps determine what type of treatment is appropriate. A bone scan may also be performed to monitor the response of a cancer to therapy.

This test is also useful in evaluating unexplained bone pain or abnormalities found on regular bone x-rays. A bone scan

may also reveal the cause for an elevated blood level of alkaline phosphatase (see p. 45), an enzyme that can suggest abnormal bone metabolism.

### Preparation:
Tell your doctor if
    You are breast-feeding
    You might be pregnant

If you have recently had barium x-ray studies of your stomach or colon, you may be asked to take laxatives or an enema the day before the test to remove any remaining barium, since the barium can interfere with the scan.

Remove all jewelry and metal objects before the test. Since you will be asked to drink several glasses of fluid during the test, don't eat or drink too much before the test. It is important to empty your bladder just before the test.

Since the test involves a long waiting period, you may wish to bring along some reading material or plan some other quiet activity to keep you occupied.

### Procedure:
The test is done in a hospital radiology or nuclear medicine department by a nuclear medicine physician and a technician. It does not usually require overnight hospitalization.

A tourniquet will be placed on your upper arm, and a tiny amount of radioactive substance will be injected into a vein on the inside of your elbow. You will then be asked to wait 2–3 hours while the radioactive tracer distributes throughout your body. While waiting you will be asked to drink 4–6 glasses of fluid to help clear your body of the radioactive material that is not picked up by the bone tissue. During the wait you may resume regular activities. Just before the actual scan is to begin, you will need to empty your bladder. Otherwise the collection of radioactive substance in your bladder can block the view on the scan of some of your pelvic bones.

When the waiting period is over, you will be asked to lie on your back on a table with a very large scanning camera positioned above you. The camera will move slowly back and forth about 6 inches above your body. The camera detects the radiation emitted by the radioactive tracer which has temporarily accumulated in your bones. The machine itself is not an x-ray device and does not expose you to any additional radiation.

The scan takes approximately one hour. You will have to lie very still during the procedure. You may be asked to lie in other positions so that different views may be taken. You may resume usual activities after the test.

## How Does It Feel?

You will feel a brief, pricking sensation similar to that of having your blood drawn when the needle is inserted into your arm to inject the radioactive tracer. Otherwise the procedure is painless. You may find it tiring and a bit uncomfortable to lie completely still for nearly an hour during the scan. Be sure to make yourself as comfortable as possible before the scan begins. You may wish to ask for blankets, a pillow, or a mattress pad for the hard table.

## Risks:

There is always some concern about the potential health effects of any radiation exposure, including nuclear scans. Radiation exposure has been shown to cause various diseases and birth defects—however, at levels far greater than those involved in this test (see p. 227). When this test is necessary, the risk from radiation exposure is generally very low compared with the benefits of the test. Since fetuses and infants are far more sensitive to radiation, nuclear scans are not usually recommended for pregnant or breast-feeding women or for young children. The total body radiation dose with a bone scan is approximately 110 millirads (the equivalent of 5 chest x-rays). Most of the radioactive material is eliminated from your body within a day. Allergic reactions to the radioactive tracer are very rare.

Occasionally, as with any blood drawing or injection, some soreness and swelling may develop at the injection site. This can usually be managed with moist, warm compresses applied every few hours.

## Results:

The results of the bone scan are usually available within a day or two. Areas of increased bone metabolism will pick up more of the radioactive tracer and will show up as "hot spots" on the scan. These hot spots may represent normal growing bone in children or the healing of a fracture, but they are also found with bone tumors (cancerous as well as benign), bone infections (osteomyelitis), arthritis, and disorders of bone metabolism such as Paget's disease. Both primary bone cancers and metastatic cancers (cancers which have spread to bone from elsewhere in the body) can often be detected on a scan 3 to 6 months before they can be seen on regular bone x-rays.

"Cold spots" are abnormal areas of decreased radioactive labeling and may suggest tumors such as multiple myeloma or lack of blood supply to the bone (bone infarction).

The findings on a bone scan must always be interpreted in light of x-ray and blood tests as well as of clinical examination and history.

**Cost:**
$250 to $400

# Brain Scan
## (Cerebral Perfusion and Brain Scintigraphy)

In this test an image of the brain is made to detect abnormalities in brain blood flow and structure. A very small amount of radioactive substance, injected into a vein, travels to the brain. A scanning camera detects where the radioactive substance has accumulated in the brain. If an abnormality exists in the brain, such as a tumor or abnormality of the blood vessels, the abnormal area may show up on the brain scan image as a concentration of the radioactive substance.

### Why Performed:
Brain scans are sometimes performed when there is a suspicion of a mass or other abnormality in the brain. Symptoms such as seizures, dizziness, numbness, or weakness in an arm or a leg might be further evaluated with a brain scan. Brain scans are also sometimes used in monitoring the response of a brain tumor to surgery, radiation, or chemotherapy. However, in most cases, the CT scan (see p. 256) is now used instead of this test.

### Preparation:
Tell your doctor if
> You are breast-feeding
> You might be pregnant

It is not necessary to restrict food or fluids before the test. Remove all jewelry, metal objects, and glasses before the test.

Sometimes a capsule or solution of a "blocking agent" may be given to you 15 minutes to several hours before the test. This blocking agent will prevent the radioactive substance from accumulating in other tissues (salivary glands and thyroid), which can interfere with a clear picture of the brain.

Since there will be some waiting time during the test you may wish to bring along some reading material or plan some other quiet activity to keep you occupied.

### Procedure:
The test is done in a hospital radiology or nuclear medicine department by a nuclear medicine physician and a technician. It does not usually require overnight hospitalization.

You will be asked to lie on your back on a table or sit with a very large camera above your head. A tourniquet will be placed on your upper arm, and a small amount of radioactive substance will be injected into an arm vein.

The camera will then detect the radioactive substance as it flows through the arteries in your neck into the brain. The camera itself is not an x-ray device and does not expose your body to any additional radiation. This cerebral flow or perfusion scan takes about 5 minutes. You may then resume normal activities during the following 1- to 2-hour waiting period.

Another set of pictures is taken 1 to 2 hours after the initial injection. Five or six different views of your head will be made. For each view either you or the large camera may be repositioned. During each scan, which takes approximately 5 minutes, you must hold completely still. Try not to move or cough during the scan, and be sure to keep your hands away from your face and head. In rare instances you may be called back 24 hours later for additional pictures.

## How Does It Feel?

You will feel a brief, pricking sensation similar to having your blood drawn when the needle is inserted into your arm and the radioactive tracer is injected. Otherwise, the procedure is painless. You may find it a bit uncomfortable and tiring to lie completely still during the scan. Be sure to get as comfortable as possible before the scan begins. You may wish to ask for blankets, a pillow, or a mattress pad for the table.

## Risks:

There is always some concern about the potential health effects of any radiation exposure, including nuclear scans. Radiation exposure has been shown to cause various diseases and birth defects—however, at levels far greater than those involved in this test (see p. 227). When this test is necessary, the risk from radiation exposure is generally very low compared with the benefits of the test. Since fetuses and infants are far more sensitive to radiation, nuclear scans are not usually recommended for pregnant or breast-feeding women or for young children. The total body radiation dose with a brain scan is approximately 120 millirads (the equivalent of 5 chest x-rays). Most of the radioactive material is eliminated from your body within a day. Allergic reactions to the radioactive tracer are very rare.

Occasionally, as with any blood drawing or injection, some soreness and swelling may develop at the injection site. This can usually be managed with moist, warm compresses applied every few hours.

## Results:

The results from a brain scan are usually available in a day or two. The perfusion scan done immediately after the injection of radioactive tracer may reveal an uneven, abnormal blood flow to the brain due to a narrowing or blockage of the arteries. Normally the radioactive substance cannot get out of the blood vessels into the brain tissue. However, damage to the "blood-brain barrier" allows the radioactive substance to leak into abnormal areas. Therefore, radioactively labeled areas may represent brain tumors (benign or malignant), metastases (cancers that have spread to the brain), infections, malformations of the arteries and veins, leakage of blood following trauma (subdural hematoma), or areas of brain deprived of normal blood flow because of a stroke. If an abnormality is detected, other tests such as a CT scan or arteriogram may be necessary to determine the exact type of abnormality.

## Cost:

$300 to $400

# Gallbladder and Biliary Tract Scans (Cholescintigraphy)

In this test the function of the liver, gallbladder, and biliary tract is assessed. A very small amount of radioactive material is injected in a vein in the arm and circulates through the bloodstream to the liver. The substance is excreted along with bile into the gallbladder for storage (see illustration, p. 281). By following the course of this radioactive material with a scanning camera it is possible to identify blockages in the system.

## Why Performed:

A nuclear scan is one of several tests (see pp. 266 and 304) available to evaluate suspected gallbladder and biliary tract disease.

It is often performed to evaluate pain in the upper right side of the abdomen or jaundice (a condition in which the skin turns yellow). It can also be used to evaluate abdominal trauma when injury to the liver or biliary tract is suspected.

### Preparation:

Tell your doctor if
> You are breast-feeding
> You might be pregnant

You should not eat or drink anything except clear liquids (water, tea, or black coffee) for at least 2 hours before the test. Remove all jewelry and metal objects before the test.

### Procedure:

The test is performed in a hospital nuclear medicine or radiology department by a nuclear medicine physician and a technician. An overnight stay in the hospital is usually not required.

A tourniquet is placed around your upper arm to help locate the vein at the bend of your arm. After the area is cleansed, a small amount of radioactive material is injected.

You will be lying on your back on a table with a very large camera positioned above your abdomen. This camera detects the radioactive material as it circulates through your liver and is excreted into the biliary tract, gallbladder, and eventually into the small intestine. The camera itself is not an x-ray device and does not expose you to any additional radiation.

Pictures will be taken every 5 minutes or so for the first 30 minutes. Depending upon what is seen in earlier pictures, additional scans may be taken several hours or 24 hours after the injection. Each scan takes only a few minutes.

### How Does It Feel?

You will feel a brief, pricking sensation similar to having your blood drawn when the needle is inserted into your arm to inject the radioactive tracer. Otherwise, the procedure is painless. You may find it a bit uncomfortable and tiring to lie completely still during the scan, especially if you are already experiencing abdominal pain. Try to relax by taking slow deep breaths. Be sure to get as comfortable as possible before the scan starts. You may wish to ask for blankets, a pillow, or a mattress pad for the table.

### Risks:

There is always some concern about the potential health effects of any radiation exposure, including nuclear scans. Radiation exposure has been shown to cause various diseases and birth defects—however, at levels far greater than those involved in this test (see p. 227). When this test is necessary, the risk from radiation exposure is generally very low compared with the benefits of the test. Since fetuses and infants are far more sensitive to radiation, nuclear scans are not usually recommended for pregnant or breast-feeding women or for young children. The total body radiation dose with a gallbladder scan is approximately 120 millirads (the equivalent of 5 chest x-rays). Most of the radioactive material is eliminated from your body within a day. Allergic reactions to the radioactive tracer are very rare.

Occasionally, as with any blood drawing or injection, some soreness and swelling may develop at the injection site. This can usually be managed with moist, warm compresses applied every few hours.

### Results:

The results from a gallbladder scan are usually available within hours or the next day.

The failure of the radioactive material to be excreted into bile by the liver suggests a disorder of the liver cells (hepatocellular disease). If the material is excreted but never shows up in the gallbladder, this demonstrates a blockage of the cystic duct leading to the gallbladder, either by a gallstone or by inflammation (cholecystitis). If the radioactive tracer never appears in the small intestine, this shows that the common bile duct is blocked (biliary obstruction).

## Cost:
$300 to $400

# Gallium Scan
## (Body Scan)

This test provides an overall image of the body to help detect tumors and inflammation. A very small amount of a radioactive substance (gallium citrate) is injected. Hours later a special camera detects areas in which this radioactive tracer has concentrated. Gallium tends to accumulate in areas where cells are rapidly growing and metabolizing. Therefore, gallium scans can highlight cancers and areas of inflammation due to infection, irritation, or injury.

### Why Performed:
Gallium scans are used to detect primary cancers, cancers that have spread (metastases), or areas of inflammation such as bone infections or localized collections of pus (abscesses). They are often performed to determine the spread of cancers like Hodgkin's lymphoma as well as to follow the response of tumors to radiation and chemotherapy. They are occasionally used to detect a hidden infection in a person with persistent unexplained fever or to evaluate an unexplained mass.

### Preparation:
Tell your doctor if
> You are breast-feeding
> You might be pregnant

There is no need to restrict food or fluids before the test. However, because the gallium is excreted in the stool, your bowel must be cleaned out so that stool doesn't interfere with the reading of the test. This usually involves taking a laxative the night before the test and an enema 1 to 2 hours before the scan. You will be asked to remove all jewelry and metal objects before the scan.

Since the test involves some long waiting periods, you may wish to bring along some reading material or plan some other quiet activity to keep you occupied.

### Procedure:
This test is done in a hospital nuclear medicine or radiology department by a nuclear medicine physician and a technician. The test itself does not usually require an overnight stay in the hospital.

A tourniquet will be placed around your upper arm to help locate the vein at the bend of your arm. After this area is cleansed, a small amount of the radioactive material (gallium citrate) will be injected into your arm. You will then have to wait. The scans are usually taken at 6 hours, 24 hours, 48 hours, and sometimes 72 hours after the injection.

During each scan you will lie on your back on a table with a very large camera poised over you. This camera, as it scans your body, will detect the radioactive gallium. The camera itself is not an x-ray machine and does not expose you to any additional radiation. During the scan you must lie completely still. It usually takes 30–60 minutes for each scan. After the first scan at 6 hours, you can usually return home and resume normal activities and diet, returning to the hospital for the later scans.

### How Does It Feel?

You will feel a brief, pricking sensation similar to having your blood drawn when the needle is inserted into the vein in your arm to inject the radioactive material. Otherwise, the procedure is painless. You may find it somewhat uncomfortable and tiring to lie completely still while each scan is being taken. Try to get as comfortable as possible before the scan begins. You might want to ask for blankets, pillows, or a mattress pad for the table.

### Risks:

There is always some concern about the potential health effects of any radiation exposure, including nuclear scans. Radiation exposure has been shown to cause various diseases and birth defects—however, at levels far greater than those involved in this test (see p. 227). When this test is necessary, the risk from radiation exposure is generally very low compared with the benefits of the test. Since fetuses and infants are far more sensitive to radiation, nuclear scans are not usually recommended for pregnant or breast-feeding women or for young children. The total body radiation dose with a gallium scan is approximately 80 millirads (the equivalent of 4 chest x-rays). Most of the radioactive material is eliminated from your body within a day. Allergic reactions to the radioactive tracer are very rare.

Occasionally, as with any blood drawing or injection, some soreness and swelling may develop at the injection site. This can usually be managed with moist, warm compresses applied every few hours.

### Results:

The results of a gallium scan are usually available within a day or two. Gallium is normally picked up by bones, liver, spleen, breast tissue, and the large bowel. Therefore, these areas are highlighted on a normal scan. If other areas show increased gallium concentrations, an abnormality may be present. The abnormality may be a cancer, such as lymphoma, sarcoma, or lung, liver, colon, stomach, uterine, or testicular cancer.

Unfortunately, not all cancers show up on a gallium scan, so a normal or "negative" scan doesn't exclude the possibility of cancer. Highlighted areas on the scan may also be due to inflammation, such as the accumulation of pus in an infected abscess, pneumonia, inflammatory bowel disease, or bone infection (osteomyelitis). The findings on a gallium scan must be interpreted in light of other tests, symptoms, and physical examination.

### Cost:
$400 to $500

# Liver/Spleen Scan

This test examines the size, shape, position, and function of the liver and spleen. The liver is a large organ tucked up under the lower rib cage on the right side of the abdomen (see illustration, p. 281). It plays a central role in metabolism, digestion, and detoxification. The spleen is located under the lower rib cage on the left side. One of the main functions of the spleen is to remove old red blood cells from the bloodstream.

A very small amount of a radioactive

substance (radionuclide or radioisotope tracer) is injected into the bloodstream and is concentrated by the liver and spleen. A scanning camera then measures the amount of radioactive substance in these organs and produces an image of the liver and spleen which may reveal abnormalities.

## Why Performed:

Liver/spleen scans are most often done to determine whether a known cancer, such as lung or colon cancer, has spread (metastasized) to the liver. This "staging" of cancer helps in the selection of the appropriate treatment. The scan can also be helpful in determining the response of liver metastases or tumors to treatment.

Liver/spleen scans are sometimes used to evaluate an enlarged liver (hepatomegaly) or spleen (splenomegaly) or unexplained abdominal masses (lumps) or pain. A scan may also be performed after abdominal injury to find out whether the liver or spleen has been damaged. It is also occasionally performed to look for a liver infection (abscess) in a person with persistent, unexplained fever.

## Preparation:

Tell your doctor if
>You are breast-feeding
>You might be pregnant

There is no need to restrict food or fluids before the test. You will be asked to remove all jewelry and metal objects before the scan is taken.

## Procedure:

The test is performed in a hospital nuclear medicine or radiology department by a nuclear medicine physician and a technician. An overnight stay in the hospital is not usually required.

A tourniquet is placed around your up-

per arm to help locate the vein at the bend in your arm. A very small amount of radioactive substance is injected into the vein. After waiting 10 minutes, you will be asked to lie on your back on a table with a very large camera above your abdomen or to sit in front of the camera.

The camera detects the low level radiation emitted by the radioactive tracer as it is absorbed by your liver and spleen. The camera itself is not an x-ray machine and does not expose you to any additional radiation. During the scan you must hold very still and breathe quietly. You may be asked to hold your breath briefly or to turn onto your side or stomach to check additional views. The entire procedure takes about one hour. After the test you can resume your usual activities and diet.

## How Does It Feel?

You will feel a brief, pricking sensation similar to having your blood drawn when the needle is inserted into your arm to inject the radioactive tracer. Otherwise, the procedure is painless. You may find it a bit uncomfortable and tiring to lie completely still during the scan. Be sure to get as comfortable as possible before the scan begins. You may wish to ask for blankets, a pillow, or a mattress pad for the table.

## Risks:

There is always some concern about the potential health effects of any radiation exposure, including nuclear scans. Radiation exposure has been shown to cause various diseases and birth defects—however, at levels far greater than those involved in this test (see p. 227). When this test is necessary, the risk from radiation exposure is generally very low compared with the benefits of the test. Since fetuses and infants are far more sensitive to radiation, nuclear scans are not usually recommended for pregnant or breast-feeding women or for young children. The total body radiation dose with a liver/spleen scan is approximately 20 millirads (the equivalent of one chest x-ray). Most of the radioactive material is eliminated from your body within a day. Allergic reactions to the radioactive tracer are very rare.

Occasionally, as with any blood drawing or injection, some soreness and swelling may develop at the injection site, but this can usually be managed with moist, warm compresses applied every few hours.

### Results:

The results of a liver/spleen scan are usually available within a day or two. Normal liver and spleen tissue picks up the radioactive tracer from the bloodstream and appears as a smooth, uniformly labeled image. Decreased radioactivity or a patchy image suggests liver disease, such as cirrhosis or hepatitis. Specific areas of decreased uptake appear as a "cold spot" or "focal defect" and may represent a tumor (cancerous or benign), cyst, abscess, or an area of diminished blood supply. Further tests such as biopsies, ultrasound, gallium or CT scans are usually required to clarify the nature of the defect revealed in the scan.

### Cost:

$250 to $350

### Special Considerations:

★A special type of nuclear scan can be done to specifically evaluate the spleen using a sample of the patient's own blood which has been mixed with a radioisotope. These "tagged" red blood cells are reinjected into the patient and are removed from the bloodstream by a normally functioning spleen.

# Lung Scans
## (Ventilation and Perfusion Scans)

There are two separate types of lung scans which test respiratory function: a perfusion scan and a ventilation scan. A *perfusion scan* detects blockages in the flow of *blood* from the heart to the lungs. In this test a very small amount of radioactive material is injected into an arm and travels through the bloodstream to the lungs. A picture is then taken of the lungs by a special camera which measures the radioactivity in the lungs and can highlight areas not receiving adequate blood.

A *ventilation scan* measures the flow of *air* in and out of the lungs. You inhale a radioactive gas, and the camera detects those areas of the lungs not receiving air. These tests can be done separately or together to aid in the diagnosis of lung disease by comparing the flow of blood and air to the lungs.

### Why Performed:

Lung scans are most frequently performed when it is suspected that a blood clot may have lodged in one or more of the arteries that flow to the lungs. This is called a *pulmonary embolism*. A pulmonary embolism is a very serious disorder which requires prompt treatment. Unfortunately, it is difficult to diagnose an embolism from symptoms or chest x-rays alone. The symptoms of chest pain, shortness of breath, rapid breathing, and rapid heart rate could be caused by a pulmonary embolism or by some other disorder. A lung scan can help determine the cause of such symptoms.

Ventilation scans are also sometimes

performed to determine the severity of chronic lung disease.

### Preparation:
Tell your doctor if
>You are breast-feeding
>You might be pregnant

You need not restrict food or fluids prior to the test. You should remove all jewelry and metal objects before the test.

### Procedure:
These scans are performed in a hospital nuclear medicine or radiology department by a nuclear medicine physician and a technician. The test itself does not usually require overnight hospitalization.

*Perfusion Scan:* You will be asked to lie on your back on a table. A tourniquet will be placed on your upper arm to help locate the vein at the bend of your arm. After the area is cleansed, a tiny amount of a radioactive substance is injected. This radioactive material travels through the bloodstream to the lungs where it is detected by a large scanning camera. The camera itself is not an x-ray machine and does not expose you to any additional radiation. Pictures will be taken with you lying on your back or sitting upright. You will need to hold quite still during the scan. The scan itself usually takes 15–30 minutes.

*Ventilation Scan:* For this test you will be asked to inhale a radioactive gas (xenon or krypton). The gas is administered through a mask (which fits over your mouth and nose) or through a mouthpiece (in which case noseclips are used to pinch your nostrils closed). You will be asked to take a deep breath and hold it and then re-breathe the gas in and out through your mouth for 3 to 5 minutes while a large camera measures the radioactivity in your lungs. During the scan you may be sitting or be lying on your back on a table. The scan itself takes about 5–10 minutes.

### How Does It Feel?
You will feel a brief, pricking sensation similar to any blood drawing when the needle is inserted in your arm. Otherwise, the tests are painless. You may find that breathing through the mask or mouthpiece is uncomfortable, especially if you feel very short of breath. Don't worry—you will be given plenty of oxygen through the mask.

*Patient Comments:*
"At first I was afraid I wouldn't be able to get enough air through the mask, but after a few practice breaths I found that I could breathe just fine."

### Risks:
There is always some concern about the potential health effects of any radiation exposure, including nuclear scans. Radiation exposure has been shown to cause various diseases and birth defects—however, at levels far greater than those involved in these tests (see p. 227). When this test is necessary, the risk from radiation exposure is generally very low compared with the benefits of the test. Since fetuses and infants are far more sensitive to radiation, nuclear scans are not usually recommended for pregnant or breast-feeding women or for young children, unless the situation is life-threatening. The total body radiation dose with a ventilation-perfusion scan is approximately 10 millirads (the equivalent of a chest x-ray). Most of the radioactive material is eliminated from your body within a day. Allergic reactions to the radioactive tracer are extremely rare.

Occasionally, as with any blood drawing or injection, some soreness and swelling may develop at the injection site. This can usually be managed with moist, warm compresses applied every few hours.

**Results:**

The results of a lung scan are usually available within minutes to hours. In a normal perfusion scan the radioactive material should spread to all areas of the lungs. If the perfusion scan is normal, a significant blood clot within the arteries to the lungs (pulmonary embolism) is extremely unlikely. If the perfusion scan is "positive"—that is, areas appear without radioactivity—these abnormalities could be due to a pulmonary embolism, inflammation of the blood vessels (vasculitis), a tumor, or a pneumonia.

Comparing the perfusion scan with the ventilation scan and chest x-ray can help determine the cause of such defects. For example, if the ventilation scan and chest x-ray are normal, but the perfusion scan is abnormal, a pulmonary embolism is the likely diagnosis. The ventilation scan detects airway obstruction which blocks the flow of air to certain areas of the lung. Sometimes it is necessary to perform an additional test, pulmonary arteriography (see p. 241), to discover whether a blood clot is present.

**Cost:**

Perfusion scan: $250 to $400
Ventilation scan: $300 to $450

# Renal Scans
## (Renogram, Renal Scintigraphy, Renography, Kidney Scan)

Renal scans are one way of studying the structure and function of the kidneys and urinary system. A very small amount of various radioactive materials (radionuclides) is injected into the bloodstream through a vein. A special scanning camera which detects radioactivity records the radioactive tracer as it circulates through the kidneys.

These studies can reveal abnormalities in the blood flow into the kidneys, the size, shape, location, and function of the kidneys, as well as blockages in the collecting system which conducts urine from the kidneys to the bladder (see illustration, p. 261). Nuclear renal scans are very safe and can often eliminate the need for more dangerous and invasive procedures.

**Why Performed:**

Renal scans are performed to evaluate kidney function, renal blood flow, kidney transplants, kidney diseases (such as pyelonephritis or glomerulonephritis) or suspected kidney masses, stones, or injury. They are also sometimes used to detect narrowing of the arteries supplying the kidneys, a condition that can cause high blood pressure. Kidney scans can also be helpful when other contrast x-rays (see IVP, p. 269) cannot be used because of allergies to the iodine contrast dyes.

**Preparation:**

Tell your doctor if
> You are breast-feeding
> You might be pregnant

There is no need to restrict food or fluids before the test. In fact, you should drink two or more glasses of water an hour or two before the test to prevent dehydration, which can interfere with test results. Remove all jewelry and metal objects and empty your bladder before the test begins.

**Procedure:**

Renal scans are done in a hospital nuclear medicine or radiology department by a nuclear medicine physician and a technician. An overnight stay in the hospital is usually not necessary. Often two or more of the different types of renal scan are performed one after the other.

A tourniquet will be placed on your upper arm to help locate the vein at the bend of your arm. The area is cleansed and then a small amount of the radioactive tracer is injected into the vein. The material travels through the bloodstream to the kidneys. A very large camera records the radioactive material as it courses through your kidneys (perfusion scan). The camera itself is not an x-ray machine and does not expose you to any additional radiation.

Another injection will be made of a different type of radioactive material, and a series of pictures will be made every few minutes for the next 30 minutes. These images trace the flow of the material through the kidney, into the collecting system and ureter, and into the bladder. When each of the pictures is being taken you must lie on your back completely still. Sometimes the test is done in the sitting position.

The entire series of scans usually takes about an hour to complete. However, sometimes you may need to come back in 4 hours and then again later for additional scans. When the scans are finished you will be asked to empty your bladder. You may then resume normal activities and diet, but you should flush the toilet immediately after urinating for the next 24 hours to reduce exposure to the trace amounts of radioactivity in your urine.

**How Does It Feel?**

When the needle is inserted into your arm to inject the radioactive material, you will feel a brief, pricking sensation similar to any blood drawing. Otherwise, the procedure is painless. You may find it somewhat uncomfortable and tiring to lie completely still during the scan. Make yourself as comfortable as possible before the scan begins. You may wish to ask for blankets, pillows, or a mattress pad for the table.

**Risks:**

There is always some concern about the potential health effects of any radiation exposure, including nuclear scans. Radiation exposure has been shown to cause various diseases and birth defects—however, at levels far greater than those involved in this test (see p. 227). When this test is necessary, the risk from radiation exposure is generally very low compared with the benefits of the test. Since fetuses and infants are far more sensitive to radiation, nuclear scans are not usually recommended for pregnant or breast-feeding women or for young children. The total body radiation dose with renal scanning is approximately 120 millirads (the equivalent of 5 chest x-rays). Most of the radioactive material is eliminated from your body within a day. Allergic reactions to the radioactive tracer are extremely rare.

Occasionally, as with any blood drawing or injection, some soreness and swelling may develop at the injection site. This can usually be managed with moist, warm compresses applied every few hours.

**Results:**

The results for renal scans are usually available within a day or two. The scans may reveal a decreased blood flow to the whole kidney or to part of a kidney. Blockage of the ureter may be seen, or it may be noted that one kidney is absent or nonfunctioning. Areas on the scan that fail to take up the radioactive tracer ("cold spots") may represent tumors, cysts, infections, or the result of trauma.

The findings on renal scans should always be interpreted in light of symptoms, history, physical examination, and other laboratory tests. Sometimes additional tests are required to clarify abnormalities found on a renal scan.

**Cost:**

$250 to $600

# Thyroid Scan and Radioactive Iodine (RAI) Uptake Test

The thyroid is the butterfly-shaped gland located in the front of the neck below the Adam's apple. This gland extracts iodine from the bloodstream and uses it to make hormones which help regulate the body's metabolism.

There are two tests that use radioactive iodine to detect abnormalities in the thyroid gland. In the *radioactive iodine uptake test* (RAIU test), a very small amount of radioactive iodine is swallowed. The amount of this radioactive tracer taken up by the thyroid gland is then measured to evaluate the overall function of the gland. The other test is a *thyroid scan*, which creates a picture of the thyroid gland from the radioactive iodine taken up by the gland. The thyroid scan indicates the size, position, and function of the thyroid. One or both of these tests may be performed to check thyroid gland function.

**Why Performed:**

These tests are most often done to evaluate a swelling of the neck, an enlarged thyroid gland (goiter), or a lump (nodule) found in the thyroid gland during a physical examination.

These tests are also used to determine the cause of excessive thyroid hormone production (hyperthyroidism, see p. 108). Thyroid scans are sometimes performed to check residual gland function following surgery done to remove part or all of a diseased thyroid gland, and they are sometimes recommended to check for thyroid cancer in people who were exposed to radiation treatment of the head and neck as children.

**Preparation:**

Tell your doctor if

You are taking any medications, including thyroid medication, antithyroid drugs, or iodine-containing preparations (iodized salt, kelp, cough syrups, or multivitamins)

You have had any recent nuclear medicine tests involving radioactive materials or x-ray tests that used an iodine-containing contrast dye such as kidney x-rays (IVP), angiography, or gallbladder x-rays (OCG)

You are breast-feeding

You might be pregnant

You should not eat or drink anything for 8–12 hours before the tests (before swallowing the radioactive material). Remove jewelry or metal objects from the neck and upper chest area.

## Procedure:

The tests are done in a hospital nuclear medicine or radiology department by a nuclear medicine physician and a technician. An overnight stay in the hospital is not usually required. You will be given a capsule or liquid containing a small amount of radioactive iodine and asked to swallow it 6 hours before the test is scheduled to begin. You may resume a normal diet 1–2 hours after swallowing the radioactive iodine.

The RAI uptake study is done by measuring the radioactivity in your neck area with a special camera 6 hours after swallowing the radioactive iodine. Occasionally, another measurement is made 24 hours after taking the iodine. Each uptake measurement takes about 10 minutes. During the measurements you will be asked to hold completely still.

The thyroid scan is done 6 hours (and sometimes 24 hours) after swallowing the radioactive material. You will be asked to lie on your back on a table with your head extended all the way back. A large detecting instrument will then scan your neck to detect the radioactive iodine picked up by your thyroid gland. The scan takes about 30 mintues.

## How Does It Feel?

Both these tests are painless. Holding completely still with your head extended back during the scan may be slightly uncomfortable.

## Risks:

There is always some concern about the potential health effects of any radiation exposure, including nuclear scans. Radiation exposure has been shown to cause various diseases and birth defects—however, at levels far greater than those involved in this test (see p. 227). When this test is necessary, the risk from radiation exposure is generally very low compared with the benefits of the test. Since fetuses and infants are far more sensitive to radiation, nuclear scans are not usually recommended for pregnant or breast-feeding women or for young children. The total body radiation dose with a scan approximately 18 millirads (the equivalent of a chest x-ray) although the radiation dose to the thyroid gland is much greater. Most of the radioactive material is eliminated from your body within a day.

## Results:

The radioactive iodine uptake test measures the percentage of the iodine that accumulates in the gland after swallowing the radioactive test material. Normal values are 1%–13% after 2 hours, 2%–25% after 6 hours, and 15%–45% after 24 hours. Less than normal uptake suggests an underactive thyroid (hypothyroidism), inflammation of the thyroid (subacute thyroiditis), or suppression of the gland's activity by thyroid medication. Greater than normal uptake values indicate an overactive thyroid (hyperthyroidism) or iodine deficiency.

A normal thyroid scan shows a butterfly-shaped thyroid with evenly distributed radioactivity throughout the gland. An enlarged gland with increased radioactive labeling usually represents hyperthyroidism (Graves' disease). An enlarged gland with decreased labeling usually suggests a hypothyroid goiter, inflammation of the gland, or suppression of the gland with thyroid medication. Specific areas of decreased activity ("cold nodules") are seen on the scan as white or light-gray areas of decreased uptake of iodine. These cold nodules may be due to a thyroid cancer, benign tumor, or cyst. Further testing, including thyroid needle biopsy (see p. 359) and/or ultrasound (see p. 306), is necessary to determine the nature of cold nodules. Areas of increased activity are seen as dark areas ("hot nodules") and usually represent hyperfunctioning thyroid nodules.

Many factors, including thyroid medications and previous nuclear medicine or contrast x-ray tests, can interfere with iodine utilization and cause inaccurate test results.

**Cost:**

RAI uptake: $100 to $150
Thyroid scan: $100 to $200

# Other Scans

## Salivary Gland Scan

In this test a very small amount of radioactive material is injected into a vein in your arm in order to examine the parotid salivary glands located in each cheek and the submandibular salivary glands located underneath the jaw. The radioactive tracer travels through the bloodstream to the salivary glands where it is concentrated and then normally excreted into the mouth. A special scanning camera is used to measure the radioactivity and to provide an image of the glands. The test is sometimes performed to evaluate a complaint of dry mouth (xerostomia) or swelling in the area of the glands. The scan is essentially painless and without risk. It takes less than 30 minutes. Results may indicate the presence of a tumor or blockage of the salivary ducts by a stone or infection. The cost is approximately $300.

# Testicular or Scrotal Scan

The rapid onset of pain and swelling in the scrotum is usually due to one of two different conditions which require very different treatments. Epididymitis is an infection in the tubular structure connected to each testicle. It requires antibiotic treatment. Torsion or twisting of the testicle results in a blockage of the blood supply to the testicle and requires immediate surgery to save the testicle. To help distinguish between these two different conditions a testicular or scrotal scan can be performed.

A tiny amount of a radioactive material, injected into a vein in your arm, travels through the bloodstream to the testicles. A special scanning camera detects the radioactivity and thereby measures the blood flow to each testicle. In epididymitis there is increased blood flow to the infected testicle, whereas in torsion of the testicle the blood flow is decreased. The scan itself is painless and with very little risk compared with the conditions being diagnosed. It takes less than 15 minutes. The cost is approximately $250.

# Vein Scan

The formation of blood clots in the deep veins of the legs (deep vein thrombosis or thrombophlebitis) is a serious condition. Such blood clots can break loose and travel through the bloodstream to the lungs and block blood flow to a portion of the lungs. (This condition is called pulmonary embolism.) To prevent pulmonary embolism in a person with deep vein thrombosis, anticoagulant medication is given. But this medication is itself hazardous, so it is important to give it only to people who actually have blood clots in the leg veins. Unfortunately, it is difficult to diagnose this condition without laboratory tests. The definitive test for blood clots in the leg veins is contrast venography (see p. 283). However, there are two alternative types of vein scan using small amounts of radioactive material and a scanning camera or probe.

Fibrinogen is a protein found in blood which helps form blood clots. Fibrinogen labeled with radioactive iodine can be injected into a vein in the arm. This material circulates through the bloodstream and is incorporated into any actively forming blood clots. The radioactivity labeled clots can then be detected by measurements made 6 hours, 24 hours, 48 hours, and sometimes 72 hours after the injection.

In another type of nuclear scan, a radioactivity labeled material is injected into the veins on the top of the feet. As the radioactivity tagged blood flows through the veins in the legs back toward the heart, blockage due to clots can be viewed with the aid of a special scanning camera. The cost of a vein scan is approximately $300.

# 8 Ultrasound

Ultrasound produces a picture of the inside of your body using high-frequency sound waves (like those used in submarine sonar systems) instead of x-rays.

A small instrument (transducer) which emits high-pitched sounds is moved back and forth over the part of your body to be examined. The sounds produced are of very high frequency—well above the human hearing range. A microphone on the transducer records and analyzes the sound waves reflected back from inside your body. The resulting image is displayed on a screen like a TV.

Ultrasound can be used to examine many different parts of the body, including the heart (see Echocardiogram, p. 160), a baby in the mother's uterus (see Fetal Ultrasound, p. 205), and the abdominal and pelvic organs. The picture produced by an ultrasound exam is called a sonogram, an echogram, or a scan.

## Advantages of Ultrasound

Ultrasound is quick, painless, and relatively inexpensive. Even though ultrasound scans are frequently done in an x-ray department, these procedures do not involve the use of x-rays. These tests require little or no special preparation and do not require that a scope or needle be inserted into your body.

## Limitations of Ultrasound

Ultrasound cannot be used to examine bones, the lungs, or the brain. Some patients may be difficult to scan, especially those who are obese (a thick layer of fat may block sound waves), or those with unhealed incisions or large scars over the area to be studied.

## What Are the Risks?

There are no proven ill effects of exposure to sound waves at the intensity used in most ultrasound procedures. However, this does not mean that ultrasound has been proven safe.

Although many researchers feel that ultrasound is completely safe, others believe that there could be some as yet undiscovered risk, particularly with fetal ultrasound—even though there is at present no evidence of such risk. But even the most cautious researchers seem to have very little concern about the risk of procedures other than fetal ultrasound.

# Abdominal Ultrasound
## (Abdominal Aorta, Liver, Gallbladder, Spleen, Pancreas, Kidneys)

In this test a small instrument (transducer), which emits high-frequency sound, will be passed back and forth over your abdomen. A microphone on the transducer will pick up the reflected sound waves. This information will then be processed by a computer, and an image of the organs within your abdomen will be displayed on a TV screen (see illustrations, pp. 281 and 206).

**Preparation:**
Tell your doctor if you have had a recent barium enema or upper GI series (residual air or barium can interfere with the exam), if you might be pregnant, or if you are taking any medications. You may be asked to take an enema or a drug (simethicone) to reduce the amount of gas in your intestine.

**Procedure:**
This test is done in an ultrasound room in a hospital or doctor's office by a radiologist and an ultrasound technician. You will be asked to lie on your back on an examining table. A water-soluble gel will be applied to your abdomen to improve the transmission of the sound waves.

A small instrument which emits high-frequency sounds will be passed back and forth across your abdomen a number of times. A microphone on the instrument will pick up the sound waves as they are reflected back from the organs inside your body. This information will be processed by a computer, and an image of the inside of your abdomen will be displayed on a TV screen. You will be asked to hold still and hold your breath while each picture (sonogram) is done.

As the scan progresses, an outline of the organ being studied may be drawn on your abdomen with a marking pen. You may be asked to change positions so that additional scans can be made.

The test usually takes about 15–30 minutes. The gel will be wiped off immediately. You may resume your normal diet as soon as the test is finished.

**How Does It Feel?**
The gel may feel cold and slippery. You will feel only a light pressure as the instrument passes over your abdomen. If this test is done to investigate the extent of damage from a recent abdominal injury, the slight pressure of the instrument may be somewhat painful.

**Risks:**
There are no known risks of ultrasound.

**Cost:**
The cost of an ultrasound examination of any abdominal organ is $100 to $180

## Abdominal Aorta

This is the large artery that passes down the back of the chest and abdominal cavity, just to the left of the backbone. It is examined when an abdominal pulsating bulge (aneurysm) of the aorta is suspected.

*Results*—If the aorta is enlarged or if a bulging outpocketing is seen on the sonogram, an aneurysm may be present. The bulge may be filled with either fluid or clotted blood.

## Liver

This is the large dome-shaped organ that lies under the rib cage on the right side of the abdomen. Its upper tip is behind the right nipple, and its base is at the level of the lowest right rib. The liver secretes bile, stores sugars from digested foods, and breaks down many of the body's waste products.

Liver ultrasound is sometimes done to determine whether jaundice (a condition in which a yellow pigment called bilirubin accumulates in the blood) is caused by a blocked bile tract. This test is also done to screen for liver disease, including tumors, abscesses, and cysts.

*Results*—A normal liver appears light, with dark spots (bile ducts) throughout and a dark outline. If there is a blockage in bile flow, the bile ducts may be enlarged. If there is increased blood pressure in the veins leading to the liver (portal hypertension, a frequent complication of cirrhosis of the liver), they will be enlarged. Areas of infection (abscesses) usually appear as round, hollow structures with thin walls. In hepatitis the entire liver may be enlarged.

## Gallbladder

This is the saclike organ beneath the liver. The gallbladder stores bile, which helps digest fat. When you eat fatty foods it contracts, squeezing the bile into your intestine. This test is used when gallstones or inflammation of the gallbladder is suspected and to determine whether jaundice is caused by a blocked bile tract.

You will be asked to eat a fat-free meal on the evening before the test and to fast for 8–12 hours before the test. An empty bowel and a gallbladder filled with bile help make the sonogram clearer.

You may be given an injection to make your gallbladder contract during the test. This drug may produce some abdominal cramping, nausea, dizziness, flushing, or sweating. This medication should not be given to children, pregnant women, or people with allergies to the drug or related compounds.

*Results*—Gallstones usually show up as movable objects within the gallbladder. Polyps and tumors do not move when you change position. Infections and inflammation of the gallbladder (cholecystitis) usually produce an enlarged organ with thickened walls, although in some long-standing infections the organ may be smaller than normal.

## Spleen

This is the soft, round organ that recycles old blood cells. The spleen is located to the left of the stomach, just behind the lowest left rib.

This test is used to investigate unexplained pain or swelling in the left upper abdomen, to determine the effects of abdominal injury, and to check for other disorders of the spleen. You will be asked to eat a fat-free meal on the evening before the test and to fast for 8–12 hours before the test. An empty bowel and a gallbladder filled with bile help make the sonogram clearer.

*Results*—A normal spleen shows up uniformly light, with indentations from the surrounding organs—the stomach, the pancreas, and the left kidney. The point at which the blood vessels enter and leave the spleen is normally dark. If the spleen has been ruptured, there may be a dark area which represents free fluid. Abscesses usually appear as irregular hollow structures with thickened walls. Cysts usually appear as round hollow structures with thin walls. In some conditions (e.g., mononucleosis, endocarditis, parasitic infections) the spleen may be enlarged.

## Pancreas

This is the gland located in the upper abdomen that secretes digestive enzymes into the intestine and insulin into the bloodstream. Pancreatic ultrasound is used to evaluate suspected pancreatic disease, to investigate unexplained pain or masses in the upper abdomen, to evaluate the effects of upper abdominal injury.

You will be asked to eat a fat-free meal on the evening before the test and then to fast for 8–12 hours. An empty bowel and a gallbladder filled with bile help make the sonogram clearer.

*Results*—An enlarged pancreas with a distinct border may indicate pancreatitis. A mass with smooth edges may indicate a pseudocyst. A poorly defined mass near the head of the pancreas may indicate cancer. Test results may also suggest abscesses or inflammation of the pancreas.

## Kidneys

The kidneys are the pair of bean-shaped organs located in the back of the abdominal cavity. The kidneys remove wastes from the blood and produce urine.

This test is used to determine the cause of blocked urine flow, to evaluate abnor-malities found in an IVP (see p. 269), and to follow the progress of transplanted kidneys.

You will be asked to lie on your back for most of the test.

*Results*—Normal kidneys will appear as sharply outlined bean-shaped organs. The collecting system (the network of tubes through which the urine flows) will appear as a dark area near the center of each kidney. A circular structure with a smooth, regular border may indicate a cyst. A displaced kidney or a fluid-filled structure with an irregular border may indicate an abscess.

# Thyroid Ultrasound

The thyroid is a butterfly-shaped gland located in the front of the neck, with the two "wings" on either side of the Adam's apple. The thyroid secretes hormones which regulate the rate of many metabolic processes in the body's cells.

In this test a small instrument (transducer) which emits high-frequency sound will be passed back and forth over your neck. A microphone on the transducer will pick up the sound waves as they are reflected from your thyroid. This information will be processed by a computer, and an image of the inside of the thyroid and adjacent structures will be displayed on a TV screen.

### Why Performed:

This test is used to evaluate lumps (nodules) in the thyroid and to monitor the size of the thyroid during therapy. Many doctors now use thin needle biopsy of the thyroid (see p. 359) in place of ultrasound, since it frequently provides more exact information.

This test is easier to perform and less expensive than a thyroid scan (p. 299). In addition, since it does not expose you to radiation, it is safer. For these reasons it is sometimes preferred to the scan for certain abnormalities, especially in pregnant women.

### Preparation:

You should remove any jewelry from your head and neck. You will be asked to remove all clothing above the waist and to put on a hospital gown.

### Procedure:

This test is done in an ultrasound room in a hospital or doctor's office by a radiologist and an ultrasound technician. You will be asked to lie on your back on a high table with your neck extended and a pillow beneath your shoulders. An ultrasound technician will apply a gel or oil to your neck and will pass an ultrasound transducer lightly over the skin of your neck. In some facilities, a small water-filled bag may be placed over your throat to help conduct the sound waves. If so, the transducer is applied to the bag during part of the scan.

Reflected sound waves will be converted to an image which will be displayed on a TV screen. A photograph of the scan will be taken to provide a permanent record.

This procedure usually takes 15–30 minutes.

### How Does It Feel?

You will feel no discomfort, only a light pressure on your neck. Maintaining the neck-extended position for 15 minutes or more may be slightly uncomfortable.

### Risks:

There is no known risk of this test.

### Results:

This test may reveal an enlarged thyroid (goiter), cyst, or tumor of the thyroid gland. Cysts normally appear as smooth-bordered masses with echo-free centers. Tumors usually appear solid, and may be either sharply outlined or irregular.

If the thyroid lump is larger than one centimeter (about half an inch), this test can usually distinguish a hard tumor from a fluid-filled lump (cyst). It cannot distinguish a benign tumor from a cancerous one. If a tumor is detected, a biopsy (p. 359) will probably be needed to determine whether it is malignant.

### Cost:

This test usually costs $100 to $200

### Special Considerations:

★The parathyroid glands lie within the thyroid, so abnormalities of the parathyroid glands can sometimes be detected by this test. Normal parathyroids usually cannot be distinguished from normal thyroid tissue.

# Pelvic Ultrasound

In this test a small instrument (transducer) which emits high-frequency sound waves will be passed back and forth across your abdomen a number of times. A microphone on the instrument will pick up the sound waves reflected from the organs within your pelvis: the bladder, ovaries, uterus, fallopian tubes, and prostate. This information will be processed by a computer and an image of your pelvic organs will be displayed on a TV screen.

## When Performed:

*Ovaries and Uterus*—These organs are frequently examined to help evaluate persistent painful cramps and other pain in the pelvic area, unexplained vaginal bleeding, or lack of menstrual flow. This test is also used to examine pelvic masses and to locate lost intrauterine devices (IUDs).

*Bladder*—This test may be used to help determine the cause of unexplained blood in the urine or difficulty in urinating or to look for bladder stones.

*Other Organs*—This test is occasionally used to investigate problems of the prostate and fallopian tubes.

## Preparation:

Tell your doctor if
You are taking any medications
You might be pregnant
You have an intrauterine device (IUD)
You have had difficulty in urinating
You have had a barium enema or upper
GI series within the past two days
or a proctoscopy or sigmoidoscopy
within the past day. Barium or air
in the colon can interfere with this
test.

As a full bladder is usually required, you will be asked to drink several glasses of water (about 32 ounces) about an hour before the test. You will be asked not to urinate until the test is finished. A full bladder pushes the bowel up out of the pelvic area, makes it easier to identify the surrounding structures, and ensures better transmission of the sound waves. If you are unable to drink the required fluids, your bladder may be filled through a thin tube (catheter) inserted through your urethra (the passage by which urine leaves your body).

You will be asked to undress and to put on a hospital gown.

## Procedure:

This test is performed by a specially trained physician (radiologist or obstetrician) or an ultrasound technician. It is done in an ultrasound room in a hospital or doctor's office.

You will be asked to lie on your back on a padded examining table. The technician will apply a gel or oil to your abdomen. This improves transmission of the sound waves.

The examiner will move the transducer up and down your abdomen a number of times and then repeat the process in a back-and-forth direction. Scans at other angles may also be done.

The reflected sound waves will be converted to an image on a TV screen. Photos of the TV image will be taken to create a permanent record.

After the test the gel will be wiped off and you will be able to return home (or to your hospital room). The test usually takes 20 minutes, but may take longer if additional scans are needed. You can urinate as soon as the test is finished.

## How Does It Feel?

The gel may feel cold and slippery. You will feel only a light pressure as the instrument passes over your skin.

## Risks:

There are no known risks of ultrasound.

## Results:

*Ovaries and Uterus*—Normal ovaries are small and may not be seen. The results of this test may suggest the presence of infection, bleeding, cyst, or tumor. It may also suggest enlargement or congenital abnormality of the ovaries or uterus. The proper position of an IUD in the uterus can also be checked.

*Bladder*—This test can often identify tumors, stones, or thickening of the bladder wall.

This test cannot distinguish between benign and malignant tumors.

### Cost:
$120 to $200

# Doppler Ultrasound

This procedure is used to evaluate blood flow through the major arteries and veins of the arms, legs, and neck. A hand-held ultrasound instrument called a transducer is passed lightly over the skin overlying the blood vessel to be examined. The transducer sends out and receives high-frequency sound waves. If blood is flowing through the vessel, the reflected sound waves create a swooshing sound on the speaker used to monitor the procedure. If blood flow is rapid, the sound is high-pitched. Low blood flow produces a low-pitched sound. If there is no blood flow, no sound is heard.

### Why Performed:
This test is used to detect blockages, narrowings, and clots within the arteries and veins. It may be performed to look for narrowing (stenosis) of the carotid arteries in the neck, which supply blood to the brain. Blockage of these arteries can cause symptoms such as dizziness, loss of vision, paralysis, weakness, or numbness. It is also sometimes done to evaluate leg pain and swelling when blood clots in the deep veins of the leg (thrombophlebitis) are suspected.

This test was developed as a noninvasive alternative to arteriography (p. 234) and venography (p. 283). It is quicker, safer, less painful, and less expensive than these procedures, but not always as accurate in identifying minor blockages to blood flow.

### Preparation:
No restriction of food or drink is necessary; however, you will be asked not to smoke for 30 minutes before the test because nicotine can constrict the arteries.

If your legs are to be examined, you will be asked to remove all clothing below the waist. If your arms or neck is to be examined, you will be asked to remove all clothing above the waist and to put on a hospital gown.

### Procedure:
This procedure is performed by a specially trained physician or an ultrasound technician. It can be done at bedside for hospitalized patients or in a vascular studies laboratory or doctor's office.

You will be asked to lie on your back. A blood pressure cuff may be wrapped around one or both legs or arms so that blood pressures can be taken at several different places. The places chosen will vary with the vessels to be examined.

A conductive gel will be placed over the vessel or vessels to be studied to improve the transmission of sound waves. The transducer will then be passed back and forth along the skin overlying the target vessels in your legs, arms, or neck. You will need to lie very still during the procedure.

The test may be repeated while the examiner presses on blood vessels close to the surface to block blood flow and/or with your legs or arms in different positions, to be sure that the blood supply is not blocked in these positions.

You will be able to listen to the amplified sound waves which reflect the flow of blood in the vessels being studied.

This test usually takes 15–20 minutes.

### How Does It Feel?

There is no discomfort associated with this test. You may feel some pressure when the blood pressure cuffs are inflated.

### Risks:

There is no known risk from this procedure.

### Results:

Doppler ultrasound is about 95% accurate in detecting massive blockages of blood flow (those in which blood flow is reduced by at least half). It may not detect smaller obstructions.

Normal, uniform readings on both sides indicate open vessels with normal blood flow. Drops in blood flow, differences on the right and left sides, or irregular variations in flow may indicate a partially or totally blocked vessel.

Doppler ultrasound may demonstrate blockage of blood flow in the carotid arteries of the neck (which may cause strokes) or blood clots in leg veins (thrombophlebitis), which may break off and lodge in the lungs (pulmonary embolism).

### Cost:

$140 to $160

# 9 Scoping Procedures: Looking Inside Your Body

**U**ntil recently, if your doctor wanted to look inside your stomach, intestines, lungs, bladder, or knee to diagnose a disease, it usually required surgery. A large incision had to be made to create access to the organ or body space in question. These exploratory operations were often risky and expensive, and recovery was often slow.

Today, many such operations can be avoided through the use of a variety of viewing instruments. These devices vary from rather simple magnifying lenses (ophthalmoscopes for looking into eyes) to lighted telescopes (laparoscopes for the abdominal cavity) to complex fiberoptic viewing systems (colonoscopes for viewing the interior of the large bowel).

The latter fiberoptic instruments can now be used to examine your upper and lower gastrointestinal tract (upper GI endoscopy, sigmoidoscopy, and colonoscopy) and your airways (bronchoscopy). These fiberoptic devices are thin flexible tubes containing bundles of glass filaments which can transmit light from a powerful source around bends and curves to illuminate the inside of the body. The internal images are transmitted back to the examiner's eye. The result is an unparalleled view of the inside of your body without the risk of more invasive procedures. Photographs, even video pictures, can also be taken through some viewing instruments to offer a more permanent record of the inside view.

Some scoping devices offer more than just a look inside. Tiny instruments such as forceps, snares, and scissors can be threaded through channels in the scope to allow surgical procedures to be performed: tissue samples can be collected (biopsy); polyps, foreign bodies, or torn cartilage removed; bladder stones crushed.

In the following section the major scoping procedures (endoscopies or "oscopies") are described. The description of colposcopy is found in the section Tests for Women (p. 183) and otoscopic exams are found under Home Ear Exam in the Home Medical Tests section (p. 409).

# Arthroscopy

In arthroscopy the interior of a joint is viewed directly with a specially lighted, pencil-thin tube (arthroscope) inserted through a small incision in the skin. This often permits diagnosis of problems not revealed by physical examination or other diagnostic tests such as x-rays.

In addition to being used in diagnosis, arthroscopy can also be used for certain types of surgical treatment. Torn cartilage can sometimes be removed, and the joint surfaces can be shaved and smoothed through a tiny hole instead of a large surgical incision. Arthroscopy is less painful, less costly and allows much quicker recovery than more extensive surgical procedures. Arthroscopy is usually done on an outpatient basis, allowing you to come and go home within hours of the procedure.

Arthroscopy is most commonly performed on the knee but is sometimes used on shoulders, ankles, elbows, wrists, hips, and even fingers.

## Why Performed:
Most joint pains and injuries get better on their own. The remainder can often be diagnosed by your doctor on the basis of a careful history, physical examination, and perhaps x-rays. However, if you have persistent unexplained joint pain, swelling, instability, or limited motion, either arthroscopy or a special contrast x-ray (see arthrogram p. 243) may be useful. Arthroscopy is also frequently performed immediately before open knee surgery (arthrotomy) to confirm the diagnosis and plan the appropriate surgical approach.

## Preparation:
Tell your doctor if
> You have allergies to any medications or anesthetics
> You are taking any medications
> You have had any bleeding problems
> You might be pregnant

You will be asked to sign a consent form. Use this opportunity to discuss with your doctor any concerns you have about the need for the test, the procedure, or the risks.

Arthroscopy can be done by putting you asleep under general anesthesia, using a spinal anesthetic, or numbing the joint area with a local anesthetic injection (see p. 465). You should discuss with your doctor which is the best method for you.

If a general or spinal anesthetic is planned, you should not eat or drink anything for 8–12 hours before the test. You will need someone to drive you home after the test. Bring along clothing roomy enough to accommodate a bulky bandage around the joint being examined. Remove all jewelry and, for your comfort, empty your bladder before the exam begins. You will be given a hospital gown to put on.

## Procedure:
The most common type of arthroscopy is performed on the knee. It is done by a specially trained orthopedic surgeon in the operating room or a special procedure room. The doctor and several assistants will wear

sterile gowns, masks, and gloves during the procedure.

You may be given a sedative medication shortly before the procedure to help you relax. You will lie on your back on a table with your leg supported and, sometimes, with a tourniquet wrapped tightly around your upper thigh. The area around your knee is shaved, scrubbed with an antiseptic solution, and draped with sterile towels.

If a general anesthetic is used, you will be put to sleep with a medication given through an IV in your arm or inhaled gases or both. If a local anesthetic is used, it will be injected into the skin and joint space.

After the anesthetic takes effect a small incision (less than one-half inch) will be made at one or more sites around your knee. A long pointed instrument called a trocar is then placed into one of the small incision sites to make way for the arthroscope, which is then inserted into the joint space. A saline (salt) solution is pumped

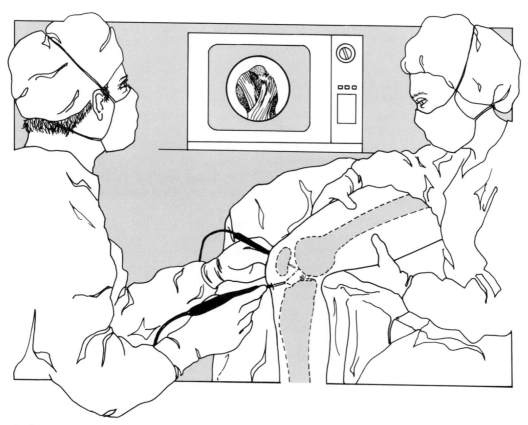

**Arthroscopy.** *The arthroscope is inserted into the joint, and the interior of the joint can be viewed on a television screen.*

into the joint through the arthroscope to expand the knee capsule and permit clear vision inside the joint.

The physician will then view the interior structures of your knee through the eyepiece of the arthroscope or on a TV monitor connected to the arthroscope. You may even be able to get a glimpse of the inside of your own knee on this screen. Assistants will bend, extend, and reposition your knee so that the doctor can view different areas inside the joint. Sometimes other instruments such as forceps and probes are inserted into the joint. The arthroscope may be reinserted through other small skin incisions for better viewing.

After the examination has been completed, the arthroscope will be removed (unless corrective surgery using the arthroscope is planned at that time). The joint is washed out with saline solution, the incisions are closed with stitches or tape, and the knee is bandaged. This diagnostic test usually takes about 30 minutes, but may last longer if treatment is also performed through the scope.

If a general anesthetic is used, you will awaken slowly in the recovery room. When fully awake, usually within a few hours, you will be allowed to go home.

You should be able to walk immediately after the procedure, although you may be asked to use crutches for a day or two and to keep your leg elevated as much as possible. Do not get the wound or bandages wet for a week, as advised. Ask your doctor for advice on knee strengthening exercises and when you can begin vigorous activity.

### How Does It Feel?

If a general anesthetic is used, you won't feel anything during the procedure. If a local anesthetic is used, you will feel a burning or stinging sensation as the anesthetic is injected. You may feel a brief, sharp pain

as the trocar is inserted to make way for the arthroscope. There may be some mild to severe discomfort when your leg is manipulated and repositioned during the examination. After the test it is normal to feel some mild soreness and a slight grinding sensation in your knee for a day or two. Notify your doctor if the pain is severe or persistent, if you cannot bend your knee, or if you develop a fever.

*Patient comments:*

"I was able to walk immediately after the arthroscopy and was back to my normal activities within a few days."

"I was able to see inside my own knee on the TV screen. I didn't really understand everything I was seeing but it was exciting."

### Risks:

Arthroscopy is generally quite safe when performed by a skilled, experienced physician. If a general anesthetic is used, the average risk of death from the anesthetic is less than 1 in 3000. Fewer than 1 in 1000 patients develop complications such as serious joint infections, bleeding into the joint, or blood clots in the leg. Very rarely, injury to one of the nerves surrounding the joint can lead to an area of persistent numbness or pain. The specific risks in your case should be discussed with your physician.

### Results:

Usually your doctor will be able to discuss the results with you right after the test. The condition of the ligaments and surface cartilage can be reviewed. A torn ligament or meniscus (the crescent-shaped cartilage overlying the bones) may be seen. Roughened or eroded cartilage covering the leg bones and patella (kneecap) or loose fragments of cartilage known as loose bodies may be identified. Depending on the damage seen, medication, physical therapy, or surgery may be recommended.

**Cost:**
Diagnostic arthroscopy: $400 to $1000
Operative or surgical arthroscopy:
    $1500 to $2500

# Bronchoscopy

In bronchoscopy the interior of your major air passages is viewed directly through a lighted viewing instrument (bronchoscope) inserted through your mouth or nose. This procedure is usually performed to gather specimens for laboratory analysis, to diagnose tumors or other lung diseases, as well as to remove blockages from the airways. Bronchoscopy can often make more extensive exploratory surgery unnecessary.

One of two types of viewing instruments can be used: the *rigid* bronchoscope, which is a straight hollow metal tube, or the *flexible* bronchoscope, which is a long thin tube containing a fiberoptic lighting system that can transmit images around bends.

The type of bronchoscope used depends largely on the reason for the test. The flexible bronchoscope is generally safer, more comfortable for the patient, and offers a better view of the smaller airways. However, the rigid bronchoscope may make it easier to remove tissue samples (biopsy). The rigid bronchoscope is also used to clear the air passages of thick mucous plugs or foreign bodies, such as when a child inhales a coin, button, or food. The rigid broncho-

scope is also useful when there is considerable bleeding in the airways which could obscure the view with the flexible scope.

**Why Performed:**
Bronchoscopy is used both for diagnosis and treatment. It is helpful in locating the cause of symptoms such as coughing up blood-tinged sputum (hemoptysis), localized wheezing in the chest, or difficult breathing due to compression of the upper airway (stridor). It is also used to further evaluate abnormalities found on chest x-rays such as nodules, lesions, masses, collapsed airways (atelectasis), paralysis of the diaphragm, or poorly resolving pneumonias. Bronchoscopy is often performed to search for lung cancer if suspicious lesions are seen on chest x-rays or if cancerous cells are found in the sputum or elsewhere in the body. Bronchoscopy can also be useful in discovering the location and extent of a lung cancer in order to determine whether surgery would be the best treatment.

Bronchoscopy may be used to clear the airways of obstructing foreign bodies or secretions.

**Preparation:**
Tell your doctor if
    You have allergies to any medications
        or anesthetics
    You are taking any medications
    You have had bleeding problems
    You have any loose teeth
    You might be pregnant

You will be asked to sign a consent form. Use this opportunity to discuss with your doctor any concerns you have about the need for the test, how it is performed, or the risks. Bronchoscopy can be performed with a rigid or flexible scope, under local or general anesthesia. We suggest that you discuss with your doctor which is the best method for you.

You will be asked not to eat or drink for at least 6–8 hours before the test. An empty stomach helps prevent vomiting during the procedure and reduces the risk of choking or a pneumonia developing from the accidental inhalation of vomited material. Smokers are strongly advised to abstain from smoking for a minimum of 24 hours before and after the test to help reduce the risks of complications. If the test is scheduled as an outpatient, bring someone to drive you home after the test.

Before the test remove dentures, eye-glasses, and all jewelry, and for your comfort empty your bladder. You will be given a hospital gown to put on.

## Procedure:

Bronchoscopy is usually done in a procedure room, in an operating room, or at your bedside. The test is performed by a specially trained physician or surgeon and several assistants.

Several blood tests are usually ordered before the procedure is done. You may be given medications by injection about an hour before the test to relax you and dry up the secretions in your mouth and air-

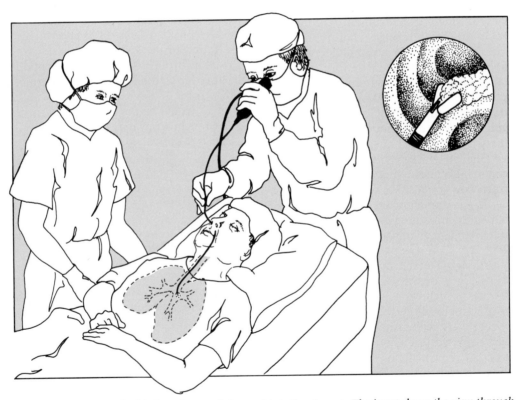

**Bronchoscopy.** *The flexible bronchoscope is inserted into the airways. The insert shows the view through the scope as a biopsy forceps collects a tissue specimen from an abnormal growth.*

ways. An intravenous (IV) line may also be placed in a vein, usually in your arm.

*Flexible Bronchoscopy:* This procedure is most often performed with local, rather than general anesthetic. Before insertion of the flexible bronchoscope, an anesthetic solution is sprayed into the back of your throat and the vocal cord area. This is to numb your throat and to inhibit your gag reflex, which might cause you to gag or vomit during the passage of the instrument. If the bronchoscope is to be inserted through your nose, an anesthetic ointment may be swabbed onto your nasal passages. Sometimes the anesthetic for the vocal cord area is injected directly into the windpipe through a needle inserted through the skin just above the Adam's apple. The local anesthetic takes a few minutes to begin to work.

Flexible bronchoscopy is usually performed while you lie on your back on a table with your shoulders and neck supported by a pillow, though it is sometimes done in a sitting position. The physician gently inserts the thin bronchoscope through your mouth (or nose) and advances it slowly to the area of your vocal cords. Some additional anesthetic is applied through the bronchoscope to the vocal cords. You may be asked to make a high-pitched vocal sound or pant like a dog to help ease the scope past your vocal cords. The bronchoscope is then moved down your major airways to investigate the lower air passages. The lights in the room may be dimmed to allow the physician to see the light of the bronchoscope more clearly. A large x-ray machine (fluoroscope) may be positioned above you to transmit pictures to a TV monitor. The image on the monitor helps the doctor to move the bronchoscope into different sections of the lung.

A tiny biopsy forceps or a brush may be inserted through the scope to collect small bits of tissue from suspicious areas for laboratory analysis. A saline solution may be washed into some of the airways where the scope can't reach. These washings are sent to the lab to be examined for cancer cells or bacteria.

*Rigid Bronchoscopy:* This test is often performed under general anesthesia (see p. 465). You will lie on your back on a table and be put to sleep with an injection through an IV in your arm or an inhaled gas or both. Sometimes a muscle relaxant is also given.

Once you are asleep, your head is carefully positioned with your neck extended, and the hollow bronchoscope is gently inserted through your mouth and into your windpipe. A guard may be placed over your teeth to protect them. Your head will be repositioned periodically as the bronchoscope is moved to examine different areas. Tiny forceps or a brush may be inserted through the bronchoscope to gather small biopsy specimens.

Bronchoscopy by either procedure usually takes between 30 to 60 minutes. You will be frequently checked by a nurse for several hours after the test. A chest x-ray may be taken sometime after the procedure to look for signs of complications or improvement. After the procedure you should not eat or drink anything until the numbness in your throat wears off (usually about 2 hours) and your gag reflex recovers.

### How Does It Feel?

If you are given a sedative, you may feel very drowsy during and shortly after the procedure. If you have a general anesthetic you will feel nothing during the procedure, but afterward you may feel general tiredness and muscle aching for a day or so.

If a local anesthetic is used, the anesthetic may taste slightly medicinal and cause you to gag and cough when it is first sprayed into your throat. After a few minutes you may notice a feeling that your tongue and throat are swollen and that you can't swallow (you actually can). Your mouth may also feel very dry for several hours due to the medication given before the procedure.

The most uncomfortable sensation associated with bronchoscopy is usually the fear that you might not be able to breathe. Remember that the bronchoscope will not block your breathing even though it may feel as though it will. Try taking slow, deep breaths through your nose with your mouth open. You may feel an unpleasant sensation of pressure in different areas of your chest as the bronchoscope is moved from place to place. If the procedure becomes very uncomfortable, let your physician or one of the assistants know. You will have to use hand signals, since you will not be able to talk with the instrument in place. Try not to cough during the examination unless asked to do so.

Following the procedure you can expect to have some hoarseness or voice loss for several days. You will also have a sore throat which may be helped by throat lozenges and/or warm salt-water gargles. You may notice some blood-tinged sputum for a few days, especially if a biopsy is done. If the bleeding is heavy and persistent or if you experience increased difficulty in breathing, chest pain, or fever after the bronchoscopy, notify your physician immediately.

*Patient Comments:*

"I admit it. I was scared of the test. I was worried that my airway was going to be blocked off, but actually I was able to breathe quite well. I just kept thinking 're-lax,' 'breathe,' and it was over before I knew it."

## Risks:

Bronchoscopy is generally a safe procedure. The risk of a major complication such as profuse bleeding, respiratory arrest, serious heart rhythm abnormality, and death is less than 1 in 1000 with bronchoscopy alone and 2 in 1000 with transbronchial opsy. When a biopsy is performed, collapse of a small portion of the lung (pneumothorax) due to puncture of the airway occurs in about 3 in 100 cases. A pneumothorax usually heals on its own but may require the help of a small tube placed through the chest wall. Infections such as pneumonia occur about 5% of the time but usually can be cured with antibiotic treatment. There is some risk of damage to or loss of teeth, mainly if you have loose teeth or the rigid scope is used. Very rarely the bronchoscope may cause damage to the airways or vocal cords. If the test is performed under general anesthesia, the average risk of death from the anesthetic itself is less than 1 in 3000. The risks of bronchoscopy vary from patient to patient, so you should discuss your specific risks with your doctor.

## Results:

Your physician may be able to discuss the preliminary results with you after the test, though biopsy results may take several days, and tests for infection may take as long as several weeks. Your doctor will carefully examine your airways for evidence of infection or obstruction due to mucous plugs, foreign bodies, or tumors. Cancers located in very small airways cannot be directly seen, but suspicious growths or irregularities in the mucous membranes lining the larger airways can be sampled and sent to the laboratory to look for cancer and other lung diseases.

**Cost:**
$300 to $500 (more if a hospital stay is included)

# Colonoscopy

Colonoscopy is a procedure in which a physician views the interior lining of the large intestine (colon) through a long, flexible instrument called a colonoscope. This instrument is a tube, about half an inch thick, composed of fine filaments of fiberglass which can transmit light around curves from the tip of the instrument to the viewing lens at the other end. The colonoscope is inserted through the anus and then gently advanced through the colon. Colonoscopy permits visual examination of the entire colon, while sigmoidoscopy (p. 335) permits viewing of only the 10 to 12 inches closest to the anus.

Sources of bleeding can be identified, polyps can be removed through the colonoscope, and tissue samples (biopsies) can be taken of areas suspicious for colon cancer. In many instances colonoscopy allows accurate diagnosis and treatment without the need for a major abdominal operation.

**Why Performed:**
Colonoscopy is most often performed to evaluate unexplained blood in the stool, abdominal pain, persistent diarrhea, or abnormalities (such as polyps) found on contrast x-rays (see barium enema, p. 245). Colonoscopy is sometimes used to determine the type and extent of inflammatory bowel disease (ulcerative colitis and Crohn's disease). When a bowel cancer is known to exist, the rest of the colon can be checked through a colonoscope for other cancers.

Following surgery to remove a cancer or polyp, colonoscopy or a barium enema is often recommended on a yearly basis to check for recurrence. Colonoscopy is also used to screen patients who are at particularly high risk for colon cancer, such as patients with a long history of ulcerative colitis or a family history of colonic polyps and cancer.

**Preparation:**
Tell your doctor if
    You have allergies to any medications or anesthetics
    You are taking any medications
    You have had bleeding problems
    You have a history of disease of your heart valves
    You have had a recent barium x-ray examination
    You might be pregnant

Before the exam you will be asked to sign a consent form. Use this opportunity to discuss with your doctor any concerns you have about the need for the test, how it is performed, or the risks.

A clean colon is essential to an adequate examination, so before the exam considerable preparation is necessary to clear the colon of all stool. Usually it is recommended that for 2 or 3 days before the test you abstain from all solid foods and take in only clear liquids, such as juices, broths, and Jell-O. This low-residue diet reduces the amount of stool in your colon. During this preparatory diet, drink plenty of liquids to avoid dehydration, and continue taking any regularly prescribed medications unless otherwise instructed.

You will be asked to take a strong laxative, such as castor oil, magnesium citrate, and/or bisacodyl (Dulcolax), the evening before the test. You may be instructed to take several 1-quart enemas of warm tap

319

water on the morning of the exam. Lie on your left side while letting the first half of the enema drain in. Then roll onto your back and empty the remainder. Finally, roll onto your right side for a few minutes before going to the toilet to expel the enema as completely as possible. Repeat the procedure until the return from the enema is clear of stool particles. The morning of the exam you should not eat or drink anything.

These preparatory procedures are extremely important. Since each physician may modify the cleansing procedure, check with your doctor for specific instructions. If your colon is not thoroughly clean, the exam cannot be done or may need to be repeated. If you are not staying in the hospital, you should arrange for someone to drive you home after the test.

You will be asked to put on a hospital gown. You may wish to leave your socks on to stay warm. During the exam you will be covered with a drape, but if you are cold, ask for a blanket. For your comfort, empty your bladder just before the exam.

**Procedure:**

Colonoscopy is usually done in an x-ray department or special procedure room of a hospital or doctor's office on an outpatient basis. The test is performed by a specially trained physician with an assistant.

An intravenous (IV) line will be started in a vein, usually in your arm. During the procedure you will be given a pain reliever (usually Demerol) and a sedative (usually Valium) through the IV. You should feel relaxed and drowsy, but alert enough to cooperate.

You will be asked to lie on your left side with your knees drawn up toward your abdomen. First, your doctor will insert a gloved, lubricated finger into your anus to check for tenderness or obstructions. Next the doctor will insert the thin, well-lubri-

cated colonoscope and gently advance it while examining the intestinal lining through the scope. At times some air will be instilled through the colonoscope to help clear a path. Suction through the instrument may also be used to help remove excessive secretions, stool, or blood. The doctor may press on your abdomen or ask you to change positions to help advance the scope through the twists and turns of your colon. The doctor may also view your abdomen on an x-ray screen (fluoroscope) to occasionally check the position of the colonoscope.

Your doctor will attempt to examine the entire length of your large intestine. If suspicious growths are observed, tissue samples will be taken with tiny biopsy forceps or brushes inserted through the colonoscope. Small polyps (growths on the intestinal lining) can also be removed through the colonoscope. The colonoscope is then slowly withdrawn and the instilled air allowed to escape. Your anal area will then be cleaned with tissues.

The procedure may take from 30 minutes to 2 hours or more, depending upon how easy it is to advance the colonoscope. After the procedure you will be observed for several hours until the medications wear off. When you are fully recovered someone may drive you home, and you may resume your usual diet and activities unless otherwise advised. Drink lots of liquids after the exam to replace the fluids you may have lost due to the laxatives and fasting.

**How Does It Feel?**

Colonoscopy can be a long, tiring, and uncomfortable procedure. The bowel cleaning preparation, especially the strong laxative taken the night before, can produce diarrhea and cramping, which may keep you visiting the bathroom for the better part of the night. For this reason you may prefer

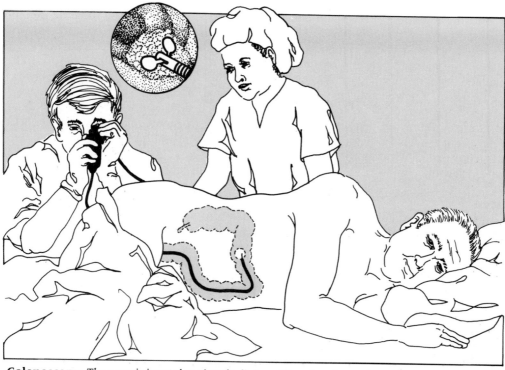

**Colonoscopy.** *The scope is inserted to view the lining of the colon. Insert shows the view through the scope as a biopsy forceps collects a tissue specimen from an abnormal growth.*

to take the laxative the afternoon before the day of the exam.

During the exam you may feel very drowsy and relaxed from the sedative and pain medications. When the lubricant and colonoscope are first inserted they may feel slightly cool. At times you may feel pressure from the colonoscope moving inside. As it is advanced or air is instilled, you may feel some brief cramping gas pains and the urge to have a bowel movement and expel gas. Taking slow, deep breaths in and out through your mouth will help relax your abdominal muscles and lessen any discomfort. However, if you are experiencing pain,

signal your doctor. More pain medication or sedative may be administered.

You will probably feel and hear some of the instilled air escape around the scope. Don't try to control it and don't be embarrassed. The passing of air is expected and necessary.

The suction machine used to remove stool and secretions is noisy but painless. The removal of biopsy specimens and polyps is also painless, since the lining of your intestine does not contain pain nerves.

You will feel groggy after the procedure until the medication wears off—this usually takes a few hours. Many patients report that they remember very little of the exam. This is an aftereffect of the medications.

After the exam you may notice some mild abdominal cramping and pass a considerable amount of air. If a biopsy was performed or a polyp removed, you may see small amounts of blood in your stool for a few days. However, if you notice heavy or persistent rectal bleeding, severe abdominal pain, or a fever, report this to your doctor immediately.

### Risks:

Complications from colonoscopy are rare. A perforation in the intestinal wall from the colonoscope or biopsy occurs in fewer than 2 in 1000 tests. If a perforation does occur, an operation to repair the hole is usually necessary. Heavy bleeding from biopsy or polypectomy sites occurs infrequently (1 in 1000), and seldom requires transfusions or surgery to stop the bleeding. An adverse reaction to the sedative medication is very rare (4 in 10,000) but may cause respiratory arrest and shock. Rarely does an infection result from colonoscopy and require antibiotic therapy. Patients with artificial or abnormal heart valves are usually given antibiotics before and after the procedure to prevent an infection. Since risks vary from patient to patient, you should discuss with your doctor the specific risks of the procedure for you.

### Results:

Your doctor will examine the lining of your colon and will be able to discuss some of the findings with you immediately after the procedure. Suspicious masses or lesions will be biopsied and sent to the laboratory. It may take several days to find out whether a cancer is present. If detected early, most colon cancers can be treated successfully. Polyps are not usually cancerous and can

often be treated by removal through the colonoscope. Sources of bleeding from polyps, tumors, ulcers, or hemorrhoids may be identified. The presence, extent, and type of inflammatory bowel disease (ulcerative colitis or Crohn's disease) may be determined. A common finding, particularly in older people, is diverticulosis, a condition in which many small, fingerlike pouches protrude from the colon wall.

### Cost:

$300 to $700 (more if a hospital stay is included)

# Cystoscopy
## (Cystourethroscopy)

In cystoscopy the interior lining of the bladder and urethra (the tube that conducts urine from the bladder) is visually examined. This examination is done with a cystoscope, a pencil-thin, lighted tube with telescopic lenses which is inserted into the urethra and advanced into the bladder (see illustration, p. 261).

In addition to viewing the urethra, bladder, and, in men, the prostate, small bladder stones or lesions can be removed through the cystoscope and specimens of tissues and urine collected. Thin, flexible tubes called catheters can also be inserted through the cystoscope in order to perform special x-ray studies. Cystoscopy can often eliminate the need for more extensive surgery.

### Why Performed:

Cystoscopy is frequently used to diagnose problems in the urinary system. It is most often done to evaluate unexplained blood in the urine (hematuria), persistent painful urination (dysuria), difficulty in urinating (hesitancy), urgency and frequency of urination. Cystoscopy may also be helpful in identifying the cause of frequent and recurrent urinary tract infections. It is also used to further investigate abnormalities found on x-ray studies of the kidney and ureters (see IVP, p. 269) or to identify problems which cannot be seen on x-rays.

**Preparation:**

Tell your doctor if

> You have allergies to any medications or anesthetics
>
> You are taking any medications
>
> You have had bleeding problems
>
> You might be pregnant

You will be asked to sign a consent form before the procedure. Use this opportunity to discuss with your doctor any concerns you have about the need for the test, how it is performed or the risks.

Cystoscopy can be performed with a local anesthetic (numbing medicine), spinal anesthetic, or general anesthetic (see p. 465). Discuss with your doctor which method is best for you and whether you should plan on staying overnight in the hospital. If hospitalization is not required, you may need to bring someone to drive you home after the test.

If a local anesthetic is used, there is no need to restrict food or fluids. In fact, you should drink plenty of liquids before the test to ensure a good flow of urine. However, if a general anesthetic is to be given, you should not eat or drink for at least 8 hours before the test unless otherwise advised.

You may or may not be asked to empty your bladder just before the procedure. You may also be given some antibiotic tablets to take before and for several days after the test to prevent infection due to the insertion of the instruments. Just before the test you will be given a hospital gown to put on.

**Procedure:**

Cystoscopy is performed by a specially trained physican (urologist) with one or more assistants. The procedure is done in a procedure room, office, x-ray department, or operating room. You may be given a sedative medication about an hour before the test to help you relax. An intravenous (IV) line may be placed in a vein in your arm to give you medications and fluids.

You will lie on your back on a special table with your knees bent, legs apart, and your feet or thighs supported by stirrups. Your genital area will be cleansed with an antiseptic solution, and your abdomen and thighs will be covered with sterile drapes. If a general anesthetic is used, you will be put to sleep with a medication given through an IV or inhaled gases or both. If a local anesthetic is used, the anesthetic solution or jelly will be gently instilled into your urethra. After waiting a few minutes for the anesthetic to numb your urethra, the thin, well-lubricated cystoscope will be gently inserted into the urethra and slowly advanced into your bladder. If the urethra is too narrow to allow the scope to pass, other smaller instruments may first be inserted to gradually enlarge the passageway.

Once the scope is inside the bladder, a sterile saline solution will be instilled through the cystoscope to help expand your bladder and create a clear view. Tiny instruments such as forceps, scissors, and tubes may be inserted through the scope to collect urine specimens and small tissue samples (biopsy specimens), which are sent to the laboratory. After a thorough inspection of your urethra and bladder lining, the cystoscope is removed. The instrument is usually in your bladder for only 5–10 minutes, but the entire procedure may take from 15 to 45 minutes or longer if x-ray contrast studies are also performed (see later). Sometimes a tube (catheter) is left in the bladder to help drain the urine until the swelling in the urethra has decreased.

If a local anesthetic is used, you will be asked to lie or sit down and rest for 15–30 minutes after the test. If general anesthesia is used, you will be taken to the recovery room until you are awake and able to walk (usually a few hours). You will be allowed to eat and drink as soon as you are fully awake and your gag reflex has recovered from the anesthetic.

## How Does It Feel?

Most patients report after the procedure that it was not nearly as uncomfortable as they had feared.

If a general anesthetic is used, you will feel nothing during the procedure but may notice some tiredness and aching of your muscles throughout your body after the anesthetic wears off. If a local anesthetic is used, you may feel a brief burning sensation or urge to urinate as the instrument is inserted and removed. Also, when the sterile solution is added to your bladder you may feel a cool sensation, an uncomfortable fullness, and an urgent need to urinate. Try to relax during the procedure by taking slow deep breaths. If the procedure is a lengthy one, lying on the table can become tiring and uncomfortable.

After the procedure it is common to experience frequent urination with some burning during and after urination for several days. Drink lots of fluids to help minimize the burning and prevent infection. It's also common to notice a pinkish tinge to your urine for several days after cystoscopy, particularly when a biopsy was performed. However, if you notice reddish urine with blood clots that persists for several voidings, or if you are unable to pass urine within 8 hours of the procedure, notify your doctor immediately. Also, if you develop a high fever, chills, severe flank or abdominal pain after the procedure, let your doctor know right away.

*Patient Comments:*

"I was somewhat anxious about the exam. Aside from a slight feeling of pressure as the instrument was moved in and out, there wasn't actually any pain. And it was over pretty quickly."

## Risks:

Cystoscopy is generally a very safe procedure. If a general anesthetic is used, the risk of death from the anesthetic is less than 1 in 3000. There is no risk of loss of sexual function with the procedure. The most common complication is a temporary swelling of the urethra which makes it difficult to pass urine. It may be necessary to insert a tube (catheter) into your bladder temporarily to help drain the urine. Bleeding sometimes occurs, but usually stops on its own.

Cystoscopy is usually not performed when you have an acute infection of the urethra, bladder, or prostate gland. A mild infection may occur after cystoscopy but can usually be prevented or managed by the use of antibiotics before and after the procedure. Occasionally the infection can spread through the body, and in very rare circumstances (usually with seriously ill patients), the infection can be life-threatening. Another rare complication is damage or perforation of the urethra or bladder. If this occurs a surgical repair is sometimes necessary. The specific risks in your case should be discussed with your doctor.

## Results:

Your doctor may be able to discuss the preliminary results with you right after the cystoscopy, although the results from biopsies of suspicious areas usually take several days. A cystoscopic examination may reveal inflammation or narrowing of the urethra due to previous infections or an enlarged prostate. Bladder tumors (cancerous or benign), polyps, ulcers, stones (calculi), or inflammation of the bladder walls may also be observed. Sometimes abnormalities in the structure of the urinary tract that have been present from birth are seen.

## Cost:

Office cystoscopy with local anesthesia: $150 to $300

Operating-room cystoscopy with general anesthesia: $500 to $1000

## Special Considerations:

★*Retrograde Ureteropyelography:* This contrast x-ray study may be done during cystoscopy to outline the kidney and ureters. This test is performed when the more common test known as an IVP (Intravenous Pyelogram, p. 269) is inconclusive or cannot be performed due to poor kidney function or allergies to iodine contrast materials. Looking through the cystoscope into the bladder, the doctor threads a thin tube (catheter) through the cystoscope and into one or both of the ureters (see illustration, p. 261). A contrast material which shows up on x-rays is then injected through the catheter to fill and outline the ureter and kidney collecting system. Blockage of the flow of contrast material, dilation of the ureters, or displacement of the kidney may suggest the presence of kidney stones, tumors, abscesses (localized infections), blood clots, or strictures.

# Laparoscopy
## (Peritoneoscopy, Pelvic or Abdominal Endoscopy)

The laparoscope is a thin, lighted viewing instrument which is inserted through a small incision in the abdominal wall. Laparoscopy permits direct visual examination of the outer surface of the abdominal organs (intestines, liver, and spleen) and pelvic organs (uterus, fallopian tubes, and ovaries). In many cases, laparoscopy can eliminate the need for a more extensive surgical procedure (laparotomy) in which a larger incision is made in the abdomen. Laparoscopy is less risky, stressful, and costly than laparotomy and can often be performed on an outpatient basis, allowing you to return home the same day as the procedure.

## Why Performed:

Laparoscopy is often done when the diagnosis for abdominal or pelvic complaints is not clear after a thorough history, physical exam, ultrasound, and x-ray studies. It can help evaluate abdominal or pelvic masses or pain, abnormal menstrual periods, and female infertility. In cases of known cancer, laparoscopy is sometimes helpful in determining whether the cancer has spread to the abdominal organs. Laparoscopy may also be used to look for damage to internal organs following abdominal trauma.

In addition to its use as a diagnostic tool, laparoscopy is used for treatment such as sterilization by tubal ligation in women.

**Preparation:**

Tell your doctor if

> You have allergies to any medications or anesthetics
>
> You are taking any medications
>
> You have had bleeding problems
>
> You might be pregnant

You will be asked to sign a consent form. Use this as an opportunity to discuss with your doctor any concerns you have about the need for the test, how it is performed, or the risks.

You should not eat or drink for at least 8–12 hours before the test. Make arrangements to have someone drive you home after the test. Just before the test, remove all jewelry, dentures, eyeglasses. A hospital gown will be given to you to wear. For your comfort, empty your bladder just before the procedure.

**Procedure:**

Laparoscopy is performed by a specially trained physician (gynecologist or surgeon), usually in a hospital operating room or outpatient surgical center. Usually you can go home the same day as the procedure, although sometimes it may be necessary to stay overnight in the hospital. The procedure is most often done under general anesthesia (see p. 465). However, a local or spinal anesthetic is possible. Discuss this with your doctor.

About an hour before the procedure you may be given an injection of a sedative medication to help you relax. A small area of the upper part of your pubic hair may be shaved before the test.

You will lie on a table which will be tilted so that your feet are higher than your head. Your abdomen and pelvic area will be scrubbed with an antiseptic solution and covered with sterile drapes. A tube, called a catheter, may be inserted through the urethra into your bladder to completely empty the bladder. A blunt instrument known as a cannula may be inserted through your vagina into the uterus, making it possible for the doctor to move the uterus and allow a better view.

The anesthetic is usually given through an intravenous (IV) line placed in a vein in your arm, as well as by anesthetic gases inhaled through a mask over your nose and mouth. When you are asleep, a small one-inch incision is made in the abdominal wall in or just below your navel. A needle is then inserted through the incision. Gas (carbon dioxide or nitrous oxide) is slowly injected through the needle to inflate your abdomen. The gas creates a viewing space by lifting the abdominal wall away from the organs below.

Next the laparoscope, which is a lighted tube about one-half-inch thick, is inserted through the incision, and the doctor looks at the abdominal and pelvic organs. Other instruments such as small scissors, forceps, or probes may also be inserted through a separate, smaller incision usually at the pubic hairline.

In addition to examining the internal organs, fluid specimens and small tissue samples (biopsies) may be collected, ovarian cysts may be drained, fibrous bands of tissue (adhesions) may be cut, and abnormal endometrial tissue may be treated with electrocautery.

At the end of the procedure the laparoscope is removed and the gas is released. The small incision may be closed with a few stitches and a Band-Aid or with adhesive strips alone. This is why laparoscopy is sometime referred to as "Band-Aid" surgery. The stitches are usually the type that dissolve and do not need to be removed. Keep the incision area dry for about 3 to 4 days. There is usually little or no visible scar after the incision heals.

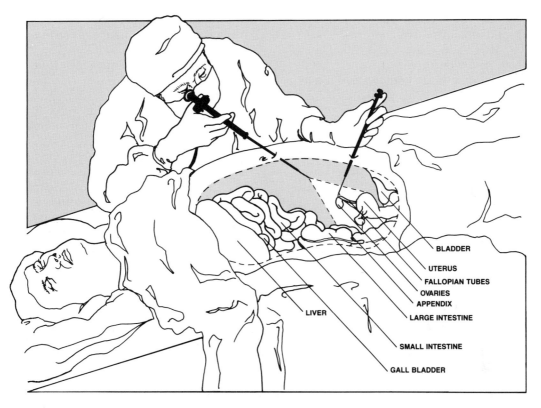

**Laparoscopy.** *During laparoscopy a viewing instrument is inserted into the abdomen and the internal organs are examined.*

The entire procedure usually takes 30–45 minutes, after which you will be taken to the recovery room and closely observed for a few hours, until you are fully awake and able to walk. If there are no complications you will then be able to return home. When you are able to resume your normal daily activities will depend upon the nature of the problem. Unless otherwise advised, you can resume normal activities within a day but should avoid strenuous activity or exercise for about a week.

## How Does It Feel?

When a general anesthetic is used, you will be asleep and feel nothing during the procedure. For a day or two after the test you may feel some tiredness, general body aching from the general anesthetic, a mild sore throat if a breathing tube was placed in your throat, mild soreness at the incision site, and some abdominal bloating. There may be a dark discoloration around your navel for a few days. You may also notice an aching in your shoulders. This is due to the remaining gas in your abdomen, which can irritate your diaphragm, causing a pain that is referred to your shoulders. Some of the gas that was injected into your abdomen may leak into the skin. This may cause a crackling sound if you rub the skin surrounding the incision. This is harmless and subsides in a few days.

If you notice severe abdominal or back pain, fever, or increasing redness, tenderness, and drainage from the incision after the procedure, notify your doctor immediately.

## Risks:

Laparoscopy is generally a safe procedure. The risk of death from the general anesthetic is less than 1 in 3000. Infection inside the abdomen or pelvis is rare (less than 1.5 in 1000). The risk of puncturing an internal organ is slight (less than 3 in 1000), and serious bleeding occurs in fewer than 6 per 1000. Although these complications are rare, when they do occur they may require transfusions or surgery to correct. The risks may vary depending upon your individual condition. You should discuss the specific risks for you with your doctor.

## Results:

Your doctor will examine your internal organs directly and should be able to discuss some of the findings with you right after the procedure. Laboratory results from tissue specimens and cultures for infection may take several days.

The source of abdominal or pelvic pain may be identified and, sometimes, treated. Fibrous bands of scar tissue (adhesions) from previous surgery or infections can sometimes be cut during laparoscopy. If tissue that is normally found inside the uterus is seen growing outside the uterus (endometriosis), it can be identified and, sometimes, cauterized. Internal bleeding from a ruptured organ such as a spleen or ovarian cyst may be located. An ectopic or tubal pregnancy (a pregnancy occurring outside the uterus) may also be seen. The fallopian tubes can be examined for scarring, which may account for infertility. Abdominal masses such as fibroid tumors of the uterus, ovarian tumors, or ovarian cysts can be examined. Sometimes the source of pain may be found to be due to appendicitis or an infection.

Fluid samples collected during laparoscopy may be analyzed for infection or for the cause of fluid accumulation in the abdominal cavity (ascites). Biopsies of suspicious areas may demonstrate benign tumors or malignant tumors. Cancers may be either primary tumors or metastases (cancers that have spread to the abdomen from cancers located elsewhere in the body).

## Cost:

$500 to $1000

## Special Considerations:

★*Open Laparoscopy:* Sometimes in obese patients or those who have had previous abdominal surgery, a modified procedure is used. This calls for making a slightly larger incision below the navel to open the abdominal wall to ease the insertion of the laparoscope.

★*Culdoscopy:* A thin, lighted instrument may be inserted through an incision in the vagina to view the uterus, fallopian tubes, and rectal wall from another approach. This procedure has been largely replaced by laparoscopy.

# Laryngoscopy

By looking into your mouth with a tongue blade and a light, your doctor can see your tongue, cheeks, teeth and gums, palate, and back of the throat (pharnyx). But there is much more to see. In order to examine the base of the tongue, epiglottis, larnyx, and vocal cords, which are located deeper in the throat, your doctor may perform laryngoscopy.

There are two basic types of laryngoscopy: *office laryngoscopy*, which uses a hand-held mirror, laryngeal telescope, or a flexible fiberoptic instrument, and *operative (direct) laryngoscopy*, which is usually performed under general anesthesia in an operating room using a straight, hollow, lighted laryngoscope.

## Why Performed:

Office laryngoscopy is part of a routine examination for ear, nose, and throat problems. It is particularly helpful in evaluating hoarseness or voice change which lasts more than two weeks. It can be used to investigate the source of blood-tinged sputum, difficulty in swallowing, a persistent sensation of a lump in your throat, or stridor (a harsh, high-pitched whistling sound produced when the airway is blocked in the larynx). Operative laryngoscopy permits removal of foreign objects like fish bones which may get caught in your throat and can be used for the collection of tissue samples from possibly cancerous lesions.

## Preparation:

Tell your doctor if
  You have allergies to any medications
    or anesthetics
  You are taking any medications
  You have had any bleeding problems
  You might be pregnant

Office laryngoscopy requires no special preparation although it may be helpful to avoid eating or drinking for several hours before the exam to avoid vomiting. If you wear dentures, remove them just before the exam.

The preparation for operative laryngoscopy involving a general anesthetic requires that you not eat or drink anything for at least 6 to 8 hours before the procedure. If you are scheduled for the test as an outpatient, bring someone to drive you home after the exam. With operative laryngoscopy you will be asked to sign a consent form. Use this opportunity to discuss with your doctor any concerns you have about the need for the test, how it is performed, and the risks. Just before the procedure, remove all jewelry, dentures, and eyeglasses and, for your comfort, empty your bladder. You will be given a hospital gown to wear.

## Procedure:

*Office Laryngoscopy:* Your doctor can perform this examination using a hand-held mirror and lighted laryngeal telescope or a flexible fiberoptic instrument. With mirror laryngoscopy your doctor will sit face to face with you and will wear a head mirror to direct the light into your throat. You will be asked to sit upright and lean forward, with your chin thrust out as if sniffing a flower. This position helps make the larynx visible, so it is important to hold this posture throughout the exam. You will then be asked to stick your tongue out as far as possible. It will be wrapped in gauze for protection and gently pulled forward. A small, hand-held mirror or laryngeal telescope will be inserted and held at the back of your throat.

You will be asked to breathe through your mouth, taking quick, short, panting breaths. You may be asked to utter a prolonged, steady, high-pitched "e-e-e-e" sound or a low-pitched "a-a-a-a" sound to move and make visible your vocal cords. If you are having problems with gagging during the exam, concentrate on the panting breaths. Relaxation is the key. The exam will not block your breathing. If the gagging interferes, a local anesthetic may be spread into the back of your throat to numb it. Ask the doctor to wait a few minutes for the anesthetic to take effect. The entire exam takes only 5 to 10 minutes.

Another way to perform this exam is with the aid of a pencil-thin fiberoptic viewing instrument with a self-contained light. A local anesthetic ointment is applied to the nasal passages and an anesthetic solution is sprayed into the back of your throat to numb these areas. Then the flexible instrument, a nasopharyngoscope, is inserted through one of your nostrils and advanced down the back of your throat. Again, you will be asked to make various sounds while your vocal cords are examined. The exam usually takes 10–15 minutes.

If a local anesthetic is used with the exam, you should not eat or drink anything until your gag reflex has recovered, which is usually about 2 hours.

*Operative (Direct) Laryngoscopy:* This procedure is usually performed by a specially trained physician and several assistants in an operating room with the use of general anesthesia (see p. 465). About an hour before the test you may be given an injection of a sedative medication to help you relax. An intravenous (IV) line may be placed in a vein in your arm to give you fluids and medications.

You will lie on your back with your head positioned by an assistant. After you are asleep, a lighted laryngoscope will be inserted through your mouth, down your throat. Your larynx and vocal cords can then be viewed either directly or under magnification. If necessary, foreign objects can be removed or small tissue samples of suspicious areas can be collected for laboratory analysis. Benign polyps can also be removed from the vocal cords by cutting or laser treatment during operative laryngoscopy. The examination usually takes 15–30 minutes, after which you will be closely observed for several hours until fully awake and able to swallow.

If biopsy or other tissue is removed, you should avoid clearing your throat or coughing vigorously for several hours after the procedure. In addition, you may be asked to maintain absolute voice rest after the procedure for 7–10 days. If so, you will need to use a pencil and pad to communicate.

### How Does It Feel?

In office laryngoscopy you may feel like gagging as the mirror or fiberoptic laryngoscope is placed in your throat. With the fiberoptic instrument you may feel a slight warmth from the heat of the light in the instrument. If a local anesthetic is used, it usually tastes bitter and may cause a sensation of swelling in the back of your throat and difficulty in swallowing. With the mirror exam, the pulling on your tongue may be somewhat uncomfortable. If it becomes painful, signal your doctor by pointing at your tongue; you won't be able to speak.

When a general anesthetic is used you will be asleep and feel nothing during the procedure, but afterward may experience a day or two of tiredness and generalized muscle aching. You may have a sore throat and some hoarseness for a few days. Throat lozenges or gargling with warm salt water may help soothe the sore throat.

If a biopsy is taken, you may spit up a

small amount of blood after the procedure. This is normal. However, if the bleeding is substantial or persistent, or if you begin having difficulty breathing after the procedure, notify your doctor immediately.

### Risks:

Laryngoscopy is generally a very safe procedure. However, with all types of laryngoscopy there is a slight risk of triggering a life-threatening obstruction of the airway. This may occur because the airway is already partially obstructed by tumors, polyps, or a swollen epiglottis (inflammation of the tissues at the back of the throat). If obstruction should occur, it may be necessary to create an alternative airway by making an emergency incision (tracheotomy) in your neck. This complication is very rare. With operative laryngoscopy the risk of a fatality is about 1 in 3000 due to the general anesthetic. If a biopsy is performed there is a very slight risk of prolonged bleeding, infection, or perforation of the airway. Although complications are infrequent, you should discuss the risks in your particular case with your doctor.

### Results:

During the examination the doctor will look for causes of obstruction, foreign bodies, inflammation, strictures, or lesions. Your vocal cords will be examined to look for nodules, tumors, polyps, scars, abnormal movement, or paralysis. If suspicious areas or growths are biopsied or specimens are sent to the laboratory to look for infection, the results will take at least several days.

### Cost:

Office laryngoscopy: $30 to $75 (as part of a complete ear, nose, and throat examination)
Operative laryngoscopy: $300 to $700

# Mediastinoscopy

The mediastinum is the space behind the sternum (breastbone) and between the lungs. It contains the heart and its major blood vessels, the windpipe (trachea), the esophagus, and lymph nodes. The structures of the mediastinum can be viewed through a mediastinoscope, a thin, hollow lighted tube which is inserted through a small incision made above the breastbone. The lymph nodes in the mediastinum receive lymph fluid from the lungs. Therefore, it is often possible to determine the type and extent of certain lung diseases such as cancer by removing sample lymph nodes during mediastinoscopy.

With mediastinoscopy the expense, discomfort, and risks of more extensive surgical procedures can sometimes be spared.

### Why Performed:

Mediastinoscopy is often performed to determine whether a lung cancer has spread (metastasized) to the lymph nodes in the mediastinum. This can help in selecting the most appropriate treatment. Mediastinoscopy is also useful in evaluating certain abnormalities found on chest x-rays, such as a possible mass in the mediastinal area.

### Preparation:

Tell your doctor if
You have any allergies to any medications or anesthetics
You are taking any medications
You have had any bleeding problems
You might be pregnant

You will be asked to sign a consent form. Use this opportunity to discuss with your doctor any concerns you have about the

331

need for the test, how it is performed, or the risks.

The procedure is usually done under general anesthesia (see p. 465). Therefore, you should not eat or drink anything for at least 12 hours before the test. An empty stomach helps prevent vomiting during the procedure and reduces the risk of complications. Plan to have someone drive you home after the test if you are not staying overnight in the hospital.

Before the test remove dentures, eyeglasses, and jewelry, and, for your comfort, empty your bladder. You will be given a hospital gown to wear.

**Procedure:**

Mediastinoscopy is performed by a surgeon and assistants in an operating room. Several blood tests are usually performed before the procedure to check your blood clotting and blood type in case you should need a transfusion. About an hour before the procedure you will be given an injection of a sedative to help you relax. An intravenous (IV) line will be placed in a vein, usually in your arm, to give you fluids and medications. Your neck and chest will be scrubbed with an antiseptic solution and covered with sterile drapes.

You will be put to sleep with a general anesthetic and given a mixture of oxygen and anesthetic gases to breath through a hollow endotracheal tube placed in your throat.

After you are asleep, a 2- to 3-inch incision will be made at the base of your neck just above the breastbone. The long, thin mediastinoscope is then carefully inserted through the incision into the space behind your breastbone. Your doctor will examine the mediastinal space, and suspicious lymph nodes or abnormal tissues are removed (biopsied) through the scope. The instrument is then withdrawn and the incision is closed with a few stitches and covered with a bandage.

The entire procedure usually takes about an hour. You will then be taken to the recovery room and closely observed for several hours until you are fully awake and your gag reflex has recovered. You can then return home or to your hospital room and resume normal activities and diet unless otherwise advised. The stitches will be removed in 10 to 14 days, and usually only a tiny scar remains.

**How Does It Feel?**

The sedative injection will make you feel very drowsy and relaxed. During the procedure itself you will be asleep and feel nothing. After the procedure you may feel some mild soreness at the incision site for one to two days. You may also have some generalized muscle aching from the anesthetic and a sore throat from the endotracheal tube for a day or so. Throat lozenges and gargling may help with the sore throat. If you notice bleeding from the incision, fever, severe chest pain, shortness of breath, difficulty in swallowing, or persistent hoarseness, notify your physician immediately.

**Risks:**

The risk of death during mediastinoscopy, including the general anesthesia, is less than 1 in 3000. Complications are rare and include bleeding from damage of one of the blood vessels near the heart, collapse of a lung (pneumothorax), perforation of the esophagus, infection, and injury to the recurrent laryngeal nerve which can cause permanent hoarseness. Some of these complications, if they occur, may require transfusions and surgery. Although these complications are rare, you should discuss your specific risks with your physician.

**Results:**

In the evaluation of lung cancer, the lymph nodes removed during mediastinoscopy are sent to the laboratory. Sometimes these lymph nodes are analyzed by "frozen section" and the results are available immediately. If the nodes are free of cancer, a more extensive operation to open the chest and remove the lung segment with the primary cancer may be performed while you are still in the operating room. This avoids the need to have general anesthesia again for the lung surgery. In approximately one third of cases, cancerous lymph nodes are found in the mediastinum, which usually means that the lung cancer is not curable by surgery. In these cases, nonsurgical treatments may be used.

Mediastinoscopy may also reveal other types of chest diseases such as lymphoma (Hodgkin's disease), cysts, sarcoidosis, or granulomatous diseases like tuberculosis.

**Cost:**

$1200 to $1500

**Special Considerations:**

★If you have had a previous mediastinoscopy or open-heart surgery, this test will probably not be done, since the scarring from the first procedure may make the second difficult if not impossible.

# Ophthalmoscopy
## (Funduscopy)

The eye has been called the "window of the body," because a careful eye exam can reveal valuable information, not only about the health of the eye but about the health of the whole body. In this test an examiner views the interior and back portion of the eye with the aid of a hand-held, lighted, magnifying instrument called an ophthalmoscope. The back portion of the eye, known as the fundus, contains the retina, blood vessels, and the optic nerve. Examining the fundus provides a unique opportunity to directly view living nerves and blood vessels.

**Why Performed:**

Ophthalmoscopy is a valuable part of a routine physical or complete eye exam. It is useful in evaluating symptoms such as visual disturbance or headaches which may be due to diseases of the eye itself or diseases that affect the whole body, including the eye. Diseases such as hypertension, diabetes, arteriosclerosis, or even head injury or brain tumors may produce important clues which can be detected during this exam.

**Preparation:**

Tell your doctor if
>You have allergies to any medications
>You are taking any medications
>You have glaucoma or a family history of glaucoma

Usually no preparation is necessary. However, eye drops are sometimes used to dilate the pupil and make it easier to see the back of the eye. These eye drops take about 15–20 minutes to fully dilate the pupil.

The dilating drops may make it difficult to focus your eyes for several hours. So if you know your eyes will be dilated for the exam, you may wish to arrange to have someone drive you home afterward.

**Procedure:**

There are two types of ophthalmoscopy.

*Direct Ophthalmoscopy*: This is the common type of exam performed by most physicians. In the procedure the doctor uses a lighted instrument, about the size of a flashlight, with rotating lenses on top which can magnify up to 15 times. You will be seated in a darkened room and asked to stare straight ahead at some distant spot in the room. The examiner, looking through the ophthalmoscope, will move very close to your face and shine a bright light into one of your eyes. Try to hold your eyes steady without blinking. The examiner may ask you to look up and down, right and left, and to stare directly into the light. Each eye is examined separately. The exam takes 3 to 5 minutes.

*Indirect Ophthalmoscopy*: This type of exam gives a more complete view of the retina and is useful in further evaluating abnormalities in the back part of your eye. It also enables the examiner to view the fundus even through some cataracts. This exam requires special equipment and is usually performed by an eye specialist (ophthalmologist) in his or her office. You will be asked to sit in a semireclining position in a darkened room. The examiner wears an instrument on the head like a miner's light. The doctor will hold your eye open and direct a very bright light into your eye with a hand-held lens. During the exam you will be asked to look in a number of different directions. Pressure may be exerted on your eyeball through the skin of the eyelids with a small, blunt instrument to help bring the edges of your fundus into view. The indirect exam takes between 5 and 10 minutes.

### How Does It Feel?

In direct ophthalmoscopy you will hear a clicking sound as the instrument is focused. The light is sometimes very intense and you may see afterimages for a short time after the exam. Some people report seeing light spots or colorful branching images. These are actually the outlines of the blood vessels of the retina. With indirect ophthalmoscopy the light is much more intense and may even be somewhat uncomfortable. If pressure is put on your eyeball with the blunt instrument, this may also be uncomfortable. If it is painful, let the examiner know.

If eye drops are used, you may notice a brief stinging sensation when they are instilled, followed by a medicinal taste in your mouth. The taste is from the medication draining from the tear ducts into the back of your throat. For 4–6 hours after having the dilating drops, you will have trouble focusing your eyes. Near vision (reading and close vision work) is mainly affected. Your distance vision is usually little disturbed, although your eyes may be very sensitive to light, making it somewhat difficult to drive. Wearing sunglasses may make it more comfortable until the drops wear off in a few hours.

### Risks:

Ophthalmoscopy itself involves no risk. However, the dilating drops that are used can, in rare instances, produce a brief episode of nausea, vomiting, dryness of the mouth, flushing, and dizziness. The drops can also trigger an attack of narrow-angle glaucoma; however, if this is suspected, the drops are usually not used. Acute- or narrow-angle glaucoma may produce intense eye pain, visual disturbance (halos may appear around light), and loss of vision, which is usually not permanent. If you should experience any of these symptoms after the exam, contact your doctor immediately.

### Results:

Many eye disorders can be detected by ophthalmoscopy, including clouding of the lenses (cataracts), cloudy vitreous material inside the eyeball, detached retinas, optic nerve degeneration (atrophy) or swelling (papilledema), and changes due to glaucoma. Diabetes, hypertension, and other systemic diseases can produce characteristic changes in the back of the eye such as hemorrhages, exudates, or vessel abnormalities (retinopathy).

### Cost:

Direct ophthalmoscopy is usually included without separate charge as part of the physical exam. A complete eye exam by an ophthalmologist, which includes ophthalmoscopy, costs $40–$60.

### Special Considerations:

★*Slit-Lamp Examination (Biomicroscopy)*: In ophthalmoscopy, just described, the main focus is the retina and optic nerve at the back of the eye. To view the structures at the front of the eye more thoroughly, a slit lamp is used. You sit facing the slit-lamp instrument, place your chin on a rest and your forehead against a support bar, and stare straight ahead. Your doctor looks through a binocular magnifying instrument, while a narrow beam of bright light is directed into your eye. The doctor looks for abnormalities in your eyelids, the whites of your eyes (sclerae), the membranes that line your eyelids and sclerae (conjunctiva), the colored portion of your eyes (iris), the thin transparent membrane (cornea) which overlies the iris, and your lens.

★*Fluorescein Eye Staining*: The cornea is the thin, transparent membrane that covers the dark parts of the eye (the pupil and iris). When an injury or infection of the cornea is suspected, your doctor may put fluorescein, an orange dye, into your eye. The dye is applied by gently touching a sterile, fluorescein-impregnated paper strip to the inside of your lower eyelid. The dye coats your cornea and temporarily accumulates in any irregularities on the corneal surface; the rest of the dye is rapidly washed away by tears. Next your doctor looks at your cornea under a blue-colored ultraviolet light. The fluorescein stain glows bright green, highlighting corneal abrasions, ulcers, burns, or irritations due to scratches, foreign bodies, infections, excessive sun exposure, or trauma from contact lenses.

★For information on other eye tests see Vision Tests (p. 390), Home Vision Tests (p. 403), and Glaucoma Tests (p. 379).

# Sigmoidoscopy
## (Anoscopy, Protoscopy, Proctosigmoidoscopy)

In this test your doctor visually examines the inside lining of your lower gastrointestinal tract (sigmoid colon, rectum, and anus) for tumors, polyps, inflammation, hemorrhoids, and other bowel diseases (see illustration, p. 281).

This exam is done with the aid of several different viewing instruments which are inserted through the anus. The *anoscope*, a short hollow tube with a light, is used to examine the last few inches of your digestive tract (anal canal). A *proctoscope* is slightly longer and used to view the inside of the rectum. The standard, *rigid sigmoidoscope* is a 10- to 12-inch-long, hollow, lighted tube about 1 inch in diameter which allows viewing of the rectum and a portion of the lower large intestine. A *flexible fiberoptic sigmoidoscope* allows a more complete view of the lower colon. This instrument is a 2-foot-long tube containing a powerful light source and thin threads of fiberglass which can transmit light around bends. Despite the longer length, the flexibility of the fiberoptic scope usually makes the exam more comfortable. This new flexible sigmoidoscope requires special training for its use and is not yet available at all facilities. Another even longer flexible fiberoptic scope has been developed to examine the entire colon (see Colonoscopy, p. 319).

In addition to viewing the lining of the lower gastrointestinal tract, your doctor can remove small polyps and tissue samples (biopsies) through the sigmoidoscope.

## Why Performed:

Sigmoidoscopy is usually the first test done to evaluate unexplained rectal bleeding, change in bowel habits (unaccustomed diarrhea, constipation, or pencil-thin stools), or rectal pain. It can be performed to determine the cause of hidden (occult) blood in the stool when this is detected on screening tests (see p. 443) or to evaluate abnormalities found on a barium enema x-ray (see p. 245). Sigmoidoscopy allows careful examination of the lower colon and rectum, areas often not seen well with a barium enema x-ray. This test is also used to monitor the progress of polyps or inflammatory bowel disease.

The usefulness and cost effectiveness of doing routine sigmoidoscopies as a screening test for people without symptoms are matters of some debate. The American Cancer Society recommends an annual sigmoidoscopy for everyone over the age of 50. If the first two exams are normal, then the exam may be done every 3 to 5 years. High-risk patients with a history of colonic polyps, ulcerative colitis, or a strong family history of colorectal cancer or polyps might benefit from more frequent and intensive examination. We recommend that you discuss periodic screening with your physician.

## Preparation:

Tell your doctor if

> You have had a recent barium x-ray examination
>
> You have an artificial heart valve or a history of disease of your heart valves
>
> You might be pregnant

You may be asked to sign a consent form for this exam. Use this as an opportunity to discuss with your physician any concerns you have about the need for the test, how it is performed, or the risks.

Stool in the colon and rectum may make an adequate exam difficult if not impossible. Recommendations on how to prepare the bowel vary considerably. Some doctors suggest only a tap-water or bottle enema (Fleet enema) an hour before the exam. Others request that you eat a clear liquid diet of juices, broths, and gelatin for 1 to 2 days before the test in addition to an enema the night before and another enema an hour before the exam. Still other doctors require no special preparation at all, especially in patients with bloody diarrhea or severe abdominal cramping. Check with your doctor for specific instructions.

You will be asked to undress from the waist down and put on a hospital gown. You can leave your socks on to help stay warm. For your comfort, empty your bladder just before the exam.

## Procedure:

The test is done by a physician and an assistant in an office, special procedure room, or, if you are hospitalized, at your bedside.

During the exam you will either be lying on your left side with your knees drawn up toward your chest or be resting on your elbows and knees with your buttocks raised. Many offices have tilting exam tables which will support you in a head-down, buttocks-up position.

Once you are in position, the doctor will gently insert a well-lubricated, gloved finger into your anus to check for tenderness, obstructions and, in men, the condition of the prostate gland. Next, a lubricated anoscope may be inserted several inches into the anal canal. To relax your anal muscles and ease the entry of the scope, bear down as though having a bowel movement. The anoscope is then slowly withdrawn while your physician examines your anal canal.

Next the physician will insert the sigmoidoscope through the anus into your rectum. Again, bear down gently as the scope is first inserted. The examiner will gradually advance the scope through your rectum into the lower colon. Sometimes puffs of air are blown through the scope to help clear a path and permit better viewing of the bowel lining. A suction device may be used to remove stool, mucus, or blood through the sigmoidoscope to improve the view. Once the doctor has advanced the scope as far as possible, it is slowly withdrawn while the mucosal lining of your bowel is carefully inspected. Your doctor may also insert tiny instruments such as forceps, snares, and swabs through the sigmoidoscope to collect biopsy tissue samples, remove polyps, or gather specimens for culture.

After the scope is removed, your anal area will be cleaned with tissues. If you have been in a head-down position, you may feel lightheaded if you try to stand up immediately after the exam, so it is best to rest for a few minutes lying flat on the table. The entire exam usually takes 5–10 minutes, slightly longer if biopsies are taken or polyps removed. You will be able to resume your normal diet and activities after the exam unless otherwise advised.

## How Does It Feel?

This exam can be somewhat embarrassing and uncomfortable, but most patients report that the *thought* of the exam is worse than the experience itself. Knowing what to expect helps ease most of the discomfort. Remembering that your doctor has done many of these exams and will approach the procedure professionally can be reassuring.

When the lubricant and the scope are first inserted they may feel slightly cool. As the scope is advanced and air instilled, you may feel some brief cramping (gas pains) and the urge to defecate. Taking slow, deep breaths in and out through your mouth will help relax your abdominal muscles and lessen any discomfort.

You will probably feel and hear some of the instilled air escape through and around the scope. Don't try to control it and don't be embarrassed. The passing of air is expected and necessary.

The suction machine used to remove stool and secretions is noisy but painless. Biopsies are also painless, since the lining of the intestine contains no pain nerves.

Lying in a head-down position can produce a sensation of fullness and pressure in your head and face. You may feel dizzy if you try to stand up too quickly. If so, lie down again or sit with your head between your knees.

After the procedure you may experience mild lower abdominal gas pains and may pass some gas. If a biopsy was performed or a polyp removed, you may notice traces of blood in your stool for a few days. If you experience heavy rectal bleeding, severe abdominal pain, or a fever, notify your doctor immediately.

*Patient Comments:*

"The position during the exam is a bit awkward. It felt like I was going to fall forward. When the tube was put in I felt like I had to have a bowel movement. I could feel the scope moving inside. Not really painful, just a pressure. It wasn't half as bad as I expected."

**Risks:**

Sigmoidoscopy is a very safe procedure, with few serious complications. Perforation of the intestinal wall or substantial bleeding caused by the scope or biopsy is extremely rare (less than 1 in 10,000). These rare complications may result in infection or blood loss severe enough to be life-threatening but usually can be managed safely with antibiotics, surgery, or transfusions. Patients with abnormal or artificial heart valves are usually treated with antibiotics before and after the procedure to prevent serious infections. Irregular heartbeats may also occur but nearly always subside quickly without treatment. Although complications are rare, you should discuss your specific risks with your doctor.

**Results:**

Your doctor should be able to discuss some of the findings with you immediately after the test. However, the laboratory results from biopsies and tests for infection may take several days. The normal lining of the bowel appears as folds of smooth, semi-translucent, pinkish membrane (mucosa). The examination may reveal hemorrhoids (the most common cause of blood in the stool), tumors, polyps, ulcers, or inflammation. A reddened, swollen, inflamed bowel lining may be due to infection or inflammatory bowel disease (ulcerative colitis or Crohn's disease). Suspicious growths will be biopsied and sent to the lab to determine if they are cancerous or benign. It is estimated that 30%–40% of all cancers of the colon and rectum can be diagnosed with the sigmoidoscope.

**Cost:**

$75 to $150

# Upper Gastrointestinal Endoscopy
## (Esophagoscopy, Gastroscopy, Duodenoscopy)

Endoscopy is a procedure that allows direct visual examination of the interior lining of the upper gastrointestinal (GI) tract (see p. 281). The examination is performed using a thin, lighted viewing instrument which is inserted through the mouth. When the primary area examined is the esophagus (the tube that leads from the mouth to the stomach), the procedure is known as *esophagoscopy*. In *gastroscopy* the stomach is viewed, and in *duodenoscopy* the duodenum (the first portion of the small intestine) is examined. Often all of these areas are viewed during a combined procedure.

The fiberoptic endoscope that makes these examinations possible is a 3-foot-long flexible tube about a half-inch thick. It contains bundles of fine, fiberglass filaments which can transmit images around bends from the lighted tip of the instrument to the viewing lens at the other end. The lighted tip is inserted through your mouth and then gently advanced down into the esophagus, stomach, and duodenum.

Through the endoscope your doctor can look for ulcers, inflammation, tumors, or bleeding. Also tissue specimens from suspicious lesions can be collected (biopsies), polyps can be removed, and bleeding can often be stopped through the scope. Endoscopy can reveal lesions missed by x-ray tests, and it sometimes can eliminate the need for extensive exploratory surgery.

### Why Performed:

If you vomit blood or pass blood in your stool, endoscopy may help locate the source of bleeding. Endoscopy is sometimes performed to evaluate persistent upper abdominal pain or bloating, difficulty in swallowing (dysphagia), and vomiting. Endoscopy may also be used to further investigate abnormalities such as ulcers or masses found on x-ray contrast tests (see UGI Series, p. 280) or to document the healing of known gastric ulcers.

### Preparation:

Tell your doctor if

> You have allergies to any medications or anesthetics
>
> You are taking any medications
>
> You have had bleeding problems
>
> You have had problems with your heart valves
>
> You might be pregnant

You will be asked to sign a consent form before the test. Use this opportunity to discuss with your doctor any questions you have about the need for the test, how it is performed, and the risks.

Having an empty stomach before the exam is important to help ensure a clear view and prevent vomiting. Therefore, you should not eat or drink anything for 6 to 8 hours before the test. If the test is done on an emergency basis, a tube may be inserted through your nose or mouth to empty your stomach.

Bring someone with you to drive you home after the test unless you will be staying overnight in the hospital. Before the test you will put on a hospital gown, remove dentures, jewelry, and glasses, and, for your own comfort, empty your bladder.

### Procedure:

Endoscopy is usually done in a special procedure room or operating room in a hospital or office. An overnight stay in the hospital is not usually necessary. The procedure is performed by a specially trained physician (gastroenterologist or surgeon) with the help of one or two assistants.

Before the procedure some blood tests may be done to check for low blood count or clotting problems. Shortly before the procedure an intravenous (IV) line will be placed in a vein in your arm. You will also be given an injection of a medication to relax you and reduce discomfort and sometimes a drug to decrease gastrointestinal secretions. A pain medication and sedative are given to you through the IV in your arm during the procedure. You should feel relaxed and drowsy but still alert enough to cooperate.

Your throat may be numbed with an anesthetic spray, gargle, or lozenge. The anesthetic dulls your gag reflex, making it easier to pass the endoscope. You will be asked to lie on your left side with your head slightly bent forward. A mouth guard may be inserted to protect your teeth from the endoscope (and the endoscope from your teeth). Next the lubricated tip of the endoscope is guided into your mouth while the examiner gently presses your tongue out of the way. You may be asked to swallow to help move the tube alone. It is helpful to remember that the instrument is no thicker than many foods you swallow without difficulty. During the procedure, try not to swallow unless requested to. An assistant may remove the saliva from your mouth with a suction device, or you can just let the saliva drain from the side of your mouth.

The lights in the room will be dimmed. Your doctor will then slowly advance the endoscope while looking through the eye-

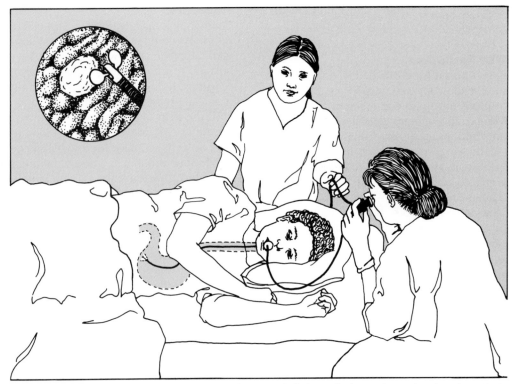

**UGI Endoscopy.** *The scope is inserted to view the stomach lining. The insert shows the view through the scope as a biopsy forceps collects a tissue specimen from the edge of an ulcer.*

piece to examine the walls of your esophagus, stomach, and duodenum. Air or water may be instilled through the scope to help clear a path for the scope or to clear the lens. A camera may be used to take pictures of certain areas. Tiny biopsy forceps or brushes may also be inserted through the endoscope to collect specimens. You may be repositioned during the exam, or gentle pressure may be applied to your abdomen. When the examination is completed, the endoscope will be removed.

The procedure itself usually takes 15–30 minutes. Afterward you will be closely observed for an hour or two. You should not eat or drink until your throat is no longer numb and your gag reflex has returned to normal. This usually takes an hour or two. You can then resume your normal diet and activities and have someone drive you home unless otherwise instructed.

### How Does It Feel?

You may notice a brief, sharp pain when the IV is started in your arm. The local anesthetic usually tastes slightly bitter and will make your tongue and throat feel numb and swollen. Some patients report that they feel at times as if they can't breathe because of the tube in their throat. This is a false sensation caused by the anesthetic. There will always be plenty of room to breathe around the tube. Remember to relax and take slow deep breaths.

You may experience some gagging, nausea, bloating, or mild abdominal cramping as the tube is moved or as air is instilled. If the discomfort is severe, alert your physician with an agreed-upon signal or tap on the arm. Even though you will be unable to talk during the exam, you can still communicate and can retain a good deal of control.

The IV medications will make you feel very sleepy. Your eyelids will feel heavy, and you may have difficulty speaking, a dry mouth, and/or blurred vision. These effects may last for several hours after the test. The medications may also cause you not to remember much about what went on during the test.

After the test you may belch and feel bloated from the instilled air. You may also have a tickling, dry cough, a slight hoarseness, or a mild sore throat, all of which can last several days. Throat lozenges and warm salt-water gargles can help.

If you vomit blood or notice black or bloody stools, or if you have difficulty swallowing, shortness of breath, increased chest or abdominal pain, or a fever, notify your doctor immediately.

*Patient Comments:*

"The exam wasn't nearly as bad as I thought. As long as I remembered to relax and breathe slowly around the tube, I was fine."

"I arranged with my doctor before the test to look through the scope myself. Even though I was a little drowsy, at one point I was given a brief look at the inside of my own stomach. That was truly fascinating!"

**Risks:**

Endoscopy is generally a very safe procedure, with an overall complication rate of less than 1 in 1000. There is a very slight chance (1 in 3000) that the instrument might perforate the gastrointestinal wall. This could require surgical repair. Bleeding may also occur from instrument injury or from the biopsy site, but this usually stops on its own without treatment. If vomiting occurs during the exam and any material is then inhaled into the lungs, an aspiration pneumonia may develop. This would require antibiotic treatment. Patients with disease of the heart valves or an artificial heart valve usually receive antibiotics before and after the procedure to prevent infection. Although complications are extremely rare, you should discuss your specific risks with your doctor. We should also mention that there is some risk to the doctor of a bitten finger when the scope is inserted!

**Results:**

Your doctor will be able to discuss some of the findings with you immediately after the procedure. Endoscopy sometimes reveals lesions such as ulcers which were missed on x-ray studies. Inflammation of the esophagus, stomach, or duodenum is a common finding. Endoscopy may also reveal a source of bleeding, which may be due to inflammation, an ulcer, a tumor, a tear in the esophagus, or dilated veins (varices) in the esophagus or stomach. A hiatal hernia (which is a bulging of the stomach through the diaphragm) or a narrowing (stenosis or stricture) or widening (dilation) of the esophagus may be identified. Tumors and ulcers may be seen and biopsied to determine whether the lesion is cancerous or benign. Biopsy results may take several days.

**Cost:**

$200 to $500 (more if a hospital stay is included)

**Special Considerations:**

★*Endoscopic Retrograde Cholangiopancreatogram (ERCP)*: This is an x-ray test of the ducts draining the liver, gallbladder, and pancreas which is performed using an upper gastrointestinal endoscope. This test is usually done to evaluate jaundice (yellowing of the skin) when blockage of the bile or pancreatic ducts is suspected, and other tests such as ultrasound, liver scan, and x-ray studies are not conclusive. This test sometimes eliminates the need for more expensive, riskier abdominal surgery. The preparation and procedure for an ERCP are very similar to the routine endoscopy just described.

The endoscope is passed into the duodenum and a small, hollow tube (catheter) is threaded into the opening of the common duct, which drains the secretions from the liver and pancreas. A contrast material is then injected through the endoscope, and x-ray pictures are taken of the duct system. Stones, strictures, obstructing tumors, and cysts are looked for. The procedure requires an experienced physician (gastroenterologist) and takes about 30–60 minutes to perform. Complications, including infection or inflammation of the pancreas and liver, occur in about 2 in 100 patients. The cost is approximately $800 –$1000.

# 10. Biopsies and Taps

## Biopsies

Sometimes the only way to get the information needed to diagnose a known or suspected abnormality is to remove a small sample of tissue from the body and send it to the laboratory to be examined under a microscope. The procedure by which the tissue sample is collected is called a biopsy.

A biopsy is the single most important test for helping to decide whether cancer is present. Biopsies are also used to help diagnose and follow conditions involving inflammation and certain other abnormalities of tissues and organs.

Biopsies may be done during surgery, during endoscopy (see p. 311), or as a separate procedure. Those done as a separate procedure are described in this section.

There are three types of biopsy: exci-

sional, incisional, and needle biopsies.

- *Excisional biopsy*—The entire lump, node, or suspicious area and some of the surrounding tissue are removed.
- *Incisional biopsy*—Only a slice or wedge of the suspicious area is removed.
- *Needle biopsy*—A long, thin needle is inserted into the suspect tissue, and a core of tissue removed.

In incisional and needle biopsies, the amount of tissue removed is usually very small. In excisional biopsies, it may be larger. Biopsies rarely have any effect on the overall function of the organ or tissue from which the sample is taken.

The tissue removed is sent to the pathology laboratory, where it is first closely inspected. It is then either cut into thin slices, which are placed on a glass slide, or smeared directly onto a slide. The slide is then closely examined under a microscope.

### Frozen Sections

Sometimes a special kind of biopsy, a *frozen section*, is performed during surgery. The surgeon makes an incision, exposing the target organ. A biopsy is taken and is rushed to the pathology lab, where it is quick-frozen, sliced, and examined under a microscope. The patient remains under anesthesia and the surgical team stands by while the pathologist examines the tissue, makes a diagnosis, and phones it back to the operating room. Results are usually ready in about 10–20 minutes. The surgeon can then decide whether to remove further tissue.

For instance, a frozen section might be done of a suspected lung cancer. If the diagnosis is positive for cancer, the surgeon might remove the affected lung. If it is negative, the lung is left in place.

### Frozen vs. Permanent Section

Sometimes it is necessary to decide whether to have a frozen section done during an operation or a *permanent section* done later. Each has its advantages.

If a frozen section is done, and surgical removal of an organ or tissue is needed, this can be done at once. Thus a cancer may be removed before it spreads further, and a second operation can be avoided.

A permanent section, on the other hand, offers slightly greater accuracy; frozen sections occasionally turn out, on further study, to be inaccurate. A permanent section also makes it possible to obtain a second or third opinion before making a decision about having further surgery. The tissue from a frozen section deteriorates shortly after it is examined.

# Bone Biopsy

In this test a small piece of bone is removed for examination under a microscope. The bone may be obtained by a *closed biopsy* (also called a *needle* or *drill biopsy*), in which a needle is inserted through a small incision in the skin and into the bone, or by an *open biopsy*, in which a sample of bone is removed through a larger surgical incision. This test can be performed on any bone in which an abnormality is suspected. It is often performed on the vertebrae. If the bone to be sampled is in the lower spine, a needle biopsy is usually done. In the upper spine, an open biopsy is most commonly used.

### Why Performed:

Bone biopsies are most often done to evaluate abnormal findings from another test, usually an x-ray or CT scan. This test can also help evaluate persistent bone pain and tenderness. It can help diagnose bone cancer, infections, and metabolic disorders that affect bone.

### Preparation:

Tell your doctor if
    You have a history of allergies to any medications or anesthetics
    You are taking any medications
    You have had bleeding problems
    You might be pregnant

You will be asked to sign a consent form authorizing this procedure. Use this opportunity to discuss with your doctor any concerns you may have about the need for the test, the risks of the test, or how it will be performed.

*Needle Biopsy*—If the procedure will be done under local anesthesia, no special preparation is needed. General anesthesia is sometimes used for children and occasionally for very anxious adults. If your biopsy will be done under general anesthesia, you should not eat anything for 8–12 hours before the test.

*Open Biopsy*—If this test is done under general anesthesia, you will be asked to eat nothing for 8–12 hours before the test. If your stomach is empty, there is less risk of vomiting and other complications of anesthesia.

## Procedure:

*Needle Biopsy*—This procedure is done in a hospital radiology department or in an operating room by an orthopedic surgeon. You will be positioned on an examining table or firm bed. The skin overlying the bone to be biopsied will be cleansed and shaved if necessary. A local anesthetic will be injected to numb the skin over the bone. In some cases, general anesthesia is used.

The surgeon will then make a small incision (less than 1 inch long) and will insert the hollow biopsy needle through the incision into the bone. He or she will rotate the needle and then remove it, carrying with it a small sample of bone. Pressure will then be applied to the biopsy site to stop the bleeding and the incision will be closed with a few stitches. An antiseptic and a bandage will be applied. This test usually takes 15–30 minutes.

*Open Biopsy*—This test is done in an operating room by an orthopedic surgeon. You will be given either a regional or a general anesthetic (see p. 465). An injection containing a sedative medication is usually given by injection about an hour before the procedure begins. An intravenous (IV) line will be placed in a vein, usually in your arm.

If general anesthesia is used, you will be given a mixture of anesthetic gases and oxygen through a hollow endotracheal tube which is inserted through your mouth into the airway (trachea) which leads to your lungs. Once you are asleep, the biopsy site will be shaved and cleansed. The surgeon will make an incision several inches long over the bone to be sampled, remove a small piece of bone, and close the incision with stitches.

Depending on the course of action you and your doctor have agreed on, the surgeon may send a frozen section for immediate microscopic inspection and perform further surgery if microscopic exam reveals cancer (see p. 334). This procedure usually takes 30–60 minutes, but may take longer if a frozen section is required.

The stitches will be removed in 5–14 days after the procedure.

## How Does It Feel?

*Needle Biopsy*—You will feel a needle prick and a mild stinging sensation as the local anesthetic is injected and will feel pressure and perhaps a brief, sharp pain when the needle enters the bone. You may feel a brief, aching pain as the sample is withdrawn. The biopsy site may be sore and tender for 1–3 days after the procedure. You may be given pain medication to use as needed.

*Open Biopsy*—You will be asleep and will feel nothing during the procedure. You may feel sleepy and mildly disoriented for 1–2 hours after waking. (See Anesthesia, p. 465.) You may be given pain medication to use as needed. You will probably feel some pain and tenderness at the biopsy site for 2–6 days.

In the days immediately after the bone biopsy, watch for prolonged bleeding, increasing tissue redness or tenderness, excessive drainage from the biopsy site, fever, or increasing pain on movement. If any of these occur, notify your doctor immediately.

**Risks:**

There is a very slight chance that the needle could either fracture the bone being sampled or injure one of the nerves, vessels, or organs near the biopsy site. For example, if one of the back vertebrae is the biopsy site, there could be some injury to the kidneys or to the large artery (aorta) that runs just in front of the backbone. Such complications are rare, but may require an operation to repair. If general anesthesia is used, the risk of death from the anesthetic itself is less than 1 in 3000.

There is some risk of prolonged bleeding in patients with bleeding disorders. Persons with a low platelet count may need a platelet transfusion before this test is done.

There is a slight chance that the biopsy site might become infected, delaying healing and possibly leading to further complications, such as bone infection (osteomyelitis).

**Results:**

The main concern with a bone biopsy is usually whether cancer is present. Biopsy results frequently reveal normal bone or a benign (noncancerous) condition such as a bone cyst or osteoma. However, sometimes a cancerous (malignant) condition such as osteosarcoma, Ewing's sarcoma, or multiple myeloma is found. Results may also indicate infections or metabolic disorders of the bones.

**Cost:**

> Needle biopsy: $300 to $500
> Open biopsy: $700 to $1200

# Bone Marrow Biopsy and Aspiration

Bone marrow is the soft tissue inside some of the longer bones. The marrow produces red and white blood cells and platelets (particles that help your blood clot). In certain diseases the marrow produces too many or too few of these vital blood cells. In this test, a small sample of bone marrow is removed through a needle inserted into a bone—most frequently the hip or the breastbone. The sample is then examined under a microscope. In a *bone marrow aspiration*, a fluid specimen is drawn out. In a *needle biopsy*, a core of solid cells is removed.

**Why Performed:**

This test is most frequently ordered after an abnormal type or number of red blood cells, white blood cells, or platelets is found in a complete blood count (see p. 61). For example, if you have recurrent bleeding or bruising and a low platelet count (thrombocytopenia), a bone marrow examination may reveal the cause.

This test is sometimes used to diagnose the cause of certain types of anemia (decreased red blood cells) or to evaluate abnormal white blood cells due to a cancer of the bone marrow (leukemia). It can be used to monitor the extent and response to therapy of such cancers as multiple myeloma and Hodgkin's disease and may also help to determine the cause of decreased immunity to infection.

**Preparation:**

Tell your doctor if
> You are allergic to any medications or
> anesthetics

You are taking any medications
You have had bleeding problems
You might be pregnant

You will be asked to sign a consent form authorizing this procedure. Use the opportunity to discuss with your doctor any concerns you may have about the need for the test, the risks of the test, or how and when it will be performed.

If you are to be given a sedative, you should bring someone to drive you home after the test.

## Procedure:

A bone marrow biopsy is performed by a physician—frequently a hematologist (blood specialist)—and an assistant. A laboratory technician may also be present to help prepare the specimen. This test may be done in a physician's office or at your bedside if you are in the hospital.

You may be given an injection containing a mild sedative about an hour before this test.

Bone marrow samples are usually taken from your hip, though the breastbone (sternum) may be used as an alternative site. In infants and young children, bone marrow samples are sometimes taken from the tibia (shinbone) just below the knee.

*Bone Marrow Aspiration*—The skin over the biopsy site is cleansed with antiseptic solution, and local anesthetic is injected to numb the skin. After a few minutes to let the anesthetic take effect, the biopsy needle is inserted into the bone. The metal core is removed from the needle, and a sample of bone marrow is drawn back up into the syringe. The needle is then withdrawn. Pressure is applied to the biopsy site to stop any bleeding, and a bandage is applied.

*Needle Biopsy*—The skin is cleansed with antiseptic solution and is injected with a local anesthetic to numb the skin over the biopsy site. After a few minutes to let the anesthetic take effect, the biopsy needle is inserted into the bone. The core of the needle is removed and the needle is advanced and rotated in both directions, forcing a tiny core of bone into the needle. The needle is then removed. Pressure is applied to the biopsy site. When the bleeding has stopped a bandage is applied.

Each test takes about 10–20 minutes. You will be asked to lie down for 10–15 minutes after the test. If the bleeding has stopped and your blood pressure is normal at the end of that time, you may resume your normal activities. If you have been given a sedative, you may need more time— as long as several hours—to fully recover.

## How Does It Feel?

*Bone Marrow Aspiration*—You will feel a stinging sensation as the anesthetic is injected and will feel pressure when the needle is inserted. You may feel a brief, sharp pain as the sample is drawn out. If you do feel pain, it will stop in a few seconds, as soon as the suction stops.

*Needle Biopsy*—You will feel a stinging pain from the anesthetic injection and a dull to sharp pain that will last as long as the needle is being advanced and removed. This pain may occasionally be fairly severe in some people. The local anesthetic doesn't affect this deeper bone pain, but the pain lasts a minute or less.

There may be some soreness at the biopsy site for several days. If it is very painful, you may wish to ask your doctor for a pain medication.

## Risks:

Complications of this test are extremely rare, and problems such as persistent bleeding or infection can almost always be controlled.

For people with bleeding problems,

pressure on the biopsy site after the procedure should be continued for 10 to 20 minutes or longer. If necessary, a person may be transfused with the necessary clotting factors before the test to prevent prolonged bleeding.

If the marrow sample is taken from the breastbone, there is an extremely remote risk of accidental puncture of the heart, lung, or a major blood vessel. This may require emergency surgery.

**Results:**
Test results will be available in several days. The various types and numbers of maturing blood cells will be determined. This can help reveal whether the bone marrow is producing cells and, if so, whether the cells are normal or abnormal. The cause of such conditions as anemia (too few red blood cells), thrombocytopenia (too few platelets), or abnormal white blood cells can frequently be determined. Cancers of the bone marrow (such as leukemia or Hodgkin's disease) may be detected.

**Cost:**
$200 to $300 including laboratory fees

# Kidney Biopsy
## (Renal Biopsy)

The kidneys are two fist-sized organs which manufacture urine. They are located on either side of the backbone at the bottom of the rib cage, a few inches above the waist (see p. 261).

In this test a sample of kidney tissue is removed through a needle inserted through your back just beneath the lowest rib, several inches to the side of the backbone. The tissue sample is then sent to a pathology laboratory, where it is examined under a microscope.

**Why Performed:**
This test is most frequently ordered when there is unexplained, persistent blood or protein in the urine or unexplained decreased kidney function. It is also sometimes used to evaluate a transplanted kidney for evidence of a rejection reaction.

**Preparation:**
Tell your doctor if
    You have allergies to any medications
      or anesthetics
    You are taking any medications
    You have had bleeding problems
    You might be pregnant

You will be asked to sign a consent form authorizing this procedure. Take this opportunity to discuss with your doctor any concerns you may have about the need for the test, the risks of the test, or how it will be performed.

Blood tests to evaluate your blood's ability to clot will probably be done, usually several days before the test. You may be asked to abstain from all food and drink for 8 hours before the test.

**Procedure:**
You will usually be admitted to the hospital the day before the test, and can expect to be in the hospital 2–3 days. You may be asked to take a mild sedative and/or a pain medication one-half to one hour before the test.

This test is usually performed in a hospital special procedures room or in an x-ray or ultrasound laboratory. It is performed by a physician and an assistant.

Blood and urine specimens are usually collected immediately before the test. This is to establish a baseline to compare with later tests.

It is particularly important that you follow the physician's directions about breathing and keeping still while the test is being performed.

You will be asked to lie face down on a firm surface. A sandbag, a firm pillow, or a rolled towel will be placed beneath your body to support your abdomen. Be sure you make yourself as comfortable as possible so you can hold still during the biopsy.

The doctor will examine your back and may mark the biopsy site by making a slight indentation in your skin with a pencil or blunt instrument. In some hospitals, ultrasound or x-ray is used to help locate the proper site. The biopsy may be done on either the right or the left side, though the majority are done on the right to avoid injury to the spleen and large blood vessels that lie on the left. The chosen site will then be cleansed with an antiseptic solution and draped with sterile sheets.

A local anesthetic will be injected to numb the skin at the chosen site. The doctor will then make a tiny (about one-eighth inch) incision in the skin. You will then be asked to take another deep breath and hold it and to stay very still. A short (3- to 4-inch) very thin needle (the locating needle) is then inserted through the incision and into the kidney. You will then be asked to take several deep breaths, so that the doctor can verify proper placement of the needle: if the needle is in the kidney, it will move back and forth with each breath.

Once the locating needle is properly placed, the doctor will mark the desired depth on the needle shaft. The needle will then be removed.

The doctor will then insert a longer (8"–10"), thicker (about one-eighth-inch) biopsy needle through the incision and along the path of the first needle. You will again be asked to hold your breath and stay very still. The needle is then advanced into the kidney to the same depth the first needle was. You will then be asked to breathe in and out. Again, the needle will move with each breath if it is properly placed. If not, it will be readjusted.

Once the needle is properly positioned, the solid core is removed and the inner biopsy needle is inserted. You will again be asked to take a deep breath and hold very still. The inner needle is then pushed into the kidney and immediately pulled out. The specimen is then examined to make sure it is adequate. Sometimes a second sample is taken.

When an adequate sample has been obtained, pressure will be placed on the biopsy site for several minutes to stop the bleeding and a bandage will be applied. The part of the test involving the needles takes only about 5 minutes. The entire procedure takes about 30 minutes.

You will remain in the hospital on the night following the test and will be asked to lie on your back for the next 12–24 hours. During this time you will be observed closely to make sure that your kidney function is normal and that there are no complications. Urine specimens will be collected and blood samples will be drawn. The nursing staff will check your pulse, blood pressure, and temperature. You should drink all the fluids you can during this period.

You may return to your normal diet immediately after the test. For 2 weeks after this test you should avoid such strenuous activities as heavy lifting, hard running, motorcycle riding, contact sports, or other activities which might jar or jolt the kidney.

### How Does It Feel?

When the biopsy area is cleansed, the antiseptic solution may feel very cold. When the local anesthetic is injected, you will feel a brief stinging sensation.

You may feel a brief, sharp pain as the locating needle is inserted through the back and into the kidney; and when the biopsy specimen is taken, you will feel an intense sudden aching sensation. (Many patients describe it as being kicked in the back or having the wind knocked out of them.) This will last only about 5 seconds.

For 2–3 days after the procedure it is normal to feel mild muscle soreness in the area of the biopsy. However, if you experience severe deep pain in the back, belly, or groin, or notice bleeding from the biopsy site, let your nurse or doctor know. Many patients experience bright red blood in the urine within the first 24 hours after this test. This is expected. However, let your doctor know if you notice blood in your urine 24 hours or more after the test.

*Patient Comments*:

"The most remarkable thing was the way they used ultrasound to locate my kidney. The most surprising thing is how quickly the whole thing was completed. The most distressing thing was the feeling of having the air knocked out of you when the needle was inserted and removed."

### Risks:

There is a very slight risk of infection of the skin at the biopsy site. There may be some bleeding into the muscle, which can cause soreness. The main complication of this test is prolonged bleeding into the kidney itself. In less than 1 in 1000 cases, injury caused by the biopsy results in the loss of the kidney.

Very rarely, a major blood vessel may be ruptured by the biopsy needle. This may require transfusion or emergency surgery.

You should discuss with your doctor the specific risks of the procedure in your case.

### Results:

The specimens are placed on slides and observed under a light microscope and an electron microscope. Results are usually available in 7–10 days.

Test results may indicate scarring due to infection, poor blood flow (e.g., renal vein thrombosis), or signs of multiorgan disease (e.g., systemic lupus erythematosus affecting the kidney). Kidney biopsies rarely show malignancies.

About 20%–30% of the time, the results of this test will be inconclusive. Sometimes a repeat biopsy is necessary.

### Cost:

$800 to $1500 (including hospital stay)

### Special Considerations:

★A sample of kidney tissue may also be obtained by *open biopsy*. This is a surgical procedure performed in an operating room under general anesthesia. Open biopsy is the method of choice when a tumor is suspected. It may also be done when a patient has one functioning kidney, to reduce the chance of injuring the remaining kidney. (However, there is the additional risk of the general anesthetic and major surgery.)

In this procedure an incision is made through the back and a small wedge of kidney tissue is cut out with a scalpel.

# Liver Biopsy

The liver is a pyramid-shaped organ which lies within the upper right side of the abdomen. The tip of the pyramid lies behind the right nipple, its base at the level of the lowest rib (see p. 281). It is the body's largest internal organ and performs many functions: it converts newly digested food to energy and stores it for later use, removes waste products from the blood, helps regulate blood sugar levels, stores iron, builds proteins, and produces cholesterol and bile.

In this test a needle is inserted through the rib cage and into the liver to obtain a tissue specimen. The tissue is then examined by microscope. This test is used to help diagnose a wide variety of disorders of the liver.

### Why Performed:

This test is most commonly used to help determine the cause of unexplained enlargement of the liver (hepatomegaly); persistent abnormal liver enzymes as detected by blood tests such as alkaline phosphatase, bilirubin, SGOT, and SGPT; unexplained yellowing of the skin (jaundice); or an abnormality found on ultrasound, CT scan, or nuclear scan. In addition to its use in diagnosing a wide variety of liver diseases, this test is used to follow response to treatment and to assess the effects of certain medications on the liver.

### Preparation:

Tell your doctor if
    You have allergies to any medications or anesthetics
    You are taking any medications
    You have had bleeding problems
    You might be pregnant

You will be asked to sign a consent form authorizing this procedure. Use this opportunity to discuss with your doctor any concerns you may have about the need for the test, the risks of the test, or how it will be performed.

Blood tests are often done before this biopsy to evaluate your blood's ability to clot. An ultrasound or nuclear scan of the liver is sometimes done to help determine the best biopsy point.

You may be asked to abstain from all food and liquids after midnight on the night before this test is to be done, or as instructed by your physician. Unless you will be staying overnight in the hospital, you should arrange to have someone drive you home when the test is finished.

For your own comfort, be sure to empty your bladder immediately before the test.

### Procedure:

This test does not in itself require overnight hospitalization. The test may be done on an inpatient or an outpatient basis, and is usually done by a physician and an assistant, either in a hospital special procedures room or at your bedside if you are hospitalized. You will be given a sedative and/or a pain medication by injection about an hour before the procedure.

You will be asked to lie on your back with your right elbow out to the side and your right hand under your head. It is important that you remain as still as possible throughout this procedure.

The doctor will first examine your liver. The examination may include some thumping and pressing at the bottom of your ribs on the right side. The doctor will then mark a spot between two of your ribs or below your lowest rib. This is the point at which the biopsy needle will be inserted. The area will be cleaned with an antiseptic solution and draped with sterile towels.

A small needle will be used to inject a local anesthetic at the biopsy site. The skin, the underlying tissue, and the diaphragm (the thin sheet of muscle just below the lungs) will be numbed.

Your doctor will then make a small incision (about one-quarter inch) at the site and will insert the biopsy needle. You may be instructed to take a deep breath, blow all the air out, and then hold your breath while the biopsy is taken. (Some doctors will have you take a full breath and hold it.) This reduces the chance of the needle puncturing your lung or tearing your liver. It is extremely important not to move during the 1–2 seconds it takes to do the biopsy.

The biopsy needle will be inserted and withdrawn quickly—within 2 seconds or less. As soon as the needle is withdrawn, you can begin breathing normally again. Pressure will be applied to help stop the bleeding, and a bandage will be placed over the site. The entire procedure usually takes less than 20 minutes.

You will be asked to rest in bed at the hospital for 6–8 hours after the procedure. You should lie on your right side with a firm pillow under your waist for the first 2 hours to help stop any bleeding. A nurse will check your pulse, blood pressure, and temperature at regular intervals following the test. If you had the test as an outpatient and no complications develop in 6–8 hours, you will be allowed to go home. You may resume your regular diet and activities but should avoid strenuous activities for several days.

### How Does It Feel?

You may feel a stinging pain as the anesthetic needle is inserted, and another brief pain as the anesthetic itself is injected. When the biopsy needle is inserted you may feel a deep pressure and a dull pain in your abdomen. You may feel a dull pain after the anesthetic wears off. This rarely lasts more than 12 hours and is usually well controlled by a mild pain medication. Pain from this area is occasionally felt in the right shoulder—this is called referred pain.

Be sure to tell your nurse or doctor if you notice chills and fever, difficulty in breathing, increasing tenderness at the biopsy site, or severe pain at the biopsy site or in the chest, shoulder, or abdomen.

### Risks:

A liver biopsy involves some risk. However, if a definitive diagnosis of a liver problem cannot be obtained by such other tests as blood tests, liver scan, and x-rays, this risk is small compared with the risk associated with many of the diseases it is used to diagnose.

The most serious side effect is prolonged internal bleeding. Some bleeding occurs in about 1 case in 600. In about 1 case in 1200, the bleeding is serious enough to require a transfusion. In about 1 case in 2400, it is serious enough to require emergency surgery.

Other possible complications include collapsed lung (pneumothorax) and injury to the gallbladder or the kidney. Some complications may require immediate surgery. Death due to complications of this test occurs in about 2–3 of every 10,000 cases.

### Results:

Results will be available in 7–10 days. Liver biopsies can help diagnose a wide variety of liver diseases, including bacterial and viral infections (hepatitis, liver abscess, tuberculosis), cirrhosis, liver damage caused by alcohol and other toxic substances, and tumors (benign and malignant). The most common form of malignant liver tumor is a hepatic metastasis—a tumor seeded in the liver from a preexisting cancer elsewhere in the body.

**Cost:**
$200 to $300

**Special Considerations:**

★If a more extensive sample of liver tissue is needed, it can be obtained by an *open biopsy* of the liver—which can be done either by an exploratory operation with a 3"–4" incision in the abdomen or through laparoscopy (see p. 325). A small slice of tissue is cut from the liver, and the biopsy site is closed with stitches. These procedures are performed in an operating room, usually under general anesthesia (see p. 465).

# Lung Biopsy

In this test a small piece of tissue is removed from the lung and sent to the lab for analysis. The tissue may be removed by one of three methods: by a needle inserted between two ribs (*needle biopsy*), through an instrument passed through your mouth or nose and down your throat (*bronchoscopic biopsy*), or through a surgical incision in the chest (*open biopsy*). The specimen is then examined for cancer, infection, and other lung diseases.

**Why Performed:**
Lung biopsies are most frequently performed to evaluate abnormalities detected by x-ray, especially single round spots or "coin lesions" which could be cancers. They can also be used to help diagnose a wide variety of other lung diseases.

If the suspect area is located deep within the chest, bronchoscopic biopsy (p. 315) is often the method of choice. If the area is close to the chest wall, a needle biopsy is usually done. When the suspect areas are spread throughout the lungs, either needle biopsy or bronchoscopy may be used. Open biopsy is usually reserved for situations in which neither of the other two methods has yielded a diagnosis.

**Preparation:**
Tell your doctor if
> You have allergies to any medications or anesthetics
> You are taking any medications
> You have had bleeding problems
> You might be pregnant

You will be asked to sign a consent form authorizing this procedure. Use this opportunity to discuss with your doctor any concerns you may have about the need for the test, its risks, or how and when it will be performed.

If a general anesthetic will be used, you will be asked to take nothing by mouth for 8–12 hours before this test. In some instances you may be allowed clear fluids. If you are taking medication, ask your doctor whether you should continue it.

**Procedure:**
A needle biopsy or bronchoscopic biopsy can be done on an outpatient basis. An open lung biopsy will require a hospital stay of at least several days. A chest x-ray and several blood tests will be performed before the test to make sure your clotting mechanism is working well. You will be asked to undress and put on a hospital gown.

*Bronchoscopic Biopsy*—See p. 315.

*Needle Biopsy*—This procedure may be done in a hospital x-ray room or a special procedures room by a surgeon or radiologist. You may be given an injection containing a sedative about half an hour before the test begins.

You will be asked to sit in a chair with your arms folded on a table in front of you. X-rays will be taken to locate the suspicious area (lesion), and small metal markers will be attached to the overlying skin to help mark its position. These markers will help the doctor position the needle correctly.

The skin over the biopsy site will be cleansed with an antiseptic solution and the area around it draped with sterile towels. It is very important that you do not touch this sterile area.

A local anesthetic will be injected to numb your skin and the underlying tissues at the place the biopsy needle will be inserted. The doctor will then make a small (less than one-half inch) incision with a scalpel. You will be asked to hold your breath, while the doctor inserts the biopsy needle through the incision and into the lung.

When an adequate sample of lung tissue has been obtained, the needle will be removed. Try not to cough or move while the needle is in your chest. A sterile dressing will be applied to the biopsy site. An x-ray may then be taken to check for lung damage. The test takes about 30−45 minutes.

Following the test you will be checked regularly by a nurse for 2−4 hours. If no complications develop, you can return home or to your hospital room. Unless advised otherwise, you should rest for a day or two, and may then resume your regular activities, but should avoid strenuous activities for a week.

*Open Biopsy*—This test is usually done under general anesthesia (see p. 465) in an operating room by a surgeon, an anesthesiologist, and one or more assistants. A sed-ative medication is usually given by injection about an hour before the procedure begins. An intravenous (IV) line will be placed in a vein, usually in your arm. During the procedure you will be given a mixture of anesthetic gases and oxygen through a hollow endotracheal tube which is inserted through your mouth into the airway (trachea) which leads to your lungs.

An incision is made over the area of lung to be sampled. A wedge of lung tissue is removed, the incision in the overlying muscles is closed with stitches, and the skin incision is closed with an additional row of stitches. The procedure usually takes about one hour.

A chest tube is usually left in place, with one end inside your lung and the other end protruding out through the closed incision. The chest tube will remain for 1−2 days to prevent the collapse of your lung. A chest x-ray is usually taken after the procedure.

After the biopsy is completed, you will be taken to the recovery room and observed until you are fully awake and your gag reflex has recovered. You can then return to your hospital room.

The stitches will be removed in 7−14 days.

### How Does It Feel?

*Needle Biopsy*—If you receive a sedative, it will make you feel drowsy and relaxed. You will feel some burning or stinging for a few seconds as the local anesthetic is injected. You may feel a brief, sharp pain and some pressure as the biopsy needle is inserted into the lung.

*Open Biopsy*—The sedative injection will make you feel very sleepy and relaxed. During the procedure itself you will be asleep and feel nothing. After you wake up you will feel drowsy for several hours. For a day or two after the procedure you may notice some general tiredness and muscle aches from the anesthetic and a mild sore throat from the endotracheal tube. If your throat is sore, throat lozenges and warm salt-water gargles may help.

You may also feel some discomfort at the biopsy site when you breathe and mild pain or itching along the incision for 3–4 days. You may be given pain medication to use as needed.

Notify your doctor or nurse if you notice any of the following after the lung biopsy: extreme chest pain, lightheadedness, difficulty in breathing, or cyanosis (a very pale or slightly bluish tinge to your skin). You may notice a small amount of blood in your sputum for a day or two after the biopsy. If the bleeding continues or is very heavy, notify your doctor.

### Risks:
*Needle Biopsy*—A needle biopsy is safer than an open biopsy, mainly because no general anesthetic is used. Sometimes air leaks in through the hole made by the biopsy needle. This usually causes no problem, but can lead to a collapse of the lung. If this occurs, it may be necessary to insert a tube into the chest to remove the air.

Coughing of blood occurs in about 1 of 20 people having needle biopsies. This is usually mild and stops on its own. Other possible, but rare, side effects include prolonged bleeding or infection.

*Open Biopsy*—The average risk of death from general anesthetic itself is less than 1 in 3000. Possible complications of an open lung biopsy include infection or an air leak into the chest. Such a leak may result in a partially or totally collapsed lung (pneumothorax) and may require the insertion of a chest tube to remove the air.

The overall risk of this test depends on the severity of preexisting lung disease. If you have severe respiratory problems, your breathing may be somewhat impaired while you are recovering from this test. If your breathing capacity is relatively normal, there is very little risk of serious complication from the test.

The risks of this test vary greatly from person to person. Discuss the risks in your particular circumstances with your physician.

### Results:
Samples of lung tissue will be sent to the pathology laboratory where the cells will be examined under a microscope. Another sample may be sent to the microbiology lab to be examined for infection. Results are usually available in 2–4 days, although some cultures, like tuberculosis, may take up to 6 weeks.

Lumps (nodules) in the lung may be due to active infection, scars from previous infections, benign tumors, or several different types of cancer. If a lung cancer is present, determining the type will help determine the appropriate therapy (surgery, radiation, and/or chemotherapy). The biopsy may also reveal such lung diseases as pulmonary fibrosis, sarcoidosis, or certain infections.

The results of a lung biopsy should always be considered along with your history, physical examination, and the results of such tests as sputum cytology, cultures, and bronchoscopy before a final diagnosis is made.

### Cost:
Needle biopsy: $200 to $300
Open biopsy: $1000 to $1500

### Special Considerations:
★*Pleural Tap*—See p. 365.

# Lymph Node Biopsy

The lymph channels (lymphatics) are an extensive system of branching vessels which carry the lymphatic fluid formed in the tissues back to the bloodstream. Along the channels of the larger lymph vessels are clusters of lymph nodes. There are hundreds of lymph nodes in the body.

Lymph nodes are normally small, soft, and flat. The majority of nodes in most healthy people can't be felt, though in some healthy individuals, especially in children, small nodes in the neck, armpit, or groin may be palpable.

The lymph nodes help fight disease by filtering invading organisms out of the lymph fluid and by producing cells and antibodies which attack them. Thus in the presence of certain infections and some other diseases, the lymph nodes may enlarge as part of the body's defense reaction.

Most of the time swollen nodes (commonly called "swollen glands," though they are not really glands) are the result of such infections as an infected scratch or a sore throat. But there are a number of other conditions, including some forms of cancer, which can produce lymph node enlargement.

In this test an entire lymph node or a piece of tissue from a lymph node is removed for microscopic examination. The sample may be obtained either by inserting a needle into a node (*needle biopsy*) or by surgically removing part or all of a node (*open biopsy*). Some lymph nodes may be biopsied by special scoping procedures (see Mediastinoscopy, p. 331). If infection is suspected, lymph nodes may be cultured as well.

## Why Performed:

This test is done to determine the cause of enlarged lymph nodes, especially when enlarged nodes are accompanied by such persistent signs and symptoms as swollen arms or legs, breathing difficulties, backache, difficulty in swallowing, weight loss, itching, hoarseness, fever, night sweats, or coughing of blood. This test is sometimes used to help diagnose suspected cancer and to determine the extent to which cancer has spread.

## Preparation:

Tell your doctor if
> You are allergic to any medications or anesthetics
> You are taking any medications
> You have had bleeding problems
> You might be pregnant

You will be asked to sign a consent form authorizing this procedure. Take this opportunity to discuss with your doctor any concerns you may have about the need for the test, the risks of the test, or how it will be performed.

Sometimes a sedative injection is given about an hour before the test to help you relax. If a needle biopsy is done, no special preparation is necessary.

If an open biopsy is done under general anesthesia, you will be asked to refrain from food and drink after midnight the night before the test.

## Procedure:

This test is done in a hospital operating room by a physician and an assistant.

*Needle Biopsy:* You will be asked to lie on an examining table. The surgeon will cleanse the biopsy site, inject a local anesthetic, and insert a biopsy needle into the node. A sample of tissue is removed through the needle, pressure is applied to the biopsy site to stop the bleeding, and a bandage is placed over the site.

This test takes about 15–30 minutes. You may resume your regular diet and activities as soon as the test is over.

*Open Biopsy:* You will be asked to lie on an examining table. The skin over the lymph node to be biopsied will be cleansed, and the site draped with a sterile sheet. Sometimes a general anesthetic is given (see p. 465), but usually a local anesthetic is adequate.

A small incision (usually only 1–2 inches) is made, and the surgeon removes the entire lymph node or a slice of it, closes the wound with stitches, and applies a bandage.

## How Does It Feel?

If a local anesthetic is used, you should feel little or no pain during the procedure, though you may feel a mild stinging when the anesthetic itself is injected. If you do feel pain during the procedure, let your doctor know.

The biopsy site may be somewhat tender for 1 to 2 days after the needle biopsy and for 3 to 4 days after an open biopsy. Notify your doctor if you notice any increased tenderness or swelling, bleeding at the biopsy site, or a pus discharge at the biopsy site.

## Risks:

If general anesthesia is used, the average risk of death from the anesthetic itself is less than 1 in 3000. The degree of risk depends on which lymph nodes are being biopsied. For example, the risk of bleeding is somewhat greater if the node to be biopsied lies near the large blood vessels at the base of the neck. There is also a small risk of infection, but on the whole the risks of this procedure—other than the risk of general anesthesia—are few and minor. Ask your doctor about the risk of this procedure in your particular circumstances.

## Results:

Most results should be available in several days, but identification of some infections may take longer. Results of tuberculosis cultures may not be available for several weeks.

Microscopic examination of the tissue removed can usually distinguish between malignant and nonmalignant causes of lymph node enlargement. The most frequent benign result of this test is normal lymph node or enlargement due to chronic infection. The most frequent malignant results are lymphoma, Hodgkin's disease, and metastasis of a preexisting cancer elsewhere in the body.

It is sometimes impossible to make a diagnosis from the sample obtained. When the results of this test are inconclusive, other diagnostic procedures such as laparoscopy, laparotomy, or mediastinoscopy may be able to provide additional information.

## Cost:

$200 to $500 (more if anesthesia is used)

# Skin Biopsy

In this test a small piece of the skin is removed and sent to a laboratory, where it is examined by microscope and may be cultured to look for infection. Samples may be taken of a suspected cancerous growth or sore or to help in diagnosing other skin conditions.

There are three kinds of skin biopsy: In a *punch biopsy*, a small cylinder of skin, sometimes involving only a portion of the suspect area, is removed with a skin punch. In a *shave biopsy*, the outer part of the suspect skin area is removed. In an *excisional biopsy*, the entire suspect area is taken out.

## Why Performed:

A skin biopsy is used to diagnose skin conditions that cannot be identified by their appearance or fail to respond to treatment. Without a biopsy it is often impossible to determine whether an abnormality of the skin—particularly a mole or other skin problem that has changed in size or color, or a sore that has not healed—is cancerous. It is also used to diagnose some bacterial and fungal skin infections and a number of other skin conditions.

## Preparation:

Tell your doctor if

> You are allergic to any medications or anesthetics
>
> You are taking any medications
>
> You have had bleeding problems
>
> You might be pregnant

You will be asked to sign a consent form authorizing this procedure. Take this opportunity to discuss with your doctor any concerns you may have about the need for the test, the risks of the test, or how it will be performed.

## Procedure:

This test is usually performed in an office by a physician, often a skin specialist (dermatologist).

*Punch Biopsy*—After a local anesthetic is injected, the skin around the area to be sampled is pulled taut. A hollow instrument (punch) is inserted into the skin and rotated to free a "plug" of skin and underlying fat. The punch is then removed, and the plug is lifted out with forceps or a needle. If a large punch specimen is taken, the skin

may be closed with one or two stitches. If stitches are not used, bleeding will be controlled by pressure or cautery.

*Shave Biopsy*—A local anesthetic is injected. The physician then uses a sharp scalpel to cut the protruding growth off flush with the skin. Bleeding is controlled by pressure or cautery.

*Excisional Biopsy*—A local anesthetic is injected. The entire lump, spot, or sore is cut out with a scalpel. The incision is then closed with stitches. Bleeding is controlled by pressure or cautery. If the biopsy site is large, a skin graft may be used to cover it.

Keep the area as dry and clean as possible until healing is complete. Stitches in your face are usually removed in 3–5 days. Stitches in other parts of your body are usually removed in 7–14 days.

## How Does It Feel?

You will feel a brief stinging when the local anesthetic is injected. You should not feel anything at the biopsy site at the time the sample is taken.

Notify your doctor if you notice extensive swelling, tenderness, redness, or pus discharge at the biopsy site.

## Risks:

There is a slight risk of infection and a slight risk of continued bleeding. If you have a history of forming large scars (keloids) in response to skin wounds, there is a fair chance that keloids will appear in response to the biopsy.

## Results:

Results are usually available in 7–10 days.

Results may indicate a benign (noncancerous) or malignant (cancerous) condition. Common benign growths include cysts, warts, moles, keloids, dermatofibromas, and neurofibromas.

Skin cancers are the most common

cancers in humans: about 300,000 new skin cancers occur each year in the United States. Over 75% are cases of basal-cell carcinoma, a nonlife-threatening skin cancer which most frequently appears on the head and neck, especially in the folds of the nose. Other malignant results include squamous-cell carcinoma and malignant melanoma.

Squamous-cell carcinoma is a slow-growing, slow-spreading cancer. It is most frequently found on the lips, in the mouth, and on the genitals.

Malignant melanoma is the most serious skin cancer—mainly because it can spread (metastasize) to other areas of the body. It can originate anywhere on the body, and usually appears as a spreading, darkly pigmented, flat spot with irregular borders.

Biopsy specimens can also help detect bacterial and fungal infections as well as some inflammatory diseases of the skin.

## Cost:
$80 to $200

## Special Considerations:
★If the biopsy is to be done on an area where the cosmetic result is important to you (face, hands, etc.), you may wish to have the biopsy done by a physician with special training or experience in plastic surgery techniques which can minimize scarring.

# Thyroid Biopsy

The thyroid is a butterfly-shaped gland that lies in front of the windpipe (trachea) at the top of the neck, with its wings (lobes) extending back on either side of the Adam's apple. A thyroid biopsy is a test for thyroid cancer.

There are three different types of thyroid biopsy: the *large-needle* (or *core*) *biopsy*, the *fine-needle* (also sometimes called an *aspiration* or *skinny-needle*) *biopsy*, and the *open biopsy*. In the first two procedures, a needle is introduced through the skin of the neck and into the thyroid gland. A sample of thyroid tissue is removed and sent to a laboratory for microscopic examination. In the open biopsy a sample of thyroid tissue is taken through a surgical incision.

## Why Performed:
There are three indications for biopsy of the thyroid: a palpable lump (nodule), a "cold" nodule in the thyroid detected by thyroid scan (p. 229), or a diffusely enlarged thyroid gland due to unknown causes.

Many thyroid specialists now recommend a skinny-needle thyroid biopsy as the test of first choice if a thyroid lump is discovered.

## Preparation:
Tell your doctor if
   You have allergies to any medications or anesthetics
   You are taking any medications
   You have had bleeding problems
   You might be pregnant

You will be asked to sign a consent form authorizing this procedure. Use this opportunity to discuss with your doctor any concerns you may have about the need for the test, the risks of the test, or how it will be performed.

If a needle biopsy is to be done, no special preparation is needed. If a large-needle biopsy is planned, your doctor may order tests to evaluate your blood's ability to clot. If general anesthesia is to be used, you should not eat or drink anything for 8−12 hours before the test. If your stomach is empty, there is less risk of vomiting and complications.

## Procedure:

*Fine-Needle Biopsy*—This test is done in a doctor's office, in a hospital treatment room, or at hospital bedside by a physician. No anesthetic is used, since the biopsy needle is about the same size as the needle that would be used to inject the anesthetic.

You will be asked to lie on your back with a pillow under your shoulders and your neck extended. The biopsy site is cleansed. The thin needle is then inserted into the thyroid. A sample of thyroid cells and fluid is drawn into the needle. The needle is then quickly withdrawn. Try not to cough or swallow while the needle is in place. Pressure is applied to the biopsy site to stop the bleeding, and the site is covered with a small bandage.

This test takes about 3–5 minutes.

*Large-Needle Biopsy*—This test is done in a doctor's office, in a hospital treatment room, or at hospital bedside by a physician.

You will probably be given an injection containing a mild sedative shortly before the procedure. You will be asked to lie on your back, with a pillow under your shoulders, your head tipped back, and your neck extended. The physician will cleanse the biopsy site and will inject a local anesthetic. Then a small incision (less than one inch long) will be made in the skin, and the biopsy needle will be inserted through the incision and into your thyroid. Do not cough or swallow when the needle is in place.

A sample of tissue is removed in the needle as the needle is quickly withdrawn. Pressure is applied to the biopsy site. Sometimes the pressure must be continued for 15 minutes to stop the bleeding. A bandage is then applied.

This test takes about 5–10 minutes.

*Open Incisional Biopsy*—This test is done in an operating room by a surgeon and an assistant. It is usually done under general anesthesia (see p. 465). A sedative medication is often given by injection about an hour before the procedure begins. An intravenous (IV) line will be placed in a vein, usually in your arm. During the procedure you will be given a mixture of anesthetic gases and oxygen through a hollow endotracheal tube, which is inserted through your mouth into the airway (trachea) which leads to your lungs.

After you are anesthetized, the surgeon makes a small incision in your neck. The whole thyroid lump or a portion of it is removed. The surgeon may send a sample of thyroid tissue to the laboratory while you are still on the operating table, then wait for the pathologist's report before continuing. (See Frozen Sections, p. 334). If cancer is present, part or all of the thyroid gland may be removed. The incision is then closed with stitches.

This test takes about 1 hour.

## How Does It Feel?

*Fine-Needle Biopsy*—The needle used in this test is so thin that even though no anesthetic is used, the whole thing feels as though you are receiving a quick injection. There is little or no tenderness after the test.

*Large-Needle Biopsy*—You will feel a stinging needle-prick when the local anesthetic is injected. While the sample is being taken you may feel a sharp sensation of pressure in your neck. This will last only a few seconds. The site may be sore for a few hours and tender for a day or two after the test.

*Open Biopsy*—The sedative injection will make you feel very sleepy and relaxed. During the procedure itself you will feel nothing, since you will be asleep (anesthetized). After you wake up, you will feel drowsy for several hours. For a day or two after the procedure you may notice some tiredness and some general aches and pains (the aftereffects of the anesthetic) and a mild sore throat (the result of the endotracheal tube). Throat lozenges and salt-water gargling may help with the sore throat. The incision site may be sore and tender for 3–4 days after the test.

If you experience pain or tenderness at the biopsy site after the test, you may be more comfortable lying with your head partially raised. You can avoid strain at the biopsy site by supporting the back of your neck with both hands when you sit up.

Keep the biopsy site clean and dry. Notify your doctor if you notice moderate to severe swelling or pain at the biopsy site or if you develop a fever.

### Risks:

If general anesthesia is used, there is a small but significant risk of death from complications of anesthesia (see p. 466).

The main complication is the risk of bleeding into the thyroid gland. This is more common with the large-needle biopsy, much less common with the skinny-needle biopsy.

If bleeding or swelling occurs, it can usually be managed by treating with cold compresses. Very rarely, surgery may be required to stop the bleeding.

### Results:

Results are usually available in 7–10 days.

A thyroid cyst can usually be diagnosed at the time of the biopsy—as the fluid is drawn back into the syringe, the nodule disappears.

Common results of this test include normal thyroid tissue, diffuse thyroid disease (e.g., thyroiditis, Graves' disease), or thyroid cancer.

Thyroid cancers are more frequent in women than in men. The three most common kinds of thyroid cancer are the slow-growing papillary carcinoma (60%–70% of all thyroid cancers), follicular carcinoma (15%–20%), and anaplastic carcinomas (10%–12%).

As it is not possible to sample all parts of the thyroid, a negative report on this test does not entirely rule out the possibility of thyroid cancer.

### Cost:

Fine-needle biopsy: $150 to $250
Large-needle biopsy: $200 to $300
Open-biopsy: $1000 to 1500

### Special Considerations:

★Some cases of thyroid cancer develop as a side effect of medical treatment. From the 1920s through the 1950s, one to two million U.S. children received radiation to the neck as a treatment for tonsillitis and other conditions. Recent studies show that about 1 in 4 of those so treated now have thyroid abnormalities. About 1 in 12 of those who received radiation now have thyroid cancer.

Most thyroid cancers are slow-growing and easily treated once they are detected. But it is most important that persons who received neck radiation as children be examined by a thyroid specialist every year or two. Those with positive findings on a physical exam should have a thyroid scan or thyroid biopsy.

# Taps

A *tap* (also known as *centesis*) is a test in which a long, thin needle is introduced into one of the internal cavities of the body in order to remove a sample of a fluid. The fluid obtained is analyzed under a microscope and may also be subjected to chemical testing or cultures. Analysis of the fluid obtained by a tap can frequently help determine whether infection, inflammation, or cancer is present.

A *dry tap* is a tap in which no fluid is obtained. A dry tap means either that there is no fluid in the target body cavity or that the fluid was missed.

## Abdominal Tap
### (Peritoneal Tap, Abdominal Paracentesis)

The abdominal cavity normally contains little or no free fluid, but in certain conditions fluid can accumulate. Fluid in the abdomen is called *ascites*.

In this procedure, a needle is inserted through the wall of the abdomen to obtain a sample of any free fluid that may be present. The fluid is then sent to the laboratory for analysis.

### Why Performed:

This test is performed to help determine the nature and cause of fluid in the abdomen. This test is also frequently done to check for internal bleeding after an injury to the abdomen.

### Preparation:

Tell your doctor if
>   You have allergies to any medications or anesthetics
>   You are taking any medications
>   You have had bleeding problems
>   You might be pregnant

You will be asked to sign a consent form authorizing this procedure. Take this opportunity to discuss with your doctor any concerns you may have about the need for the test, the risks of the test, or how it will be performed.

A blood sample may be taken for laboratory analysis before this test is done.

You will be asked to put on a hospital gown. For your own comfort and to decrease the chance of puncturing the bladder, you should empty your bladder immediately before the test.

### Procedure:

This test is done by a physician at your hospital bedside or in an office, treatment room, or emergency room. You will be either lying on your back or sitting up.

The puncture site or sites will be cleaned and shaved if necessary. A local anesthetic will be injected. The tap needle will then be inserted. The point of insertion is usually 1–2 inches below the navel, but other locations may be used. The needle is inserted 1 to 2 inches into your abdomen. A small incision (approximately one-quarter inch) may be made to help the doctor insert the needle.

A sample of fluid is withdrawn with a syringe. You may be asked to change positions to help the fluid drain out. Sometimes a sterile salt solution is introduced, then withdrawn and analyzed for cancer cells or blood. In some cases antibiotics may be introduced through the needle. Multiple punctures may be needed to locate and remove fluid.

The needle is then removed and a thick gauze dressing is applied to the tap site. If an incision was made, one or two stitches may be used to close it.

This procedure usually takes about 10–15 minutes, but may take longer if a large quantity of fluid must be removed.

Your pulse, blood pressure, and temperature may be checked regularly after the test to be sure that there are no complications. Shortly after the procedure is completed, you may be weighed and the distance around your abdomen may be measured. You may resume normal activities unless instructed otherwise.

### How Does It Feel?

You will feel a brief stinging sensation from the local anesthetic. You should feel only pressure when the tap needle is inserted. You may feel dizzy or lightheaded if a large quantity of fluid is withdrawn. Be sure to describe any such symptoms to your doctor during the test.

The tap site or sites may be sore for a day or two after the procedure. Be sure to let your doctor know if you experience fever, severe abdominal pain, or increasing abdominal redness or tenderness, or if you notice blood in the urine or bleeding or discharge from the tap site.

### Risks:

There is a very slight risk that the needle might puncture the bowel, the bladder, or a blood vessel within the abdomen. In rare cases this may require emergency surgery.

There is a slight risk that removal of a large quantity of fluid may produce shock, resulting in a sharp drop in your blood pressure after the test. This is rare and can be treated. Signs of shock include rapid heartbeat, dizziness, paleness, perspiration, and increased anxiety. There is also a slight risk of introducing an infection into the abdomen, which would require antibiotic treatment. This test is usually not performed on pregnant women, to avoid injuring the fetus.

### Results:

Preliminary results will be available within hours or by the next day. The abdominal fluid is examined and sent to the laboratory for microscopic examination, chemical testing, and, in some cases, culture. The presence of bloody fluid after an abdominal injury suggests internal bleeding from a ruptured organ or blood vessel.

Other findings may suggest infection, tumor (cancerous or noncancerous), appendicitis, damaged bowel, cirrhosis of the liver, or disease of the pancreas, kidneys, or heart.

### Cost:

$60 to $100

# Joint Tap
## (Synovial Fluid Analysis, Arthrocentesis, Joint Aspiration)

Within the capsule of most joints in the body there is a small amount of fluid which acts as a lubricant. Sometimes, due to injury, infection, or other disorder, the amount of fluid increases and the joint becomes swollen and painful. In such cases the cause of the swelling (effusion) can often be determined by analyzing a sample of the joint fluid (synovial fluid).

In this test a small hollow needle is inserted into a joint to remove a sample of the joint fluid. This test is most frequently performed on the knee, but can be done on almost any joint in the body. It is usually done under local anesthesia, but occasionally (e.g., in children and in tapping hip joints) a general anesthetic may be needed.

## Why Performed:

A painful, red, hot, swollen joint can have many causes. Your doctor may perform this tap to help distinguish among infection, gout, arthritis resulting from an injury (traumatic arthritis), rheumatoid arthritis, and other types of joint problems. This procedure is also sometimes used to inject a local anesthetic or other medication into the joint to ease a painful joint.

## Preparation:

Tell your doctor if
> You have allergies to any medications or anesthetics
> You are taking any medications
> You have had bleeding problems
> You might be pregnant

You will be asked to sign a consent form authorizing this procedure. Take this opportunity to discuss with your doctor any concerns you may have about the need for the test, the risks of the test, or how it will be performed.

## Procedure:

This test is done by a physician in an office, special procedures room, operating room, or emergency room. You will be asked to assume a position that will allow your doctor easy access to the joint to be examined. The joints most commonly tapped are the knee, hip, elbow, shoulder, wrist, ankle, and big toe.

Your doctor will examine and move the joint and determine the location at which the needle should be inserted. The skin over the joint will be cleansed with antiseptic solution.

If a local anesthetic is to be used, it will be injected or sprayed on. The tap needle will then be slowly inserted into the joint. If the needle comes in contact with bone or cartilage, the needle will be withdrawn slightly and gently redirected.

Once the needle is in place, a syringe will be used to remove a sample of fluid. The needle may have to be repositioned several times to enter different "pockets" of fluid.

The procedure usually takes 5–10 minutes. After the test is completed, the joint may be wrapped in an elastic bandage. You will be asked to avoid excessive use of the joint for several days.

## How Does It Feel?

If a local anesthetic is used, you will feel a slight needle-prick and a brief burning as it is injected. If a spray is used, it will feel very cold. You will also feel a brief, sharp discomfort as the needle penetrates the joint capsule.

If no anesthetic is used, you may feel a mild discomfort as the needle is inserted and brief, sharp discomfort as the needle penetrates the joint capsule.

If the joint is already tender and inflamed, the movement of the joint during the exam may prove painful.

You may feel an unfamiliar grating sensation in the joint for a few days after the test. This will gradually disappear as your body secretes new joint fluid.

You may experience some pain and

swelling in the joint for a few days after the procedure. This may be very minor if the tap was an easy one, or more extensive if many repeat attempts were required.

If the joint becomes sore or inflamed, prop it up comfortably with pillows and keep it elevated and immobile. Ice packs applied intermittently for 15–20 minutes every few hours will help reduce swelling and discomfort.

Notify your doctor if you notice fever or increasing redness, tenderness, persistent bleeding, or drainage at the tap site.

**Risks:**
There is a very small risk of infection and a small risk of continued bleeding from the tap site (especially in persons with bleeding problems). There is also a slight risk that the needle will strike a nerve, producing nerve injury, or a blood vessel, producing bleeding into the joint, but both are exceedingly rare.

**Results:**
Your doctor will use one portion of the joint fluid sample to do a series of immediate tests for bacteria, blood cells, and crystals in the joint fluid. Another portion will be sent to the lab for other tests, which may take several days.

Lab examination of the joint fluid may reveal a number of joint conditions, including various kinds of inflammatory diseases (such as rheumatoid arthritis, gout, and systemic lupus erythmatosus), non-inflammatory diseases (traumatic arthritis or osteoarthritis), and infections (septic arthritis).

Normal joint fluid is straw-colored and transparent. Joint fluid that is yellow, green, gray, or cloudy may indicate infection or inflammation. Red fluid is due to bleeding. The presence of uric acid crystals in the joint fluid establishes the diagnosis of gout,

while crystals of calcium pyrophosphate indicate pseudogout.

In most joint infections or inflammations due to crystal deposits in the joint, a joint tap will provide a definitive diagnosis. In other conditions, it will provide useful evidence which must be weighed with the results of other tests in making a diagnosis.

**Cost:**
$50 to $100, depending on which tests are done on the joint fluid. (It may cost more if performed in an operating room.)

**Special Considerations:**
★A contrast medium can be injected after the joint fluid is withdrawn so that x-rays of the joint can be taken (see Arthrogram, p. 243).

★*Synovial Biopsy*—Sometimes it may be necessary to remove a small piece of tissue from a joint lining (synovium) and examine it under a microscope. This can be done by inserting a needle or by a surgical incision.

# Pleural Tap (Thoracentesis, Pleural Fluid Analysis)

The lungs normally press tightly against the membrane (pleura) which lines the inside of the chest cavity. But in some disorders fluid accumulates in the space between the lungs and the pleura. This is called a pleural effusion. It can be caused by an infection, a tumor, bleeding, or other conditions.

In this test a needle is inserted through the chest wall to remove accumulated fluid from the space around the lungs. The fluid is then sent to the laboratory for analysis.

## Why Performed:

This test is done to determine the cause of a persistent pleural effusion after it has been detected by a physical examination and chest x-ray. It is also performed to relieve breathing difficulties caused by an accumulation of fluid in the space around the lungs. It may also be used to inject medications into the space between the lung and the chest wall.

## Preparation:

Tell your doctor if

> You have allergies to any medications or anesthetics
> You are taking any medications
> You have had bleeding problems
> You might be pregnant

You will be asked to sign a consent form authorizing this procedure. Take this opportunity to discuss with your doctor any concerns you may have about the need for the test, the risks of the test, or how and when it will be performed.

Tests may be done to make sure your blood can clot normally. X-rays of your chest are taken to guide your doctor. As coughing may make the needle jerk and possibly injure the lung, you may be given a pill or syrup to suppress coughing before the procedure.

## Procedure:

This test may be done in a doctor's office, a treatment room, an emergency room, or at your bedside in the hospital. It is performed by a physician and an assistant.

You will be asked to sit up and lean forward, resting your arms on a pillow placed on a table. The doctor will examine your back and chest to help determine the proper tap site. Occasionally the sample is collected while you lie on your side. The location of the tap site will depend upon where the fluid has collected.

The skin over the tap site will be cleaned with antiseptic solution, shaved if necessary, and draped with sterile towels.

A local anesthetic will be injected. After the area has become numb, a larger needle will be inserted between your ribs and into the fluid pocket. To avoid damage to the lung, hold very still and try not to cough when the tap needle is inserted. A syringe will be used to remove the fluid. The needle may need to be repositioned as the fluid is drawn out.

If there is a large volume of fluid to be removed, a suction device may be used. The amount of fluid removed at one time is usually limited to 1 to 2 liters (roughly 1 to 2 quarts). If additional fluid is present, another tap will be done later. The needle is then withdrawn and a bandage applied to the tap site.

You must not cough, move, or breathe deeply during the procedure: these actions increase the risk of puncturing a lung. An x-ray is usually taken immediately after the procedure to be sure that there was not an accidental puncture of the lung, which results in air leaking into the pleural space (pneumothorax).

This procedure takes 10–15 minutes. If a great deal of fluid needs to be removed, it may take longer.

## How Does It Feel?

The antiseptic solution may feel cold when applied to your chest. You will feel a brief stinging sensation as the local anesthetic is injected. You should feel mostly pressure and little or no pain from the tap needle. As the needle is removed, you may feel an urge to cough.

After the test you will be asked to tell your doctor or nurse if you feel faint. If so, you may be given oxygen to breathe. You will also be asked to report any increased difficulty in breathing, chest pain, or uncontrollable cough. This could be a symptom of a collapsed lung.

If a large volume of fluid is removed, you should find it much easier to breathe afterward.

### Risks:

There are some risks associated with this test. The needle can tear the wall of the lung, allowing air to flow into the pleural space. This can produce a partial collapse of the lung (pneumothorax). This usually resolves on its own, but sometimes requires the placement of a tube through the chest wall. There may be bleeding into the pleural space. This is usually reabsorbed quickly. There is also a slight risk that the needle could injure the liver or spleen. In a very few severely ill persons, the insertion of the needle can trigger a shock reaction. This can usually be treated. You should discuss the risks in your particular situation with your physician.

This test is not usually done on persons with only one good lung or on persons with uncontrolled bleeding disorders.

### Results:

Results are usually available in 1 to 2 days. The results of some tests may take much longer—up to several weeks for tuberculosis cultures.

The fluid is tested to determine whether it is just the fluid portion of the blood (transudate), a pussy fluid accumulated as the result of an infection (exudate), or blood (hemorrhage). The results of lab analysis will help determine whether the pleural fluid is the result of infection, heart or lung disease, cancer, or inflammation.

The most common cause of pleural effusion is infection; however, some effusions are due to cancers. Therefore, the pleural fluid is examined for the presence of cancer cells.

### Cost:
$100 to $150

### Special Considerations:

★*Pleural Biopsy*—Sometimes a sample of the pleura (the lining of the chest cavity) is obtained as part of a pleural tap. A long, hooklike instrument is inserted through the same needle as that used to obtain the fluid sample, and a small sample of the pleura is taken.

# Spinal Tap
## (Lumbar Puncture, Spinal Puncture, Spinal Fluid Tap, Cerebrospinal Fluid (CSF) Analysis)

Spinal fluid (also known as cerebrospinal fluid or CSF) is a clear fluid which surrounds and cushions the brain and spinal cord. Since spinal fluid bathes the brain and spinal cord, analysis of its contents can reveal a variety of disorders affecting these organs.

In this test a doctor inserts a needle between two vertebrae of your lower back and into the spinal canal to obtain a sample of spinal fluid. This sample is then sent to the laboratory for analysis.

### Why Performed:

A spinal tap may be done when an infection or bleeding in the area around the brain or spinal cord is suspected. Symptoms might include numbness or paralysis, stiff neck with a high fever, delirium, or sudden onset of severe headache. The test may also be done to diagnose other suspected diseases affecting the brain or spinal cord.

In addition, this procedure is sometimes used to administer anesthetics, contrast media, chemotherapy, or other medications, to evaluate the effects of treatment, or as part of another procedure, such as myelography (p. 275).

### Preparation:

Tell your doctor if

> You have allergies to any medications or anesthetics
>
> You are taking any medications
>
> You have had bleeding problems

You will be asked to sign a consent form authorizing this procedure. Use this opportunity to discuss with your doctor any concerns you may have about the need for the test, its risks, or how it will be performed.

This test is often done as an emergency procedure. But if the test is a scheduled one, you may be asked to refrain from eating for several hours beforehand.

### Procedure:

This procedure is usually performed by a physician, sometimes with an assistant, at the bedside of hospitalized patients or in an office or a treatment room.

You will usually receive a complete neurologic exam, including an examination of your eyes with an ophthalmoscope to check for signs of increased pressure in your brain. Several blood tests may also be performed.

You will be asked to assume one of two positions: either sitting on the edge of a chair or bed and leaning forward over a table with your head and chest bent toward your knees, or, more commonly, lying on your side, with your knees drawn up toward your chest in a "fetal" position. These positions help widen the spaces between the bones of the spine to allow insertion of the needle. The physician's assistant will help you maintain this posture. (Once the needle is in place, you may be able to assume a more comfortable position.)

The doctor will examine your back and determine the proper tap site—in your lower back (lumbar) area. Once found, the site may be marked with a marking pen. The area is then cleaned with an antiseptic and draped with sterile towels.

A local anesthetic will be injected under the skin at the chosen site. You will be asked to hold still and breathe normally.

A small needle is then inserted into the spinal canal. Once it is in place, the solid core of the needle (stylet) will be removed. If the needle is properly placed, a small amount of fluid will drip from the end of the needle. If not, it will be repositioned until fluid drips out. Sometimes (especially if you are overweight, very muscular, or have arthritis of the back), it is necessary to remove and reposition the needle several times.

Once the needle is in place, a pressure-measuring device will be attached and the CSF pressure measured. This reading is called the "opening pressure." One or more specimens of spinal fluid are then collected. Between 5 and 10 ml (1–2 teaspoons) of fluid are usually removed and sent to the lab. Occasionally the physician is unable to obtain a fluid sample. This is called a "dry tap."

If blockage of the spinal canal above the tap site is suspected, the doctor may ask an assistant to compress the veins in your neck (Queckenstedt test). This normally results in a rapid rise in CSF pressure. If such a rise does not occur, blockage is proved.

A final pressure reading (the "closing

pressure") may be taken after the fluid sample is removed. The needle is then removed. The puncture site is cleaned and a bandage is applied. Collecting the specimen takes about 10–20 minutes.

Following the tap you may be asked to lie flat in bed for anywhere from several hours to a full 24 hours, depending on your doctor's customary practice. This is done to reduce the chance of a headache. Any position is acceptable as long as your head is not raised above the rest of your body. You may turn your head from side to side, but should not raise it.

Since your brain replaces your entire supply of spinal fluid 2–3 times per day, the small amount of fluid that was removed will be rapidly replaced. Some doctors suggest that you drink additional fluids after the tap to help prevent headaches and other side effects. You will be given fluids through a bent straw so that you can drink without lifting your head.

If your spinal fluid appears abnormal, you will be closely observed and a series of brief neurologic examinations may be performed periodically for the first few hours after the test.

### How Does It Feel?

Some people find lying on their side curled up in the fetal position uncomfortable. The antiseptic solution may feel cold on your back. You will probably feel a brief stinging sensation when the local anesthetic is injected. You may feel a brief pain when the spinal needle is inserted or repositioned.

Some patients worry that the needle may damage the spinal cord. This is virtually impossible, since the needle is inserted well below the lower end of your spinal cord. However, the needle may touch one of your spinal nerves, producing a tingling sensation like a light electric shock running down one of your legs.

Roughly three quarters of patients experience no aftereffects of this test. Of those who do get headaches, only about half report that they are severe. These headaches normally last 24–48 hours but may occasionally continue longer. They can usually be controlled by pain medication.

Some doctors feel that lying flat in bed for several hours afterward can decrease the risk of headache. Experts disagree on this point, but there is general agreement that lying down can help relieve a headache once it does develop.

You may feel drowsy and tired and may experience a slight backache the day after the test. Some people experience difficulty sleeping for a day or two.

You should let your doctor know immediately if you develop a fever, stiff neck, bleeding from the puncture site, a severe headache even when lying down, or any numbness or loss of strength.

*Patient Comments:*

"The antiseptic was cold. The needle with the anesthetic stung a little. I could feel my back getting numb. With the spinal needle, there wasn't any pain—just a feeling of pressure. Lying flat in bed for 24 hours was boring, and I got a headache anyway."

### Risks:

A spinal tap is generally a very safe procedure. However, this test may be hazardous if performed on people with increased pressure within the brain. (Such increased pressure may be due to a tumor, blood clot, or other mass.) In such cases there is a risk that the brain might be displaced downward (herniation of the brain), resulting in severe injury and possible death. This is one reason your doctor should carefully examine your eyes for signs of increased pressure within the skull before performing a spinal tap.

Persons with bleeding problems and those taking a blood-thinning drug (such as heparin) are at some increased risk of continued internal bleeding after the procedure.

About 1 in 1000 people having this test suffers some nerve injury. This usually heals on its own with time. There is also a slight risk of infection of the spinal canal (meningitis) or damage to the cartilage between the vertebrae. You should discuss the risks in your particular circumstances with your doctor.

### Results:

Many different tests can be performed on the spinal fluid. Some results will be available at once, some within a few hours of the test. Others may take as long as several weeks.

Greater-than-normal spinal fluid pressure suggests increased pressure inside the skull and/or spinal cord, usually due to a tumor, bleeding, infection, or swelling (edema). Lower-than-normal spinal fluid pressure may mean a blockage in the spinal canal above the puncture site.

Bloody spinal fluid may suggest bleeding (hemorrhage) in or around the spinal cord or brain, but it may also be due to the harmless puncture of a tiny blood vessel by the spinal needle. Cloudy spinal fluid may indicate an infection (meningitis or brain abscess.) An increased level of protein may be due to bleeding into the spinal fluid, tumor, diabetes, infection, injury, or other nervous system disease. High glucose levels are frequently due to diabetes. Low glucose levels may be due to infection (meningitis), cancer, or hypoglycemia.

A white blood cell count, culture, and/or Gram stain may be performed to test for infection of the spinal cord (meningitis) or brain infection (encephalitis). The spinal fluid may also be tested for a syphilis infection. Protein electrophoresis and other special tests may be performed if multiple sclerosis is suspected.

### Cost:

$100 to $200, but may cost more if additional tests of CSF fluid are ordered.

### Special Considerations:

★*Cisternal and Ventricular Puncture*—If it is not possible to obtain spinal fluid from the lumbar area or if it is necessary to find the upper limits of a blocked spinal canal, a spinal fluid sample may be obtained from the upper spinal canal or from within the skull. This is a potentially hazardous procedure, and should be done only by a very experienced specialist and only in exceptional circumstances.

# 11    Other Tests

## Allergy Testing

Allergies result from a malfunction of the body's immune system, which usually protects us from foreign substances. With allergies, the immune system overreacts to normally harmless foreign substances such as pollens, dusts, danders, or foods. The overreaction can cause sneezing, wheezing, watery eyes, itching, rashes, and even at times life-threatening anaphylactic shock.

Allergy testing is performed to find out specifically what you are allergic to so that you can try to avoid these substances or be desensitized to them. In these tests you are exposed to a series of substances, known as allergens or antigens, which commonly cause allergic reactions. Minute quantities of these substances are applied to your skin in a variety of ways (scratch, intradermal injection, or patch). If you are sensitive to the substance a skin reaction will take place.

### Why Performed:
Allergy testing is not necessary in the management of most allergic reactions. The offending substance, whether it be cat dander, pollens, medications, cosmetics, or jewelry, is often obvious. Symptoms that typically appear with certain changes in season, diet, location, habits, or exposures can provide essential clues. Seasonal variations suggest pollen allergy. Symptoms that occur repeatedly after eating certain foods point to a food allergy. If avoiding these suspected allergens results in an improvement of symptoms, this helps confirm your suspicions. It may be useful to keep a journal of allergic symptoms for several weeks to look for a pattern. If such careful history-taking does not suggest the substance or substances responsible, allergy testing may be helpful.

Skin tests (scratch and intradermal injection) are most often done to identify inhaled allergens which may be causing the sneezing, runny noise, and nasal congestion of hay fever or the wheezing of asthma. Skin tests are occasionally performed for evaluation of hives or suspected food or drug allergies. Patch tests may be done to help diagnose unexplained rashes when chemical allergy, such as allergy to nickel, rubber, preservatives, or fragrances, is suspected.

A blood test (RAST) is also sometimes used to evaluate allergies (see later).

**Preparation:**
Tell your doctor if you are taking any medications.

You may be advised to stop certain medications, such as antihistamines, for several days before this test. Such medications can inhibit allergic reactions and interfere with the detection of allergens on the tests.

**Procedure:**
Allergy tests are usually performed by a physician or technician in a doctor's office or clinic. Depending upon the site to be tested, you may be asked to remove all clothing above the waist.

There are two different types of skin test: the scratch test and the intradermal test.

The *scratch test* is most frequently used first because the reaction it can produce in a highly allergic person is less severe. In the scratch test, very small amounts of dilute solutions of different suspected allergens (grasses, weeds, trees, molds, dusts, and foods) are placed on your arms or back. The skin beneath the sample is then lightly scratched with a sterile pin. You must then wait for 20–30 minutes. You may want to bring reading material or another activity to occupy yourself during the waiting period. Then your skin is examined for a reaction, usually marked by redness, swelling and blistering. The entire test usually takes about 30–40 minutes and may be repeated later.

With the *intradermal test* minute amounts of various suspected allergens are injected into the skin on your arms or back. The injection sites are then evaluated for reactions after waiting 20–30 minutes.

In a *patch test* dilute samples of suspected allergens are placed on small pieces of filter paper and taped to the skin on your back. It usually takes about 40 minutes to apply all the patches. They are left in place for 24–48 hours. During this time you should not bathe or engage in vigorous activity which might promote sweating and loosen the patches. You will be asked to return at a specified time so that the patches can be removed and any reactions evaluated. You may also be asked to return several days later to be examined for a delayed reaction.

**How Does It Feel?**
With scratch testing you will only feel a slight pricking sensation as the skin beneath each sample is lightly scratched.

With intradermal testing, the samples are injected very superficially into the skin with a very thin needle. You may feel a slight sting with each injection.

If an allergic reaction forms with any of the tests, you may experience some itching, tenderness, and swelling, which can be managed with cool compresses and a mild steroid creme. If you are having a patch test and notice severe itching or pain under any of the patches, remove them and notify your doctor.

**Risks:**
With skin testing the major risk is that of an extreme allergic response, an anaphylactic reaction. This may produce a serious drop in blood pressure and difficulty in breathing and must be treated immediately. An anaphylactic reaction occurs in less than 1 in 2000 cases and usually can be treated effectively with medications such as epinephrine (Adrenalin). Death is exceedingly rare.

With patch testing there may rarely be some persistent lightening or darkening of the skin where the patches were applied.

**Results:**

If any inflammation or rash develops at the test sites, the test is considered positive for that specific allergen. However, this does not necessarily mean that the specific substance is responsible for your symptoms, since a person can be allergic to more than one substance, including some that may not be tested for. If you are allergic to a substance and cannot practically avoid it, sometimes treatment involving repeated injections of minute quantities of that substance may be tried to desensitize you.

**Cost:**

$200 to $500

**Special Considerations:**

★ *RAST (Radioallergosorbent Test)*: Recently a blood test has been developed to screen for allergies. A sample of your blood is analyzed for the presence of specific antibodies (immunoglobulins, IgE) to a variety of allergens (foods, pollens, danders). The presence of specific antibodies suggests an allergy to that particular allergen. RAST tests are less dangerous and uncomfortable than skin testing, but may be less sensitive in detecting certain allergies. In addition, RAST testing is very expensive ($15–$30 per allergen, and usually 20–30 different allergens are tested at a time).

# Cystometrogram
## (Cystometry)

Cystometric tests measure how well the bladder is functioning. By instilling water or gas into the bladder, the ability of the bladder to expand and contract, to retain and expel urine, can be measured.

Urination is a very complex process. As the bladder fills, sensory nerves in the bladder send messages to the spinal cord. These messages are answered by a signal for the bladder to contract. Unless this voiding reflex is voluntarily inhibited, the urine will flow. A problem anywhere in this complex nerve pathway can cause abnormal bladder function.

**Why Performed:**

This test is used to help determine the cause of abnormal bladder function, especially involuntary urination (incontinence), inability to retain urine in a full bladder (stress incontinence), unexplained urge to void (urgency), or weak urine stream.

**Preparation:**

Tell your doctor if

You are taking any medications

You might be pregnant

Before the test begins you will be asked to put on a hospital gown. Otherwise no other preparation is necessary.

**Procedure:**

This test is performed in a doctor's office or hospital urology procedures room by a doctor (usually a urologist or gynecologist) and a technician.

At the beginning of the test you may be asked to urinate into a funnel attached to a machine which measures the amount of flow and time of urination. The time and effort needed to start the flow, the continuity of the urine stream, and the presence of dribbling after finishing will also be noted.

Then you will be asked to lie on your back on an examining table. The opening of the urethra (the tube through which the urine leaves the body) will be thoroughly cleansed. A well-lubricated, thin, flexible tube (catheter) will be gently inserted into the urethra and slowly advanced into the bladder. Any urine remaining in your bladder (residual volume) will be measured.

The catheter is then attached to a bottle which hangs above your head and contains sterile water. A measured volume of room-temperature water is then instilled through the catheter into your bladder. The catheter is also attached to a device which measures the pressure in your bladder during the instillation. The water is then allowed to drain by gravity and another infusion is made—this time with warm water. You will be asked to report any sensations (such as warmth, bladder fullness, urge to urinate). The process may be repeated. Sometimes a gas (usually carbon dioxide) is used instead of water.

You may be given a drug (bethanechol) which normally makes the bladder muscles contract in order to test your bladder's ability to do so. If this test is done, the drug will be injected under your skin.

Each time your bladder is filled, you will be asked to report your first urge to urinate. When your bladder reaches its full capacity, you will be asked to void. If no additional tests (see Special Considerations below) are required, the catheter is then removed.

This test usually takes 30–60 minutes, though it may take slightly longer if further testing is needed.

### How Does It Feel?

You may find it embarrassing to have your genitals examined and to have to urinate in front of the medical personnel performing the test. Remember that they perform this test regularly and think it nothing out of the ordinary.

You will have a strong urge to urinate at times during the test. You may find it somewhat painful to have the catheter inserted and may be sore afterward. If so, a warm tub bath may help. After the test you may notice blood in your urine and may feel some burning on urination (especially if carbon dioxide was used).

Notify your doctor if the blood in the urine persists longer than the third time you urinate after the test or if you develop chills or fever.

### Risks:

Cystometry is usually a very safe procedure. There is always a slight risk of developing a urinary tract infection when a catheter is inserted into the bladder. If an infection occurs, it will be treated with antibiotics.

### Results:

The results of the test allow your doctor to determine whether the neuromuscular and sensory function of your bladder is normal; and if it is not, the results help determine exactly what the difficulty is.

Conditions that can cause problems with bladder control include urinary tract infections, bladder stones, kidney disease, diabetes, multiple sclerosis, arteriosclerosis, Parkinson's disease, spinal cord injury, and drugs.

Since cystometry alone can sometimes give ambiguous results, such other tests as cystourethrography (p. 260), excretory urography (IVP) (p. 269), or voiding cystourethrography (p. 260) may also be needed.

### Cost:

$75 to $125

### Special Considerations:

★Other tests that may be done as part of a cystometrogram include the following:

★*Ice Water Test*—Ice water is injected into the bladder through a catheter to test the bladder reflex. Normal results: water is immediately expelled.

★*Stress Incontinence Test*—The bladder is filled with water and the catheter is withdrawn. You are then asked to cough, bend over, and/or lift a heavy object. Normal result: No urine is spilled. Dribbling of urine indicates stress incontinence.

# Electroencephalogram
## (EEG, Brain Wave Test)

Brain cells communicate by producing tiny electrical impulses. In an electroencephalogram (EEG) these impulses are detected by sensors (electrodes) placed on the scalp, amplified approximately a million times, and recorded as wavy lines on moving graph paper. Certain brain abnormalities can be detected by observing alterations in the characteristic pattern of these recorded brain waves.

### Why Performed:
The EEG is most frequently used to help diagnose the presence and type of seizure disorder (convulsions, fits, epilepsy). It may also be used to investigate periods of unconsciousness, confusion, head injuries, suspected brain tumors, infections, degenerative diseases, and metabolic disturbances affecting the brain. An EEG may be performed for legal purposes to confirm brain death in comatose patients who are being sustained on respirators. An EEG may also be included as one of the tests done to evaluate sleep disorders.

The EEG cannot be used to measure intelligence, diagnose mental illness, or "read the mind" of the patient; it simply measures the amount and type of electrical activity in the brain.

### Preparation:
Tell your doctor if you are taking any medications. Your doctor may advise you to discontinue certain medications such as anticonvulsants, tranquilizers, muscle relaxants, and sleeping medications before the test.

Avoid all caffeine-containing foods (coffee, tea, colas, chocolate) for at least 8 hours before the test. However, you should plan to eat a small meal shortly before the test; low blood sugar may produce an abnormal test.

Since the electrodes are attached to your scalp, it is important that your hair be clean, unbraided, and free of sprays, oils, creams, lotions and other hair preparations. Shampoo your hair the morning before the test.

To detect certain types of brain wave abnormality it may be necessary to have you sleep during the test. To help prepare you to sleep during the recording, you may be asked not to sleep at all the night before the test or to reduce your sleep time to 4–5 hours by going to bed later and awakening earlier. If your child is to be tested, try to keep him or her from taking naps just before the test. If a sleep-deprived EEG is planned, have someone drive you to and from the test.

### Procedure:
This test is performed by an EEG technician in a specially designed room (or at your bedside) in a hospital or doctor's office.

You will be asked to lie on your back on an examining table, reclining chair, or bed. The technician will apply between 16 and 25 flat metal discs (electrodes) in different positions on your scalp. They will be held in place with a sticky paste or a cap. Rarely, these electrodes are attached to the scalp with tiny needles. Sometimes additional small wire electrodes are placed through your nose into the back of your throat.

The electrodes are connected by wires to an amplifier and recording machine which converts the electrical signals into a series of wavy lines drawn by a row of pens on a moving piece of graph paper. During the recording it is important that you lie very still. Try to minimize blinking, swallowing, talking, or other movements, since these may produce electrical activity (artifacts) that interferes with the recording. The technician will observe you directly or through a window during the test. The recording may be stopped from time to time to allow you to stretch and reposition yourself.

Certain procedures may be done to observe how your brain responds to stimulation. You may be asked to breathe deeply and rapidly (hyperventilate) for several minutes. Or you may be asked to look at a very bright flickering light (strobe).

In some studies you will be asked to try to sleep during the recording. If you are unable to fall asleep, you may be given a medication (usually chloral hydrate) to help you sleep.

The test usually takes one to two hours. After the test you may resume normal activities. However, if you were sleep-deprived or given a sleep medication, you should plan to have someone drive you home after the test.

### How Will It Feel?

During the EEG recording you will feel nothing. If paste is used to position the electrodes, some will remain in your hair after the test, so it will be necessary to wash your hair to remove it. If needle electrodes are used (which is rare), you will feel a brief sharp, pricking sensation (about like having a hair pulled out) when each electrode is inserted. If electrodes are placed in your nose, they may produce an uncomfortable tickling sensation and, rarely, some soreness or a small amount of bleeding for a day or two after the test.

If you are asked to breathe rapidly, you may notice some lightheadedness and numbness in your fingers. This is normal and will subside within a few minutes of breathing normally again.

### Risks:

An EEG is a very safe procedure. The electrical discharges produced by your brain are detected, but at no time is any electrical current put into your body. An EEG should not be confused with electroshock therapy. If you do have a seizure disorder, a seizure may be triggered by the flashing lights or by hyperventilation. If this occurs, the technician is trained to take care of you during the episode.

### Results:

The EEG record is analyzed by a physician (neurologist) and the results are usually available within a few days.

There are several types of brain waves. *Alpha waves* have a frequency of 8–12 cycles per second. These waves are normal and tend to be more prominent when you are relaxed with your eyes closed. *Beta waves* have a frequency of 13–30 cycles per second and are normally found when you are alert and attentive. *Delta waves*, with a frequency of less than 4 cycles per second, occur normally during sleep and in young children. Delta waves found in adults who are awake may suggest brain injury. *Theta waves* have a frequency of 4–8 cycles per second and are normally found in children and, occasionally, in older people. An excess of theta waves may indicate brain injury.

The two sides of the brain normally show similar patterns of electrical activity. If they do not, it may indicate a problem in one area or side of the brain. A sudden burst of electrical activity (epileptiform abnormalities) or slowing of activity in one area of the brain may indicate the presence and type of seizures. However, in patients with seizures, the EEG may appear completely normal between seizures. Therefore, a normal EEG does not exclude a seizure disorder.

An area of abnormal discharges or slowing of brain waves may be due to a tumor, infection (brain abscess), injury, stroke, or epilepsy. A diffuse, generalized abnormality in the brain waves suggests a disorder affecting the entire brain, such as drug intoxication, metabolic abnormalities, or certain infections. The complete absence of electrical activity in the brain ("flat" or "straight-line" EEG) confirms brain death.

**Cost:**
$175 to $225

# Electromyogram and Nerve Conduction Studies
## (EMG, Electromyography, Electroneurography)

Nerves conduct messages in the form of electrical impulses. These impulses can cause muscles to contract, which itself produces electrical discharges. Measurement of the electrical discharges in nerves and muscles can help detect the presence, location, and extent of neuromuscular diseases.

Electromyography (EMG) measures the electrical activity in muscles while nerve conduction studies measure the ability of specific nerves to transmit electrical impulses. Either or both of these tests may be performed, depending upon the type of disorder suspected.

**Why Performed:**
Weakness or paralysis may be due to a problem in the muscle, the nerves supplying that muscle, the spinal cord, or the area in the brain that controls those muscles. EMG and nerve conduction studies can help distinguish which of these causes is responsible for the weakness. In addition, nerve conduction studies are sometimes used to identify the cause of abnormal sensations (numbness, tingling, or pain). EMG studies may also be helpful in evaluating involuntary muscle twitching or the finding in the blood of abnormally increased muscle enzymes (CPK, see p. 151).

**Preparation:**
Tell your doctor if

You are taking any medications. Certain muscle relaxants and other drugs that act on the nervous system can interfere with the results.
You have had bleeding problems.
You have a pacemaker.

No restriction of food or fluids is necessary. Some doctors ask that you refrain from smoking or drinking caffeine-containing beverages for at least 3 hours before the test.

You should wear loose-fitting clothing which permits access to the muscles and nerves to be tested. You may be given a hospital gown to put on.

**Procedure:**
These tests are performed in an EMG laboratory in a hospital, clinic, or doctor's of-

fice. A special copper-lined room is preferable to help screen out electrical interference. The test may be performed by an EMG technician or a physician specializing in diseases of the nervous system (neurologist) or rehabilitation (physiatrist).

If you are extremely anxious or apprehensive, a sedative medication may be offered before the examination. You will be asked to lie on a table or sit in a reclining chair in such a position that the muscles being tested are relaxed and accessible.

*Electromyography (EMG):* a flat metal disc electrode will be attached to your skin near the test area. The skin over the areas to be tested will be cleansed with an antiseptic solution. Then a thin sterile needle attached by wires to a recording machine will be inserted through the skin and into the specific muscle to be tested. The electrical activity in that muscle is recorded while you are at rest and then as you slowly and progressively contract that muscle as directed by the examiner. The electrical activity in the muscle is displayed as electrical waves on a TV-like screen and may also be heard on a loudspeaker as machine-gunlike popping sounds as you contract the muscle. The needle may be repositioned many times to record different areas in the muscle or different muscles. When the testing is completed, the needle and skin electrode are removed.

*Nerve Conduction Studies:* In this test several flat metal disc electrodes are attached to your skin. A shock-emitting electrode is placed directly over the nerve to be studied, and a recording electrode is placed over the muscles supplied by that nerve. Repeated brief electrical shocks are administered to the nerve, and the time it takes for the muscle to contract in response to the stimulus is recorded. In this way the conduction velocity (speed) of nerve impulse transmission is calculated. The cor-responding nerves on the other side of the body are also usually studied for comparison. When the testing is completed, the skin electrodes are removed.

The testing may take from 15 minutes to an hour or more, depending upon how many areas are studied. After the testing you may immediately resume normal activities.

### How Does It Feel?

With the EMG testing you will feel a brief, sharp pain each time the needle electrode is inserted into the muscle. After EMG testing some soreness and a tingling sensation may persist for a day or two. However, if you notice increasing pain, swelling, tenderness, or pus at any of the needle insertion sites, notify your doctor.

With the nerve conduction studies, you will feel a brief, burning pain, tingling sensation, and involuntary twitching of the muscle each time the electrical shock is applied. This can be quite uncomfortable.

### Risks:

These tests are very safe. There is no risk of allergic reaction, since nothing is injected. With the EMG you may develop small bruises at some of the needle insertion sites. The needles are sterilized so that the chance of an infection is remote. There is no risk of electrocution with nerve conduction studies, since the electrical current used is very low-voltage.

### Results:

Your doctor may be able to discuss the preliminary findings with you immediately after the tests, although full analysis of the results may take several days. The EMG recording should show no activity at rest, and there should be smooth wavelike forms with each muscle contraction. The nerve conduction studies should show normal speed of nerve impulse transmission (the precise velocity varies from nerve to nerve).

Abnormalities involving the muscles (*myopathy*) may include such disorders as muscular dystrophy or myasthenia gravis. Disorders of the nerves (*neuropathy*) may be due to nerve injury, trauma, toxins (such as alcohol), vitamin deficiencies, diabetes, polio, or amyotropic lateral sclerosis (ALS, Lou Gehrig's disease). Carpal tunnel syndrome is a common example of a nerve injury due to compression of the median nerve as it passes through the wrist. This damage to the median nerve causes numbness and tingling in some of the fingers, a weak grip, and a characteristically slowed nerve conduction velocity.

The results from EMG and nerve conduction studies must be interpreted in light of your history, symptoms, physical examination, and the results of other tests.

## Cost:
$100 to $300 (depending upon how many nerves and muscles are tested)

# Glaucoma Tests (Tonometry)

This test measures the pressure inside the eyes (intraocular pressure). It is used to screen for glaucoma, a disease in which the pressure inside the eye increases to abnormal levels and may impair vision.

Glaucoma accounts for 12% to 15% of all blindness in the United States. There are usually no symptoms during the early stages of this disease. It can go unrecognized for years, and then quickly progress to rapid loss of vision. Glaucoma can be treated if detected early.

## Why Performed:
People over 40 are at highest risk for glaucoma and should have this test every 3 to 5 years. People with a family history of glaucoma, blacks, and diabetics should be tested regularly beginning at age 25. People with borderline test results should be tested every year or two. Glaucoma screening is often performed during routine eye examinations and refractions, but you may have to ask for the test.

## Preparation:
Tell your doctor if
> Anyone in your family has ever had glaucoma
> You are taking any drugs
> You have an eye infection or ulcer of the eye

If you wear contact lenses, you will be asked to remove them.

## Procedure:
Glaucoma testing is usually performed by optometrists, ophthalmologists (eye doctors), or regular physicians in their office. There are three different ways to test for glaucoma: the Schiotz method, the applanation method, and the noncontact ("air-puff") method.

*Schiotz Method*—You will be asked to lie on your back on an examining table. Relax as much as possible. Loosen or remove any tight clothing around your neck—constriction of the veins in the neck can increase the pressure inside your eyes.

Try not to squeeze your eyelids during the test, as this can artifically increase the pressure inside your eyes.

You will be asked to look down while the examiner raises your upper eyelid. A drop of anesthetic will be placed in your eye. You will then be asked to look up at a spot on the ceiling.

The examiner will lower a small, smooth metal instrument (tonometer) onto the surface of your eye. It will remain there only a few seconds. The procedure is then repeated on the other eye.

You should be careful not to rub your eyes for 20 minutes after the test, until the anesthetic drops have worn off. If you wear contacts you will need to wait at least 2 hours after the test before putting them back in.

*Applanation Method*—This test is done by an ophthalmologist and is the most precise test of pressure inside the eyes. It measures the force required to flatten a certain area of your cornea.

The device required for this test is mounted on a slit-lamp biomicroscope. This examination is frequently done as part of a slit-lamp examination (p. 335).

An anesthetic drop is placed in the eye. The corneal fluid is then stained with a moistened strip of fluorescein paper to make the cornea visible for examination. You are seated as for a slit-lamp exam and are asked to look straight ahead.

The examiner moves the lamp forward until the tonometer comes into contact with your cornea. The examiner, looking through the eyepiece of the slit lamp, adjusts a dial controlling the tension on the tonometer.

This test is sometimes done to obtain a more precise reading after an earlier exam has detected increased pressure inside the eye.

You should not rub your eyes for 20 minutes after this test, until the anesthetic wears off. If you wear contacts you should wait 2 hours before putting them in.

*Noncontact ("Air Puff") Method*—In this method you will be asked to rest your chin on a padded stand and to stare straight into the examining instrument. The examiner will sit opposite you and will shine a bright light into your eye.

When the instrument is properly aligned, a brief puff of air will be blown at your eye. The instrument calculates the intraocular pressure from the change in the light reflected off the cornea as it is momentarily indented by the puff of air. This may be done several times for each eye. No anesthetic is used.

Each test takes only a few minutes.

### How Does It Feel?

*Schiotz Method*—You should feel no pain because of the anesthetic. If the tonometer moved across the eye during the test, your eye may feel slightly scratched, but this should last no longer than 24 hours.

*Applanation Method*—You should feel no pain because of the anesthetic.

*Noncontact ("Air-Puff") Method*—You will hear a pufflike sound and will feel a cool sensation or mild pressure on your eye. The instrument never touches your eye.

You should not notice any eye pain or visual problems after tonometry. If you do, notify your doctor.

### Risk:

With the Schiotz and applanation methods, there is a very slight risk that your cornea may be scratched by the tonometer. The cornea will normally heal itself in 1–2 days. There is also a very slight risk of an eye infection.

There is no risk with the noncontact method.

### Results:

Normal values are 12 to 22 millimeters of mercury (mm/Hg). However, some people with pressures up to 30 mm Hg do not have glaucoma.

If your pressure is higher than normal, further testing, including funduscopy (p. 333) and visual field testing (p. 392), may be necessary. Since the pressure inside your eyes varies at different times of the day, additional measurements should be obtained at different times.

## Cost:

$40 to $60 as part of a complete exam by an ophthalmologist

# Hair Analysis

The chemical analysis of hair is an exciting research and diagnostic tool whose full potential is still to be realized. Hair can be easily collected without any discomfort, stored without deterioration, and analyzed without difficulty. Hair also contains higher concentrations of trace elements than blood or urine, making it a good complement to blood and urine analysis.

Currently the most accepted use of hair analysis is in documenting heavy-metal poisoning and monitoring other environmental pollutants. Lead, mercury, cadmium, and arsenic can be easily detected in hair, and these measurements correlate well with concentrations in the internal organs. Unlike blood and urine samples, which may give only short-term evidence of toxic exposure to heavy metals, hair analysis can reveal cumulative exposure over a period of many months.

The use of hair analysis as a tool for nutritional assessment is extremely controversial. Many physicians, nutritionists, chiropractors, naturopaths, and others use the results of hair analysis to prescribe dietary changes, vitamin and mineral supplements, and even detoxifying drugs. However, the accuracy and scientific validity of hair analysis for these purposes has not been proved.

## Why Performed:

Hair analysis can be a reliable method of testing for suspected toxic exposures to lead, mercury, arsenic, and other heavy metals. Its role, if any, in nutritional assessment or the diagnosis of other diseases remains to be established.

## Procedure:

A small sample, usually about 3 teaspoons' worth, of hair is cut from the nape of the neck. The hair sample should be 1 to 1½ inches long and include the new growth closest to the scalp. The samples are sent to a special laboratory along with information on the type of hair treatments the person has used, including shampoos, conditioners, colorings, bleaches, and permanents. At the laboratory the hair sample is washed and analyzed for heavy metals such as lead, mercury, cadmium, aluminum, and arsenic and for minerals such as zinc, selenium, magnesium, and copper.

## Risks:

Hair analysis itself has no risk. However, if you take high doses of potentially toxic vitamins, minerals, or chelating agents (drugs that bind and remove toxic metals) based on the results of this test, you may be at risk for the side effects associated with those substances.

## Results:

Within several weeks of sending the sample, you or your doctor will receive a computer printout of the mineral and heavy-metal levels in your hair sample.

Interpreting the report is difficult. There is no widely accepted standardization of procedures for cutting, washing, and analyzing the hair. Therefore, different labs may report different results from the same hair sample, and, in fact, the same lab may report different results for separate specimens from the same hair.

The significance of most of the findings is also unclear. How well does the presence or absence of certain elements in the hair actually reflect what's happening inside the body? The composition of hair is determined not only by our nutrition and internal metabolism but also by external contamination. Air pollution, shampoos, hair dyes, sprays, permanents, and bleaching may increase or decrease certain minerals in the hair. The use of medications such as oral contraceptives can change the mineral concentration of hair. The location of the hair sample, age, sex, hair color, and rate of hair growth may also influence the results. For most of the trace minerals, we do not yet know what really constitutes normal or significant deviations from normal. Any interpretation of hair analysis regarding the presence or absence of trace minerals or toxic metals in the body, therefore, should be confirmed with analysis of blood and urine specimens.

**Cost:**
$25 to $50

**Special Considerations:**

★Hair analysis is performed by some companies that offer this service to customers by mail order. The reports are mailed back to the customer along with recommendations for taking various vitamin and mineral supplements. Frequently the same companies that offer the hair analysis also sell the vitamin and mineral supplements. While such potential conflict of interest does not in itself invalidate the results, you should critically evaluate the claims made by such companies as you would the claimed benefits of any procedure, orthodox or unorthodox.

# Hearing Tests (Audiometry)

Sounds are vibrations of different frequencies and intensities in the air around us. The outer ear collects these sound waves and channels them down the ear canal to the eardrum (tympanic membrane). The eardrum then begins to vibrate. These mechanical vibrations are conducted across the middle ear by a series of tiny bones, producing pulsed waves in the fluid-filled inner ear. Finally these waves are transformed into electrical impulses by tiny hair cells which line the inner ear. The auditory nerve carries these impulses to the brain. A problem anywhere in this complex auditory chain can produce partial or complete hearing loss (see illustration, p. 411).

Hearing (audiometric) tests are done to detect the presence, degree, and type of hearing loss. In these tests you will be asked to respond to a series of tones and words presented to you through earphones.

**Why Performed:**
Hearing tests are recommended for anyone who has noticed a persistent decrease in hearing in one or both ears or has had problems understanding words in conversation. These tests are also useful in screening young children for hearing problems which might interfere with learning, speech, and language development or older people who may gradually develop hearing loss which may, at times, be mistaken for loss of mental capacities. In addition, people exposed to loud noises or taking certain antibiotics should be screened periodically.

**Preparation:**
Tell your doctor if

You have been recently exposed to any painfully loud noise or to noise that made your ears ring

You are taking any antibiotics (certain antibiotics are potentially toxic to the hearing mechanisms)

You may be asked to remove your eyeglasses, earrings, or hairclips which might interfere with the placement of the earphones.

## Procedure:

This test is performed in an audiometry laboratory by an audiologist or in a doctor's office, school, or workplace by a nurse, physician, psychologist, or audiometric technician.

The examiner will first check your ear canal for earwax and will determine whether pressure on the outer ear tends to constrict the ear canal. (If so, a thin plastic tube may be placed in the ear canal before the testing.) The examiner will then put the earphones on you and adjust the fit.

You will hear a series of tones of different pitches and intensity. You will be instructed to signal with your hand or by pressing a button every time you hear a tone. You should respond even if the tone is very faint. Each ear will be tested.

Speech reception and discrimination tests may also be performed to test your ability to hear and understand sounds used in normal conversation. You will be asked to repeat a series of simple words presented to you with different degrees of loudness.

These tests evaluate your ability to hear sounds that reach your inner ear through the ear canal. This is known as air conduction. However, sound waves may also be conducted through the bones of your skull. To test bone conduction, the earphones are removed and a vibrating device is placed on the bony area behind each ear.

Again, you will be asked to signal when you hear the vibrations.

Audiometric testing takes anywhere from 5 minutes for a simple screening to an hour for a full evaluation.

## Results:

Sound can be described in terms of both frequency and intensity. Frequency, or pitch, is measured in vibrations per second, or hertz (Hz). The human ear can normally hear sounds from a very low rumble of 16 Hz to a high-pitched whine of 20,000 Hz. Dogs can hear much higher frequencies.

Sound intensity of loudness is measured in decibels (db). The loudness levels of some common sounds are 15–25 db for a whisper, 40–60 db for background noise in the home or office, 100–120 db for loud music, and 140–180 db for a jet airplane.

If you have a hearing loss, you will be able to hear sounds only when they are at higher decibel levels. An audiogram records how loud a sound of a certain frequency must be for you to hear it; this level is called the hearing threshold. For example, a person may be able to hear low-frequency sounds at 10 decibels but may require 70 decibels to hear high-frequency sounds. This high-frequency hearing loss pattern is common with aging and with exposure to loud noises.

| Hearing Threshold | Degree of Hearing Loss |
|---|---|
| 0–25 db | Normal |
| 26–40 db | Mild |
| 41–55 db | Moderate |
| 56–70 db | Moderate to severe |
| 71–90 db | Severe |
| 91+ db | Profound |

Hearing tests may also help determine the type of hearing impairment. A *conductive* type of hearing loss occurs when sound is not conducted efficiently through the ear canal, eardrum, or middle ear due to blockage, damage, or malformation. A *sensorineural* type occurs when there is damage or malformation in the structures of the inner ear that convert sound energy into nerve impulses or in the auditory nerve, which conducts the nerve impulses to the brain. A *mixed* type of impairment occurs when there is a combination of conductive and sensorineural defects. Finally, hearing impairment may be *central* due to damage or malformation of the nervous structures in the brain.

These types of hearing impairment may be caused by heredity, birth defects, repeated exposure to loud noise, aging, head injury, earwax, middle ear infections or fluid accumulations, tumors, or drugs such as antibiotics.

### Cost:

Screening tests: $10 to $20
Full evaluation: $60 to $100

### Special Considerations:

★*Impedance Audiometry:* This test evaluates the function of the middle ear by measuring the amount of sound energy that is reflected back from the eardrum instead of being conducted on to the inner ear. The soft tip of a small instrument is inserted into your ear canal and adjusted to achieve a tight seal. Either a tone or air pressure is directed toward the eardrum. The test is not painful. You may feel slight changes in pressure or hear the tone. The test usually takes only 2–3 minutes.

# Impedance Plethysmography
## (IPG, Occlusive Impedance Phlebography)

Blood clots in the veins of the leg (thrombophlebitis) can be potentially life-threatening because one or more clots can detach and be carried through the bloodstream to the lungs, where they can cause a blockage of blood flow (pulmonary embolism). This test is used to detect blood clots (also called deep vein thromboses or DVT) in the legs.

### Why Performed:

This test is most frequently used to evaluate swelling, redness, or tenderness of the leg that could be caused by a blood clot in the deep veins. It may also be used to screen people who are at high risk of blood clots in the leg—especially after leg injuries, surgery, or long periods of bed rest or inactivity. And it is used to evaluate the leg veins when a blood clot in the lungs is suspected, since the leg veins are the source of most such clots.

This test is sometimes an alternative to a vein scan (p. 302) or venography (p. 283), which is the more definitive test for blood clots in the legs. Venography requires the injection of contrast material into the leg veins, exposes the patient to a moderate dose of radiation, and cannot be successfully performed on all patients.

### Preparation:

No restriction of food, fluid, or medication is necessary. You will be asked to undress and put on a hospital gown. You should empty your bladder just before the procedure.

**Procedure:**

This test is performed in a specially equipped hospital laboratory by a technician and a physician. You will be asked to lie on your back. The leg to be tested will be outstretched and raised at an angle of approximately 30 degrees. A conductive jelly will be applied to your leg. (This helps the electrodes make good contact.) Two straps containing electrodes are then wrapped around your leg about 8–10 inches apart.

A blood pressure cuff will then be wrapped around your upper leg just above your knee. The cuff will be inflated to a low pressure for 1 to 2 minutes and then deflated, while the plethysmograph (an instrument that measures blood volume) measures the blood volume in your leg veins. It is important that you relax your leg completely and breathe normally during this procedure.

As many as 3–5 tracings may be made. The process is then repeated on the other leg.

The test usually takes about 30–45 minutes.

**How Does It Feel?**

The conductive jelly may feel cold. You will feel a mild pressure as the cuff is inflated.

If the room is cold and you feel chilled, be sure to ask for a blanket. Being too chilly can prevent relaxation and interfere with test results.

This test is usually painless, but can be painful if the blood pressure cuff constricts an inflamed or tender place on your leg. If this occurs, you may wish to request a mild pain medication.

**Risks:**

There is little or no risk with this test.

**Results:**

In a normal leg without blood clots, the blood volume in the leg veins increases gradually after the cuff is pumped up, then rapidly drops black to normal when the cuff is released. When a clot or other blockage to blood flow exists, the resting blood volume is increased and the blood flow out of the veins is slowed, so the volume takes much longer to return to normal after the cuff is deflated.

The increased time taken to return to normal after the cuff is deflated may indicate the existence of a blood clot, but may also be due to compression of veins in the pelvic area due to tumors, tight bandages, or restrictive clothing.

**Cost:**

$50 to $100

# Magnetic Resonance Imaging (MR, MRI, Nuclear Magnetic Resonance, NMR)

Magnetic Resonance Imaging (MRI, NMR) is one of the newest and most promising of the new medical imaging devices. It can produce detailed images of the body's internal structures—in many cases revealing information not available with any other imaging technique. And it does all this *without* the use of potentially hazardous x-rays or injected contrast materials. Future MRI devices may also be able to distinguish healthy tissues from those that are weakened, damaged, or diseased.

The heart of an MRI scanner is a massive cylindrical magnet which weighs from 5 to 100 tons and is large enough to encircle a patient's body. The patient lies inside the cylinder while a quick magnetic pulse is applied to the magnet. When subjected to a powerful magnetic field, the nuclei of the hydrogen atoms in the body line up in parallel, like so many little compasses, all pointing in the same direction. When the pulse stops, the nuclei "relax" back to their previous positions. As they do so they emit a faint electrical "echo." This echo is picked up by sensitive detectors and converted into an image of the tested area.

This image is similar to, though not identical with, that produced by a CT scan. MRI has been mainly used to produce images of the brain and spinal cord but has recently been applied to other body parts as well.

This new test has generated a great deal of excitement within the medical community: it is completely painless, has no known harmful effects, and can produce more detailed images of the soft tissues of the body than any x-ray.

Some researchers feel that MRI has already established itself as the most useful and versatile diagnostic imaging tool ever developed. It seems quite likely that it will soon come into much more widespread use. However, this test is quite expensive and is not available in many communities.

### Why Performed:

To investigate suspected disease of the soft tissues of the brain and spinal cord. It can also be used to investigate suspected disorders of the heart, blood vessels, gallbladder, kidneys, pelvis, and other organs and tissues.

### Preparation:

You must remove all metal or metallic objects from your body, since such objects may be attracted to the powerful magnet used in the procedure. If you have a cardiac pacemaker, artificial limb, or any other implanted or prosthetic medical device,

discuss appropriate preparation and precautions with your doctor. This test cannot be done on women with intrauterine devices (IUDs).

### Procedure:

This test is performed in a hospital radiology department by a radiologist and an MRI technician. You will be asked to put on a hospital gown and to remove all metallic objects from your body. You will lie on a table inside the cylindrical magnet. The table will be moved so that the part of your body to be examined lies in the center of the magnet. It is important that you hold still while the test is in progress. You will feel nothing from the test.

The test usually takes about 30 minutes, but because of occasional delays and because further evaluations are sometimes necessary, you should allow an hour or more.

There are no aftereffects of MRI. No special aftercare is necessary.

### Risks:

The magnetic field used in MRI is so powerful that it can send metal objects flying across the room and pull stethoscopes out of physicians' pockets. The magnet may affect pacemakers, artificial limbs, and other implanted or prosthetic medical devices that contain metal. There is also a risk that metal objects coming within the field may become flying projectiles as they are pulled toward the powerful magnet. The magnetic field will stop watches several yards away.

Other than its effect on metallic objects, no harmful effects of MRI are known. However, this is a new method of testing and it is possible, though unlikely, that harmful effects might be discovered at a later date.

**Results:**

Results are usually available in 1–2 days. The radiologist will analyze the scans and review them with your doctor, who will explain them and discuss them with you.

The radiologist reading the scan will compare your findings with the normal appearance of the organs under investigation. MRI can sometimes detect tissue abnormalities even when the size and shape of the suspect organs or tissue are normal. Since MRI "sees through" such dense objects as bone, calcifications, or kidney stones, it cannot be used to examine these substances.

**Cost:**

$600 to $1000 (Costs vary considerably from facility to facility and depend on the specific test performed.)

# Pulmonary Function Tests (PFT)

Pulmonary function tests evaluate your ability to breathe in and out. You will be asked to breathe into a mouthpiece connected to a machine that measures the rate and amount of air inhaled and exhaled. Pulmonary function tests are used to help diagnose lung disease and to measure the extent of respiratory impairment.

Some tests of lung function can be done at home (p. 418).

**Why Performed:**

These tests can help determine the cause of shortness of breath and other breathing difficulties, and especially help to distinguish between restrictive forms of lung disease (e.g., pulmonary fibrosis) and obstructive diseases (e.g., asthma, bronchitis, or emphysema). These tests are also used to determine the extent of known respiratory disease and to determine the effectiveness of treatment with bronchodilator drugs.

Pulmonary function tests are sometimes performed before chest surgery to determine how much lung tissue can be safely removed. These tests may also be used to monitor workers who are exposed to certain chemical or other lung hazards.

**Preparation:**

Tell your doctor if
> You have ever had angina or other chest pain or a recent heart attack
> You have allergies to any medications
> You are taking any medications

You should eat no solid food for 4 hours before the test, as a full stomach may limit full expansion of your lungs. Small quantities of liquids are fine.

You should not smoke, exercise, or use bronchodilator drugs for 4 hours before the test, unless advised otherwise by your doctor. You should wear loose clothing that does not in any way restrict your breathing.

If you wear dentures, you should have them in during the test, since they will help you form a tight seal around the rubber mouthpiece.

**Procedure:**

Some of the simpler pulmonary function tests, such as vital capacity and forced expiratory volume, can be performed in a doctor's office or at your bedside. However, complete lung function testing is usually done in a pulmonary function laboratory or respiratory therapy department by a specially trained technician or therapist.

You will be asked to put on a noseclip to make sure that no air passes in or out of your nose during the breathing tests. You will then place your lips tightly around a mouthpiece which is connected to a machine that measures the air you inhale and exhale. Sometimes these tests are performed with you sitting inside a small telephone-boothlike enclosure which has a regulated atmosphere.

The exact instructions will depend upon the type of test being performed. For example, you will be asked to inhale as deeply as possible and then to blow all the air out as fast and hard as possible. You may also be asked to breathe in and out as deeply and rapidly as possible for 15 seconds. It is essential for the accuracy of the tests that you give these tests your full effort.

Some of the tests may be repeated after you have inhaled a spray containing a bronchodilator medication which acts to expand the airways in your lungs. You may also be given a special mixture of air and carbon dioxide to breathe to measure the ability of your lungs to exchange gases. Sometimes it is also necessary to take one or more samples of blood from an artery in your wrist to measure blood gases (see pp. 37 and 50).

The testing may take from 5 to 30 minutes depending upon how many tests are performed.

## How Does It Feel?

All the required procedures (except the arterial blood gas sample, if required) will be painless, though some may be tiring to those with severe respiratory disease. You may feel lightheaded after breathing in or out rapidly. You will be given a chance to rest between tests.

Some people find the noseclip uncomfortable, and some people with severely restricted breathing report that the apparatus gives them a "suffocating" feeling. Breathing through a mouthpiece for a long period of time can be uncomfortable. Some people

find the sealed, phone-boothlike enclosure unpleasantly confining.

## Risks:

These tests present little or no risk to a healthy individual. If you have a severe or unstable heart or lung condition, or any other severe medical problem, you should discuss the risks in your particular case with your doctor.

## Results:

These tests show how rapidly you can fill and empty your lungs and how much air your lungs can hold.

There are two principal kinds of lung disease—obstructive and restrictive. In obstructive conditions (e.g., asthma and bronchitis) the passageways through which the air flows are narrowed. In these conditions, the time it takes to fill and empty your lungs is increased.

In restrictive lung disease (e.g., pulmonary fibrosis), there is a loss of lung tissue, a loss in the lung's ability to expand, or a loss in its ability to transfer oxygen to the blood. In such conditions, either the lung volume or the transfer of oxygen from air to blood may be reduced.

The following are some of the more frequently used pulmonary function tests:

*Forced Vital Capacity (FVC)*—This measures the maximum amount of air you can exhale after inhaling as deeply as possible. This volume is less than normal in people with either restrictive or obstructive lung disease.

*Forced Expiratory Volume in One Second (FEV$_1$)*—This is the amount of air breathed out during the first second of a forced exhalation. This volume is usually substantially reduced in those with obstructive lung disease. It may be somewhat reduced in people with restrictive lung disease. The FEV$_1$ will increase after bronchodilator drugs in some people with reversible obstructive disease like asthma.

*Maximum Midexpiratory Flow (MMEF)*—This is the maximum rate at which air flows through the airway during forced exhalation. It is usually reduced in obstructive disease and normal in restrictive disease.

*Maximum Voluntary Ventilation (MVV)*—This is the greatest amount of air you can breathe out during 1 minute. It is decreased in both restrictive and obstructive disease.

Persons in pain may not be able to breathe fully because of it. Thus the results of their tests may be misleading.

Pregnancy or enlargement of the stomach (such as that resulting from a large meal) can significantly restrict lung volume, and thus interfere with the results of this test.

## Cost:

If a few tests are done in a doctor's office, there is usually no additional charge beyond the usual office visit fee. For tests done in a pulmonary function lab, charges range from $30 to $50 for 3−4 basic tests to $150 to $250 for a more elaborate sequence of studies.

# Sweat Test

This test measures the sodium and chloride concentrations in sweat. It is used to diagnose cystic fibrosis in children (and rarely in adults).

Cystic fibrosis is an inherited disease affecting the sweat glands. It also affects the glands in the lungs, intestines, bile duct, and pancreas. Early diagnosis of this condition is important, as early treatment can help reduce the severity of symptoms. Therapy includes a diet high in calories,

protein, and salt and low in fat; digestive enzyme supplements; vitamin supplements (A, D, and K); mist tents; expectorants; and preventive treatment with antibiotic drugs.

## Why Performed:

Children with a family history of cystic fibrosis and those suspected of having this condition (because of frequent colds, recurrent lung infections, recurrent diarrhea, difficulty absorbing food, or slower than normal growth) should have this test. Young adults with pancreatitis, cirrhosis of the liver, or unexplained chronic bronchitis should also have this test to determine whether cystic fibrosis is present.

## Preparation:

There is no need to restrict food, activity, or medications before the test. If possible one or both parents or a close adult friend should accompany a child to this test, and should bring along a favorite toy or book to occupy waiting time.

## Procedure:

This test is done in a laboratory or at a hospital bedside by a trained technician. The test is usually done on a child's right forearm. If done on an infant, the right thigh may be used.

The area is washed and dried and two metal electrodes are positioned and attached with straps. Gauze pads—one soaked in salt water, the other soaked with a drug that produces sweating (pilocarpine)—are positioned under the electrodes. A tiny electric current is then applied for 5−10 minutes. The child will feel only a light tingling or tickling. The electric current carries the pilocarpine into the skin and causes sweating.

The electrodes are then removed and the skin is again cleansed and dried. A dry gauze pad or piece of filter paper which has been previously weighed is placed on the spot where the pilocarpine was applied. It is covered with a piece of clear plastic. The edges of the plastic are taped to the child's skin.

This "sweat patch" is left in place for 30–45 minutes. The plastic is then removed, and the pad placed in a sealed bottle. The sweat on the pad is later weighed and analyzed for sodium and chloride content.

The test takes about 45–60 minutes.

**How Does It Feel?**

The child will feel a light tingling or tickling sensation when the current is applied. There should be no pain.

If the child cries or seems to be in pain, the current should be stopped and the electrodes inspected. Improperly placed electrodes can produce a burning sensation.

The test site may be red and continue to sweat for several hours after the test.

**Risks:**

Although there is almost no risk of electrical shock from this procedure, it should always be done on the right arm or leg to reduce the chance of the current affecting the heart. The chest area should be avoided. A battery-powered rather than direct-current unit is recommended to decrease any risk of shock.

**Results:**

Sweat from a normal child contains about 10–30 milliequivalents per milliliter (mEq/ml) of sodium and about 10–35 mEq/ml of chloride. A sodium level greater than 90 and a chloride level greater than 60 is diagnostic of cystic fibrosis.

Some other conditions can also produce increased sodium and chloride levels in sweat. These include adrenal insuffi-

ciency, glycogen storage disease, diabetes insipidus, and kidney failure.

Salt depletion due to hot weather may result in false normal test results in infants who do have cystic fibrosis.

**Cost:**

This test usually costs about $30 to $50

**Special Considerations:**

★ *Kiss Test*—To perform a simple sweat test, kiss or lightly lick your baby's skin and then your own and see whether your baby's skin tastes highly salty. This is a crude way to screen for cystic fibrosis at home. However, this "test" is not conclusive for or against the diagnosis of cystic fibrosis.

# Vision Tests
## (Visual Acuity Test, Refraction, Visual Fields, Color Vision Test)

The basic test of visual function is the *visual acuity test*. In this test you are asked to read letters from a chart (Snellen chart). Another chart, using the letter E or pictures of small objects in various positions and sizes, is used for young children. The smaller the letter you can distinguish, the better your visual acuity. A near-vision test is also usually done for persons over 40 and for those with eyestrain or reading difficulties.

Other vision tests can also be performed (see Special Considerations).

**Why Performed:**

Visual acuity testing should be performed whenever you experience any problems or changes in your vision. It is also routinely performed as part of a complete physical examination, in schools, and by some employers.

### Preparation:

No special preparation is required. If you wear glasses or contact lenses, bring them with you to the examination; the test cannot be properly performed without them.

### Procedure:

This test is usually performed by a nurse or medical assistant. It may also be performed by a physician, optometrist, teacher, or some other trained person. It may be performed at a doctor's or optometrist's office, a school, a workplace, a health fair, or elsewhere. The test for visual acuity can also be done at home (see Home Vision Tests, p. 403).

You will be asked to stand behind a line 20 feet from the eye chart. If you are wearing glasses or contacts, you will be asked to remove them. You will be asked to cover one eye and to read the smallest line of letters you can on the chart. If you are not sure of a letter, you should feel free to guess.

When you have read all you can with the first eye, cover your other eye and repeat the process. You may be asked to read a different chart or to read the lines backward to make sure that you did not remember the sequence of letters from the previous trial.

If you wear glasses or contacts, you will be asked to repeat the test while wearing them.

If you are unable to read the largest letters on the chart, another test will be used to determine what you can see.

If you are over 40 or if you have had problems reading or with eyestrain, you will be asked to read from a small chart held at your normal reading distance.

### Results:

Visual acuity is expressed as a fraction, such as 20/20, 20/40, or 20/100. The top number is the distance you stood from the chart. This is usually 20 feet. The bottom number is the distance from which a person with good eyesight could read the smallest line you were able to read.

For example, if the vision in your right eye is 20/20, it means that a person with normal vision could read the smallest line you could read while standing at the same distance from the chart that you were standing. If your vision is 20/40, it means that a person with normal vision could read the smallest line you were able to read while standing 40 feet from the chart—twice as far away.

It is possible to have vision better than 20/20. If the vision in your right eye is 20/15, it means that a normal person would have to stand 5 feet closer to the chart to read the smallest line you were able to read.

Vision of 20/20 is considered normal; 20/10 or 20/15 vision is better than normal. Vision between 20/25 and 20/60 is worse than normal. A person with 20/60 vision or worse is considered partially sighted. A person with 20/200 vision or less in his or her best corrected eye is considered legally blind.

If you have difficulty reading the letters on one side of the line, or if some letters disappear while you are looking at other letters, a *visual field defect* may be present. Let the examiner know if you notice this. Further testing may be needed.

### Cost:

A visual acuity test is usually included as part of a regular checkup or a routine eye examination.

### Special Considerations:

★*Refraction*—In this test the examiner determines the exact extent of your nearsightedness, farsightedness, and/or astigmatism (an irregular curvature of the cornea). The resulting measurement is called your *refractive error*. The examiner first looks into your eyes with a lighted scope to observe the path that light rays take when they enter your eyes. He or she then places a series of trial lenses before your eyes and adjusts them until the light rays are properly focused on your retina (the back of the eyeball). You will then be asked to read an eye chart through various trial lenses.

★*Visual Field Test (Tangent Screen Exam)*—The total area within which objects can be seen while the eye is focused on a central point is called the visual field. In this test the visual field of each of your eyes will be mapped. This test is used to detect and measure loss in your visual field.

You will be asked to sit about 3 feet from a screen with a target in the center. While you focus on the target, the examiner will move another target to various parts of the screen. You will be asked to let the examiner know when you see the moving target and when it disappears.

If the special equipment required for this test is not available, a rough evaluation of the visual field may be made by the *confrontation test*. In this test the examiner sits directly in front of you and moves his hand up and down and to each side. You are asked to look the examiner in the eye and to say when you can see the hand.

★*Color Vision Test (Color Blindness Test)*—This test measures your ability to recognize different colors. Color blindness affects about 8%–10% of males and less than 1% of females.

In the most common color vision test you will be asked to look at color plates made up of dots of various colors. A person with normal color vision will see patterns in the dots. A person who is color-blind will not be able to see the patterns.

★Also see Ophthalmoscopy, p. 333.

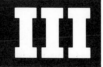

# III

# Home Medical Tests

**H**ome medical testing is not new. Self-diagnosis and self-treatment have always been the foundation of health care. Even today, when professional care is widely available, over 80% of all symptoms are completely self-managed. Those who do consult a health professional have usually practiced some form of self-care prior to the visit and often have a working diagnosis in mind.

Until recently, though, health consumers have had few diagnostic tools to help with this task. Now simple tools like the home thermometer are being supplemented by a growing number of other home medical tests: pregnancy tests, blood pressure cuffs, blood glucose monitoring systems, at-home screening tests for colon cancer, and many others. These tests, and others yet to come, hold great promise for aiding earlier, more accurate diagnoses, for improving home self-monitoring of chronic diseases, and for substituting cost-effective self-care for more expensive professional care.

The business of home health care products is rapidly expanding. Analysts estimate that there were $825 million in sales in 1984 and forecast sales as high as $1.8 billion by 1988.

## The Uses of Home Medical Tests

Home medical tests can be used for screening, diagnosis, and monitoring.

- *Screening* ("I feel well, but is something wrong?"): Screening tests are performed to detect hidden disorders before symptoms develop. Regular breast self-examination by women, testicular self-examination by men, and stool testing for hidden blood can be valuable aids in the early detection of cancer. Home screening can sometimes alert you to diseases at an early stage when prompt treatment can be invaluable.

- *Diagnosis* ("I feel sick. What is it?"): Home diagnostic tests such as those for strep throat, pregnancy, or ear problems can help you evaluate symptoms and decide whether professional advice is needed.

Home medical tests rarely provide a definitive diagnosis, but they can often give valuable information to be evaluated along with your symptoms and medical history, and, when appropriate, discussed with your health care provider.

- *Monitoring* ("I have a health problem. How well am I managing it?"): Home monitoring aids such as those for blood pressure or blood glucose can help you evaluate a continuing health problem and determine the effects of various treatments. Having access to home testing information can help you manage certain conditions on your own and participate actively with your health professional in the management of others.

### Benefits of Testing at Home
Home medical testing can offer many advantages: cost savings, improved accuracy, convenience, privacy, and an increased sense of control. Home blood pressure monitoring can be done when you are more relaxed or at different times of the day, providing more accurate and more representative readings than the measurements taken only in a doctor's office. Home blood glucose monitoring can be safer and less expensive, since it allows frequent, rapid determinations of blood glucose levels during normal daily activities without having to go to a laboratory. Home pregnancy tests can be more private and convenient than professional testing. Finally, all home medical tests offer you the opportunity to participate more actively in your own health care. Many people find this sense of empowerment makes them better, more informed, more responsible health consumers.

### Which Tests Are for You?
Virtually anyone could, with appropriate training, learn to perform any of the diagnostic tests done by health professionals. After all, health professionals are only lay people with specialized training. In practice, however, home diagnostics are limited by laws, by the expense of the equipment, and by the interest and motivation of the person doing the test. It makes little sense to spend a great deal of time learning a procedure that you may use only once or twice. Although you could, with a great deal of training, learn to examine the fundus of the eye with an ophthalmoscope (see p. 333), few lay people would have the need to use the skill frequently enough to justify the time and expense involved. However, if your child gets frequent ear infections, it probably would be worth the time and effort needed to learn to use an otoscope (p. 409) to examine your child's ears at home. The medical skills you choose to develop depend on the conditions you need to deal with.

### Limitations of Do-It-Yourself Medical Tests
Home medical tests are not without potential problems. No tests, including those performed in medical laboratories, are 100% accurate (see p. 26). Some tests may show abnormal results even though you are quite healthy (false-positives), while others may fail to detect abnormalities (false-negatives). In the discussion of each test we try to inform you of the limits of the test, the potential problems in performing it, and when to seek professional advice. For many home tests it is useful to have a health professional review with you the proper use and method the first time you do them.

Knowing when and when not to use a test is important. Many symptoms require prompt medical attention, not home testing. For instance, if you notice blood in your stool or urine or significant difficulty in breathing, home testing should not be used as a substitute for medical consultation.

It is essential to follow the instructions exactly. If the instructions in this book differ somewhat from those you receive with the test kits or device, be sure to follow the manufacturer's instructions.

Practicing some test procedures when you are healthy will help you learn what normal is for you and your family. It is then easier to spot an abnormality. If you do find an abnormal result, repeat the test. If it is still abnormal, if you are at all doubtful about the test results, or if your symptoms persist, you should consult your health professional. Finally, if you become excessively concerned about your health as a result of self-testing, or find yourself using these tests more frequently than is recommended, you may wish to discuss this with a sympathetic health professional. In this situation, home medical testing can do more harm than good.

## Equipment for Home Medical Testing

Most of the devices and tests discussed in this book can be obtained from your local pharmacy or from your doctor. Sometimes you may need to contact a local medical and surgical supply store (see your Yellow Pages) or write for the equipment (we list mail-order sources in most sections). In addition, we suggest that you send for a free copy of The Self-Care Catalog, a mail-order service specializing in home medical tests (The Self-Care Catalog, P.O. Box 999, Pt. Reyes, California 94956; 415-663-8464). Some tests are designed for use in physicians' offices and laboratories and are not packaged for the lay consumer. And some suppliers may be uneasy about selling these items to nonprofessionals even though they do not, by law, require a doctor's prescription. Showing them this book and explaining that you know how to properly use the test may be helpful. Be persistent, and if necessary, look elsewhere.

The cost of the equipment varies widely, so it pays to shop around. Your health insurance company may reimburse you for the cost of some of these tests, but a letter from your doctor recommending the specific test may be required.

The cost of some self-testing equipment may seem quite high, but most of these devices pay for themselves many times over by eliminating the need for some visits to a health professional, saving time, and providing increased peace of mind.

If you notice any problem with the tests or devices, check with the supplier, manufacturer, your doctor, or the federal Food and Drug Administration (FDA). The FDA maintains a toll-free telephone number (800-638-6725, in Maryland call collect 301-881-0256) which you can call to report problems with hazardous products, mislabeling, incomplete or confusing instructions, defective materials, or inaccurate results. Every year the FDA has to recall scores of products and devices. While we have not performed formal consumer tests on each of the tests or devices listed in this book, we have used them and found them generally reliable.

The field of home diagnostic testing is growing and changing rapidly. Currently under development are tests for monitoring blood cholesterol, urinary sodium, and therapeutic drug levels; screening tests for sexually transmitted diseases and breast cancer; home strep throat detection kits; and many others. With the new advances in microelectronics and laboratory chemistry, more accurate, convenient, and easy to interpret tests will soon be available.

But remember, no matter what tests you use, home medical testing is only one part of the picture of your health. Test results must be viewed in the context of your symptoms, past medical history, physical exam, and perhaps other tests. In many situations this is most appropriately done in a cooperative relationship with a health professional. More and more doctors and other health professionals are welcoming this type of partnership.

# Self-Examination

## Body Temperature Measurement

Breathing, digesting, moving, even thinking, all generate body heat. Your temperature is a reflection of this overall body metabolism and muscular activity. The body has evolved a remarkable mechanism to keep its temperature within a narrow, safe range in spite of considerable variations in environmental temperatures.

When you're too hot, the blood vessels in your skin dilate, carrying the excess heat to the surface. You then begin to sweat, and the evaporating sweat helps dissipate heat. If you are too cold, you may put on extra clothing or may start shivering. This involuntary, rapid contraction of the muscles generates enormous heat.

Sometimes this remarkable thermoregulatory mechanism goes awry. The result can be an abnormally high temperature, a fever, which is most often due to an infection. During the infection chemicals called pyrogens are released into the bloodstream. These pyrogens disrupt the thermostat in the brain. The message goes out to the body, "Quick, turn up the heat!" So you curl up to reduce surface heat loss, you begin to shiver, and you put on extra blankets to keep warm.

A fever may not be all bad; it may even help us fight infections. High body temperature appears to bolster the immune system and may inhibit the growth of infectious organisms. When temperature goes up, for example, blood levels of iron go down. This reduction of availability of a vital nutrient may, in effect, starve out the invading germs.

A temperature of 98.6 degrees Fahrenheit is often given as *the* normal temperature, but there is really nothing sacred about this figure. Many perfectly healthy people normally run a temperature a degree or more above or below the classic 98.6°F. Therefore, it is important to know what is normal for *you*.

### Why Performed:

It is a good idea to measure your temperature a few times when you're feeling well to establish your normal baseline. Be sure to include both morning and evening readings, since body temperature typically varies by 0.5 to 1 degree throughout the day. Body temperature is a useful measurement to make whenever you're sick. Temperature measurement may be helpful in evaluating symptoms like cough, earache, headache, abdominal pain, diarrhea, vomiting, back pain, painful urination, cold symptoms, weight loss, malaise, rashes, and skin infections. It can provide a clue to the cause of the symptoms and can help monitor whether a treatment is working, especially antibiotic treatment of infections. Measuring body temperature may also be used to estimate time of ovulation in women (see p. 195).

### Equipment:

The first thermometer was probably the back of a mother's hand, and this can still provide a rough indication of an elevated temperature. However, several types of more precise instrument are available to measure body temperature.

*Glass Thermometers:* These are the most common home diagnostic tool. Glass thermometers are usually filled with mercury or a red fluid. There are two types: oral (with a thin bulb tip) and rectal (with a thicker tip). The rectal thermometer can be used orally, but oral thermometers should not be used in the rectum, since the thinner tip may break. Glass thermometers are available at most pharmacies for $1–$2.

*Plastic Strip Thermometers:* Several new plastic strip thermometers are now available in many pharmacies for $2–$3: for example, Fever Scan Digital Thermometer (American Thermometer Co., Dayton, Ohio) or Clinitemp Fever Detector (Clinitemp Inc., Indianapolis, Indiana). These plastic strips contain a heat-sensitive liquid crystal which changes color to indicate the temperature. The strip is placed on the forehead (not in the mouth) and read after one minute. The readings must be made while the strip is in place. To take your own temperature with this device, you will have to look in a mirror.

Fever strips have several advantages. They can be left in place for continuous monitoring. They are quick, fun to watch, and easier to read than glass thermometers. However, the fever strips are considerably less accurate in detecting fevers. In one study the fever strips missed more than 20% of clinically significant fevers. We recommend the glass thermometer for general home use.

*Electronic Thermometers:* Several electronic thermometers with digital visual displays are now available. One company even offers a "talking" thermometer. In general, the electronic thermometers are quick, easy to use, very easy to read, and highly accurate. The major drawbacks are the expense ($18–$25) and the fact that they need batteries, which may run down just when you need them. Digital electronic thermometers are available from Marshall Electronics, Inc., 5425 W. Fargo Ave., Skokie, Illinois 60077, or from The Self-Care Catalog, P.O. Box 999, Pt. Reyes, California 94956.

### Preparation:

Temperatures should not be measured for at least 20–30 minutes after smoking, eating, or drinking a hot or cold liquid. You should also wait at least one hour after vigorous exercise or a hot bath.

### Procedure:

When using a glass thermometer, first clean it with rubbing alcohol or cool (hot water may break it) soapy water. Then grip the end opposite the bulb and shake vigorously as though trying to shake drops of water off the tip. Hold tightly; too many thermometers have been sent flying across the

**Body Temperature Measurement.** *QUESTION: Can you read this thermometer? What is the temperature?*
*ANSWER: 100.8°F.*

room by this maneuver. Shake it down until it reads 95°F or less.

Temperature can be measured in three locations:

*Oral:* The thermometer is placed under the tongue and enclosed tightly by the lips. This requires breathing through the nose. If this is impossible because of a stuffy nose or lack of cooperation, try one of the alternative locations. For an oral temperature, leave the thermometer in the mouth for a full *3 minutes*. If left in for only 2 minutes nearly a third of temperature readings will be in error by at least half a degree.

*Rectal:* This is the most accurate location to measure internal body temperature. It is recommended for infants, small children, and others unable to safely hold a thermometer in their mouth. Small children can be turned face down on a lap or flat surface. Spread the buttocks with one hand, then gently insert the bulb end of a well-lubricated rectal thermometer about ½ to 1 inch into the anal canal. After *3 minutes* remove and read.

*Axillary:* Placing the thermometer under the armpit is the least accurate method. The thermometer is positioned in the armpit (axilla) with the arm pressed against the body for a *full 5 minutes* before reading.

*How to Read a Thermometer:* Grip the thermometer at the end opposite the bulb and hold it in good light so that the numbers are facing you. Roll the thermometer slowly back and forth between your fingers until you see the silver or red reflection of the column. See where the column ends and compare it with the degrees marked in lines on the thermometer. Begin by noting the first long line immediately to the left of where the mercury stopped. This long line will tell you the full degree. Then count the number of short lines to the end of the mercury column. Each short line counts as an additional 0.2 (two-tenths) degree. Most thermometers have a special mark, usually an arrow, indicating a "normal" temperature of 98.6 degrees (see illustration). Most thermometers for home use are calibrated in degrees Fahrenheit (°F), but some may have the alternative scale of degrees centigrade (°C).

## Results:

Remember, "normal" temperature varies from person to person, so it is important to know your own usual temperature. Your temperature will also vary throughout the day, lowest in the early morning and rising by ½ to 1 degree in the early evening. Your temperature may also rise by a degree or more if you exercise on a hot day. In women, body temperature typically varies by a degree or more through the menstrual cycle, peaking around the time of ovulation.

Rectal temperatures normally run about ½ to 1 degree higher than oral temperatures, while axillary (armpit) temperatures are usually about ½ to 1 degree below oral temperatures. Therefore, if your oral temperature is 99°F, your rectal temperature should be about 100°F and your axillary temperature about 98°F. It is always important to note not only the temperature but also the location at which it was taken.

If your recorded temperature is more than 1–1.5 degrees above your "normal" baseline temperature, you have a fever.

Most fevers are the sign of an infection and are often accompanied by other symptoms (sore throat, cough, urinary symptoms, etc.) which may give a clue to the type of infection. But abnormally high temperatures may also occur as so-called drug fevers caused by reactions to antibiotics, narcotics, barbiturates, antihistamines, salicylates, and many other drugs. Fevers may also occur in severe injuries (such as burns), heart attacks, strokes, heatstroke, transfusion reactions, arthritis, excess thyroid hormone production (hyperthyroidism), and even some cancers such as leukemia, Hodgkin's disease, liver and lung cancer.

The pattern of the fever from hour to hour and day to day may give an important clue to its cause. For example, a fever that stays elevated for several days may suggest a flu or pneumonia. An intermittent fever, which rises each day only to fall dramatically to normal levels, may mean a hidden localized infection (abscess). Relapsing fevers occurring every few days may suggest an infection such as malaria. Temperature is only one of many signs, symptoms, and tests that help diagnose a disease, but it can be an important one. Therefore, keeping your own daily chart of temperature with multiple recordings may help determine the cause of the illness as well as the response to therapy.

In most healthy people, a temperature below 103°F does not in itself require treatment other than drinking lots of fluids to replace losses from evaporation. In most instances a fever can be considered a part of your body's natural defense against infection. However, a call or visit to a health professional would be advised in the following circumstances:

> A fever greater than 103°F
> A fever lasting more than 3 days or recurring every few days
> A fever in an infant less than 3 months old
> A fever in a child with a history of convulsions or fits associated with fever (febrile seizures)
> A fever accompanied by a rash, stiff neck, earache, trouble breathing, or extreme lethargy
> A fever in a person who is very old or ill with other serious diseases
> A fever that begins shortly after starting a new medication

Abnormally low temperatures can also be serious, even life-threatening. Low body temperature, usually a degree or more below 97°F, may occur in cold exposure, shock, alcohol or drug use, certain metabolic disorders (diabetes, hypothyroidism), and paradoxically in certain infections, particularly in newborns, the elderly, or the frail. If you discover an abnormally low temperature, seek medical advice.

**Special Considerations:**

★Hand-warming with temperature biofeedback has been suggested as a way to treat migraine headache and reduce overall levels of stress. By lightly holding a small thermometer between your thumb and index finger, you can learn to increase the warmth of your hands by dilating the blood vessels. Small, inexpensive thermometers with a wide temperature range can be ordered from Conscious Living Foundation, Box 520, Manhattan, Kansas 66502, for $.95 each or $.35 each for 100 or more. Information about more sophisticated temperature biofeedback instruments can be requested from the Conscious

Living Foundation, or from Thought Technology, Ltd., 2180 Belgrave Ave., Montreal, Canada H4A 2L8.

# Pulse Measurement and Fitness Testing

Pulse is a measurement of the number of heartbeats per minute. Normally each time the heart contracts, a wave of blood is sent through the arteries. This pulse wave can be felt wherever an artery is located near the skin. Veins, the blood vessels that return blood from the body to the heart, do not pulsate.

Pulse rate normally varies from minute to minute. When you exercise, have a fever, or are under stress your heart rate (and therefore pulse rate) speeds up to meet the increased body demand for oxygen and nutrients carried in the blood.

**Why Performed:**
Pulse-taking can be useful for monitoring medical conditions. For example, in evaluating certain symptoms such as palpitations, dizziness, fainting, chest pain, or shortness of breath, the pulse rate can provide important clues as to the function of the heart. In an emergency situation where a person has collapsed, the pulse rate can help you determine if the person's heart is pumping at all. People who are taking certain medications that can slow the heart rate such as digitalis (Digoxin) or beta-blocking agents (propranolol, atenolol, etc.) may find it useful to periodically check their pulse rate and report the results to their doctor.

Measuring the pulse rate at rest, during exercise, or immediately after vigorous exercise can also give important information about your fitness level and health.

**Equipment:**
All that is needed is a watch with a second hand or digital display. A variety of electronic pulse meters are available to automatically measure pulse and heart rate from your finger, wrist, or chest. These devices cost $30 to $150 and are mainly useful if you have difficulty measuring your pulse or if you wish to monitor your pulse during an exercise program without stopping to feel it.

**Procedure:**
You can measure your pulse anywhere in the body where an artery passes close to the skin: the wrist, neck, temple area, groin, behind the knees, or top of the foot. Place your index and middle finger over the underside of the opposite wrist, below the base of the thumb. With the flat of your fingers, rather than the tips, press firmly, but not so hard that you obliterate the pulse. Alternatively, you can place your index and middle finger just to the side of your Adam's apple, in the soft hollow area at the side of your neck (see illustration). Again, press firmly until you locate the pulse. Do not use your thumb to feel for the pulse, since the thumb has a pulse of its own.

*Resting Heart Rate:* To determine your heart rate at rest, measure your pulse when you first awaken or after you have been resting for at least 10 minutes. You can count your pulse for a full minute, or for 30 seconds and multiply by 2, or for 15 seconds and multiply by 4, to get the number of beats per minute.

*Exercise Heart Rate:* Your pulse rate during exercise can provide a good guide to how much work your heart is doing. This

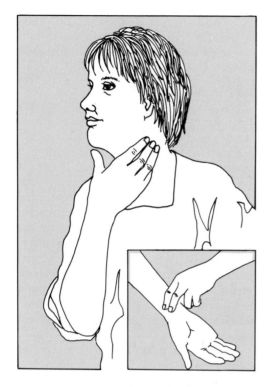

**Pulse Measurement and Fitness Testing.**
*Your pulse can be measured by placing your fingers at the side of your neck or on the thumb side of your wrist.*

can help you be sure that you are exercising with enough intensity to assure a good training effect, but not too hard. While you are exercising (stopping for a few seconds if necessary), measure your pulse rate for 6 seconds and multiply by 10, or for 10 seconds and multiply by 6, to get the number of beats per minute.

*3-Minute Step Test for Fitness:* This simple test allows you to roughly estimate the exercise capacity of your heart and your fitness level.

Before taking this test, answer these questions:

1. Has your doctor ever said you have heart trouble?

    Yes_____  No_____

2. Do you frequently have pains in your heart or chest?

    Yes_____  No_____

3. Do you often feel faint or have spells of severe dizziness?

    Yes_____  No_____

4. Has your doctor ever told you that you have a bone or joint problem, such as arthritis, that has been aggravated by exercise or might be made worse by exercise?

    Yes_____  No_____

5. Has a doctor ever said your blood pressure was too high?

    Yes_____  No_____

6. Are you taking any medication for your heart or high blood pressure?

    Yes_____  No_____

7. Is there a good physical reason, not mentioned here, why you should not engage in exercise if you wanted to?

    Yes_____  No_____

8. Are you over age 69 and not accustomed to vigorous exercise?

Yes_____ No_____

If you answered yes to any one of these questions, we suggest that you check with your doctor *before* trying this step test for fitness.

Find a 12-inch step (a bench, sturdy box, chair, or stack of newspapers tied in a secure bundle). Facing the step, first step up with one foot, then the other. Next step down with one foot, then the other. Each sequence of getting up and down from the step counts as one step. The pace is critical. You must make 24 full steps each minute (that's 2 every 5 seconds). Go for 3 minutes, then sit down immediately. Starting 5 seconds after you finish the exercise and sit down, start to count your pulse (at your wrist or neck) for a full minute. Compare your rate with the chart given under Results. If at any time during the stepping you feel chest pain, extreme shortness of breath, dizziness, unsteadiness, or are otherwise unable to continue, stop the test immediately and sit down.

## Results:

When measuring your pulse you should notice not only the rate (beats per minute) but also the rhythm. Is it steady and regular or are there pauses or extra beats? If you notice more than an occasional skipped or extra beat, discuss this with your doctor. Normally your heart rate will increase slightly when you take a deep inhalation and decrease slightly as you exhale. You can check this normal response on yourself.

| RESTING HEART RATE | beats per minute |
|---|---|
| Newborn infants | 100–160 |
| Children 1–10 years | 70–120 |
| Children over 10 and adults | 60–100 |
| Well-trained athletes | 40–60 |

Resting heart rates above these levels may be due to activity, fever, stress, overactive thyroid, low blood count or blood loss, stimulants (caffeine, amphetamines, decongestants, asthma medications, diet pills, and cigarettes), and various forms of heart disease. If your heart rate is consistently high, medical consultation is advised.

Resting heart rates below these rough guidelines may be due to an underactive thyroid gland, heart medications, or various types of heart disease and should be discussed with your doctor. Fitness programs that include endurance (aerobic) exercise lower resting heart rate. In general, the lower the resting heart rate, the more efficient your heart and the healthier you are.

*Exercise Heart Rate:* During exercise your heart should be working hard enough to

## Target Heart Rates for Exercise

| Age Range | Minimum–Maximum |
|---|---|
| 16–20 | 142–171 |
| 21–25 | 138–167 |
| 26–30 | 134–163 |
| 31–35 | 131–159 |
| 36–40 | 127–155 |
| 41–45 | 124–151 |
| 46–50 | 120–146 |
| 51–55 | 117–142 |
| 56–60 | 113–138 |
| 61–65 | 110–134 |
| 66–70 | 106–130 |
| 71–75 | 103–126 |

obtain a good training effect but not so hard as to be unsafe. There are recommended target pulse rates based on your age (see chart). During exercise you should attempt to keep your heart rate somewhere in the target range. Exercising with your heart rate in this target range for at least 20–30 minutes continuously three or more times a week is all that is required to keep your heart fit.

The ranges listed in the chart are based on a formula that estimates your maximum heart rate as 220 minus your age. The minimum heart rate of the target range is 70% of 220 minus your age, and the maximum heart rate of the target range is 85% of 220 minus your age. These recommended target ranges may not apply if you are taking medications (such as beta blockers) that slow your heart rate, if you have an artificial pacemaker, or if you have certain forms of heart disease. In these cases consult your physician for the appropriate exercise heart rates.

The chart below will allow you to make a rough estimate of your cardiovascular fitness level based on a 3-minute step test.

## 3-Minute Step Test for Fitness

| Age | 18–29 | | 30–39 | | 40–49 | |
|---|---|---|---|---|---|---|
| Sex | F | M | F | M | F | M |
| Excellent | to 79 | to 74 | to 83 | to 77 | to 87 | to 79 |
| Average | 80–110 | 75–100 | 84–115 | 78–109 | 88–118 | 80–112 |
| Poor | 111+ | 101+ | 116+ | 110+ | 119+ | 113+ |

| Age | 50–59 | | 68 & Over | |
|---|---|---|---|---|
| Sex | F | M | F | M |
| Excellent | to 91 | to 84 | to 94 | to 89 |
| Average | 92–123 | 85–115 | 95–127 | 90–118 |
| Poor | 124+ | 116+ | 128+ | 119+ |

# Home Vision Tests

Over 10 million people age 25 and older have some trouble seeing with one or both eyes even when wearing glasses. It is also estimated that 1 in every 20 preschool children and 1 in 4 schoolchildren have a vision problem which, if uncorrected, can lead to needless learning problems or loss of sight.

For some adults, a change in vision may be the only sign of a serious eye problem (such as cataract, glaucoma, diabetic retinopathy, or macular degeneration) which requires professional attention. Fortunately, for most adults corrective lenses (or a change in their present prescription) is all that is needed to improve their vision.

Regular professional eye examinations are important. But you can also help detect early vision problems and eye diseases by simple, at-home eye testing. You can test for distance vision, near vision, and macular degeneration, a condition that destroys the most sensitive part of the retina which is responsible for fine or distant vision.

## Why Performed:

Performing these home vision tests every year or two is useful for early detection of eye and vision problems. Many times we adjust to gradual changes in our vision and, without regular testing, often don't notice a vision problem. This can be especially true for children, who do not know how well they should see and, therefore, do not know if they have a vision problem. The discovery of "lazy eye" (amblyopia) before the age of 6 or 7 is particularly important for successful treatment.

While the home vision tests to be de-

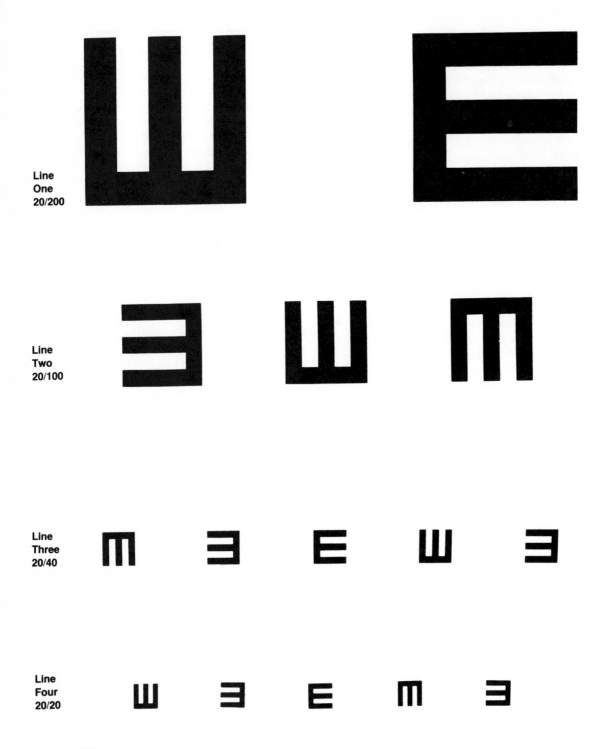

**Line
One
20/200**

**Line
Two
20/100**

**Line
Three
20/40**

**Line
Four
20/20**

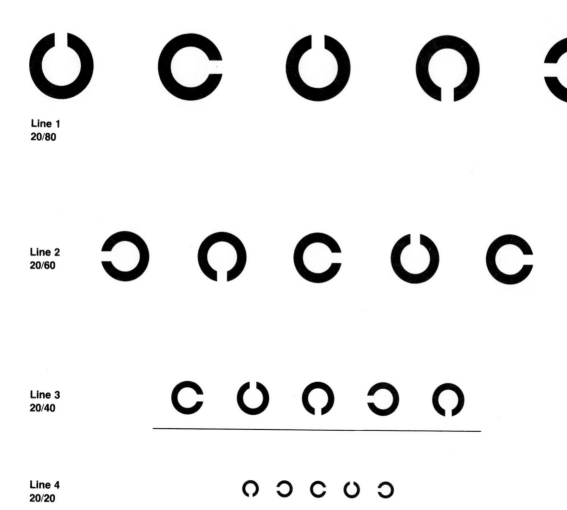

Line 1
20/80

Line 2
20/60

Line 3
20/40

Line 4
20/20

scribed are very helpful, remember that they do not replace periodic professional eye examinations, which should be done every 2 to 3 years if you wear corrective lenses or every 5 years if you don't.

### Equipment:

Well-lit area at least 10 feet long
Measuring tape or yardstick
Eye charts ( see pp. 404–405)
Tape or tack to hang the eye charts on the wall
Pencil or pen to record results
Paper or plastic cup
Another person to assist you, if possible

### Procedure for Distance-Vision Test:

*Adults and School-Age Children*: Remove the vision chart printed on p. 405 by cutting along the dotted line or make a clear copy on a photocopy machine. Tape or tack the chart to a wall (with no windows) or the back of a door in a very well-lit area. Line 3 of the chart should be at eye level. Measure exactly 10 feet from the chart and mark this spot on the floor with a piece of tape.

The object of the test is to tell where the opening is in each "C" on the chart. You will say whether the opening is at the top, bottom, right, or left, or you may point in those directions. Do not study or try to memorize the chart before the test.

Stand or sit facing the chart at a distance of 10 feet. Have the person helping you stand next to the eye chart.

Important: If you wear glasses or contact lenses for distance seeing, wear these to do the test. If you wear bifocals, look through the top part of the lenses. Do not wear your glasses if they are only for reading.

You are going to check your vision in each eye separately, first the right and then the left. Cover your left eye with your left hand. Keep both eyes open.

Start with line 1 (the largest "C's") and move down to the line of the smallest "C's" that you can read, starting where the opening is in all the "C's." Continue until you have read all the "C's" or until the openings are too difficult to see clearly. The person assisting you should point one by one to each "C" on the chart, pointing just underneath, not on, each letter.

Now write down or have your helper record the number of the smallest line for which you were able to tell where the opening was in *all* the "C's."

Repeat the test for the left eye by covering the right eye and write down the smallest line you could see with your left eye.

If you have no one to assist you, write down your answers on a piece of paper for each line or draw each "C" with the opening where you think it is. Check the answers against the chart.

*Preschool Children*: Distance-vision testing can be adapted for young children. Use the alternative "E" chart on p. 404. First, explain to the child that you are going to play a "pointing" game. Avoid coaxing or insisting. If the child doesn't want to play, choose another time. Teach the child to point up, down, right, and left when shown the large "E" of the chart in four different positions. Demonstrate how it is done and have the child practice pointing in each direction as you turn the chart.

Have the child stand 10 feet from the chart on the wall and cover one eye with a paper or plastic cup. If the child cannot hold the cup over his or her eye, you may need to have someone assist. Don't let the child peek.

Point to each "E," starting with the largest and have the child point to indicate the direction of the "E." Praise the child each time he or she points. Record the number of the smallest line on which the child can correctly identify *all* the "E's." Cover the other eye and repeat the test.

## Procedure for Near-Vision Test:

This test is to determine how good your vision is for reading and close work. If you wear glasses for reading, wear them for this test. If they are bifocals, look through the bottom part of the lenses.

Hold this book about 14 inches from your eyes, as you would for reading any newspaper or book. Be sure there is good light on the page. Using *both* eyes, read the small type on the Near-Vision Test below. Read it out loud to the person assisting you or write what you see on a piece of paper. Do not bring the paper closer to your eyes so you can see better!

---

Half of all blindness can be prevented. Everyone over 35 should have an eye examination every two years.

○ ⊃ ○ ∪ ⊂  ∪ ⊃ ⊂ ∪ ∩

---

Could you read the sentences without difficulty? ____Yes ____No

Could you tell where the opening was in *all* "C's" correctly? ____Yes ____No

## Procedure for Amsler Grid Test:

This test can detect macular degeneration, an eye disorder that causes blurred vision, distortion, and blank spots. Use the Amsler Grid which is reproduced here, p. 408.

If you normally wear glasses for reading, do the test with your glasses on. If they are bifocals, look through the bottom reading portion of the lenses.

Hold the grid directly in front of you about 14 inches from your eyes and look

at the dot in the center of the grid. Now cover your left eye and continue to look at the dot with your right eye. Repeat the test by covering your right eye.

You should be able to see the four corners of the square and to see that the large square is made up of many smaller squares.

Did any of the lines disappear or look wavy, instead of straight, when you covered either of your eyes? ____Yes ____No

## Results:

*Distance-Vision Test*: If you cannot read correctly all the figures in line 3 of the eye chart, you should repeat the test on another day. If you still cannot correctly read line 3 with each eye, arrange for a professional eye examination. This may be a sign of nearsightedness (myopia), in which near objects are seen better than distant objects.

Most people can normally read correctly all the figures in line 3 (next to the bottom line) with one or both eyes. This roughly corresponds to "20/40" vision (see later). Being able to read correctly all the figures in line 4 roughly corresponds to "20/20" vision.

*Near-Vision Test*: If you cannot correctly read the small type and identify the openings in all the "C's," repeat the test on another day. If you still cannot pass this test, arrange for a professional eye examination. Problems with near vision may be due to presbyopia or hyperopia (farsightedness), in which far objects are seen better than near objects.

*Amsler Grid Test for Macular Degeneration*: If your answer was yes for either eye—that is, if the lines of the grid disappear or appear wavy—you should have an eye examination immediately by an ophthalmologist, a medical eye specialist. The doctor will be able to carefully examine the macular area of your retina, which is responsible for your sharpest vision. Prompt diagnosis and treatment may help preserve your vision.

### Special Considerations:

★Passing any or all of these eye tests does not guarantee that you do not have an eye problem. If you have any of the following symptoms, you should have a professional eye exam:

Difficulty in focusing on near objects
Faces or objects look blurred or foggy
Double vision
Impression of a "film" or "skin" over the eyes
Frequent changes in glasses, none of which are satisfactory

Trouble adjusting to darkened rooms, as at movies, or seeing at night
Halos (rainbow-colored rings around lights)
Light flashes, dark spots, or ghostlike images
Vertical lines look distorted or wavy
Experiencing a curtainlike blotting out of vision
Eye pain or discharge

★Children who have any of the following symptoms or behaviors should also have a professional eye exam no matter what the results on the home test.

Thrusting head forward
Tilting head
Eyes watering

## Amsler Grid Test for macular degeneration

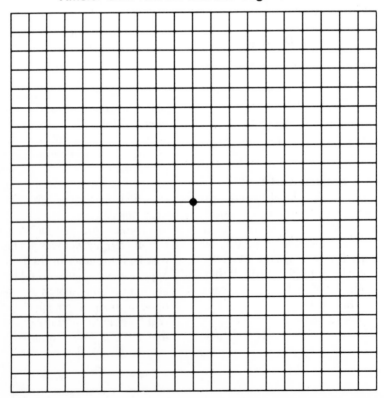

Frowning, scowling, or squinting
Puckering the face
Excessive blinking
Crossed eyes

★One of the earliest and most popular tests for distance vision used a Snellen chart. This is the familiar chart with letters, starting with a big "E," which progressively get smaller. These charts were designed to be viewed at a distance of 20 feet. If you can read the line marked 20/20, it means you can see as clearly at 20 feet as most people who have "normal" vision. However, if you can read down to only the 20/40 line or the 20/200 line, it means you can see at 20 feet what "normal" vision people can see at 40 feet or 200 feet, respectively. If you can see the smallest letters (20/15 line), then you have better than average visual acuity.

★These home eye tests have been adapted with the permission of the National Society to Prevent Blindness. For more information on eye care and eye diseases, write to the National Society to Prevent Blindness, 79 Madison Avenue, New York, NY 10016, or one of its local affiliates.

★A more elaborate home test kit, called Visionalysis, is available from Vision Research Institute (1724 Sacramento St., Suite 555, San Francisco, California 94109) for $50. This kit contains instructions and materials for 9 separate tests of visual health, including visual acuity, near vision, peripheral vision, depth perception, and color vision.

★For more information on eye tests, see Vision Tests (p. 390), Ophthalmoscopy (p. 333), and Glaucoma Tests (p. 379).

# Home Ear Examination

The ear is a wonder to behold. Just beyond the earlobe and outer ear is the external ear canal, which leads to the eardrum or tympanic membrane. This taut, delicate membrane marks the boundary between the outer ear and the middle ear, which contains three tiny bones, the smallest in the body. These bones are an engineering marvel. They attach to the eardrum and conduct sound waves to the sensitive hearing receptors in the inner ear. The middle ear also contains the upper end of the eustachian tube, a narrow passageway leading to the back of the throat. If the eustachian tube becomes congested, as it often does during a cold, pressure and fluid may collect in the middle ear, causing a sensation of fullness, pain and sometimes a partial hearing loss. When you feel your ears "pop," it is because some air is being forced through the eustachian tube.

So why is it important to know about the ear? Because ear infections are a common problem, especially among young children, as nearly any parent can testify. The infection may involve only the external ear canal (external otitis) or the middle ear behind the eardrum (otitis media). You can learn to examine the ear at home with the aid of an instrument called an otoscope. While not all ear problems can be diagnosed at home, home ear examinations can be quite useful in initially evaluating ear problems or following the progress of treatment. Further, if children become accustomed to being examined at home, they may be less afraid of ear exams in the doctor's office.

## Why Performed:

A home ear examination can give important clues to the cause of symptoms such as earache, ear fullness, or hearing loss. Sometimes a young child may have an ear infection in which the only clue may be crankiness, a fever, or tugging at the ear. A home exam may quickly reveal the cause of this "silent" infection. An otoscopic exam is also useful in monitoring the effectiveness of treatments prescribed for ear problems.

## Equipment:

An otoscope is a hand-held instrument with a built-in light supply, a magnifying lens, and a cone-shaped viewing piece called a speculum. An otoscope for home use costs between $15 and $50 and can be purchased at some pharmacies, medical supply stores, or by mail. For example, an Earscope costs about $22 from Nash & Associates, P.O. Box 300, 504 Shaw Avenue, Ferndale, California 95536, or from The Self-Care Catalog, P.O. Box 999, Pt. Reyes, California 94956. The Lighted Orotoscope is available for $25 from Sears Roebuck Home Health Care Catalog, Sears Tower, Chicago, Illinois 60684. The ear specula come in a set of different sizes. In a pinch, an ear speculum can be used with just an ordinary flashlight to catch a glimpse of the ear canal and, perhaps, the eardrum. Still, we recommend the magnifying otoscope for a better examination.

## Preparation:

The ear speculum should be cleaned and disinfected in hot soapy water or soaked for 10 minutes (preferably overnight) in rubbing alcohol.

## Procedure:

Dim the lights in the room. This makes it easier to see into the lighted ear canal.

Correct positioning of the person being examined is very important. Young children can be examined while they are lying down with head turned to the side or sitting on the lap of an adult with the head resting securely on the adult's chest. Older children or adults can sit with the head tilted slightly toward the opposite shoulder.

Start by examining the "good" ear, the one without symptoms. This is less painful, reduces the risk of spreading infection from the bad to the good ear, and may offer a basis for comparison. Begin by selecting the largest-size ear speculum that will fit comfortably in the ear canal. Hold the otoscope in the right hand to examine the right ear and in the left hand for the left ear. Brace the hand holding the otoscope securely against the side of the head so that any sudden movement is absorbed by your hand and not the instrument. With your free hand, grasp the outer ear and gently pull it up, back and slightly forward. This helps straighten out the ear canal for a better view. In infants, pulling the outer ear gently backward and down accomplishes the same thing.

Now slowly insert the ear speculum into the ear canal while looking into the otoscope. *Never advance the speculum without looking to see if the path is clear.* Angle the speculum slightly toward the person's nose to follow the normal angle of the canal. You need not insert it deeply. The light beam extends well beyond the viewing tip. The speculum is used mainly to center the light at the entrance of the canal.

Now while looking through the otoscope, move the instrument gently at different angles to view the canal walls and eardrum. *Stop at any sign of increased pain.* If your view is blocked by some yellowish-brown earwax, see the directions later for removing the wax.

Ask your health professional to review

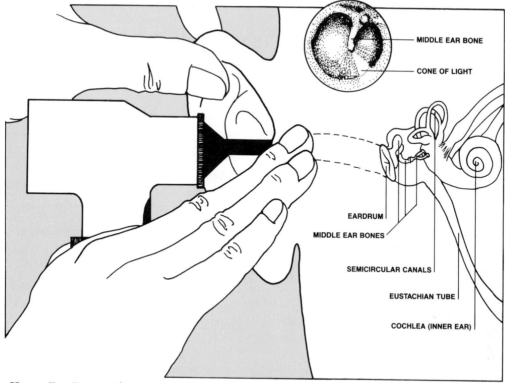

**Home Ear Exam.** *The otoscope is inserted into the external ear canal. Insert shows the view of the eardrum through the instrument. Structures behind the eardrum are not visible through the instrument.*

this technique with you and to observe while you do an exam. Then practice on some healthy, willing adults so that you can learn what a normal canal and eardrum look like. Don't be discouraged if you can't see the drum at first. It is a tricky exam and takes some practice and experience.

### Results:

Ear canals vary in size, shape, and color. Normally, the ear canal is skin-colored with small hairs and usually some yellowish-brown earwax. If wiggling or pulling on the outer ear produces pain, an external ear infection (external otitis or "swimmer's ear") may be present. A canal that is red,

tender, swollen, or filled with yellowish-green pus may also indicate an external ear infection.

The eardrum is normally a glistening pearly-white or light-gray color. On the surface of a normal drum you can also usually see the small bones of the middle ear pushing on the membrane like tent poles. You should also be able to see a cone of light, known as the "light reflex," reflecting off the surface of the eardrum (see illustration). If a middle ear infection (otitis media) is present, this light reflex may be dull or absent and the drum may be red and bulging. If fluid collects in the middle ear (serous otitis media), you can often see an

411

amber liquid or bubbles behind the eardrum.

You may notice a hole in the eardrum (perforation) or whitish scars on the surface of the drum, which are signs of previous infections. You may also see a tiny, colored, plastic tube. Doctors sometimes place these through the eardrum to help manage recurrent ear infections.

If you see an inflamed canal, pus, a dull or red eardrum, fluid behind the drum, or a perforation, report these abnormal findings to your doctor. Remember, not all ear problems can be seen with the otoscope, even by a trained professional. Therefore, no matter what you see with an otoscope, if symptoms of severe ear pain, fever, hearing loss, dizziness, ringing in the ear, or ear discharge are present, consult a health professional promptly.

### Special Considerations:

★*Removing Earwax*: Earwax, or cerumen, is a normal protective secretion of the ear canal. It is not a dangerous or dirty substance to be removed at any cost. Cleaning the ear canals daily with Q-tips, hairpins, or paper clips may be inviting trouble. Besides potentially damaging the canal or drum, the wax may be pushed farther into the canal. There are several products (e.g., Debrox or Cerumenex) available at any drugstore which can be used to dissolve and soften accumulated earwax. Place 5–10 drops of these solutions into the canal and wait 15–20 minutes. Then flush the ear canal in a shower or with warm water using a soft rubber bulb syringe. Do not completely block the opening of the ear canal with the tip of the syringe. The water pressure can damage the eardrum if flushing is done too vigorously. Just gently spray the walls of the canal with the water to loosen the wax. You may need to repeat the drops and flushing procedure in several days to clear the canal. If the procedure is painful or unsuccessful, seek professional assistance. Do not use this cleaning technique if you have an earache and discharge or if you know you have a hole or perforation in your eardrum.

# Self-Exam for Dental Plaque

Dental disease is the most common chronic disease; nearly 95% of all Americans suffer from tooth decay (dental caries) and/or gum disease (periodontal disease). The major culprit in both of these diseases is dental plaque, a sticky substance composed of millions of bacteria that accumulates around and between teeth. If not removed by proper daily brushing and flossing, plaque can cause tooth decay or cause the gums to become red, swollen, and bleed easily. If this inflammation of the gums is left untreated, the gums and supporting bone can be destroyed, resulting in tooth loss.

Plaque is virtually invisible, so how can you know if you are brushing and flossing adequately? Regular dental checkups will help, but you can also test at home by using either of two simple methods: disclosing tablets or a plaque light.

The disclosing tablets contain a red dye that stains food debris and dental plaque so you can spot areas not thoroughly cleaned. Similarly, a plaque light can be used to dramatically highlight areas missed during your daily brushing and flossing. These tests are safe, simple, inexpensive, and fun, which makes them ideal to use with children to reinforce good oral hygiene habits. But they are not just for children; most adults will "fail" their first few plaque tests with glowing colors!

**Why Performed:**

To improve your habits of tooth cleaning, you should test for dental plaque every day after brushing and flossing until you no longer leave areas of plaque. After that, a check every month or so will reinforce good habits.

**Equipment:**

Disclosing tablets cost about $1–$2 for a package of 30. Red-Kote and X-pose are two of many common brands. If you want to demonstrate plaque in a flashier, more dramatic fashion, try a plaque light with a supply of special fluorescent disclosing solution for about $10–$20. Disclosing tablets and plaque lights are available without prescription from most dentists or pharmacies. You should also have a small dental mirror ($1–$2) to check the hard-to-see areas.

**Procedure:**

*Disclosing Tablets*: After brushing and flossing, chew one of the tablets thoroughly, swishing the mixture of saliva and dye over your teeth and gums for about 30 seconds. Then gently rinse your mouth with water and examine your teeth in the mirror. Use a small dental mirror to check all areas. If your mirror fogs up, try running it under warm water before using.

*Plaque Light*: After brushing and flossing, swirl the special fluorescent solution around your mouth. Rinse gently with water and then examine your teeth and gums while shining the ultraviolet plaque light into your mouth.

**Results:**

With the disclosing tablets, areas of plaque and debris will be stained dark red. With the plaque light, these areas will fluoresce a brilliant orange-yellow. The stained areas, usually along gum lines and between teeth, indicate places you missed while brushing and flossing. Try brushing again to remove the highlighted areas of accumulated plaque.

After using disclosing tablets, your mouth and tongue may be temporarily stained for as long as a day. This is not harmful. Many people use the disclosing tablets at bedtime so that the stain will be gone by morning.

# Home Blood Pressure Monitoring

Blood pressure is the force exerted against the walls of the arteries as the heart pumps blood through the body. This pressure is determined by the force and amount of blood the heart pumps as well as the size and elasticity of the arteries. Blood pressure changes from day to day, even minute to minute, depending upon activity, posture, temperature, diet, drugs, emotional and physical state. Even talking has been shown to raise blood pressure.

About one in five Americans has high blood pressure (hypertension). If it is not controlled it increases a person's risk of stroke, heart failure, kidney failure, and heart attack. High blood pressure is often referred to as the "silent killer" because most of us cannot accurately sense if our own blood pressure is increased without measuring it. Thus, millions of people have high blood pressure without knowing it. The absence of symptoms is misleading. Early detection and treatment of hypertension using either drugs, life-style modifications (weight loss, sodium restriction, exercise, and relaxation), or both can reduce the health risks associated with high blood pressure.

Blood pressure is recorded as two numbers: *systolic* pressure and *diastolic* pressure. The systolic pressure is the maximum pressure exerted in the arteries when the heart contracts, forcing blood through the arteries. The diastolic pressure is the lowest pressure in the arteries and occurs when the heart is relaxing. The pressures are expressed in terms of millimeters of mercury (mm Hg) because the original blood pressure devices measured blood pressure using a column of mercury.

These two blood pressure measurements are recorded as systolic/diastolic. For example, if your systolic pressure is 120 and your diastolic pressure is 80, your blood pressure would be recorded as 120/80, which is read as "120 over 80."

### Why Performed:

You can easily learn to measure your own blood pressure at home. Self-recording of blood pressure has several advantages. First, it can offer a more accurate picture of your blood pressure throughout the day and in different environments (home, work, etc.). Some people have "white-coat hypertension"—that is, their blood pressure seems to increase only when they are in the doctor's office, perhaps because of anxiety of having their pressure taken. These people may be able to demonstrate that their blood pressures are usually normal by using home monitoring. This can dramatically change treatment.

If you *do* have high blood pressure, taking it yourself can let you see the effects of medications or habits on your blood pressure. Home monitoring can involve you more actively in your own care and help you feel more in control. One study even suggests that home blood pressure monitoring may in itself help reduce blood pressure levels, sometimes to normal.

Everyone should have their blood pressure checked, or check it themselves, at least every 2 to 3 years. If it is normal, no further testing is necessary. If you have increased blood pressure, you should check with a health professional and plan appropriate monitoring and, if necessary, treatment. If you are under treatment for high blood pressure, monitoring once a month or once a week is sufficient, though more frequent monitoring may be useful if your blood pressure is not well controlled or if your medications are being changed.

### Equipment:

Blood pressure is measured by a blood pressure cuff (sphygmomanometer). This consists of an inflatable bag (cuff) which is wrapped tightly around your arm, a device for measuring pressure (often a column of mercury or a gauge), and a device for detecting pulsations in the artery (a stethoscope or microphone).

There are three types of blood pressure measuring instruments:

*Mercury Column Blood Pressure Devices*: A column of mercury rises and falls in a clear tube with the units of measurement marked along the side. As the cuff pressure increases, the mercury rises. As the cuff pressure falls, so does the mercury column. Mercury blood pressure devices sell for about $50–$75. A stethoscope is also required to listen for sounds over the artery. Mercury column blood pressure cuffs are the most accurate of the blood pressure devices, but they are bulky, easily broken, and may be harder to use and read. Another potential disadvantage is that if the tube leaks or breaks, small amounts of toxic mercury and/or mercury vapor may be released. This may pose a slight hazard, especially for children.

*Aneroid Blood Pressure Devices*: This type of device displays the pressures on a circular dial with a needle. As the pressure in the cuff rises, the needle moves clockwise on the dial, and as it falls, the needle moves counterclockwise. Again a stethoscope is required; some models have the stethoscope head permanently attached to the cuff. The aneroid devices are compact, inexpensive ($20–$75), but somewhat difficult to use. Also the dial gauges may lose their accuracy. This can often be detected if the needle does not measure zero when the cuff is fully deflated. Unfortunately, some of these devices have a hidden stop-pin which prevents the needle from dropping below zero. Therefore, they can read zero even when they are inaccurate. Do not buy a blood pressure device with a stop-pin.

*Electronic Blood Pressure Devices*: These are newer, battery-operated, automated devices which use a microphone to detect the pulsations in the artery instead of having to listen with a stethoscope. Your blood pressure (and usually your pulse as well) is automatically recorded and displayed as a number (digital readout) or on a dial. Some of the electronic devices even inflate automatically and produce a printed record of your blood pressure. The electronic devices are by far the easiest to use. They are also the most expensive ($50–$250). While the electronic devices are highly accurate, they may not work well on some people with arterial sounds that are difficult for the machine to detect.

Blood pressure devices are now widely available in pharmacies, medical supply stores, and department stores. There are many different models and manufacturers, including Marshall Electronics, Inc., 7440 N. Long Ave., Skokie, Illinois 60077; Lumiscope Co., 836 Broadway, New York, N.Y. 10003; Tycos, 25 Old Shoals Road, Arden, North Carolina 28704; and Sears Roebuck and Co., Sears Tower, Chicago, Illinois 60684. The Self-Care Catalog (P.O. Box 999, Pt. Reyes, California 94956) lists several blood pressure devices that can be ordered by mail.

The length of the blood pressure cuff can affect the accuracy of blood pressure readings. If the cuff is too small, the measurements will be falsely elevated. One study showed that as many as 37% of obese people will be falsely labeled as hypertensive if a special extra-large cuff is not used. Unfortunately, most of the home monitoring blood pressure devices come equipped with standard-size cuffs, which are too small for larger people. As a general guideline, if your arm measures more than 13 inches (33 cm) around at its widest point, you will need a larger cuff, in which the inflatable bag portion of the cuff is at least 33 centimeters long. These large adult cuffs are available at most hospital and medical supply stores.

**Preparation:**
You can measure your blood pressure at any time, but standard measurements for comparison should be performed after resting for at least 5 minutes.

**Procedure:**
The instructions for how to take your blood pressure will vary depending upon the specific blood pressure device you get. Here are the basic principles.

Sit with your arm slightly bent and resting comfortably on a table so that the upper arm is on the same level as your heart. Expose your upper arm (roll up your sleeve, but not so tight as to constrict blood flow). Wrap the blood pressure cuff snugly around your upper arm so that the lower edge of the cuff is about 1 inch above the bend of your elbow.

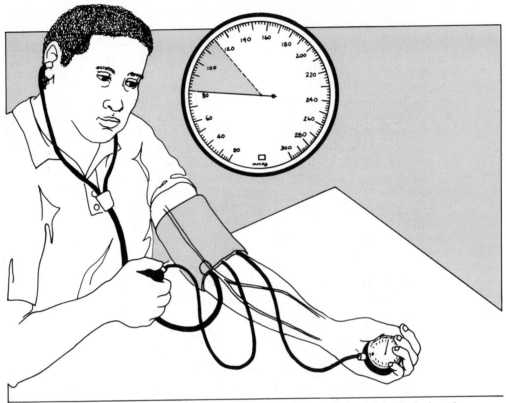

**Home Blood Pressure Monitoring.** *One type of blood pressure device (aneroid) displays the pressure on a circular dial with a needle indicator.*

A large artery (brachial artery) is located slightly above the inside of your elbow. You can check the location by feeling for the pulse in the artery with the fingers of your other hand. If you are using a stethoscope, place the earpieces in your ears and the head over the artery just below the cuff. The stethoscope should not rub on the cuff or clothing, as this can cause noises that can make your pulse hard to hear. If the cuff has the stethoscope head built in, be sure the part of the cuff with the stethoscope is positioned just over the artery. The accuracy of blood pressure recording de-

pends on the correct positioning of the stethoscope over the artery.

Close the valve on the rubber inflating bulb. Squeeze the bulb rapidly with your opposite hand. Inflate the cuff until the dial or column of mercury reads about 30 mm Hg higher than your usual systolic pressure. (If you don't know your pressure, inflate the cuff to 210 mm Hg.) The pressure in the cuff will temporarily stop all blood flow within the artery.

Now open the pressure valve just slightly by twisting or pressing the valve on the bulb. The pressure should fall gradually at about 2–3 mm Hg per second. Some blood pressure devices have a valve that automatically controls the fall at this rate. As you watch the pressure slowly fall, note the level on the dial or mercury tube at which you first start to hear a pulsing or tapping sound through the stethoscope. The sound is caused by the blood starting to be pushed through the closed artery. The pressure noted when this occurs is the systolic pressure.

Continue letting the air out slowly. The sounds will become muffled and will finally disappear. Note the pressure when the sounds completely disappear. Record this as the diastolic pressure. Finally, let out all the remaining air to relieve the pressure on your arm.

Repeat the same procedure twice, for a total of three readings. Wait 1–2 minutes between recordings while the blood flows unimpeded in your arm. Record the diastolic and systolic pressures, the date, the time, arm (left or right), and position (sitting, standing, lying). Once you become accustomed to taking your own blood pressure, you will probably need to take it only once or twice.

When you first get a blood pressure device, check its accuracy by comparing it with readings obtained by a doctor or nurse taken on a professional mercury column device. Ask your doctor or nurse to observe your technique to make sure that you are doing it correctly. It is a good idea to have your device rechecked every 6–12 months by comparing it with a mercury device.

Inspect your blood pressure cuff frequently to see that the rubber tubing, bulb, valves, and cuff are in good condition. Even a small hole or crack in the tubing can lead to inaccurate results. (This applies to all devices, including those in a doctor's office or hospital. One study showed that nearly a third of doctors' blood pressure devices had defects which could cause inaccuracies.)

**Results:**

There is no "magic number" for normal blood pressure, but there are some rough guidelines. If your systolic pressure is below 140 mm Hg and your diastolic pressure is below 90, this is considered "normal" even though lower pressures are actually healthier. Some doctors consider systolic pressures up to 160 mm Hg acceptable in people older than 60 years of age.

If your diastolic pressure is consistently between 90 and 104 mm Hg, this is considered mild hypertension, and you should discuss these findings with a health professional.

If your systolic pressure is greater than 200 mm Hg or your diastolic pressure is above 100 mm Hg on several repeated recordings, consult your doctor.

As a general rule, as long as you don't have symptoms such a lightheadedness or faintness, the lower your blood pressure the better. If your blood pressure is usually below 90/60 and you feel well, don't worry. However, if your blood pressure usually runs higher and suddenly drops to a lower level, consult a health professional.

Remember, your blood pressure may vary considerably from day to day and moment to moment. Stress, smoking, eating, exercise, cold, pain, noise, medications, even talking can affect it. A single elevated reading does not mean you have hypertension. Conversely, a single normal reading does not necessarily mean you don't have high blood pressure. Repeated measurements are important, and the results should be discussed with your doctor.

Do not adjust your blood pressure medications based upon home blood pressure readings without first discussing this with your doctor.

**Special Considerations:**

★Ambulatory monitoring over 24 hours is the most accurate way to determine blood pressure. This involves wearing a cuff attached to a small machine about the size of a tape recorder. The device automatically records your blood pressure every 15 to 30 minutes. The result is a record of how your blood pressure changes over a full day. However, this test is expensive ($225 per day) and is not yet widely available. Frequent self-recording at home can provide you with almost as complete a record.

# Self-Testing For Lung Function

The amount of air you can take into your lungs with a deep breath and how quickly you can expel it can be important in evaluating different kinds of breathing problems. Doctors will often order elaborate tests of pulmonary or lung function (see p. 387), but it is now possible to do some of the screening tests for lung function at home.

There are six lung function tests you can do at home. Two can be performed without special equipment.

*Match Test*: By trying to blow out a lighted match you can roughly check the force of your exhalation.

*Forced Expiratory Time (FET)*: This test measures how long it takes to exhale all the air out of your lungs after a deep inhalation.

Four other more precise tests can also be performed with the aid of inexpensive, hand-held instruments (spirometers and peak flow meters).

*Peak Expiratory Flow Rate (PEFR)*: This measures how fast you can blow the air out of your lungs during a vigorous exhalation.

*Forced Vital Capacity (FVC)*: This measures how much air you can expel from your lungs after a maximally deep breath.

*Forced Expiratory Volume in One Second (FEV$_1$)*: This measures the maximum amount of air you can expel in one second after taking as deep a breath as possible.

*Maximum Voluntary Ventilation (MVV)*: This measures the greatest amount of air you can breathe in and out in one minute.

**Why Performed:**

Home testing of lung function may be particularly useful if you have such chronic lung diseases as asthma, emphysema, or chronic bronchitis. These tests can help monitor the progress of the disease and assess the effectiveness of various treatments.

Home testing may also be a way to screen yourself for some lung diseases. Also, if you are starting an exercise program or stopping smoking, you may be able to measure your gradual improvement in lung function. Home spirometry has also been advocated as a way to encourage maximal deep breathing after an operation, so-called incentive spirometry, to help prevent collapse of the small airways during the period of bedrest after surgery.

**Equipment:**

All you need is a paper match for the match test and a watch with a second hand for the forced expiratory time test.

To measure your peak expiratory flow rate (PEFR) you will need one of the inexpensive peak flow monitors, such as

Peak Flow Monitor or Whistle ($5 from Biotrine Corporation, 175X New Boston Street, Woburn, Massachusetts 01801)

ASSESS Peak Flow Meter ($20 from HealthScan Products, Inc., Valley Road at Cooper Avenue, Upper Montclair, New Jersey 07043)

Vitalograph Pulmonary Monitor ($22 from Vitalograph, 8347 Quivira Road, Lenexa, Kansas 66215)

Armstrong Mini-Wright Peak Flow Meter ($70 from Armstrong Industries, Inc., P.O. Box 7, Northbrook, Illinois 60062)

To measure your FVC, $FEV_1$, and MVV you will need one of the hand-held spirometers, such as

Windmill ($85 from Kinetics Measurement Corp., Sterling Lake Road, Tuxedo, New York 10987)

Spirometer ($100–$140 from Propper Manufacturing Co., Inc., 36-04 Skillman Ave., Long Island City, New York 11101)

**Preparation:**

Loosen any tight clothing which might restrict your breathing. Sit up straight or stand when performing the tests to ensure that you can take as large a breath as possible.

**Procedure:**

*Match Test*: Hold a lighted paper match 6 inches in front of your open mouth. Take in as deep a breath as possible, open your mouth wide, then try to blow out the match with as forceful an exhalation as possible through your open mouth. Do not pucker or purse your lips to try to increase the force of the flow of air.

*Forced Expiratory Time (FET)*: Breathe in as deeply as possible, open your mouth wide, and then exhale as fast and completely as you can through an open mouth. Use a watch (with a second hand or digital display) or a stopwatch to measure the number of seconds it takes from when you first start to exhale to when you expel the last amount of air. Repeat the test for a total of three exhalations, and record the fastest (shortest) time on the three trials.

*Peak Expiratory Flow Rate (PEFR)*: Using one of the peak expiratory flow monitors, take as deep a breath as possible and then blow into the instrument's mouthpiece as hard and fast as you can. Try this three times and record the best (highest flow rate) of the three trials.

*Forced Vital Capacity (FVC) and Forced Expiratory Volume in One Second ($FEV_1$)*: Using one of the hand-held spirometers, take as deep a breath as possible and then blow out into the mouthpiece of the instrument as fast, hard, and long as possible. Keep blowing until you have expelled the last bit of air in your lungs. A maximum effort is absolutely necessary for an accurate reading. The spirometer will measure your FVC, and some types will then calculate your $FEV_1$ as well. Repeat the procedure for three separate breaths and record the best (highest) numbers for FVC and $FEV_1$.

*Maximum Ventilatory Volume (MVV)*: Again using one of the hand-held spirometers, blow as hard and as fast as you can into the mouthpiece with repeated rapid in-and-out breaths for exactly 15 seconds. Try to blow as much air as possible into the mouthpiece within this time. Multiply the recorded number by 4 to determine the value of your maximum breathing volume in one minute. Rest for a few minutes and then repeat two more times; then use the highest of the three values.

The accuracy of any of the home lung function tests depends on your taking full, deep breaths and blowing all the air out through your mouth. To help prevent any air from escaping through your nose during the test, you may wish to pinch your nostrils closed. Also be certain to seal your lips tightly around the mouthpiece of the instrument.

## Results:

There are two basic types of lung disease: obstructive and restrictive. Obstructive lung disease results in a decrease in the flow of air due to narrowing or blockage of the airways. Asthma, emphysema, and chronic bronchitis are the primary examples of obstructive lung disease.

In restrictive lung disease there is a decrease in the volume of air that can be inhaled due to decrease in elasticity or amount of the lung tissue (fibrosis, tumor, surgical removal of lung) or deformities in the rib cage or chest wall.

Comparing the results on these (and other) lung function tests can help determine which type of disease is present and what type of treatment is likely to be helpful. The home lung tests can also help measure the response to various treatments.

*Match Test*: This test is a rough measurement of the force of exhalation. People with normal lung function should be able to blow out the match without difficulty. If you could not extinguish the match, you should contact your doctor for further evaluation.

*Forced Expiratory Time (FET)*: Most people with normal lung function can expel all the air after a deep breath in 2 to 5 seconds. If it took you longer than 5 seconds to blow out all the air, you should contact your doctor for evaluation.

*Peak Expiratory Flow Rate (PEFR)*: This measurement is one of the simplest and most useful for monitoring your lung function if you have asthma. Often a decrease in PEFR will take place before symptoms develop, allowing you to adjust, in consultation with your doctor, your medications. In this way an impending asthma attack can sometimes be prevented. Nor-

mal values for PEFR vary with a person's age, sex, and size. Tables of predicted or expected values (in liters per minute or liters per second) are provided with the instruments. For example, a man 6 feet tall, age 40 might have a predicted normal PEFR of 650 liters per minute (L/min.), while the value for a woman, age 40, 5'3" tall might be 470 L/min. Generally, if your recorded PEFR is 80% or more of your predicted normal value, this is considered within normal limits. Patients with asthma have a lower baseline, and these tests could be used to watch for a further decrease in PEFR. People who quit smoking may notice an increase in their PEFR.

*Forced Vital Capacity (FVC)*: Normal values for FVC also vary with age, sex, and body size. Tables of expected or predicted FVC are usually provided with the spirometers. For example, a 6-foot-tall man, age 40, would have an expected FVC of about 5 liters, while 3.5 liters would be the predicted normal value for a woman age 40, 5'3" tall. Generally, if your measured FVC is less than 75%–80% of your predicted normal FVC, this suggests some lung disorder. FVC tends to decline with age. Recent studies suggest that FVC may be a good indicator of overall vigor and general health as well as risk of developing future heart disease.

*Forced Expiratory Volume in One Second (FEV$_1$)*: Normally you should be able to expel at least 75% of your breath in one second—that is, the FEV$_1$ should equal 75% or more of your FVC. A reduced FEV$_1$/FVC ratio (less than 75%) suggests increased airway resistance due to narrowed or constricted airways.

*Maximum Voluntary Ventilation (MVV)*: This is the greatest amount of air you can inhale and exhale in one minute. As with FVC, normal values vary with age, sex, and body size. The MVV is determined by airflow resistance, muscular strength, and endurance. Therefore, it is sometimes used to measure improvement in lung function after a physical exercise and conditioning program. Normal values are usually 15–20 times your FVC.

If you find abnormal results on any of the home lung function tests, discuss these with your doctor. It is advisable to check the accuracy and calibration of the home instruments against your doctor's more sophisticated pulmonary function tests.

While these home lung function tests may be useful in screening for some lung diseases, they are not generally sensitive enough to detect early damage from cigarette smoking. Therefore, smokers should not be reassured to any great degree by "normal" results on any of these lung function tests. Lung damage could still be occurring even with "normal" test results.

# Self-Diagnostic Tests

## Home Urinalysis

Each time we urinate we perform a urine examination. Almost unconsciously we note any unusual changes in amount, frequency, color, or odor. Urine is a complex solution of hundreds of body waste products. The composition of this remarkable fluid varies with the time of day, our diet, fluid intake, exercise, posture, and the metabolic acitvity of billions of cells in our body.

Laboratories can perform over a hundred different tests on urine. A dozen of these can be done at home. Abnormalities in these can alert us to disorders in nearly every body organ, including the kidneys, liver, blood, pancreas, gallbladder, lungs, spleen, bone marrow, and endocrine glands.

You can perform several urine tests at home using dipsticks, also known as dip-and-read reagent strips. These thin plastic strips contain chemically treated test pads at one end of the strip. Changes in color on the test strip are compared with a color chart. Within minutes, at a cost of less than 50 cents a test, you can perform a urinalysis similar to the ones done in doctors' offices, hospitals, and laboratories. Dipstick tests allow you to check the acidity (pH) and density (specific gravity) of your urine as well as for the presence of glucose, ketones, protein, blood, bilirubin, urobilinogen, nitrite, leukocytes, and vitamin C.

**Why Performed:**
A home urinalysis can be done as a general screening test to check for early signs of disease, to monitor an existing disease such as diabetes or kidney disease, or to evaluate the effectiveness of therapy.

Home testing can be helpful in determining whether dark-colored urine is due to blood, bilirubin, medications, or some other cause. People with kidney stones may find it useful to check for blood in the urine or to help them keep their urine dilute (low specific gravity) in order to prevent kidney stones. Vitamin C testing can help determine whether your urine contains excessive amounts of vitamin C, which might interfere with other urine tests for glucose, blood, or nitrite.

For many years diabetics have tested their urine for glucose and ketones to help with the control of diabetes. However, home *blood* glucose monitoring is being used much more widely because of its greater accuracy (see p. 434).

Home urine testing can also be used to check for urinary tract infections. This special use is covered in a separate section (see Self-Testing for Urinary Tract Infections, p. 428).

**Equipment:**
To perform a home urinalysis you will need a clean container, a watch that can measure seconds, and one or more dip-and-read reagent strips.

The container, preferably clear glass or plastic, must be clean and dry. Even a small amount of soap or detergent residue can interfere with test results. If you wash the container, rinse it with tap water or, if possible, distilled water before using. The urine sample in the container should be at least 1–2 inches deep to allow complete immersion of the dipstick.

There are many different types of reagent strips: some containing only one test, others with up to 9 (see chart). If you will be checking repeatedly for one or two substances in the urine, the single-test strips are much less expensive. However, for general purposes we recommend a multiple-test strip like N-Multistix SG, Chemstrip 9, or Uri-TRAK 7AN, which sell for about $35 for 100 test strips.

These reagent strips can be purchased without prescription from a pharmacy, medical or hospital supply store, or the manufacturer (addresses are given below chart). If your pharmacy doesn't carry the reagent strips you want, you may wish to ask the pharmacist to order them for you.

The reagent strips are marked with an expiration date. Don't use the strips after the marked date—the results may not be accurate. Store the strips in a cool (less than 86°F), dry place away from light. Do not store them in a refrigerator. Also be sure to keep the lid tightly closed; exposure to air may destroy the reagents.

There are several ways to check the accuracy of the test strips. If you notice a discoloration of any of the reagent pads, particularly if the ketone area is darker, the strip may not provide valid results. If you dip the strip into distilled water, the test strip should not register the presence of any chemicals. Finally, the strips may also be tested against commercially prepared "simulated" urine. This simulated urine contains specified amounts of the various substances and can be used to check the accuracy of the test strips. Chek-Stix or Tek-Chek from Ames (P.O. 70, Elkhart, Indiana 46515) and QC-U tablets from General Diagnostics (Division of Warner-Lambert Co., Morris Plains, New Jersey 07950) are two such products.

There are two ways to measure the density, known as specific gravity, of your urine. You can use the N-Multistix SG from Ames, which includes a reagent pad for specific gravity on the dipstick. Alternatively, you can purchase a small device called a urinometer or densitometer for about $10 from a hospital supply store, catalog, or from E. R. Squibb and Sons, Inc.,

## Urine Reagent Strip Tests

| | Approx. Cost | Specific Gravity | pH | Glucose | Ketones | Protein | Bilirubin | Urobilinogen | Blood | Nitrite | Leukocytes | Vitamin C (Ascorbic Acid) |
|---|---|---|---|---|---|---|---|---|---|---|---|---|
| **Ames*** | | | | | | | | | | | | |
| Albustix Strips | $14 per 100 | | | | | X | | | | | | |
| Diastix Strips | $7 per 100 | | | X | | | | | | | | |
| Hema-Combistix Strips | $25 per 100 | | X | X | | X | | | X | | | |
| Keto-Diastix Strips | $12 per 100 | | | X | X | | | | | | | |
| Labstix Strips | $30 per 100 | | X | X | X | X | | | X | | | |
| Microstix-Nitrite Kit | $4 per 3 | | | | | | | | | X | | |
| N-Multistix SG Strips | $35 per 100 | X | X | X | X | X | X | X | X | X | | |
| N-Multistix-C Strips | $35 per 100 | | X | X | X | X | X | X | X | X | | X |
| N-Uristix Strips | $21 per 100 | | | X | | X | | | | X | | |
| Stix Strips | $11 per 100 | | | | | | | | | | | X |
| **BioDynamics†** | | | | | | | | | | | | |
| Chemstrip 9 | $35 per 100 | | X | X | X | X | X | X | X | X | X | |
| Chemstrip 5L | $25 per 100 | | X | X | X | X | | | X | | X | |
| Chemstrip 4 | $20 per 100 | | X | X | | X | | | X | | | |
| Chemstrip uGK | $9 per 100 | | | X | X | | | | | | | |
| Chemstrip LN | $17 per 100 | | | | | | | | | X | X | |
| **Eli Lilly‡** | | | | | | | | | | | | |
| Tes-Tape | $4 per 100 | | | X | | | | | | | | |
| **Curtin Matheson Scientific‡‡** | | | | | | | | | | | | |
| Uri-TRAK AGK | $4 per 50 | | | X | X | | | | | | | X |
| Uri-TRAK 4A | $9 per 50 | | | X | | X | | | X | | | X |
| Uri TRAK 5AN | $10 per 50 | | | X | X | X | | | X | X | | X |
| Uri-TRAK 6A | $10 per 50 | | | X | X | X | X | | X | | | X |
| Uri-TRAK 7AN | $12 per 50 | | | X | X | X | X | X | X | X | | X |

*Ames Division, Miles Laboratories, Inc., P.O. Box 70, Elkhart, Indiana 46515
†BioDynamics, 9115 Hague Rd., Indianapolis, Indiana 46250
‡Eli Lilly & Co., 740 S. Alabama St., Indianapolis, Indiana 46206
‡‡Curtin Matheson Scientific, Inc., P.O. Box 1546, Houston, Texas 77251

P.O. Box 4000, Princeton, New Jersey 08540. A urinometer is particularly useful, and less expensive, if you will be making frequent measurements of specific gravity.

**Procedure:**

Begin by collecting a urine specimen (see p. 39). In general, the first morning urine is the most concentrated and, therefore, more likely to reveal an abnormality. However, if you are specifically looking for urobilinogen, the afternoon (1–3 P.M.) urine is the best. For diabetic monitoring of glucose and ketones a "double-voided" specimen taken after a meal is often preferred (see p. 38). Testing should be postponed during the menstrual period, since menstrual blood can interfere with the test results. Also, if you notice obviously bloody urine, medical consultation rather than home testing is advisable.

Collect the urine specimen in a clean, dry container and test it as soon as possible after collection. Some components in the urine may change or disappear if testing is delayed more than 15 minutes.

Begin by holding the urine specimen up to the light. What color is it? Is it clear or cloudy?

The specific gravity of the specimen can then be measured by floating a urinometer in it or by using one of the dipsticks that has a test area for specific gravity.

To perform the dipstick portion of the urinalysis, remove one of the strips from the container, replacing the cap immediately to protect the remaining strips. Be careful not to touch the test zones (reagent pads) with your fingers. Dip the strip into the urine until all test zones are fully moistened. Keep the strip submerged for 1–2 seconds. Remove the excess urine by gently tapping the strip against the edge of the urine container. Check the time. Hold the

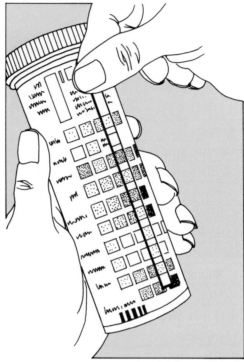

**Home Urinalysis.** *After dipping the reagent strip into a urine specimen, the color change of the reagent pads on the strip is compared with the standard color blocks on the reagent strip container.*

strip horizontally to help prevent mixing of the chemicals from adjacent test zones.

Each test is designed to be read at a specific time after dipping. These times range from immediately to 60 seconds. After waiting the specified amount of time, hold the strip close to the appropriate set of colored squares on the reagent strip container. Match the color of your test strip as closely as possible with one of the colored squares on the strip container. You will need to do the comparisons in a well-lighted area.

If you have any impairment of color

vision ("color blindness"), have someone with good color vision read the test along with you. Accurate results are dependent on good color vision.

The scoring units on the standard color chart vary depending upon the chemical being tested. Check the units on the color chart of the test strip you are using, and record your results for each reagent. Also record the date, time, use of any medications or vitamins, and any special circumstances such as fever, strenuous exercise, extreme emotional stress, menstrual bleeding, recent ejaculation, or special diet.

## Results: Color and Appearance

Many people wonder why the color of their urine varies from time to time. Some sense intuitively that changes in the color of their urine somehow reflect changes in their health—and, to some extent, this is true.

The color of urine can provide clues to certain diseases (see p. 113), but it more commonly reflects normal changes in the concentration of the urine, various foods in the diet, or medications that can color the urine. Normal urine can vary in color from almost colorless to a dark yellow, depending upon how concentrated it is. Reduced fluid intake or increased fluid losses (vigorous exercise, fevers, vomiting, diarrhea) tend to make the urine more concentrated and, therefore, darker.

Foods such as beets and blackberries can give your urine a reddish color. But so can blood and certain medications such as laxatives that contain phenolphthalein. How should you sort this out if you notice an unusually colored urine? First, review the chart on page 113–114. Second, perform a home urinalysis as described in this section. The finding of blood, bilirubin, nitrite, or leukocytes may suggest a cause. Third, consult your doctor, particularly if you have symptoms, if your home urinalysis is positive, or if the unusual color is unexplained by diet or medications.

## Specific Gravity

This test measures the ability of your kidneys to control how concentrated or dilute your urine is. Healthy kidneys should be able to adjust the amount of water excreted in urine to keep fluid output in balance with intake.

Specific gravity is a measure of the density of urine compared with pure water (see p. 115). Specific gravity of urine usually ranges between 1.006 and 1.030 (the higher the number the more concentrated the urine). It varies depending upon the time of day (usually higher after a night's sleep with no food or drink), the amount of food and liquids taken in, and the amount of exercise and sweating. For a discussion of the causes of an abnormally high or low specific gravity, see p. 115.

People with kidney stones may be advised by their physician to drink lots of fluids throughout the day to keep their urine dilute so that kidney stones are less likely to form. In this case, frequent monitoring of the specific gravity to check whether it is as low as desired can provide useful feedback.

If your urine specific gravity is consistently low (below 1.006) or high (above 1.030) on repeated measurements, or doesn't vary much at different times of the day ("fixed specific gravity"), consult your doctor.

## pH

The pH is a measurement of the acidity or alkalinity of the urine. This is influenced by the type of food you eat, the health of your lungs and kidneys, and your metabolism.

pH is measured on a dipstick and recorded on a scale in which 1.0 in strongly acid, 14 is strongly alkaline (basic), and 7.0 is neutral. Normal urine pH varies from 4.6 to 8.0, with an average of 6.0, which is slightly acid. For a discussion of the causes of very acid or alkaline urine see p. 116.

In some situations an alkaline urine is desirable. For example, kidney stones composed of uric acid, calcium oxalate, and cystine are less likely to form in alkaline urine. Also, certain antibiotics are more effective in killing bacteria in alkaline urine. Conversely, acidic urine may help prevent calcium phosphate and calcium carbonate kidney stones. Acidifying the urine by drinking large amounts of cranberry juice is also sometimes recommended to prevent the growth of certain types of bacteria in the urinary tract.

### Glucose

Urine normally contains very little glucose (sugar). However, when blood levels of glucose are very high, as in diabetes mellitus ("sugar diabetes"), some excess glucose may spill over into the urine. Glucose in the urine (glycosuria) can be detected by testing with a tablet such as Clinitest or, more conveniently, with a dipstick (either one for glucose alone or a combination strip which also contains other tests). Glucose levels are scored on the dipstick test as negative, 1/10, 1/4, 1/2, 1, and 2 grams/deciliter (%).

Urine tests for glucose are usually performed along with a test for ketones (see next). They may be performed on any urine specimen, but results are easier to interpret when performed on a "double-voided" specimen. This involves urinating once and flushing it away, urinating again 30–40 minutes later, and then collecting a sample. This second-voided specimen more accurately reflects current blood glucose levels

and metabolic acitivity. But even then, the results can be misleading. Urine glucose levels may lag well behind blood levels, and many diabetics now use home *blood* glucose monitoring (see p. 434) as a more precise and accurate method.

For a discussion of the causes of glucose in the urine other than diabetes, see p. 117. If you are diabetic, discuss with your doctor what actions to take based on the finding of glucose in your urine. If you are not diabetic and find more than a trace (1/10 gram/dl) of glucose on repeated home urine testing, medical consultation and further evaluation are advised.

### Ketones

Glucose is normally the main source of energy for your body's metabolism. However, if there is inadequate carbohydrate (sugars and starches) in your diet, or if you have diabetes mellitus (a defect in carbohydrate metabolism), your body cannot rely upon carbohydrates for energy. Instead your body burns fat. As the fat is metabolized, byproducts known as ketones or ketone bodies are produced and excreted in urine. These ketones can be detected with either a dipstick or a tablet. Ketones in the urine are scored on the dipstick test as negative, trace, small ( + ), moderate ( + + ), or large ( + + + ).

Large amounts of ketones in the urine (ketonuria) may occur in severely uncontrolled diabetes and should prompt immediate medical consultation. For a discussion of the other causes of ketonuria, see p. 118.

### Protein

Large molecules like proteins cannot normally escape through the kidney's filtering system into the urine. Therefore, finding protein in the urine is generally considered one of the best overall screening tests for kidney disease. Protein in the urine (proteinuria) is scored on the dipstick test as negative, trace, + (30 mg/dl), + + (100 mg/dl), + + + (300 mg/dl), or + + + + (over 2000 mg/dl).

There are many causes of increased protein in the urine (see p. 118). Perhaps the most common and, luckily, harmless cause of protein in the urine is a condition known as benign postural or orthostatic proteinuria. This condition, found in 3%–5% of healthy young people, results in small amounts (usually trace or +) of protein in the urine only when people are standing up, and it is not associated with any kidney disease. If you note a small amount of proteinuria, recheck the test on a urine specimen collected immediately after you get up in the morning. If protein is consistently absent when lying down and present only after standing or walking for some time, postural proteinuria is a likely cause. If you find protein on your urine test, we suggest that you discuss these findings with your doctor.

## Blood and Hemoglobin

Red blood cells and hemoglobin (the oxygen-carrying molecule in red blood cells) are not normally found in the urine. The portion of the dipstick labeled "blood" can detect blood or hemoglobin in the urine in amounts too small to be visible. The dipstick test for blood and hemoglobin is scored as + (small), + + (moderate), or + + + (large).

The finding of blood (hematuria) or hemoglobin (hemoglobinuria) in the urine may be a sign of urinary tract disease or increased destruction of red blood cells (see p. 119). However, blood or hemoglobin in the urine may also be caused by vigorous physical exercise ("march hemoglobinuria" or "jogger's hematuria"). Typically, exercise-induced hematuria appears only after vigorous exercise and disappears if retested after a day or two of rest.

If you find a positive reaction for blood in your urine which is not clearly associated with vigorous exercise, we suggest that you consult your doctor.

## Bilirubin

Bilirubin is a waste product from the breakdown of hemoglobin, the oxygen-carrying molecule in red blood cells. Normally the hemoglobin released from aged or damaged red blood cells is metabolized in your liver and excreted in bile into the intestines as bilirubin. (It is the bilirubin that gives the yellow-brown color to stools).

Bilirubin is not normally detected in the urine. Large amounts may give your urine a dark red-orange color and a yellow foam after shaking. Smaller amounts are invisible but can be detected by a change in color on the bilirubin dipstick pad. Bilirubin is scored on the dipstick test as negative, + (small), + + (moderate), or + + + (large).

Bilirubin in the urine is usually a sign of liver or bile duct disease (see p. 120). Therefore, if you find bilirubin in your urine, consult your doctor promptly.

## Urobilinogen

Urobilinogen is a pigment produced in the intestine by the action of intestinal bacteria on bilirubin. (Bilirubin is a yellowish pigment excreted by the liver in bile and derived from the breakdown of red blood cells.)

Normally a trace amount (0.1–1.0 Ehrlich units per 100 ml) of urobilinogen may be found in the urine, particularly in an afternoon urine sample (1–3 P.M.) when the excretion of urobilinogen normally tends to be higher. However, levels of urobilinogen above 1.0 Ehrlich units per 100 ml can indicate increased destruction of red blood cells (hemolysis) or liver and bile duct disease (see p. 121). So if you find more than a trace of urobilinogen on your urine test, discuss the results with your doctor.

### Nitrite and Leukocytes

These urine tests are indicators of urinary tract infections and are covered in the following section on home testing for urinary tract infections.

### Vitamin C

There is considerable debate on the optimal, as opposed to the minimal, requirements for vitamin C intake to promote and maintain health. Some proponents of megavitamin and orthomolecular medicine recommend enormous quantities of vitamin C (several grams per day) instead of the more conservative 60 mg per day of the U.S. Recommended Daily Allowance.

Whatever your daily intake of vitamin C, the amount in excess of your body's needs is excreted in your urine. Very little is stored in the body. It is, therefore, possible to test your urine to see if you are receiving an excess of vitamin C.

If you test your urine repeatedly with one of the dipstick tests and find no measurable excess vitamin C, that does not necessarily mean that your diet or body is deficient in vitamin C. If you do find a measurable excess, however, it means that the vitamin C may interfere with the results of your other urine tests. For example, excess vitamin C in the urine may cause false-positive tests for glucose or false-negative tests for blood, bilirubin, and nitrite.

# Self-Testing for Urinary Tract Infections

The healthy urinary tract (kidneys, ureters, bladder, and urethra) is normally free of bacteria. However, bladder infections (cystitis) and other urinary tract infections (UTIs) are a very common, and often uncomfortable problem, particularly in women and young children. Most of these infections are caused by bacteria that normally live in the rectum and colon but can migrate up the urethra (the tube through which you urinate) into the bladder. Bladder infections are more common in women because their urethras are shorter and closer to the bacteria-rich anal area.

Most urinary tract infections can be treated effectively with antibiotics. If not diagnosed and treated properly, however, they can spread to the kidneys, and may cause more serious infections.

There are now three types of home tests for urinary tract infections:

*Nitrite Dipsticks:* Nitrite is a chemical not normally found in the urine. Certain types of bacteria (called gram-negative bacteria) convert the nitrate from our diet into nitrite. This nitrite can be detected by dipping a special plastic strip (dipstick) into a fresh urine sample. If the reagent pad on the dipstick turns pink, nitrite is present. This suggests the presence of bacteria in the urinary tract.

*Leukocyte Dipstick:* Leukocytes (also called white blood cells) help fight infections. A special dipstick can detect leukocytes in the urine. Their presence suggests a urinary tract infection.

*Cultures:* You can also test for a urinary

tract infection by actually growing ("culturing") bacteria from a urine specimen (see p. 131). Special tubes or slides which contain a nutrient medium are available to do home cultures. If bacteria are present, they will grow and become visible on the culture medium.

Home testing for urinary tract infections is relatively easy, convenient, accurate, and economical ($1 for home testing compared with $10–$35 in a doctor's office).

## Why Performed:

This test is most useful for people with recurrent bladder infections. These infections usually produce such symptoms as pain or burning during urination, frequent urination, or the sudden, repeated urge to urinate. If you develop any of these symptoms for the first time, you should consult a doctor rather than do home testing.

But self-testing can be useful in certain circumstances. If you have had a urinary tract infection, you can test at home to see if the antibiotics you have taken have killed the bacteria. If you tend to get repeated bladder infections, you may want to screen yourself regularly at home for evidence of these infections. Further, home testing may be especially useful in young children with recurrent bladder infections who may not be able to report their symptoms.

Certain conditions lead to a higher risk of developing a urinary tract infection. If you are pregnant, have diabetes, or have some condition that may affect the flow of urine (kidney stones, stroke, or spinal cord injury), periodic home testing may also be worthwhile.

## Equipment:

Most of these "home" tests were originally designed for use in the doctor's office. Some pharmacies stock these tests or can order them for you without a prescription. Or you can ask your doctor to order them for you. You may wish to use a combination of tests.

*Nitrite Dipsticks:*
Microstix-Nitrite Reagent Strip Kit (Ames Co., Box 70, Elkhart, Indiana 46515)—$4 for kit with three nitrite strips, three cups and lay-oriented instructions.

N-Uristix (Ames Co., address as above)—$21 per 100 strips (also contain urine protein and glucose tests).

*Leukocyte Dipsticks:*
Chemstrip LN (Biodynamics, Inc., 9115 Hague Rd., Indianapolis, Indiana 46250)—$17 per 100 strips, which contain both leukocyte and nitrite tests.

*Cultures:*
Microstix-3 (Ames Co., address as above)—$40 per 25 strips, which contain a dipculture and nitrite test.

Bacturcult (Wampole Labs, Division of Carter-Wallace, Cranbury, New Jersey 80512)—$15 per 10 test kits.

Culturia (Chemical Convenience Products, Inc., Box 1493, Madison, Wisconsin 53701)—$15 per 10 test kits.

## Procedure:

A "clean-catch" or "midstream" urine sample should be used for all of these tests. Obtain a clean-catch sample as follows: Men should wipe clean the head of the penis and women should spread the inner lips of the vagina and wash the area between the lips with soapy water and rinse well. Urinate a small amount into the toilet bowl to clear the urethra of contaminants. Then catch about 1–2 ounces of urine in a clean container, remove the container from the urine stream, and finish urinating into the toilet (see p. 39).

Collecting a urine specimen from an infant can be difficult. There are special plastic bags which can be taped to a toddler to collect the urine (p. 41). Discuss how to use them with your doctor.

Be sure to perform the tests within 15 minutes of the time you collect the sample. The sooner the better. For the dipstick tests, you will need a well-lighted place to compare the test pad with its color chart.

*Nitrite Dipstick:* Since it takes several hours for any bacteria in the bladder to produce nitrite, test only urine that has been in the bladder for at least 4 hours. A first morning urine specimen (which has collected in the bladder overnight) is the best specimen to use. Dip the pad at the end of one of the plastic dipsticks into a freshly voided urine sample for a second or two, or pass the strip through the urine stream to thoroughly wet the test pad. Remove any excess urine from the pad by gently tapping the strip. After waiting 30 seconds, compare the color of the test pad with the standard color chart provided with the strips. Repeat this procedure on a fresh specimen for three mornings in a row, using a fresh dipstick each time.

*Leukocyte Dipstick:* Dip the dipstick into a freshly collected urine specimen or pass the dipstick through the urine stream, to thoroughly wet the reagent pad on the top of the dipstick. Gently tap the dipstick to remove excess urine. Wait 60 seconds and compare the color of the test pad with the standard color chart on the dipstick container. Check the results again 2 minutes after dipping.

*Cultures:* Each culture system is slightly different, so follow the instructions that come with the test kit. A slide or test strip containing a culture medium is dipped into a freshly collected "clean-catch" urine sample. The slide is then returned to its container and allowed to sit undisturbed for 24 hours at room temperature (approximately 70°F).

**Results:**

*Nitrite Dipstick:* If you have a problem with color vision, have someone assist you in reading the results. This test should be read after 30 seconds. Any color change on the reagent pad after that time should be ignored. If the test area turns uniformly pink to any degree on any one of the three consecutive morning urine samples, the result is considered positive, indicating the presence of nitrite and bacteria. Discuss any positive test results with a health professional.

False-positive results (the test is positive even though you don't have an infection) can occur if there is blood in your urine or if you are taking a urinary anesthetic drug called phenazopyridine (Pyridium), which can turn the urine and the test strip pink. False-negative test results (the test is negative even though you do have an infection) can be caused by large doses of vitamin C, if the urine has not been in the bladder for at least 4 hours before collecting the specimen, or if the infection is caused by bacteria that do not produce nitrite (only about 10% of all urinary tract infections). This means that about 10% of infections are missed by this method. So if symptoms persist, consult your clinician.

*Leukocyte Dipstick:* Compare the leukocyte dipstick with the standard color chart at 60 and 120 seconds after dipping. Look for discoloration (usually pink or purple). "Trace" results should be repeated. Results in the "+" or "++" zones are positive for leukocytes and suggest an infection. Discuss positive results with your health professional. Certain medications, including the urinary anesthetic phenazopyridine (Pyridium), certain antibiotics (cephalexin, gentamicin, and nitrofurantoin), as well as large doses of vitamin C, can cause false results. The leukocyte test can detect over

90% of urinary tract infections, and even more when combined with the nitrite test.

*Culture:* After incubating the culture slide at room temperature for 24 hours, examine the slide surface. The appearance of small dots on the slide indicates growth of colonies of bacteria. A rough estimate of the concentration of bacteria can be made by comparing the density of the dots on the slide with a standard chart supplied with the test kit. Bacterial counts of more than 100,000 colonies per milliliter ($10^5$ colonies/cc) are indicative of a urinary tract infection, and the findings should be discussed with a health professional. Colony counts below 100,000 colonies per ml may be due to infection or contamination and should be repeated.

### Special Considerations:

★Although these tests may detect the presence of a urinary infection, they cannot reveal its location. It may be in the kidney, ureters, bladder, urethra, or, in men, the prostate gland. Other tests may be necessary to determine the location and cause.

★Remember, none of these tests are 100% accurate. If you have persistent symptoms, consult your health professional. Painful urination can be caused by conditions other than a urinary tract infection, such as a vaginal infection. Symptoms like a fever or back pain may indicate a more serious kidney infection requiring prompt medical attention.

Don't treat yourself with leftover antibiotics unless specifically advised to do so by your clinician. Partial, incomplete, or incorrect treatment may do more harm than good.

# Home Pregnancy Tests

In ancient Egypt women reportedly poured their urine on papyrus leaves to tell if they were pregnant. If the plant survived, they were. If it died, they were not. Today there is another, more accurate way to test your urine to determine pregnancy.

Home pregnancy test kits can now be purchased in most drugstores without a prescription. These tests are virtually the same as the urine pregnancy tests performed in most doctors' offices and clinics. The home pregnancy tests are convenient, private, and, if performed properly, can be quite accurate.

During pregnancy a fertilized egg implants in the uterine wall. A hormone, called human chorionic gonadotropin (HCG), is then produced by the developing placenta and excreted in the urine. The amount of this hormone excreted in the urine rises rapidly during the first weeks of pregnancy. Home pregnancy tests are designed to detect this pregnancy hormone in your urine. If the hormone is present, then it is likely that you are pregnant.

### Why Performed:

Many women are able to self-diagnose pregnancy without testing by observing bodily changes. A missed menstrual period, breast tenderness, morning nausea, fatigue, and other unusual bodily sensations may be early signs of pregnancy.

The home pregnancy tests can provide confirmation and reassurance when a menstrual period is late without having to visit a doctor or laboratory. Early confirmation of pregnancy can be very useful. It may allow you to start proper prenatal care right away, during the first month of pregnancy when the risk to the fetus is greatest. This might include changes in nutrition and avoidance of cigarettes, drugs, alcohol, and x-ray exposure. Or if you decide on an abortion, this can be arranged early on, when the procedure is simpler and safer.

## Equipment:

Home pregnancy tests are available without a doctor's prescription in most pharmacies and supermarkets. There are two types of tests: the tube tests and the newer dipstick tests.

The tube tests are packaged either as a single test for $8–$12 or as a double test kit for $12–$15. The tests are not reusable. The double test kit allows you to repeat and confirm the initial test result without purchasing another kit. Several manufacturers now produce tube-type tests, including Acu-Test (Beecham Products), Answer (Carter Wallace), Daisy 2 (Ortho), e.p.t. (Warner-Lambert), and Predictor (Whitehall). If any of the liquid reagents in these kits appears cloudy, return it to the place of purchase for a new kit.

A new dipstick pregnancy test called Advance (Ortho Pharmaceutical Co.) sells for about $11 for a single test kit.

## Preparation:

The manufacturers of the tube-type tests recommend waiting at least 9 days (3–6 days for some tests) after the expected start of a missed menstrual period before testing. We recommend waiting at least 14 days after a missed period (6 weeks after the start of your last menstrual period). At that time the tests are more reliable, so false results and retesting may be avoided. If you have very irregular menstrual periods (such as often occurs in teenagers, women approaching menopause, or women who have recently stopped oral contraceptives), you should probably wait until 21 days after the expected period (7 weeks after your last period) before performing the test.

The dipstick-type tests are reported to be much more sensitive than the tube tests. The manufacturer claims that the test can detect pregnancy accurately as early as 3 days after a missed menstrual period. We still recommend waiting at least 7 days after a missed menstrual period to avoid unnecessary testing and expense.

## Procedure:

The instructions for the home pregnancy tests are fairly complicated and vary from brand to brand. Carefully read and reread the instructions that come with your test before testing and follow these directions *exactly*. One study showed that as many as two thirds of women using the tests did not follow the instructions.

*Tube Tests:* With this type of test, you take a few drops of a first morning urine specimen. This assumes that you haven't emptied your bladder for 6–8 hours overnight. This first morning sample will contain the highest concentration of the HCG hormone, and therefore should give the most reliable result. Collect the urine specimen in a clean, dry container which has been washed and rinsed thoroughly with tap water. Any traces of soap or detergent in the container can produce a false test result. If your urine is very cloudy, pink, or red, do not perform the test. It may contain excessive amounts of red blood cells, protein, or bacteria, which can interfere with the test results. Instead consult your doctor.

If at all possible, perform the test immediately. If this is not possible, cover and store the sample in the refrigerator for up to 12 hours (do not freeze). Take a few drops of the urine in the eyedropper provided and mix with the reagents in the test kit. Then let the mixture stand undisturbed for the time indicated in the instructions (usually 1 to 2 hours). Place the tube on a flat, solid surface, safe from accidental bumping or vibration—away from washing machines, refrigerators or any other source of vibration. Protect the test kit from heat or sunlight (these may cause false results). After waiting 1 to 2 hours, you can read the results. Do not attempt to interpret the results before or after the prescribed time.

*Dipstick Tests:* First, as described previously, collect a first morning urine specimen and mix a few drops of urine with the reagent solution in the test kit. Place the test pad on the end of the dipstick into the urine-reagent mixture for 15 minutes (or as instructed). Then rinse the dipstick thoroughly under cold tap water and place it into a special developing solution for another 15 minutes. Finally, read the color change on the test pad.

## Results:

*Tube Test:* At the indicated time and without moving the test tube, look at the bottom of the tube for a ring-shaped deposit with a hole in the center like a donut. If you see such a ring the test is positive, indicating the presence of pregnancy hormone and a high likelihood that you are pregnant. If there is no ring but just a hazy deposit, then there is not enough pregnancy hormone in your urine to be detected and the test is negative.

Unfortunately, these home pregnancy tests are not 100% accurate. A false-negative result (meaning the test is negative but you are actually pregnant) may occur. This may result from testing too soon after a missed menstrual period or, less commonly, from an ectopic (tubal) pregnancy

when the fertilized egg implants outside of the uterus and too little pregnancy hormone is produced to be detected. False-positive results (meaning the test is positive but you are not pregnant) occur in only 2%–3% of tests. This can be due to a detergent residue in the urine collection container, reading the test at the wrong time, exposing the test to heat, sunlight, or vibration, the presence of excess protein or blood in the urine, or HCG hormone actually being produced by a rare type of uterine cancer. Certain drugs such as thorazine tranquilizers and methadone may also interfere with the test results.

*Dipstick Tests:* Examine the test pad on the end of the dipstick at the specified time. If the test pad turns blue, pregnancy hormone is present and the result is positive. If the test pad doesn't turn blue, there is not enough pregnancy hormone in your urine to be detected and the result is negative. The manufacturer claims that the overall accuracy of the test is 95%–98%. If you have a problem with color vision, have someone help you read the test.

With either type of home pregnancy test, if the test is positive, you should see your doctor to confirm the test and arrange follow-up care. *If the test is negative, you may still be pregnant.* You should repeat the test in about one week if your menstrual period hasn't started. If it is still negative on the repeat test, you are probably not pregnant, but you should consult your doctor to determine the reasons why you are not menstruating.

If you have missed a menstrual period and are having severe lower abdominal pain, see your doctor right away even if the pregnancy test is negative. You may have an ectopic pregnancy which could rupture, leading to serious medical problems and possibly death.

**Special Considerations:**

★Pregnancy tests are sometimes available at a lower cost through community organizations. Ask local physicians, Planned Parenthood clinics, community clinics, or the health department about the availability and cost of pregnancy tests.

★There are more sensitive *blood tests* for pregnancy which can detect it within a few days of conception, even before a missed menstrual period (see p. 93). However, these blood pregnancy tests cannot be performed at home.

# Home Blood Glucose Monitoring

This test allows you to measure the concentration of glucose (sugar) in a drop of your blood. Knowing your blood glucose level can be especially important to people with diabetes, a disorder in which the body cannot properly metabolize glucose. Diabetes can be due to a failure of the pancreas to produce enough of the hormone insulin (Type I or insulin-dependent diabetes) or a lack of sensitivity in the body to insulin (Type 2 or maturity-onset diabetes). In either case, the result is an increase in blood glucose to levels that can be dangerous.

Diabetic patients have long been able to test their urine to detect glucose, but such measurements give only a very rough and delayed approximation of blood glucose. And urine measurements do not indicate when blood glucose levels fall below normal (hypoglycemia).

There are two basic methods of home blood glucose monitoring. Both involve a fingerprick and placing of a drop of blood on a reagent pad on the end of a thin plastic test strip. The pad changes color to reflect the amount of glucose in the blood. In the first method, the strip is read visually by comparing the color change on the strip with a standard color chart. With the other method, a portable glucose meter, about the size of a paperback book, is used to "read" the strip, and the blood glucose is indicated as a number on a digital display.

**Why Performed:**

Home blood glucose monitoring offers the possibility of carefully controlling blood glucose levels in the normal range. Most experts now agree that this tight control offers the best hope of reducing the major problems of diabetes—blindness, kidney disease, heart disease, and nerve damage. This test can help diabetics respond quickly to extremely low or high blood sugars and prevent life-threatening situations and hospitalizations.

In addition, home monitoring provides the opportunity for people to better understand their diabetes. In particular, the effects of diet, exercise, stress, and insulin can be observed more directly and clearly. Finally, home blood glucose monitoring enhances a person's sense of control and encourages more active participation in the effective management of the disease.

Home blood glucose monitoring is particularly useful for diabetics who use insulin, especially those with "brittle" or "unstable" diabetes, in which blood glucose fluctuates widely. It is also useful in establishing an initial insulin regimen or readjusting insulin doses according to your doctor's advice in response to illness, travel, or changes in diet or activity. Pregnant diabetics who have carefully monitored their blood glucose levels at home have been shown to have healthier babies and fewer complications during pregnancy.

Home blood glucose measurement may

sometimes be useful for the diabetic who does not need insulin, allowing direct observation of the effects of diet, exercise, and stress on blood sugar levels.

Some doctors recommend home blood glucose monitoring as a way to test non-diabetics for hypoglycemia (low blood sugar).

## Equipment:

The equipment for home blood glucose monitoring is available from some local chapters of the American Diabetes Association, medical supply stores, pharmacies, and the Self-Training Centers (1500 centers worldwide).

*Fingersticking Devices:*

Autoclix (BioDynamics, Inc., P.O. Box 50100, Indianapolis, Indiana 46250; 800-428-4674): $20

auto-Lancet (Palco Laboratories, 1595 Soquel Drive, Santa Cruz, California, 95065): $12

Autolet (Ulster Scientific, Inc., P.O. Box 902, Highland, New York 12528; 800-431-8233): $20 ($23 with built-in timer)

Monojector (Sherwood Medical, 831 Olive Street, St. Louis, Missouri 63103): $8

Penlet (Lifescan, Inc., 1025 Terra Bella Ave., Mountain View, California 94043; 800-227-8862 or 800-982-6132 in California): $15

*Fingersticking Lancets:*

Monolet lancets (Sherwood Medical, 831 Olive Street, St. Louis, Missouri 63103): fits all of the above devices, $10 for 200

*Visually Read Test Strips:*

Chemstrip bG (BioDynamics, Inc., P.O. Box 50100, Indianapolis, Indiana 46250; 800-428-4674): $45 for 100

Visidex II (Ames Co., Box 70, Elkhardt, Indiana 46250; 800-348-8100): $45 for 100

*Glucose Meters:*

Accu-Chek bG (BioDynamics, Inc., P.O. Box 50100, Indianapolis, Indiana 42650; 800-428-4674): $150 (uses Chemstrip bG test strips)

Betascan A (Orange Medical Instruments, 3183 Airway Ave., Suite F, Costa Mesa, California 92626; 213-614-5836): $250 (uses Dextrostix [Ames] reagent strips)

Glucochek II (Larken Industries, 8397 Melrose, Lenexa, Kansas 66214; 800-452-7536): $250 (uses Chemstrips bG or Dextrostix [Ames] reagent strips)

Glucometer (Ames Co., Box 70, Elkhart, Indiana 46250, 800-348-8100): $250 (uses Dextrostix reagent strips)

Glucoscan II (Lifescan, Inc., 1025 Terra Bella Ave., Mountain View, California 94043; 800-227-8862 or 800-982-6132 in California): $160 (uses Glucoscan test strips)

The glucose strips used in the different glucose meters differ and may not be interchangeable. Check the manufacturer's instructions. Expense for home blood glucose equipment and supplies are now reimbursed by some insurance programs; check with your insurer. A prescription or letter from your doctor stating the need and benefits of home blood glucose monitoring may help you secure reimbursement.

The products for home blood glucose monitoring are rapidly changing. Be sure to check for recent updates, changes, and other products not mentioned here. For continually updated information on home blood glucose monitoring equipment, contact The Sugarfree Center, P.O. Box 114,

Van Nuys, California 91408, or call (213)994-1093.

## Preparation:

This test requires precise timing, so it's important to lay out all of the test items within easy reach before starting. There won't be time to assemble the items once the test is under way.

## Procedure:

The instructions for each test system are different and must be followed precisely. Here is a general description of how the testing is done.

*Fingerstick to Draw Blood:* The days of the jab-and-cringe fingerprick are over. Several spring-loaded devices with replaceable lancets are now available to make fingerpricking easy and nearly painless. First clean the fingertip with soap and water or an alcohol swab. Be sure to dry it completely, since even a small amount of alcohol or water can interfere with test results. Select a target site along the side of the fingertip where there are fewer pain nerves and more blood vessels. The center of the fingertip may be more sensitive or calloused, which may make it more difficult to draw blood. Press the target finger against

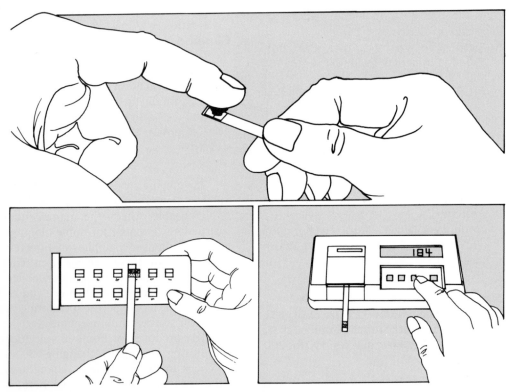

**Home Blood Glucose Monitoring.** *A drop of blood is placed on a reagent strip. The strip may be read by comparing the color change to a standard color chart or by inserting the strip into a blood glucose meter.*

the fingersticking device and release the trigger.

The lancet will lightly puncture the skin and retract immediately. Hold the pricked finger downward and "milk" it toward the puncture site. Continue the gentle massage until a large, hanging drop of blood has formed on the fingertip. If you have difficulty getting enough blood, run your finger under warm water for 10–15 seconds to stimulate blood flow before attempting the fingerprick. The disposable lancets may be reused if soaked in alcohol for several hours, but repeated use may reduce the sharpness of the point, resulting in increased pain.

*Visually Read Strips:* The instructions vary slightly, depending on the type of strip you use. Basically, you will transfer a large drop of blood onto the chemical pad at the end of one of the test strips. After waiting the specified time (usually 30–60 seconds), the blood is lightly wiped from the pad with a cotton ball or tissue or washed off and then blotted dry. After waiting another 60–90 seconds, the color of the reagent pad is matched against the standard color chart on the strip container. If the color falls between two of the standard color blocks, you can estimate the blood glucose as falling between the two values. The difference in color shades between normal and abnormal readings may be slight, so if you have difficulty with color vision, have someone else check your readings. Many people cut the strips in half lengthwise before using, after they have become experienced in reading the strips. If you test frequently, this can save a significant amount of money (and blood).

*Glucose Meters:* The instructions will vary somewhat, depending on the meter you choose. Basically, you will transfer a drop of blood onto the pad of a reagent strip. At a specified time (usually 60 seconds) the excess blood is removed from the strip and

the pad is inserted into the meter. Within seconds a number appears on the digital display indicating the blood glucose level (in milligrams per deciliter). Most meters have built-in timers.

The visual method of testing is less expensive, more portable, and more convenient. The glucose meters are somewhat more precise and easier to read, especially for people with color blindness or visual problems. Many people use the meter at home and the strips when traveling.

Home testing is not difficult to learn, but it does require proper instruction and practice. Ask your doctor or local diabetes association about individual instruction. At first, you may wish to check your blood glucose as often as 6 to 8 times per day. Later, less frequent testing may be sufficient. Home blood glucose monitoring is designed to be used in partnership with your doctor. You can work out an individualized plan with your doctor including how often to test and what actions to take based on the results.

**Results:**
Both the visually read strips and the glucose meters are highly accurate, usually falling within 10% of the blood glucose levels measured in a laboratory. Normal blood glucose levels fall between 60 to 140 milligrams per deciliter, but will vary depending upon meals, activity, and insulin administration. Most doctors recommend that for tight control, fasting blood glucose levels should not exceed 110–120 and that samples drawn 2 hours after a meal should not exceed 140–160.

If you obtain a test result that surprises you, repeat the test. If you still find the results odd or inconsistent with your body signals, check with your doctor on what actions to take, including adjusting your insulin dose if the readings are particularly high or low.

For nondiabetics, if the blood glucose level falls below 50 *at the same time* you are experiencing symptoms such as headache, lightheadedness, irritability, or extreme fatigue, then further evaluation may be warranted for hypoglycemia.

### Special Considerations:

★*Sleep Sentry:* Another device has been developed for insulin-dependent diabetics to help alert them to hypoglycemic (low blood sugar) episodes during sleep. The wristwatchlike device has sensors that detect sweating or a fall in body temperature, two common signs of hypoglycemia. If either of these signs occurs, a warning alarm sounds. You can then check for other signs and symptoms as well as measure your blood glucose to determine if hypoglycemia is present. The Sleep Sentry sells for $175 and is available from Teledyne Avionics, P.O. Box 6098, Charlottesville, Virginia 22906.

# Home Throat Cultures

Sore throats are one of the most common complaints that bring people to doctors. They are most often caused by viral infections which last 7–10 days and get better without treatment. However, between 5% and 30% of sore throats are caused by a bacteria called group A beta-hemolytic *Streptococcus* ("strep," for short). Strep throat almost always clears up without specific treatment, but a very few people may later develop rheumatic fever or glomerulonephritis, which can damage the heart

valves and kidneys. It is primarily to prevent the poststrep heart complications that treatment with antibiotics is recommended for strep throat.

You cannot tell just by looking whether a sore throat is caused by streptococci. Rather than treat every sore throat with an antibiotic and risk side effects, a throat culture can done to look for streptococci. The culture specimen is collected by swabbing the back of the throat with a cotton-tipped applicator. The procedure is quite simple and can be done at home. The specimen can then be returned to a laboratory or doctor's office to be cultured and examined for streptococci.

Collecting the culture specimen at home is inexpensive, convenient, and may save an unnecessary visit to the doctor. Leaving the sick person at home and bringing in just the specimen also reduces the risk of spreading the infection to others. Learning how to obtain a culture at home can be especially useful to parents of children who get frequent sore throats. In one study the results of cultures taken by parents agreed with those of health professionals 99% of the time, demonstrating that home throat culturing can be a highly accurate and efficient way to detect strep throat and involve parents in health care.

### Why Performed:

Most sore throats do not require a culture. A mild sore throat with a cough, hoarseness, runny nose, and little or no fever is likely to be caused by a virus, not by strep bacteria. However, if a sore throat is accompanied by any of the following symptoms, a culture should be considered:

Fever greater than 101° F (38.3° C)
White or yellow spots on the tonsils or
back of the throat

Tender, swollen lymph nodes in the neck

Recent close contact with someone with known strep throat

A history of rheumatic fever or heart disease

Consulting a health professional is advised if your sore throat is accompanied by any of the following:

Fever greater than 104° F
Rash
Earache
Stiff, rigid neck
Inability to swallow saliva
Difficulty in breathing

Repeating a throat culture after treatment of strep throat is recommended only for those with recurring strep throat infections.

## Equipment:

Since an incubator (warming oven) and culture plates are required, it is not presently possible to do the entire throat culture including incubation and interpretation at home. This now requires a laboratory, although several companies are working on the development of a home strep detection kit. For now, you will need a culture swab and an arrangement with a lab or doctor's office to drop off the specimen for culturing. The cost of a throat culture with the specimen collected at home should be about $5 as compared with $20 or more for a culture when a health professional collects the specimen (see p. 130).

## Preparation:

Before doing a culture you should check for fever and examine your (or your child's) neck and throat. Check for swollen lymph

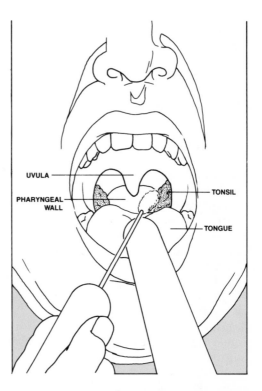

**Home Throat Culture.** *To collect a throat culture specimen, stroke the tonsils and pharyngeal wall with a cotton swab.*

nodes by pressing your fingertips gently, yet firmly, along the sides, front, and back of the neck, particularly under the jaw. Enlarged nodes may vary from about the size of a pea to that of a lima bean. They are part of the body's defense system to fight infections. The nodes may remain enlarged and slightly tender for several weeks after a throat infection.

Next look at the back of your throat in a mirror. Open your mouth wide and shine a light in or reflect the light from the mirror to illuminate the back of your throat. If your tongue blocks the view, try breathing through your mouth or gently push your tongue down with the handle of a spoon or some other smooth, clean object. Is the back of your throat red? Are there white spots on the tonsils or other structures? It is very helpful to examine yourself when you are well so that you will have a basis for comparison.

## Procedure:

With the back of the throat clearly lighted and in view, remove the cotton-tipped swab from its sterile container. Firmly stroke the cotton tip several times over both tonsils (if present) and the back of the throat (pharyngeal wall). You may notice a brief tickling sensation which may cause you to gag. Return the swab to its container, being careful not to touch the cotton tip with anything. At the end of the container there is a capsule containing liquid. Pinch this capsule firmly with your fingers to crush it and release the liquid. This keeps the swab tip moist and preserves the specimen. Some culture collection systems involve rolling the cotton swab back and forth over a special sterile filter paper, allowing it to dry and then rewrapping it. Follow the directions that pertain to the type of culture swab you get. Be sure to label the specimen with the name, date, telephone number, and, if available, medical record number or ID number before mailing or taking it to your doctor's office or lab. It is a good idea to have a health professional review the culture technique with you and observe you collecting a culture specimen.

## Results:

At the lab the culture specimen you have collected is transferred to a special culture medium and allowed to grow at a controlled temperature. Alternatively, the specimen may be tested chemically for the presence of strep. The results should be ready in about 24–48 hours. If group A beta-hemolytic strep is present, the culture will be reported as "positive," and antibiotics (usually penicillin or erythromycin) will be prescribed. If no group A beta-hemolytic strep is present, the culture is reported as "negative," and no antibiotic treatment is needed.

This test will detect about 90% of strep throat infections. Interestingly, about 10%–25% of us carry group A beta-hemolytic streptococci in our throats all the time, but the bacteria don't cause symptoms or do any harm. A negative throat culture does not necessarily mean you do not have a serious infection. If symptoms persist for more than two weeks, consult a health professional.

## Special Considerations:

★Some health professionals don't think throat cultures are needed for throat infections. They argue that it is cheaper and more efficient to treat sore throats with antibiotics and skip the culture. Others may do a culture but then start antibiotics immediately if the symptoms are very severe.

★Surprisingly, antibiotics do little to lessen the uncomfortable symptoms of a sore throat even if it is due to streptococci. Treatment with antibiotics may, at best, lessen the duration of symptoms by a day, but only if started within the first 24 hours after the onset of symptoms. If started after 48 hours, the antibiotics have virtually no effect on symptoms.

★There is no rush to start antibiotics even if you do have a strep throat. The antibiotics are effective in preventing rheumatic fever as long as they are started within 10 days of the onset of symptoms. However, it is essential to take the antibiotics for a full 10-day course even if the symptoms disappear sooner.

# Self-Test for Breath Alcohol

Within minutes of consuming an alcohol-containing drink, your blood alcohol concentration (BAC) starts to rise. When the percentage of alcohol in your bloodstream reaches .02%–.03%, you may begin to feel a relaxing "high." Between .05% and .10% you are likely to have reduced muscular coordination, decreased reaction time, and impaired judgment sufficient to make driving hazardous. At a level of about .10% you are considered legally drunk in most states. In some states the legal level is even lower.

Driving under the influence can be deadly. It is estimated that in one mile of city driving, a driver must make about 300 decisions and that even mild intoxication can significantly impair one's ability to drive. The result: alcohol is involved in nearly half of all fatal highway accidents and in over 80% of all fatalities involving pedestrians.

How much alcohol does it take to raise your blood alcohol level? This will vary depending upon the amount consumed, the speed of drinking, your body weight, the type of drink, the presence of food in your stomach, your individual body metabolism, and a number of other factors. You can roughly estimate your blood alcohol concentration by knowing your body weight and the number of drinks consumed over a 2-hour period (see chart). One drink is the equivalent of a 1.5 oz "shot" of 86 proof hard liquor, 12 oz of beer, or a 5 oz glass of wine. For example, if you weigh 180 pounds and consume 3 drinks over 2 hours, your BAC would be approximately .06%; each drink would raise your BAC roughly .02%.

This chart shows average responses. Younger people usually become impaired more easily, while older people are more likely to have vision problems at night. Tests show a wide range of responses even for people of the same age and weight. For some people, one drink may be too many.

## Estimating Blood Alcohol Concentration

| Weight (lb) | Drinks (Two-Hour Period) 1½ oz 86° Liquor or 12 oz Beer | | | | | | | | | | | |
|---|---|---|---|---|---|---|---|---|---|---|---|---|
| 100 | 1 | 2 | 3 | 4 | 5 | 6 | 7 | 8 | 9 | 10 | 11 | 12 |
| 120 | 1 | 2 | 3 | 4 | 5 | 6 | 7 | 8 | 9 | 10 | 11 | 12 |
| 140 | 1 | 2 | 3 | 4 | 5 | 6 | 7 | 8 | 9 | 10 | 11 | 12 |
| 160 | 1 | 2 | 3 | 4 | 5 | 6 | 7 | 8 | 9 | 10 | 11 | 12 |
| 180 | 1 | 2 | 3 | 4 | 5 | 6 | 7 | 8 | 9 | 10 | 11 | 12 |
| 200 | 1 | 2 | 3 | 4 | 5 | 6 | 7 | 8 | 9 | 10 | 11 | 12 |
| 220 | 1 | 2 | 3 | 4 | 5 | 6 | 7 | 8 | 9 | 10 | 11 | 12 |
| 240 | 1 | 2 | 3 | 4 | 5 | 6 | 7 | 8 | 9 | 10 | 11 | 12 |

| Be Careful Driving BAC to .05% | Driving Impaired .05%-.09% | Do Not Drive .10% & Up |
|---|---|---|
| | Risk of an Accident | |
| 2 times greater | 6 times greater | 25 times greater |

Source: NHTSA

You can now measure your *breath* alcohol level by a simple home test. This self-test is similar to, though not as precise as, the breathalyzer tests often used by the police to screen suspected drunk drivers. Breath alcohol tests roughly approximate *blood* alcohol levels (see p. 44).

## Why Performed:

People vary tremendously in their response to alcohol, but you can measure your individual response by self-testing. Knowing how much alcohol it takes to raise your blood alcohol to dangerous levels may help you make better judgments about drinking and about driving after drinking.

## Equipment:

There are two different types of self-test for breath alcohol. One uses a balloon and a glass tube filled with crystals which change color when exposed to alcohol. These disposable test kits are for one-time use only and sell for $1.50 for a two-test packet (Drink-O-Meter, from Luckey Laboratories, Inc., 7252 Osbun Road, San Bernardino, California 92404). Another single-use, disposable, breath alcohol detector called D.B.A.D. is available from Diversified Medical Technologies, P.O. Box 4793, Englewood, Colorado 80155.

There are also portable electronic breath alcohol meters available which allow repeated measurements. These pocket-sized, battery-operated devices range in price from $35 to $80. (AlcoCheck and AlcoSafe from The Continental Trading Corp., 6600 France Ave., Minneapolis, Minnesota 55435; or MICRONTA Breath Alcohol Indicator distributed by Radio Shack.)

Many bars now provide their patrons with free alcohol breath tests using one of these methods.

## Procedure:

Wait at least 15 minutes after consuming an alcoholic drink before testing. Trace amounts of residual alcohol in your mouth from a drink (or even mouthwash) can give false results. Do not blow smoke into the devices; wait at least one minute after smoking before testing.

With the glass tube tests, you first inflate the enclosed balloon with one continuous breath until it is almost full. You then attach the balloon mouthpiece to one end of the glass tube, which is filled with bands of yellow crystals. Let the air flow slowly through the tube for exactly one minute. You then count the number of bands of colored crystals in the tube that have turned from yellow to green.

If you are using one of the electronic alcohol meters, follow the specific instructions that come with the device. With most machines, you must turn them on and let them warm up for several minutes. Then take a deep breath, place your lips tightly around the mouthpiece, and blow steadily and continuously into the machine for the specified time (usually 4 to 6 seconds). Then observe the "traffic light" display or meter. After you obtain an initial reading, press the reset button and make a second test.

## Results:

To read the glass tube breath alcohol tester, count the number of yellow bands of crystals that have turned green. One green band roughly corresponds to a BAC of .00%–.05%, two green bands to .05%–.10%, and three green bands .10%–.15%.

Some of the electronic devices have a "traffic light" display. A green light indicates a BAC below .04%, a yellow light .04%–.08%, and a red light above .08%. Some devices may display the results slightly differently.

The test result reflects your approximate breath alcohol level at the time of the test. If you have consumed a drink within 30 minutes of performing the test, your blood alcohol level may continue to rise after the test.

The estimate of blood alcohol level provided with these tests is not intended to represent actual driving abilities. Your driving may be impaired even with BAC below

.05%. The degree of impairment of driving may also vary among people with the same blood alcohol levels. Recent studies also show that after heavy drinking, driving ability may be diminished by as much as 20% even after the BAC has returned to zero. The breath alcohol tests, however, do offer one added piece of information to help you make safe decisions about drinking and driving. The safest decision is not to drink at all if you are driving.

# Home Screening for Bowel Cancer

Bowel cancer is the cancer no one likes to talk about. Yet each year in the United States alone more than 130,000 people are diagnosed with this disease, and more than 60,000 people die from it.

When bowel cancer is detected in its early stages, it can be cured more than 75% of the time. However, if the cancer is detected later, after it has spread to other parts of the body, only about 25% can be successfully treated.

Early diagnosis depends on reporting to your doctor suspicious symptoms such as any visible sign of blood in your stool (bright red, burgundy, or black stools), persistent changes in bowel habits (constipation or diarrhea lasting more than two weeks), persistent abdominal pain, or unexplained weight loss. However, in the early stages, bowel cancer usually develops without symptoms, causing no pain and giving no warning signals other than slight bleeding. The amount of blood in the stool may be so small or so mixed with the stool that it cannot be seen. A simple, at-home test, sometimes called a stool guaiac or fecal occult blood test, can detect this hidden blood in the stool. If blood is detected, further diagnostic tests are necessary to locate the source of the bleeding. If a cancer is found, it is likely to be at an early stage with a better chance of cure. It is estimated that yearly screening with this test could detect nearly 90% of bowel cancers, improving the 5-year survival rate for people with these cancers from 43% to 84%.

**Why Performed:**
Men and women are at equal risk of developing bowel cancer but the disease risk increases significantly with age. Therefore, it is generally recommended that after age 50 both men and women should do the test once a year. People at higher risk for colon cancer should begin testing earlier and may benefit from performing the test more frequently. If you have a history of previous colorectal cancer, colonic polyps, ulcerative colitis or bowel irregularities, or a family history of colorectal cancer or polyps, you should discuss the appropriate screening with your health professional. Home screening for bowel cancer does not replace the need for regular examinations by your doctor, but can complement these exams.

This test can also be performed if you notice a red or black color to your stool. Is it blood or a food like beets? Home testing can help clarify this.

**Equipment:**
There are now several types of products available for at-home testing for hidden blood in the stool. They differ mainly in how the stool specimens are collected. In some tests such as Detecatest (by Fleet) or Hemoccult (by SmithKline Diagnostics), small specimens of stool are collected with a small stick, applied to a chemically treated paper, and then developed by adding a

chemical solution which highlights any hidden blood with a blue color. With Early Detector (by Warner-Lambert) a special toilet paper is used and then sprayed with a chemical which causes a blue color to appear if blood is present. CS-T (Colo-Screen Self-Test by Helena Laboratories) requires that a special test pad be dropped into the toilet bowl after a bowel movement and observed for the presence of a red-orange color change which signals the presence of blood.

These at-home tests are available in most pharmacies without a prescription and sell for $4 to $7. Alternatively, your doctor may provide you with a stool specimen collection packet and ask you to return the packet after collection for processing and interpretation.

The test kits should be protected from moisture, heat, sunlight, and fluorescent light. Check the expiration date on the test materials before use. The developing solution contains ethyl alcohol which is highly flammable so keep it away from intense heat or open flames. It is also an irritant so do not get it on your skin or in your eyes. If you do, rinse the solution off at once with water.

### Preparation:

Since colon cancers can bleed intermittently, the test is done on three consecutive bowel movements to increase the probability of detecting hidden blood. Also, to increase the accuracy of the test you should make some simple diet changes two days before starting the test and continuing until you have collected all the stool samples.

- Eat plenty of vegetables (especially lettuce, spinach, and corn), fruits (especially apples, prunes, and grapes), and a bran-containing cereal or bread, unless these foods are known to cause you problems. The increased roughage in these foods will help cause the cancers to bleed so that they can be detected.
- Avoid eating red meats, turnips, radishes, or horseradish, since these foods can cause a misleading discoloration to appear on the test (false-positive test results). Small amounts of chicken, turkey, and tuna will not interfere with test results.
- Avoid taking iron supplements, aspirin or aspirin-containing products (check the labels), antiinflammatory medications (e.g., indomethacin, phenylbutazone), or other medicines known to cause stomach irritation and bleeding. These medications can cause false-positive test results.
- Avoid taking supplements of vitamin C (ascorbic acid) in amounts greater than 250 mg per day, since this can interfere with the test for blood and produce false-negative results.

Do not do the test if you have active hemorrhoidal or menstrual bleeding. Also, do not test a stool specimen that has been in contact with toilet bowl cleaning agents that turn the water blue.

### Procedure:

The precise procedure varies depending upon the type of at-home test you select, so follow the manufacturer's detailed instructions. For all the tests, you will need to test stool samples from three consecutive bowel movements. This may take from one to several days, depending upon how often you have a bowel movement.

For tests such as Detecatest and Hemoccult you will need to obtain small samples from each of three consecutive bowel movements and apply them to the three indicated test areas on the slide packet supplied in the kits. There are various ways of collecting the samples. You might try catching the stool on some plastic wrap draped loosely over the toilet bowl and held in place by the toilet seat. If you use a container to collect the stool, first clean and rinse it well to avoid any residue which may affect test results. Using a collection stick that comes with the test kit, spread a very thin layer of stool on the marked paper test area of the cardboard packet. Do not cover the entire paper area; scrape off any excess. Reuse the collection stick to obtain a second dab from a different area of the same stool. Place this second specimen on the other test area of the first packet. Then close the front flap of the packet and discard the collection stick. Repeat the test for two additional bowel movements for a total of six specimens.

If your test kit contains developing solution, after collecting the specimens, turn each packet over and open the flap covering the development area on the back. Add two drops of developing solution to the paper test areas. Wait 30–60 seconds, then read the color (see Results). If you have difficulty with color vision, have someone help you read the test. Don't wait longer than one minute because the color may begin to fade. Some test kits have special test areas on the paper called "performance" or "control monitors." These built-in monitors show what a positive and negative test result look like and check that the test is working properly.

If you don't have the developing solution, write your name and date on the packets and give or mail them to your health care provider within 4 days.

Another test called Early Detector is designed so that the stool specimen is collected by having you wipe your anal area with a special toilet tissue supplied in the kit. The toilet tissue with specimen is then sprayed with a developing solution and observed for color change.

The simplest collection method is used in the test called CS-T (ColoScreen Self-Test). Remove all toilet cleaners and disinfectants from the toilet tank and then flush the toilet twice to remove any residual chemicals in the water. After having a bowel movement, drop the test pad into the toilet bowl and observe the test areas on the pad for 15–30 seconds to look for any color change. Then flush the toilet. With this test it is important that no urine, toilet paper, or toilet-bowl cleaner be in the toilet bowl during the test.

**Results:**

Any trace of blue color (not gray or green) that appears within 30–60 seconds after adding the developing solution is a positive result. (With the CS-T test a red-orange color change indicates a positive test.) A positive test means that blood is present in the stool; it does not necessarily mean that you have bowel cancer. The blood detected on the test could be from meat you have eaten, an inflamed colon, bleeding gums, a polyp, or possibly cancer. Between 2% and 5% of people without symptoms will have positive results on this test. Only about 10% of those people with positive tests actually have bowel cancer, and most of these will have early, highly curable cancers. Therefore, even though a positive test for hidden blood may not mean you have a cancer, a positive result on *any one* of the specimens should be discussed without delay with your doctor. Further diagnostic tests such as sigmoidoscopy (p. 335), barium enema (p. 245), and colonoscopy (p. 319) will be necessary to determine the source of the blood.

A negative test (no color change) indicates that at the time of the test there is no measurable blood in the stool samples. This does not, however, absolutely rule out the possibility of bowel cancer. Contact your physician if you have any symptoms, even if the test is negative.

# Self-Test for Bowel Transit Time

The digestive journey is a bit like going through an automatic carwash. The food is chewed, doused with a series of acids and digestive enzymes, churned in the stomach, squeezed through 20-odd feet of small intestine, propelled by rippling waves of muscular contractions through the colon, and finally expelled at the far end. The surviving food substance, usually only indigestible fibrous material, combines with water, bacteria, and various excreted substances to become stool.

The time it takes for the food to make the journey from mouth to anus is known as the *bowel transit time*. Bowel transit time, one measure of bowel function, depends largely on the type of diet we eat. People who eat large quantities of foods rich in indigestible fiber (fruits, vegetables, and whole grains) tend to have rapid transit times and heavier, bulkier stools. For example, rural African schoolchildren eating an unrefined, high-fiber diet had a mean bowel transit time of 33.5 hours and a mean stool weight of 275 grams per day. In contrast, teenage boarding school pupils in England consuming a refined diet low in fiber had to wait an average of 76 hours for a rather scant 110 grams of stool to pass through.

Because small, infrequent bowel movements are a distinct advantage during space flights, astronauts are deliberately fed a diet almost free of fiber. This typically results in a bowel transit time of 5–6 days. For the rest of us earthbound creatures, however, more bulk appears to be better.

Studies show that people who eat high-fiber diets have fewer digestive tract problems. This holds true for such diseases as constipation, diverticulosis (a condition with small outpouches from the colon), hemorrhoids, and even colon cancer.

In the case of colon cancer, it is thought that certain chemicals (carcinogens) are ingested in the diet and/or formed in the intestines. These cancer-causing chemicals can disrupt the cells lining the colon and initiate cancers. Diets high in fiber may inhibit the formation or action of these carcinogens. In addition, the rapid bowel transit time due to a high-fiber diet decreases the amount of time these carcinogens are in contact with the colonic lining. Studies suggest that people with rapid transit times, bulky stools, and high-fiber diets have lower rates of bowel cancer.

Several methods have been developed to measure bowel transit time. In most scientific experiments, subjects are asked to swallow small, undigestible pellets. Their stools are then collected and x-rayed. The pellets appear as white spots on the x-rays; this saves the researchers from the unpleasant task of sorting through the stool to find the pellets. The bowel transit time is defined as the time by which 80% of the markers have been excreted.

A simpler, but somewhat less precise method can be used for home testing. Two capsules containing a red dye are swallowed. The first and last appearance of the red color in the stool is noted. Certain other substances, including seeds, corn kernels, and beets, can also be used as stool markers.

**Why Performed:**
The major reason for doing this test is interest and curiosity. It offers an opportunity to become more aware of your bowel function and to note improvement of transit times if you start to increase the fiber in your diet.

**Equipment:**

You need two gelatin capsules filled with carmine red (cochineal), a harmless red vegetable dye. These can be obtained at most herb shops or by mail from Nature's Herb Company, 281 Ellis St., San Francisco, California 94102. You can also use a large serving of beets, seeds or corn kernels.

**Preparation:**

If you are using a food marker such as corn or beets, you will need to avoid these foods for about a week before starting the test.

**Procedure:**

Swallow two gelatin capsules filled with carmine red or the chosen food marker along with a meal. Then observe your subsequent bowel movements. Record how many hours it takes after the ingestion of the dye before the first and last appearance of red color (or other marker) in your stool. You may wish to later repeat the test after starting a high-fiber diet.

**Results:**

Bowel transit time will vary considerably even when repeated on the same person. Generally the first red color should appear in the stool about 14–24 hours after ingestion, and the last appearance of red should be within 36–48 hours. These are very rough guidelines, but if your bowel transit time is much longer, 72 hours or more, this may indicate slowed bowel function. You can speed up your bowel transit time with a high-fiber diet.

A person may have a daily bowel movement but a slow transit time. This has led to the old adage, "The person was regular but five days late!"

# Home Test for Pinworms

Pinworms are small, thin parasites that commonly infect small children, though anyone can be infested. The adult worms live inside the intestine. Each night the female adult worms migrate to deposit their eggs just outside the anus. Diagnosis depends on either seeing the worms outside the anus at night or collecting a specimen of the tiny eggs, which can be seen under a microscope.

Pinworm infection is not serious and is easily treated. Usually the only symptom is an intense itching in the anal area, particularly at night.

**Why Performed:**

Children or adults with anal itching can check for pinworms with this simple test and exam. It is not necessary for people without symptoms.

**Equipment:**

For the exam all you need is a flashlight. If a specimen of eggs is to be collected, you will need a plastic or glass microscope slide and a strip of clear cellophane tape. Kits are available for this purpose, but not absolutely necessary.

**Procedure:**

*Exam*: Sometime during the night inspect the anal area with a flashlight. Look for tiny, whitish threadlike worms. If you don't see any, check for 2–3 additional nights or try the tape test.

*Tape Test*: Since the eggs are deposited at night, the best time to collect a specimen is early morning. Simply take a 1-inch strip of cellophane tape, sticky side out, and press it firmly over the anus for a few seconds. The eggs will stick to the tape. Then transfer the tape, sticky side down, to the glass or plastic slide. If you have access to a microscope, you can look for the eggs yourself. Otherwise, take the slide to a health professional for analysis.

**Results:**

A pinworm infection can be diagnosed either by seeing the threadlike adult worms outside the anus or by seeing under the microscope the small, clear oval egg with the worm folded up inside.

**Special Considerations:**

★Treatment of pinworms consists of a one-time dose of an antiworm medicine which can be obtained without prescription from a pharmacy or from a health professional. All family members are usually treated, since pinworm infections can be easily passed back and forth between family members.

# IV

# Medical Tests
# for Healthy
# People

**M**edical tests are performed for several reasons: to help diagnose disease in people with symptoms, to follow the progress of known diseases, and to detect hidden disease in people *without* symptoms. This last use is known as *screening*.

At first glance, using batteries of tests on healthy people seems like a great idea. Diseases can be detected before symptoms develop and treatment can be done at an earlier, more curable stage. This is true in theory, but in practice very few screening tests have been shown to be of benefit.

To help you decide whether a proposed screening test is likely to be useful for you, consider the following questions:

*1. Is the disease or condition tested for an important health problem in your age group?*

Would the disease or condition have a significant effect on the quality and quantity of your life? There is no sense in screening for trivial health problems. Is the disease relatively common in your age group? For example, bowel cancer is a common health problem only after the age of 45 or 50, so in younger people there is little reason to screen for the disease unless special risk factors are present which make the disease more likely. However, screening may be helpful with a few very rare but devastating diseases such as phenylketonuria, an inherited defect in metabolism which, if not treated, can lead to severe mental retardation. Even though this condition is rare, the consequences of not diagnosing it and treating it in newborns can be extremely serious. Therefore, routine screening of all newborns is justified.

*2. Can the proposed screening test detect the disease or condition before symptoms alert you that something is wrong?:*

Most diseases announce themselves with a variety of symptoms which, when evaluated, can lead to a diagnosis. For some diseases, however, waiting for symptoms to develop can mean that the disease will spread and perhaps become incurable. Early diagnosis of cervical cancer, for example, is very desirable, since a Pap smear can detect the cancer before symptoms appear, when it is most easily cured.

On the other hand, you don't really need a screening test for appendicitis, since the condition is usually announced promptly by the symptom of abdominal pain.

*3. Do early diagnosis and treatment favorably alter the progress of the disease?*

It makes little sense to screen for a disease for which there is no effective treatment. However, even if an effective treatment is available and acceptable, it must be shown to be *more* effective when applied in the stage before symptoms develop. This is particularly important in cancer screening. For example, if an *incurable* lung cancer is discovered six months before symptoms would have announced its presence, the person doesn't actually survive any longer as a result of early diagnosis and treatment. The test merely informs the person of the cancer six months earlier. The result is that the person lives six months longer knowing that he or she has an incurable disease, but actual survival is not enhanced by the screening effort. This is one reason why chest x-rays are no longer

451

generally recommended as a screening test for lung cancer. The detection of lung cancers on routine screening x-rays has not been proven to increase the survival of lung cancer patients. Similarly, the laboratory diagnosis of arthritis before symptoms develop is not useful, since the available treatments are not any more effective in the early stages.

Fortunately, there are a few diseases that can be treated more effectively if detected early. These include high blood pressure, breast cancer, cervical cancer, and colon cancer.

*4. Is there a screening test that is reasonably accurate, acceptable, and inexpensive?*

One of the greatest stumbling blocks to effective screening programs is the lack of accuracy of the tests. If a test is not sensitive enough to identify the people with the disease in question, then many diseased people will be missed (false-negatives). On the other hand, if the test is positive in many healthy people (false-positives), mistaken diagnoses may occur and further testing is usually required to sort this out. Even with reasonably accurate tests, if you have 12 tests performed, there is a 50% chance that you will have an "abnormal" result on at least one of them even though no disease is actually present. For a further discussion of the importance of test accuracy, see p. 26.

The proposed test must also be acceptably comfortable and safe. While examination of the colon with a viewing instrument (colonoscopy) may be the most effective way to detect early colon cancer, the routine examination of healthy people by this method is not justified because of the risk, discomfort, and expense.

Since screening tests are usually applied to large numbers of people, the expense of even low-cost tests can mount

rapidly. The expense also includes the cost of follow-up investigations of those who demonstrate positive results on screening. Medical resources are not unlimited, so in a larger context, it is generally agreed that screening tests should be shown to offer significant savings in terms of prolonged life or decreased suffering to justify the effort. Otherwise, health resources would be better spent elsewhere.

■

In summary, for a screening test to be worthwhile, it must reliably detect a significant disease before symptoms develop, the treatment must be more effective when begun before symptoms arise, and the detection and treatment must be accomplished at an acceptable risk and cost. Very few tests currently meet these requirements.

In the tables that follow we offer some guidelines for medical testing in healthy people. Instead of recommending the same tests for everyone, we describe which tests should be performed depending upon your age and sex. (We also include recommendations for testing during pregnancy.) This customized approach is now favored by most health experts[1-7], though there may be differences of opinion on some specific recommendations. This is due to the lack of definitive information about the benefits of some of the tests and to a difference in interpretation of the significance of some of the research on these tests. More specific information on each recommended test can be found in the section of the book where each test is described.

These guidelines represent the minimum recommended screening for people *without symptoms*. If you are at increased risk for certain conditions, due to family history, for example, additional tests may be advised. Use these guidelines as a start-

452

ing point, and discuss your particular situation with your health professional.

Even though we recommend these screening tests for healthy people, we want to remind you that some of the most significant factors affecting your health may not show up on these tests at all. In truth, choosing not to smoke, drinking alcohol moderately or not at all, wearing seat belts, exercising regularly, eating wisely, learning to manage stress effectively, and so on, will do more to protect and promote your health than all the tests in the world.

# References

1. Council on Scientific Affairs, Division of Scientific Activities, American Medical Association, Chicago: Medical evaluations of healthy persons. *Journal of the American Medical Association* 1983;249: 1626–1633.

2. Medical Practices Committee, American College of Physicians: Periodic health examination: a guide for designing individualized preventive health care in the asymptomatic patient. *Annals of Internal Medicine* 1981;95:729–732.

3. Canadian Task Force on Periodic Health Examinations: The periodic health examination. *Canadian Medical Association Journal* 1979;121:1193.

4. American Cancer Society: ACS report on the cancer-related health check-up. *CA* 1980;30:194–240.

5. Breslow L, Somers AR: The lifetime health-monitoring program: a practical approach to preventive medicine. *New England Journal of Medicine* 1977; 296:601–608.

6. Lifetime health monitoring. *Patient Care* 1979; (February 15)162–178, (April 30)201–216, (June 15)83–153.

7. Frame PS, Carlson SJ: A critical review of periodic health screening using specific screening criteria. *Journal of Family Practice* 1975;2:29–36, 123–129, 189–194, 283–289.

## Recommended Medical Tests for Healthy Newborns:
### Birth to Age 1

| Test | Condition | Frequency |
| --- | --- | --- |
| History and physical exam | Various disorders and risks | Newborn and every 2–3 months |
| Blood test for phenylketonuria (p. 91) | Phenylketonuria | Newborn |
| Blood test for galactosemia (p. 77) | Galactosemia | Newborn |
| Blood test for thyroid function (p. 108) | Hypothyroidism | Newborn |
| Hematocrit (p. 61) | Anemia | Once at age 9–12 months |
| Tuberculin skin test (p. 133) | Tuberculosis | Once at age 9–12 months |

## Recommended Medical Tests for Healthy Infants:
### Age 1–5

| Test | Condition | Frequency |
| --- | --- | --- |
| History and physical exam | Various disorders and risks | Every 1–2 years |
| Blood pressure measurement (p. 413) | Hypertension | Once after age 3 |
| Hearing test (p. 382) | Hearing impairment | Once after age 4 |
| Vision test (p. 390) | Vision problems | Every 1–2 years after age 3 |
| Hematocrit (p. 61) | Anemia | Once at age 4–5 |
| Urinalysis (p. 112) | Diabetes, kidney disease, urinary tract infection | Once at age 4–5 |
| Tuberculin skin test (p. 133) | Tuberculosis | Once at age 4–5 or every 2–3 years |

### Recommended Medical Tests for Healthy Children and Adolescents: Age 6–17

| Test | Condition | Frequency |
| --- | --- | --- |
| History and physical exam | Various disorders and risks | Every 3–4 years |
| Blood pressure measurement (p. 413) | Hypertension | Every 3–4 years |
| Tuberculin skin test (p.133) | Tuberculosis | Every 4–5 years |
| Hematocrit (p. 61) | Anemia | Every 4–5 years |
| Urinalysis (p. 112) | Diabetes, kidney disease, urinary tract infection | Every 4–5 years |
| Hearing test (p. 382) | Hearing impairment | Once at age 12–14 |
| Vision test (p. 390) | Vision problems | Once at age 12–14 |
| *For girls add:* | | |
| Pap smear (p. 179) | Cervical cancer | Every 2–3 years if sexually active. |

## Recommended Tests for Healthy People:
### Age 18–39

| Test | Condition | Frequency |
|------|-----------|-----------|
| History and physical exam | Various disorders and risks | Every 5–10 years |
| Blood pressure measurement (p. 413) | Hypertension | Every 2–3 years |
| Vision test (p. 390) | Vision problems | Every 5 years<br>Every 2–3 years if corrective lenses are worn |
| Tuberculin skin test (p. 133) | Tuberculosis | Every 5 years until age 35 or every 1–2 years if high-risk |
| Urinalysis (p. 112) | Kidney disease, urinary tract infection, liver disease, diabetes, metabolic disorders | Every 10 years |
| Hematocrit (p. 61) | Anemia | Every 10 years (men)<br>Every 3–5 years (women) |
| Blood glucose (p. 78) | Diabetes | Every 10 years |
| Cholesterol (p. 148) | Heart disease risk | Every 5–10 years |
| *For women add:* | | |
| Pap smear (p. 179) | Cervical cancer | Every 3 years after two normal yearly exams |
| Breast self-exam (p. 187) | Breast cancer | Monthly |
| Breast exam | Breast cancer | Every 2–3 years |
| Mammography (p. 189) | Breast cancer | Once between the ages 35–39 |
| Rubella antibody titer (p. 139) | Immunity to rubella (German measles) | Once |
| *For men add:* | | |
| Testicular self-exam (p. 218) | Testicular cancer | Monthly |

## Recommended Tests for Healthy People:
## Age 40–49

| Test | Condition | Frequency |
|------|-----------|-----------|
| History and physical exam | Various disorders and risks | Every 3–5 years |
| Blood pressure measurement (p. 413) | Hypertension | Every 2–3 years |
| Vision test (p. 390) | Vision problems | Every 5 years<br>Every 2–3 years if corrective lenses are worn |
| Glaucoma test (p. 379) | Glaucoma | Every 3 years |
| Urinalysis (p. 112) | Kidney disease, urinary tract infection, liver disease, diabetes, metabolic disorders | Every 5–10 years |
| Hematocrit (P. 61) | Anemia | Every 5–10 years (men)<br>Every 3–5 years (women) |
| Blood glucose (p. 78) | Diabetes | Every 5–10 years |
| Cholesterol (p. 148) | Heart disease risk | Every 5–10 years |
| *For women add:* | | |
| Pap Smear (p. 179) | Cervical cancer | Every 3 years after two normal yearly exams |
| Breast self-exam (p. 187) | Breast cancer | Monthly |
| Breast exam | Breast cancer | Every 1–2 years |
| Mammography (p. 189) | Breast cancer | Every 1–2 years |

## Recommended Tests for Healthy People:
## Age 50–59

| Test | Condition | Frequency |
| --- | --- | --- |
| History and physical exam | Various disorders and risks | Every 2–3 years |
| Blood pressure measurement (p. 413) | Hypertension | Every 2–3 years |
| Vision test (p. 390) | Vision problems | Every 5 years<br>Every 2–3 years if corrective lenses are worn |
| Glaucoma test (p. 379) | Glaucoma | Every 3 years |
| Hearing test (p. 382) | Hearing impairment | Every 3–5 years |
| Test for blood in stool (p. 443) | Bowel cancer | Every year |
| Sigmoidoscopy (p. 335) | Bowel cancer | Every 5 years |
| Urinalysis (p. 112) | Kidney disease, urinary tract infection, liver disease, diabetes, metabolic disorders | Every 5–10 years |
| Hematocrit (p. 61) | Anemia | Every 5–10 years |
| Blood glucose (p. 78) | Diabetes | Every 5–10 years |
| Cholesterol (p. 148) | Heart disease risk | Every 5–10 years |

*For women add:*

| Test | Condition | Frequency |
| --- | --- | --- |
| Pap smear (p. 179) | Cervical cancer | Every 3 years |
| Breast self-exam (p. 187) | Breast cancer | Monthly |
| Breast exam | Breast cancer | Every 1–2 years |
| Mammography (p. 189) | Breast cancer | Every 1–2 years |

## Recommended Tests for Healthy People:
## Age 60–69

| Test | Condition | Frequency |
| --- | --- | --- |
| History and physical exam | Various disorders and risks | Every 2–3 years |
| Blood pressure measurement (p. 413) | Hypertension | Every 2–3 years |
| Vision test (p. 390) | Vision problems | Every 5 years<br>Every 2–3 years if corrective lenses are worn |
| Glaucoma test (p. 379) | Glaucoma | Every 3 years |
| Hearing test (p. 382) | Hearing impairment | Every 3–5 years |
| Test for blood in stool (p. 443) | Bowel cancer | Every year |
| Sigmoidoscopy (p. 335) | Bowel cancer | Every 5 years |
| Urinalysis (p. 112) | Kidney disease, urinary tract infection, liver disease, diabetes, metabolic disorders | Every 5–10 years |
| Hematocrit (p. 61) | Anemia | Every 5–10 years |
| Blood glucose (p. 78) | Diabetes | Every 5–10 years |

*For women add:*

| Test | Condition | Frequency |
| --- | --- | --- |
| Pap smear (p. 179) | Cervical cancer | Every 3 years |
| Breast self-exam (p. 187) | Breast cancer | Monthly |
| Breast exam | Breast cancer | Every 1–2 years |
| Mammography (p. 189) | Breast cancer | Every 1–2 years |

## Recommended Tests for Healthy People: Age 70 and Older

| Test | Condition | Frequency |
| --- | --- | --- |
| History and physical exam | Various disorders and risks | Every 2–3 years |
| Blood pressure measurement (p. 413) | Hypertension | Every 2–3 years |
| Vision test (p. 390) | Vision problems | Every 5 years Every 2–3 years if corrective lenses are worn |
| Glaucoma test (p. 379) | Glaucoma | Every 3 years |
| Hearing test (p. 382) | Hearing impairment | Every 3–5 years |
| Test for blood in stool (p. 443) | Bowel cancer | Every year |
| Sigmoidoscopy (p. 335) | Bowel cancer | Every 5 years |
| Urinalysis (p. 112) | Kidney disease, urinary tract infection, liver disease, diabetes, metabolic disorders | Every 5 years |
| Hematocrit (p. 61) | Anemia | Every 5 years |
| Blood glucose (p. 78) | Diabetes | Every 5 years |
| *For women add:* | | |
| Breast self-exam (p. 187) | Breast cancer | Monthly |
| Breast exam | Breast cancer | Every 1–2 years |
| Mammography (p. 189) | Breast cancer | Every 1–2 years |

## Recommended Medical Tests During Pregnancy

| Test | Condition | Frequency |
| --- | --- | --- |
| History and physical exam | Various disorders and risks | Every 4 weeks during months 4–6<br>Every 2 weeks during months 7–8<br>Every week during 9th month |
| Blood pressure measurement (p. 413) | Hypertension | Every visit |
| Pap smear (p. 179) | Cervical cancer | Once in months 1–3 |
| Urinalysis (p. 112) | Diabetes, kidney disease, urinary tract infection | Every visit |
| Hematocrit (p. 61) | Anemia | Once in months 1–3<br>Once in months 6–9 |
| Blood glucose (p. 78) | Diabetes | Once in months 1–3<br>Once in month 7 |
| Blood typing (ABO/Rh) and antibody screen (p. 53) | Blood group incompatibility | Once in months 1–3 |
| Rubella antibody titer (p. 139) | Rubella (German measles) immunity | Once in months 1–3 |
| Syphilis test (VDRL) (p. 144) | Syphilis | Once in months 1–3 |
| Sickle-cell test (p. 105) | Sickle-cell trait | Once in months 1–3 for blacks |
| Tay-Sachs test (p. 107) | Tay-Sachs trait | Once in months 1–3 for Ashkenazi Jews of Eastern European descent |
| Thalassemia test (p. 81) | Thalassemia trait | Once in months 1–3 for those of Mediterranean descent |

**Chart continued on next page.**

**Recommended Medical Tests During Pregnancy** (*cont'd*)

*For high-risk pregnancies\* add:*

| | | |
|---|---|---|
| Cervical culture (pp. 140, 143) | Gonorrhea and herpes infections | Once during 1st trimester Once or more during 3rd trimester |
| Toxoplasmosis test (p. 139) | Toxoplasmosis | Once in months 1–3 |
| Amniocentesis (p. 208) | Certain genetic defects Fetal maturity | Once during weeks 14–18 Once or more in 3rd trimester |
| Fetal ultrasound (p. 205) | Various fetal abnormalities | Varies |
| Estriol (p. 73) | Fetal distress | 3rd trimester |
| Fetal monitoring (p. 213) | Fetal distress | 3rd trimester |

\*High-risk pregnancies include mothers with medical conditions that might complicate pregnancy such as heart disease, diabetes, sexually transmitted diseases; mothers older than 35 or younger than 16; and mothers with a history of problem pregnancies.

# Appendices

# Appendix 1

# Anesthesia

Anesthetics are medications that dull or prevent the sensation of pain. Anesthetic medications can be used either to numb a limited part of the body (*regional* or *local anesthesia*) or to induce a state of unconsciousness (*general anesthesia*).

## Regional Anesthesia

In regional anesthesia a small amount of an anesthetic is injected directly into the area to be numbed—in the same way that a dentist might inject Novocain to numb the jaw and teeth. In some cases the anesthetic may be inserted into the spinal canal (*spinal block*). This numbs the entire lower part of the body.

If regional anesthesia is used, you will be awake throughout the procedure, although you may be given a sedative injection or intravenous medications to help you relax. The affected area may continue to be numb up to several hours after the test is finished. Occasionally a person who has had a spinal anesthetic will experience a headache for a few days after the test.

Regional anesthesia entails relatively little risk. Allergic reactions are extremely rare, and can usually be easily treated.

## General Anesthesia

In general anesthesia you are put into a drug-induced sleep. General anesthesia is usually done under the direction of an *anesthesiologist*, a physician with special training in anesthesia. Unless the test requiring general anesthesia is performed under emergency conditions, you should meet with your anesthesiologist beforehand.

If you are hospitalized, he or she will probably come to see you in your room on the afternoon or evening before the test. If you are having the test as an outpatient, you will either have a separate appointment with the anesthesiologist before the day of the test, or meet with the anesthesiologist immediately before the test begins.

The anesthesiologist will perform a brief physical examination and will ask you about any factors that could possibly be a problem while you are being anesthetized: any current medical problems, any medications you are taking, any allergies you may have, and any problems you may have had with anesthesia in the past. He or she will be particularly interested in the health of your heart and lungs. If you smoke, it is strongly advised that you stop at least 10–14 days before the procedure. This will allow some lung function to recover and will reduce the risk of anesthesia.

Whenever possible, you will be asked not to eat or drink anything for 8–12 hours before general anesthesia. This is sometimes referred to as NPO or "nothing by mouth." If you are taking prescribed medication, you will usually be permitted a small amount of water to help swallow pills. You may be advised to stop taking certain medications before anesthesia. Check with your doctor if you have any questions.

You are asked to keep your stomach empty for your own protection: If you should vomit while you are under the anesthetic, some of the vomited material may get into your airways and lungs. This can cause a lung infection (aspiration pneumonia).

On the day of the test you will be asked to come or will be brought from your hospital room to the presurgical holding area. You may receive an injected sedative to help you relax. While you are in the holding area your blood pressure will probably be taken and an intravenous line (IV) may be inserted into a vein in your hand or arm. You may experience a brief stinging sensation as the needle is inserted.

You will next be brought into the operating or procedure room and will be moved onto the operating table. If you have not yet had an IV inserted, it will be done here. A blood pressure cuff will be wrapped around your arm, and ECG leads will be placed on your arm and chest. You will then be put to sleep, either by a medication injected through your IV or by an inhaled gas from a mask placed over your nose and mouth. Sometimes a combination of IV and inhaled anesthetics is used.

The intravenous drugs used for anesthesia include narcotics, sedative-hypnotics, tranquilizers, and muscle relaxants.

Frequently used anesthetic gases include nitrous oxide, halothane, and isoflurane.

While you are asleep the anesthesiologist will constantly monitor your heart rate, blood pressure, breathing rate, and skin color. An endotracheal tube may be inserted through your mouth, down the back of your throat, and into your windpipe to help the anesthesiologist control the flow of gases to your lungs. Except in rare cases, this tube will be removed before you wake up, so that you will not be directly aware of it.

You will wake up either in the recovery room or on your way there. In some cases you may be wearing an oxygen mask. You may feel somewhat dizzy and drowsy for the first few hours. Your throat may be sore from the endotracheal tube. You may experience some nausea and possibly some vomiting. Depending on the procedure you have had, you may feel some discomfort as a result of the test procedure. If so, you may be given pain medication. A recovery room nurse will monitor your blood pressure and overall condition until you are fully awake. You may feel a bit tired, groggy, and experience some generalized muscle aches for a day or two after the test.

There is a small but significant risk of serious complications from general anesthesia. Death occurs in less than 1 in 3000 cases. Other studies suggest that the risk of death from anesthesia may be as low as 1 in 5000 or 1 in 10,000. Nevertheless, for most tests performed under general anesthesia, the anesthetic itself is the riskiest part of the procedure. Risk may be increased in the severely ill, in those with heart or lung disease, and in smokers.

Possible complications include allergic reactions to the anesthetic, difficulties with lung function after the procedure, and blood clots in the leg veins. In rare cases the teeth could be damaged when the endotracheal tube is put in place.

You can help reduce this risk by co-operating fully with your anesthesiologist. Be sure to let your doctor know of any known or suspected problems in any of your vital organs, especially your heart and lungs; any episodes of fainting or unconsciousness; any allergies; and any history of reaction to anesthetics.

# Appendix 2

# Medical Tests:
# Your Personal Record

One way to avoid unnecessary medical tests is to keep your own record of what tests you have had. This should include the test, the date, who ordered the test, the results, and where the official report or x-rays are kept. If you can locate your previous test results, sometimes you will not need to have a test repeated. Or if the test is repeated, it can be compared with your previous results; comparison often provides valuable information. Below is a sample form you can use to keep your personal record of medical tests:

| Date | Type of Test | Health Professional Who Ordered Test | Results | Address Where Records Are Kept |
|------|--------------|--------------------------------------|---------|--------------------------------|
|      |              |                                      |         |                                |
|      |              |                                      |         |                                |
|      |              |                                      |         |                                |
|      |              |                                      |         |                                |
|      |              |                                      |         |                                |
|      |              |                                      |         |                                |
|      |              |                                      |         |                                |
|      |              |                                      |         |                                |

# Appendix 3 — Reader Survey

## How You Can Help Improve This Book

The world of medical testing is changing so quickly that it won't be long before a revised edition of this book will be necessary. We're already in the process of updating our files, and we could use your help—in two ways.

*First*, we'd very much like to know how useful this book has been for you and how we could make the next edition even *more* useful. We'd specifically like to know:

- What questions did you have that this book didn't answer?
- Was there a test you were concerned about that we didn't cover—or didn't cover to your satisfaction?
- Did you find any of our sections inaccurate, misleading, or difficult to understand?
- How else could we improve the next edition?

*Second*, we invite you to share with us your own experiences with any medical tests you have had. We've prepared a step-by-step questionnaire to make it easy—feel free to make as many copies of it as you like, or if you prefer, write us a letter. We'll include your experiences and those of other readers in the next edition.

Many thanks for your help. Mail your letters and questionnaires to

David S. Sobel, M.D.
Tom Ferguson, M.D.
*The People's Book of Medical Tests*
% Summit Books
1230 Avenue of the Americas
New York, N.Y. 10020

## *The People's Book of Medical Tests:*
## Reader Feedback on Medical Test Experience

1. What test or diagnostic procedure was performed?

2. Who suggested that this test might be needed?

3. Why was the test done?

4. How were you advised to prepare for the test?

5. Describe any problems or concerns you had *before* the test. What did you do to deal with these concerns?

6. Describe exactly what happened and how it felt at each stage during the test. Please be specific and include physical sensations, tastes, smells, sounds, visual images, and how you felt at the time.

   Preparation—

   Test procedure—

   Afterward—

7. How long did the test take?

8. Describe any specific advice you were given on what to do after the test, when to resume normal activities, what symptoms to watch for, etc.

9. Describe any specific sensations, problems, or concerns you had *after* the test. Please include what happened, what you did about it, and how long it lasted.

10. What was the most surprising or the most distressing aspect of the test?

11. What was the most satisfying or reassuring thing about the test?

12. What was done (or might have been done) to make the test more comfortable and less distressing?

13. What additional information should be given to people who are going to have this test?

14. Additional comments or suggestions?

Thanks for taking the time to share your experiences with us.

DAVID S. SOBEL, M.D.
TOM FERGUSON, M.D.

# For More Information

We plan to provide continuing, updated information about recent developments in medical testing, including new home medical tests, in *Medical Self-Care Magazine* (for subscription information write to: Medical Self-Care, P.O. Box 717, Inverness, California 94937). In addition, the books described below may be useful if you want to read more about any specific test or to find out about tests which were not covered in *The People's Book of Medical Tests*.

Fischback, Frances: *A Manual of Laboratory Diagnostic Tests* (2nd edition). Philadelphia: J. B. Lippincott, 1984 (898 pages).
Written for health professionals in a clear, readable, outline format covering nearly every conceivable test, including procedures. Includes extensive discussion of medications that can interfere with blood and urine tests.

Fox, Marion Laffey; Schnabel, Truman G.: *It's Your Body: Know What the Doctor Ordered*. Bowie, Md.: The Charles Press, 1979 (279 pages).
This is one of the first books to discuss the major diagnostic tests in lay terms with background on basic anatomy and physiology. There are descriptions of the individual tests including preparation, how it is performed, and how it will feel. While it does not discuss many of the blood and urine tests, it does cover very well most x-rays, scans, scoping procedures, and biopsies.

Hamilton, Helen (editorial director): *Diagnostics*. Springhouse, Pa.: Nursing 81 Books/Intermed Communications, 1981 (1089 pages).
This is our favorite professional reference book. Although written primarily for nurses, with special focus on the nurse's role in preparing people for and assisting with the various tests, it is the most readable, comprehensive and well illustrated of the professional reference books on tests. It covers nearly every test, including procedures. We highly recommend this one.

Henry, John Bernard (editor): *Clinical Diagnosis and Management by Laboratory Methods* (17th edition). Philadelphia: W. B. Saunders Co., 1984 (1502 pages).
This is a standard comprehensive textbook for health professionals on clinical laboratory tests (blood, urine, etc.). It is highly technical, detailed, comprehensive and authoritative. We used this text as the primary source for normal values in this book.

Kliman, Bernard; Vermette, Raymond; Kolowrat, Ernest: *What You Should Know About Medical Lab Tests*. New York: Thomas Y. Crowell, Publishers, 1979 (207 pages).
This brief book on lab tests (mostly blood and urine tests) is written for the general public. Its entertaining and chatty style makes it enjoyable, informative reading.

Laws, Priscilla; Ralph Nader's Public Citizen Health Research Group: *The X-ray Information Book*. New York: Farrar Straus Giroux, 1983 (154 pages).

Written for the general public by a physicist, this short book provides an excellent overview of x-ray risks and the principles behind the medical use of x-rays. Well illustrated and referenced, this book includes questions a consumer should ask before having an x-ray examination. However, it does not include much information about specific x-ray procedures, and since it is a revision of a 1974 book, it does not contain current x-ray exposure figures for some of the procedures.

Moskowitz, Mark A.; Osband, Michael E.: *The Complete Book of Medical Tests*. New York: W. W. Norton, 1984 (386 pages).

Written for the lay person by two physicians, this book provides a very clear, though brief discussion of the major medical tests and the most common questions patients ask about medical testing. It contains an excellent section describing which tests may be useful in evaluating common symptoms and diseases. Also includes a section on several home medical tests and special sections on medical tests for athletes and pregnant women.

*National Conference on Referral Criteria for X-ray Examinations*. Washington, D.C.: Bureau of Radiological Health, October 25–27, 1978.

This technical report discusses the attempt to put the selection of x-ray examinations for patients on a more rational and scientific basis. Contains a great deal of information on the unnecessary use of x-rays.

Pagana, Kathleen Deska; Pagana, Timothy James: *Understanding Medical Testing*. St. Louis, Mo.: C. V. Mosby Co., 1983 (277 pages).

This is a clearly written popular book describing the most commonly done tests. It is organized by organ systems (tests for the heart, tests for the bones and joints, etc.) and includes several excellent case histories illustrating how a testing sequence might actually be used from first symptom to final diagnosis.

Pinckney, Cathey; Pinckney, Edward R.: *A Patient's Guide to Medical Tests*. New York: Facts on File, 1982 (297 pages).

An encyclopedia of medical tests written for the general public, this book briefly discusses over 700 medical tests. It is an excellent resource to read about some of the common and many of the less commonly performed medical tests.

Pinckney, Cathey; Pinckney, Edward R.: *Do-It-Yourself Medical Testing*. New York: Facts on File, 1983 (266 pages).

This is a very comprehensive description of medical tests you can do yourself. It is practical, clear, and offers proper warnings for the at-home performance of these tests. However, in our opinion many of the 160 tests described are not really useful for home testing, and many of them are probably more appropriately performed by a health professional.

Rumsey, Timothy; Otteson, Orlo: *A Physician's Complete Guide to Medical Self-Care*. New York: The Rutledge Press, 1981 (256 pages).

This home health guide combines a discussion of the most important tests you can perform on yourself and your family with sound advice on evaluating symptoms, treating common health problems, and taking an active role in your own health care.

Stewart, Felicia; Guest, Felicia; Stewart, Gary; Hatcher, Robert: *My Body, My Health*. New York: Bantam Books, 1981 (566 pages).

This is a clear, comprehensive and authoritative description of women's health and medical concerns. Contains excellent descriptions of symptoms and medical problems which prompt the performance of many of the tests for women.

# Index

abdominal pain:
  abdominal tap, 362–63
  abdominal x-ray, 233–34
  alkaline phosphatase, 46
  amylase, 48
  barium enema, 245
  bilirubin, 53
  body temperature measurement, 397
  calcium, 55
  colonoscopy, 319
  laparoscopy, 325–28
  liver/spleen scan, 294
  stool cultures, 129
  theophylline monitoring, 72
  upper gastrointestinal series, 281
  urine cultures, 131
abdominal pain, upper:
  abdominal ultrasound, 305–6
  cholescintigraphy, 291
  gallbladder x-rays, 266
  lipase, 88
  SGOT, 101
  SGPT, 102
  upper gastrointestinal endoscopy, 338
abdominal tap (paracentesis), 362–63
abdominal ultrasound, 304–6
ABGs (arterial blood gases), 50–51
ABO blood typing, 53–55
acetaminophen:
  lactic acid, 86
  white blood cell differential, 65
acetazolamide (Diamox):
  ammonia levels, 48
  calcium, 56

carbon dioxide, 57
phosphorus, 92
urinary protein, 119
urine pH, 116
urobilinogen, 121
acid phosphatase, 42–43, 223–24
acquired immune deficiency syndrome
  (AIDS), 136
acromegaly: growth hormone, 81
ACTH (adrenocorticotropic hormone), 43–44,
  66, 67, 68, 96
activated partial thromboplastin time (APTT),
  90–91
Addison's disease:
  adrenocorticotropic hormone, 43
  aldosterone levels, 45
  chloride, 60
  cortisol, 66
  glucose, 79
  potassium, 93
  sodium, 106
adenoma, toxic: thyroid function test, 109
adrenal gland disease:
  chloride, 60
  cortisol, 66, 67
  magnesium, 89
  sodium, 106
  testosterone, 108
  urine glucose, 117
adrenal gland tumors:
  adrenocorticotropic hormone, 43
  aldosterone, 45
  CT scan, 254, 256
  estrogens, 74

adrenal gland tumors (*cont'd*)
plasma renin activity, 97
adrenal hyperplasia (adrenogenital
syndrome): cortisol, 66
adrenaline, *see* epinephrine
adrenal insufficiency, *see* Addison's disease
adrenocorticotropic hormone (ACTH), 43–44,
66, 67, 68, 96
AFP (alpha-fetoprotein), 46–47, 212
agranulocytosis: white blood cell differential,
65
AIDS: acquired immune deficiency syndrome,
136
white blood cell differential, 65
ALA (aminolevulinic acid), 87–88
alanine aminotransferase (ALT), 102
albumin, 56, 103–5, 118–19
alcohol:
adrenocorticotropic hormone, 43
amylase, 48
arterial blood gases, 51
barbiturate monitoring, 70
bilirubin, 120
catecholamines, 59
gastrin, 78
glucose, 79
lactic acid, 86
prothrombin time, 96
SGPT, 102
uric acid, 111
urine volume, 113
alcohol, blood, 44–45
alcohol, breath, 44, 441–43
alcoholism:
alkaline phosphatase, 46
dexamethasone suppression test, 69
folic acid, 75
immunoglobulins, 83
magnesium, 89
phosphorus, 92
Aldomet, *see* methyldopa
aldosterone, 45
aldosteronism:
aldosterone, 45
carbon dioxide, 56
chloride, 60
potassium, 93
alkaline phosphatase (Alk Phos), 35, 45–46
allergic disorders:
allergy testing, 371–73
urinary hemoglobin, 120

white blood cell differential, 65
allopurinol:
alkaline phosphatase, 46
SGOT, 102
SGPT, 102
urine cells, 122
white blood cell count, 65
alpha-fetoprotein (AFP), 46–47, 212
ALS, *see* amyotropic lateral sclerosis
ALT (alanine aminotransferase), 102
Alzheimer's disease: dexamethasone
suppression test, 69
ambulatory electrocardiogram, 155, 158–60
amikacin monitoring, 69, 70
amino acids: gastrin, 78
aminoglycoside monitoring, 69, 70
aminolevulinic acid (ALA), 87–88
aminophenazone: immunoglobulins, 83
aminophylline: lithium monitoring, 71
ammonia, 47–48
ammonium chloride:
carbon dioxide, 57
urine glucose, 117
urobilinogen, 121
amniocentesis, 47, 61, 208–12
amobarbital monitoring, 70
amoebas: ova and parasite test, 130
amphetamines:
adrenocorticotropic hormone, 43
catecholamines, 59
growth hormone, 81
amphotericin B: BUN, 111
ampicillin:
estriol, 73
estrogens, 74
urine cells, 122
Amsler Grid test, 407, 408
amylase, 48–49, 88
amyotropic lateral sclerosis (ALS):
electromyogram, 379
nerve conduction studies, 379
ANA (antinuclear antibodies), 50
anemia:
acid phosphatase, 42
Bence Jones protein, 119
bone marrow examination, 346, 348
carbon monoxide, 57
folate, 124
hematocrit, 62
hemoglobin, 62–63
hemoglobin electrophoresis, 82

lactic acid, 86
LDH, 152
platelet count, 66
red blood cell count, 63
red blood cell indices, 63−64
reticulocyte count, 98
SGOT, 152
urinary protein, 119
vitamin $B_{12}$, 124
white blood cell count, 64
anemia, aplastic: white blood cell differential, 65
anemia, hemolytic:
  bilirubin, 53
  direct Coombs test, 49
  ferritin, 75
  hematocrit, 62
  reticulocyte count, 98
  SGOT, 102
  urobilinogen, 121
anemia, iron-deficiency:
  ferritin, 74−75
  hematocrit, 62
  platelet count, 66
  red blood cell indices, 64
  reticulocyte count, 63, 98
  total iron-binding capacity, 84
anemia, Mediterranean, see thalassemia
anemia, megaloblastic: folic acid and, 75
anemia, pernicious:
  gastrin, 78
  histocompatibility testing, 83
  red blood cell indices, 64
  reticulocyte count, 98
  Schilling test, 99−100
  vitamin $B_{12}$, 124
  white blood cell differential, 65
anemia, sickle-cell:
  hematocrit, 62
  hemoglobin electrophoresis, 82
  sickle-cell test, 105−6
  urine casts, 123
anencephaly:
  alpha-fetoprotein, 47, 212
  amniocentesis, 209, 212
anesthesia, 465−67
  carbon dioxide, 56
  glucose, 79
aneurisms:
  arteriogram, 234, 237, 238, 240
  CT scan, 254, 256

angina:
  carbon monoxide, 57
  infarct imaging, 171
ankle pain and swelling:
  albumin, 103
  arthroscopy, 312
  joint tap, 364
ankylosing spondylitis: histocompatibility testing, 83
anorexia nervosa:
  dexamethasone suppression test, 69
  follicle-stimulating hormone, 76
anoscopy, 335−38
antacids:
  bicarbonate, 52
  carbon dioxide, 56
  phosphorus, 92
  urine pH, 116
antibiotic monitoring, 69, 70
antibiotics:
  alkaline phosphatase, 46
  antinuclear antibodies, 50
  bilirubin, 53
  catecholamines, 59
  cholesterol, 150
  creatinine clearance, 66
  glucose, 79, 117
  platelet count, 66
  SGOT, 102
  SGPT, 102
  urinary blood, 120
  urinary hemoglobin, 120
  urinary protein, 119
  urine cells, 122
  urine odor, 115
  urine pH, 116
  urobilinogen, 121
  white blood cell count, 65
  white blood cell differential, 65
  see also specific antibiotics
antibiotic sensitivity testing, 127, 131
antibody screening tests, 49−50
antibody tests, infectious disease, 136−40
anticoagulants:
  partial thromboplastin time, 90, 91
  prothrombin time, 96
  thyroid function tests, 109
  urinary hemoglobin, 120
  urine cells and, 122
anticonvulsants:
  calcium, 56

anticonvulsants (*cont'd*)
  folic acid, 75
  immunoglobulins, 83
anti-HAV (hepatitis A virus antibody), 137
antiinflammatory drugs:
  alkaline phosphatase, 46
  bilirubin, 53
  chloride, 60
  platelet count, 66
  SGOT, 102
  SGPT, 102
antinuclear antibodies (ANA), 50
antistreptolysin-O (ASO) titer, 136
antithyroid drugs: white blood cell
    differential, 65
apexcardiogram, 161
appendicitis: abdominal tap, 363
appetite loss: potassium, 93
applanation method, 379, 380
APTT (activated partial thromboplastin time),
    90–91
arch study, 240
arginine:
  glucose, 79
  growth hormone, 81
arm swelling: lymphangiogram, 272
arsenic poisoning: hair analysis, 381
arterial blood gases (ABGs), 50–51
arteriograms:
  cardiac, 162–67
  cerebral, 237–40
  general, 234–37
  pulmonary, 241–42
arthritis:
  arthrogram, 243–44
  body temperature measurement, 399
  histocompatibility testing, 83
  x-rays, 264, 265, 280
  *see also* gout
arthritis, rheumatoid, 199
  antinuclear antibodies, 50
  joint tap, 364, 365
  platelet count, 66
  rheumatoid factor, 98–99
  sedimentation rate, 101
  serum protein, 104
  syphilis tests, 146
  white blood cell count, 64
arthritis, septic: joint tap, 365
arthritis, traumatic: joint tap, 364, 365
arthrocentesis (joint tap), 99, 363–65

arthrogram (arthrography), 243–45
arthroscopy, 243, 312–15
ascending contrast phlebography, 283–85
ascorbic acid, *see* vitamin C
ASO (antistreptolysin-O) titer, 136
aspartate aminotransferase (AST), 101–2,
    151, 152
aspirin:
  amylase, 48
  arterial blood gases, 51
  barbiturate monitoring, 70
  bilirubin, 121
  carbon dioxide, 57
  cholesterol levels, 150
  D-xylose absorption test, 72
  glucose, 79
  platelet count, 66
  prothrombin time, 96
  SGOT, 102
  SGPT, 102
  thyroid function tests, 109
  uric acid, 111
  urine cells, 122
  urine glucose, 117
  urine pH, 116
  urobilinogen, 121
  white blood cell count, 64
aspirin monitoring, 71
AST (aspartate aminotransferase), 101–2,
    151, 152
asthma:
  arterial blood gases, 51
  pulmonary function tests, 387, 388, 389
  pulse measurement, 402
Athlete's foot: fungal tests, 135
Atromid-S, *see* clofibrate
atropine: gastrin, 78
audiometry, 382–84
autoimmune diseases:
  antinuclear antibodies (ANA), 50
  sedimentation rate, 101
  white blood cell differential, 65
  *see also specific diseases*

back films, 278–80
back pain:
  body temperature measurement, 397
  lymph node biopsy, 356
  urine cultures, 131
bacterial infections:
  immunoglobulins, 83

urine casts, 123
white blood cell count, 64
white blood cell differential, 65
*see also specific infections*
balance, loss of: cerebral arteriogram, 238
barbiturate monitoring, 70
barbiturates:
bilirubin, 53
white blood cell differential, 65
barium enema, 245–48
barium swallow, 280–83
basal body temperature (BBT), 196–200, 202
basal-cell carcinoma: skin biopsy, 359
Bence Jones protein, 119
Benemid, *see* probenecid
benign prostate hypertrophy (BPH): prostate
biopsy, 223, 225
benzodiazepines: glucose, 79
beta-blocker drugs: growth hormone, 81
bethanechol (Myocholine, Urecholine): lipase,
88
bicarbonate, 51–52, 56
bile duct obstructions:
abdominal ultrasound, 305
alkaline phosphatase, 46
bilirubin, 53, 120
cholescintigraphy, 292
CT scan, 256
endoscopic retrograde
cholangiopancreatogram, 342
intravenous cholangiogram, 268
percutaneous transhepatic cholangiogram,
268–69
SGOT, 101
SGPT, 102
urobilinogen, 121
bilirubin, 35, 46, 52–53, 120–21, 427
biomicroscopy, 335
biopsies, 343–61
bone, 344–46
bone marrow, 61, 346–48
kidney, 348–50
liver, 351–53
lung, 317, 318, 353–55
lymph node, 356–57
skin, 61, 357–59
synovial, 365
thyroid, 359–61
*see also* taps
birth defects:
alpha-fetoprotein (AFP), 47, 212

amniocentesis, 47, 61, 208–12
chromosomal analysis, 61, 212
fetal ultrasound, 208
bitewing dental x-rays, 262, 263
bladder disorders:
cystometrogram, 373–74
cystoscopy, 322–25
cystourethrogram, 260–62
ice water test, 374–75
retrograde ureteropyelography, 325
stress incontinence test, 375
urine cells, 122
bladder infections:
urine cultures, 131–32
*see also* urinary tract infections
bladder (suprapubic) tap, 41
bladder tumors:
cystoscopy, 325
urinary blood, 120
urine cells, 122
bleeding, *see* hemorrhaging
blood, in sputum, *see* hemoptysis
blood, in urine, *see* hematuria
blood clots:
arteriograms, 234, 238
CT scan, 257
Doppler ultrasound, 309–10
impedance plethysmography, 384–85
venogram, 283–85
blood collection procedures, 36–37
arterial stick, 36, 37
finger stick, 36, 37
venipuncture, 36–37
blood cultures, 127–28
blood gases, arterial (ABGs), 50–51
blood pressure, high, *see* hypertension
blood pressure, low:
barbiturate monitoring, 70
potassium, 93
blood-pressure medications:
catecholamines, 59
chloride, 60
sodium, 106
*see also specific drugs*
blood-pressure monitoring, 413–18
blood testing, 35–38
blood transfusions:
antibody screening tests, 49–50, 136
blood (ABO and Rh) typing, 53–55
ferritin, 75
hemoglobin electrophoresis, 82

blood transfusions (*cont'd*)
   serum protein electrophoresis, 105
   sickle-cell test, 105–6
   urine volume, 113
blood (ABO) typing, 53–55
blood urea nitrogen (BUN), 110–11
body scan, 292–93
body temperature measurement, 396–400
bone biopsy, 344–46
bone cancer:
   bone biopsy, 344–46
   bone scan, 287–89
   *see also* multiple myeloma; myeloma
bone disease:
   alkaline phosphatase, 45–46
   x-rays, 265
bone fractures:
   bone scan, 287–89
   x-rays, 264–65
bone infection:
   bone biopsy, 344–46
   bone scan, 288
   x-rays, 265
bone marrow aspiration, 100, 346–48
bone marrow biopsy, 61, 346–48
bone pain:
   Bence Jones protein, 119
   bone biopsy, 344–46
bone scan (scintigraphy), 287–89
bone tumors:
   alkaline phosphatase, 46
   parathyroid hormone, 90
bowel habits, change in:
   barium enema, 245
   home screening for bowel cancer, 443
   sigmoidoscopy, 336
bowel transit time, self-test for, 446–47
brain disease:
   arterial blood gases, 51
   brain scan, 289–90
   CT scan, 256–60
   electroencephalogram, 375–77
   ophthalmoscopy, 333
   spinal tap, 367–70
brain injury:
   brain scan, 289–90
   electroencephalogram, 375–77
   spinal tap, 367–70
   urine glucose, 117
brain scan (scintigraphy), 289–90
brain wave test, 375–77

breast cancer:
   breast biopsy, 193–95
   breast self-examination, 187–89
   breast ultrasound, 192–93
   carcinoembryonic antigen, 59
   diaphanography, 192
   mammogram, 189–92
   thermography, 192
breast discharge: prolactin, 95
breast enlargement, male: estrogens, 74
breast swelling: pregnancy testing, 94
breast ultrasound, 192–93
breath, fruity: ketones, 85
breath, shortness of:
   cardiac blood pool imaging, 172
   cardiac catheterization, 162
   echocardiogram, 160
   electrocardiogram, 153
   heart attack enzymes, 151
   infarct imaging, 170
   lung scan, 295
   pulmonary arteriography, 241
breath, sweet-smelling: lactic acid, 86
breath analysis, 44, 45
breathing, rapid:
   chloride, 60
   lactic acid, 86
   salicylate monitoring, 71
breathing, shallow: chloride, 60
breathing, slow: barbiturate monitoring, 70
breathing difficulties:
   bicarbonate, 52
   bronchoscopy, 315
   chest x-ray, 251–53
   hematocrit, 62
   lymph node biopsy, 356
   toxicology screening, 110
bronchiectasis: bronchogram, 249–51
bronchitis:
   bronchogram, 249–51
   pulmonary function tests, 387, 388
   sputum culture, 128
bronchogram (bronchography), 249–51
bronchoscopic biopsy, 317, 318, 353
bronchoscopy, 129, 249, 250, 315–19
bronchus, cancer of: carcinoembryonic
      antigen, 59
bruising:
   bone marrow examination, 346
   platelet count, 65
BUN (blood urea nitrogen), 110–11

burns, severe:
  chloride, 60
  hematocrit, 62
  magnesium, 89
  potassium, 93
  serum protein, 104
  serum protein electrophoresis, 105
  sodium, 106
  urinary hemoglobin, 120
  white blood cell differential, 65

cadmium poisoning: hair analysis, 381
caffeine:
  bilirubin, 53
  theophylline monitoring, 72
  urine volume, 113
calcitonin: calcium, 55
calcium ($Ca^{++}$), 55–56, 90, 92
calcium carbonate: gastrin, 78
calcium chloride: gastrin, 78
calcium gluconate: adrenocorticotropic
    hormone, 43
cancer:
  abdominal tap, 363
  body scan, 292–93
  body temperature measurement, 399
  bone scan, 287–89
  carcinoembryonic antigen, 59–60
  laparoscopy, 328
  LDH, 152
  liver biopsy, 352–53
  liver/spleen scan, 294
  lymphangiogram, 272, 274
  lymph node biopsy, 356–57
  pericardial tap, 174
  platelet count, 66
  pleural tap, 367
  sedimentation rate, 100–101
  serum protein, 104
  serum protein electrophoresis, 105
  white blood cell count, 64
  white blood cell differential, 65
  *see also specific cancers*
carbamazepine: urine glucose, 117
carbon dioxide ($CO_2$), 56–57
carbon monoxide (CO), 57–58
carbon monoxide poisoning:
  bicarbonate, 52
  carbon monoxide, 57–58
  glucose, 79
  hematocrit, 62

carboxyhemoglobin, 57–58
carcinoembryonic antigen (CEA), 59–60
cardiac blood pool imaging, 171–73
cardiac catheterization, 162–67
cardiac echo, 160–61
cardiac stress test, 155–57
carotid arteriogram, 237–40
carotid artery stenosis: Doppler ultrasound,
    309–10
carpal tunnel syndrome:
  electromyogram, 379
  nerve conduction studies, 379
cartilage injuries: arthroscopy, 312, 314–15
cascara:
  estriol, 73
  estrogens, 74
cataracts: ophthalmoscopy, 334
catecholamines, 58–59
CAT scans, *see* CT scans
CBC (complete blood count), 35, 61–66
CEA (carcinoembryonic antigen), 59–60
cefoxitin: creatinine, 68
celiac disease: folic acid, 75
centesis, *see* taps
cephaloridine: BUN, 111
cephalosporins:
  creatinine clearance, 66
  urinary protein, 119
cephalothin: white blood cell differential,
    65
cerebral arteriogram, 237–40
cerebral perfusion, 289–90
cerebrospinal fluid (CSF) analysis, 146, 367–
    370
cervical biopsy, 183–84
cervical cancer:
  carcinoembryonic antigen, 59
  cervical biopsy, 183–84
  cone biopsy, 184–85
  Pap smear, 179–83
cervical conization, 184–85
cervical (C-spine) films, 278–80
cervical myelogram, 275–77
cervicitis: vaginal self-examination, 177
chain cystourethrogram, 262
chemotherapy:
  immunoglobulins, 83
  platelet count, 66
  reticulocyte count, 98
  uric acid, 111
  white blood cell differential, 65

chest injury:
 arterial blood gases, 51
 chest x-ray, 251–53
chest pain:
 cardiac blood pool imaging, 172
 cardiac catheterization, 162
 chest x-ray, 251–53
 echocardiogram, 160
 electrocardiogram, 153
 infarct imaging, 170
 lung scan, 295
 pulmonary arteriography, 241
 stress test, 155
 thallium scan, 168
chest x-ray, 241, 251–53
chlamydia, 146
chloramphenicol: white blood cell differential, 65
chlordiazepoxide (Librium): white blood cell
    differential, 65
chloride (Cl⁻), 60
chlorothiazide diuretics: carbon dioxide, 57
chlorpromazine (Thorazine):
 alkaline phosphatase, 46
 bilirubin, 121
 estrogens, 74
 follicle-stimulating hormone, 76
 growth hormone, 81
 pregnancy testing, 94
 SGOT, 102
 SGPT, 102
 urobilinogen, 121
chlorthalidone: glucose, 79
cholangiograms:
 intravenous, 268
 percutaneous transhepatic, 268–69
cholecystogram, oral (OCG), 266–68
cholera: stool cultures, 130
cholescintigraphy, 290–92
cholesterol, blood, 148–50
cholinergic drugs: lipase, 88
choriocarcinoma, 94
chorionic villi biopsy (CVB), 213
chromosomal analysis (karotype), 60–61
cigarette smoking:
 carbon monoxide, 57, 58
 carcinoembryonic antigen, 59, 60
 hematocrit, 62
 white blood cell count, 64
cineangiogram, 166
cirrhosis:
 abdominal tap, 363

alkaline phosphatase, 46
alpha-fetoprotein, 47
ammonia, 48
amylase, 48
bilirubin, 53, 120
cholesterol, 150
liver/spleen scan, 295
SGOT, 101, 152
SGPT, 102
testosterone, 108
urobilinogen, 121
white blood cell count, 64
cisternal puncture, 370
Cl⁻ (chloride), 60
clean-catch midstream specimens, 39–40
clofibrate (Atromid-S):
 acid phosphatase, 42
 glucose, 79
 thyroid function tests, 109
clotting disorders:
 partial thromboplastin time, 91
 prothrombin time, 96
CO (carbon monoxide), 57–58
CO₂ (carbon dioxide), 56–57
codeine:
 alkaline phosphatase, 46
 amylase, 48
 lipase, 88
 SGOT, 102
 SGPT, 102
coldness, feelings of: thyroid function tests,
    108
"cold spot" myocardial imaging, 167–69
colitis:
 barium enema, 246
 carcinoembryonic antigen, 59
 colonoscopy, 319, 322
 sigmoidoscopy, 336, 338
 stool cultures, 130
collagen vascular diseases:
 antinuclear antibodies, 50
 white blood cell count, 64
 white blood cell differential, 65
colon cancer:
 barium enema, 245–48
 body scan, 293
 carcinoembryonic antigen, 59
 cholesterol, 150
 colonscopy, 319, 322
 home screening, 443–45
 sigmoidoscopy, 336, 338

colonoscopy, 42, 319–22
colon polyps:
  barium enema, 245, 248
  colonoscopy, 319, 320, 322
  sigmoidoscopy, 335–38
color vision test, 392
colposcopy, 183–84
coma:
  barbiturate monitoring, 70
  carbon monoxide, 57, 58
  chloride, 60
  ketones, 85
  lithium monitoring, 71
  magnesium, 89
  sodium, 106
  toxicology screening, 110
Compazine:
  estrogens, 74
  pregnancy testing, 94
complete blood count (CBC), 35, 61–66
computerized axial tomography, see CT scans
cone biopsy, 184–85
confusion:
  barbiturate monitoring, 70
  BUN, 110
  electroencephalogram, 375
  glucose, 79, 80
  potassium, 93
  toxicology screening, 110
congestive heart failure:
  albumin, 103
  aldosterone, 45
  ammonia, 48
  cardiac blood pool imaging, 171–73
  dexamethasone suppression test, 69
  serum protein, 104
  SGPT, 102
  sodium, 106
conjugated (direct) bilirubin, 52–53
Conn's syndrome: aldosterone levels, 45
constipation:
  barium enema, 245, 246
  sigmoidoscopy, 336
  thyroid function tests, 108
convulsions:
  electroencephalogram, 375
  lithium monitoring, 71
  white blood cell count, 64
  see also seizures
Coombs test, direct and indirect, 49–50
coordination, loss of:

cerebral arteriogram, 238
  salicylate monitoring, 71
corneal disorders: fluorescein eye staining, 335
coronary angiography (arteriography), 162–167
coricosteroids:
  estriol, 73
  estrogens, 74
  glucose, 79, 117
  thyroid function tests, 109
  uric acid, 111
cortisol, 43–44, 66–67, 68
cortisone:
  adrenocorticotropic hormone, 43
  alkaline phosphatase, 46
  carbon dioxide, 57
  SGOT, 102
  SGPT, 102
cosyntropin, 43
cough:
  body temperature measurement, 397
  chest x-ray, 251–53
Coumadin, see warfarin
creatine phosphokinase (CPK), 151–52
creatinine, 67–68, 70
creatinine clearance, 67–68
cretinism: thyroid function tests, 109
Crohn's disease:
  barium enema, 246
  carcinoembryonic antigen, 59
  colonoscopy, 319, 322
  sigmoidoscopy, 338
  small bowel follow-through, 280, 283
crossmatching, blood, 54
crush injuries: urinary hemoglobin, 120
CSF (cerebrospinal fluid) analysis, 367–70
C-spine (cervical) films, 278–80
CT scans:
  body, 253–56
  head, 256–60
culdocentesis, 204–5
culdoscopy, 328
Cushing's disease:
  adrenocorticotropic hormone, 43
  cortisol, 66
  dexamethasone suppression test, 68, 69
  sodium, 106
Cushing's syndrome:
  carbon dioxide, 56
  chloride, 60

Cushing's syndrome (*cont'd*)
  cortisol, 66
  potassium, 93
  white blood cell differential, 65
CVB (chorionic villi biopsy), 213
cystic fibrosis:
  kiss test, 390
  sweat test, 60, 107, 389–90
cystinuria: kidney stone analysis, 86
cystitis: urine cells, 122
cystoscopy (cystourethroscopy), 322–25
cystourethrogram, 260–62

decongestants: catecholamines and, 59
deep vein thrombosis (DVT):
  impedance plethysmography, 384–85
  venogram, 283–85
dehydration:
  BUN, 110
  chloride, 60
  salicylate monitoring, 71
  serum osmolality, 103
  serum protein, 104
  sodium, 106
  urine pH, 116
delirium:
  salicylate monitoring, 71
  spinal tap, 367
Demerol:
  alkaline phosphatase, 46
  amylase, 48
  SGOT, 102
  SGPT, 102
dental plaque, self-exam for, 412–13
dental x-rays, 262–64
depression: dexamethasone suppression test, 68, 69
dermafibromas: skin biopsy, 358
detached retinas: ophthalmoscopy, 335
dexamethasone suppression test (DST), 68–69
dextran:
  antibody screening tests, 49
  blood typing, 55
  immunoglobulins, 83
diabetes insipidus:
  sweat test, 390
  urine specific gravity, 115
  urine volume, 113
diabetes mellitus, 38–39
  aldosterone levels, 45

arterial blood gases, 51
  cystometrogram, 374
  electromyogram, 379
  glaucoma testing, 379
  glucose, 78–80, 116–17, 422, 426, 434–438
  glycohemoglobin, 80–81
  growth hormone, 81
  ketones, 38–39, 85, 118
  lactic acid, 86
  nerve conduction studies, 379
  ophthalmoscopy, 333, 335
  potassium, 93
  serum protein, 104
  sodium, 106
  urine odor, 114–15
  urine pH, 116
  urine specific gravity, 115
  urine volume, 113
diabetic control index, 80–81
diabetic ketoacidosis:
  carbon dioxide, 57
  ketones, 85, 118
  potassium, 93
Diamox, *see* acetazolamide
diaphanography, 192
diarrhea:
  arterial blood gases, 51
  barium enema, 245, 246
  body temperature measurement, 397
  carbon dioxide, 57
  chloride, 60
  colonoscopy, 319
  D-xylose absorption test, 72
  folic acid, 75
  hematocrit, 62
  ketones, 85
  magnesium, 89
  phosphorus, 92
  potassium, 93
  serum protein, 104
  sigmoidoscopy, 336
  small bowel follow-through, 280
  sodium, 106
  stool cultures, 129
  thyroid function tests, 108
  urine color, 113
  urine pH, 116
  urine specific gravity, 115
  urine volume, 112, 113
diazepam (Valium):

bilirubin, 53
white blood cell differential, 65
diazoxide: glucose, 79
digoxin monitoring, 70
Dilantin, *see* phenytoin
dimercaprol: carbon dioxide, 57
diphenylhydantoin, *see* phenytoin
diphtheria: throat cultures, 131
direct (conjugated) bilirubin, 52–53
direct Coombs test, 49–50
disclosing tablets, 412–13
disulfiram: barbiturate monitoring, 70
diuretics:
    aldosterone levels, 45
    bicarbonate, 52
    carbon dioxide, 56, 57
    chloride, 60
    plasma renin activity, 97
    potassium, 92, 93
    sodium, 106
    uric acid, 111
    urine specific gravity, 115
    urine volume, 113
    white blood cell differential, 65
    *see also specific diuretics*
dizziness:
    aminoglycoside monitoring, 69, 70
    brain scan, 289
    carbon monoxide, 57
    cerebral arteriogram, 238
    electrocardiogram, 153
    phenytoin monitoring, 71
dopamine, 58–59
Doppler ultrasound (Doptone), 207, 208, 309–10
double-voided (second-voided) specimen, urine, 38–39, 79, 117
Down's syndrome:
    amniocentesis, 209
    chromosomal analysis, 61
drill biopsy, 344
DST (dexamethasone suppression test), 68–69
duodenoscopy, 338–42
DVT, *see* deep vein thrombosis
dwarfism: growth hormone, 81
D-xylose absorption test, 72
dysentery: stool cultures, 130

ear disorders:
    body temperature measurement, 397
    home ear examination, 409–12
ECG (electrocardiogram), 93, 153–60
echocardiogram, 160–61
eclampsia: urine casts, 123
ectopic pregnancy, *see* pregnancy, ectopic
eczema: serum protein electrophoresis, 105
edema:
    albumin, 103, 104
    urine specific gravity, 115
EEG (electroencephalogram), 375–77
EFM (electronic fetal monitoring), 213–16
EKG (electrocardiogram), 93, 153–55
elbow pain:
    arthroscopy, 312
    joint tap, 364
electrocardiogram (ECG, EKG), 93, 153–60
electroencephalogram (EEG), 375–77
electrolyte disorders: chloride, 60
electromyogram (EMG), 377–79
electronic fetal monitoring (EFM), 213–16
electrophoresis:
    hemoglobin, 62, 81–82, 105
    protein, 103, 104–5, 370
electroshock therapy: catecholamines, 59
elephantiasis: lymphangiogram, 272
EMG (electromyogram), 377–79
emphysema:
    arterial blood gases, 51
    carbon dioxide, 56
    chest x-ray, 253
    pulmonary function tests, 387
    serum protein electrophoresis, 105
    urine pH, 116
encephalitis: spinal tap, 370
endocarditis, bacterial:
    blood cultures, 127
    echocardiogram, 161
    rheumatoid factor, 99
    urine casts, 123
endometrial biopsy, 185–87, 202
endometrial cancer:
    endometrial biopsy, 185–87, 202
    vabra aspiration, 187
endometriosis: laparoscopy, 202, 328
endoscopic retrograde cholangiopancreatogram (ERCP), 342
epididymitis: testicular scan, 301
epilepsy: electroencephalogram, 375, 377
epinephrine (adrenaline), 58–59
    cholesterol, 150
    glucose, 79

epinephrine (*cont'd*)
   lactic acid, 86
   phosphorous, 92
Equanil, *see* meprobamate
ERCP (endoscopic retrograde
     cholangiopancreatogram), 342
erection problems:
   cortisol, 66
   Dacomed Snap-Gauge, 221
   nocturnal penile tumescence stamp test,
     219–21
erythroblastosis fetalis:
   ammonia, 48
   direct Coombs test, 49
   Rh antibody titer, 54
erythrocyte sedimentation rate (ESR), 100–
   101
erythromycin:
   alkaline phosphatase, 46
   SGOT, 102
   SGPT, 102
esophageal disorders:
   upper gastrointestinal endoscopy, 341
   upper gastrointestinal series, 28–83
esophagoscopy, 338–42
esophogram, 280–83
ESR (erythrocyte sedimentation rate), 100–
   101
estriol, 73
estrogens, 73–74, 76
   adrenocorticotropic hormone, 43
   calcium, 55, 56
   cortisol, 66
   estriol, 73
   follicle-stimulating hormone, 76
   glucose, 79
   growth hormone, 81
   luteinizing hormone, 89
   prolactin, 96
   testosterone, 108
   thyroid function tests, 109
ethacrynic acid:
   glucose, 79
   uric acid, 111
ethylene glycol: carbon dioxide, 57
Ewing's sarcoma: bone biopsy, 346
excretory urography, 269–72
exercise:
   CPK, 152
   creatinine clearance, 67
   glucose, 79

lactic acid, 86, 87
   platelet count, 66
   SGOT, 102
   urinary hemoglobin, 120
   urinary protein, 119
   urine casts, 123
   urine cells, 122
   urine color, 113
exercise electrocardiogram, 155–57
exercise heart rate measurement, 400–401,
   402–3
exercise thallium scan, 167–69

facial pain: sinus x-ray, 277
faintness: electrocardiogram, 153
fallopian tube disorders:
   culdoscopy, 328
   laparoscopy, 325, 328
false-negative results, 26
false-positive results, 26–27
fecal occult blood test, 443–45
ferritin, 74–75
fertility awareness, 195–201
fertility testing, 201–2
FET (forced expiratory time), 418, 419, 420
fetal testing:
   alpha-fetoprotein, 46–47
   amniocentesis, 47, 61, 208–12
   electronic fetal monitoring, 213–16
   estriol, 73
   estrogens, 74
   fetal scalp blood sampling, 216–17
   fetoscopy, 213
   oxytocin challenge test, 217
   self-monitoring of fetal movements, 217
   ultrasound, 205–8, 211
fetoscopy, 213
$FEV_1$ (forced expiratory volume in one
   second), 388–89, 418, 419, 420
fever:
   body temperature measurement, 396–400
   BUN, 110
   chest x-ray, 251–53
   dexamethasone suppression test, 69
   glucose, 79
   ketones, 118
   lymph node biopsy, 356
   pulse measurement, 402
   salicylate monitoring, 71
   sedimentation rate, 100
   uric acid, 111

urinary protein, 119
urine casts, 123
urine color, 113
urine volume, 113
white blood cell count, 64
film-screen mammography, 190–92
finger joint pain: arthroscopy, 312
first morning specimen, urine, 38
fitness testing, 400–403
flat plate, 233–34
flurazepam (Dalmane): bilirubin, 53
flushing: catecholamines, 58
folic acid (folates), 75
folic acid deficiency:
    folic acid levels, 75
    hematocrit, 62
    platelet count, 66
    red blood cell indices, 64
    white blood cell differential, 65
follicle-stimulating hormone (FSH), 76–77,
    88, 225
forced expiratory time (FET), 418, 419, 420
forced expiratory volume in one second
    (FEV$_1$), 388–89, 418, 419, 420
forced vital capacity (FVC), 388, 418, 419,
    420
four-vessel study, 240
free thyroxine index (FTI), 108–9
frozen sections, 344
FSH (follicle-stimulating hormone), 76–77,
    88
FTA-ABS (fluorescent treponemal antibody
    absorption) test, 144–46
FTI (free thyroxine index), 108–9
funduscopy (ophthalmoscopy), 333–35
fungal infections:
    fungal scrapings, 135
    skin biopsy, 358, 359
    white blood cell differential, 65
furosemide:
    ammonia levels, 48
    glucose, 79
    white blood cell differential, 65
FVC (forced vital capacity), 388, 418, 419,
    420

galaclorrhea: prolactin, 95
galactosemia screening, 77
gallbladder and biliary tract scans, 290–92
gallbladder disease:
    abdominal ultrasound, 305
    amylase, 48
    bilirubin, 53
    cholescintigraphy, 290–92
    endoscopic retrograde
        cholangiopancreatogram, 342
    intravenous cholangiogram, 268
    magnetic resonance imaging, 386
    oral cholecystogram, 266–68
    percutaneous transhepatic cholangiogram,
        268–69
    x-rays, 266–69
gallbaldder series, 266–69
gallbladder ultrasound, 268
gallium scan, 292–93
gallstones:
    abdominal ultrasound, 305
    abdominal x-ray, 234
    bilirubin, 53, 120
    cholescintigraphy, 292
    CT scan, 256
    gallbladder x-rays, 268
    intravenous cholangiogram, 268
    urobilinogen, 121
gamma globulins, 83–84
gastrin, 77–78
gastrin stimulation test, 78
gastroenteritis: stool cultures, 130
gastrointestinal bleeding:
    ammonia, 48
    BUN, 110
    platelet count, 65
    upper gastrointestinal endoscopy, 338, 341
    upper gastrointestinal series, 281
gastroscopy, 338–42
Gaucher's disease: acid phosphatase, 42
gentamicin:
    BUN, 111
    monitoring, 69, 70
German measles: rubella antibody testing, 139
gigantism: growth hormone, 81
glaucoma tests, 379–81
globulin, 103–5
glomerulonephritis:
    antistreptolysin-O (ASO) titer, 136
    BUN, 110
    creatinine clearance, 66
    renal scan, 297
    urine casts, 123
    urine cells, 122
glucagon:
    growth hormone, 81

glucagon (*cont'd*)
   lactic acid, 86
glucose, 78–80, 116–17
   home monitoring, 434–38
   potassium, 93
glucose tolerance test (GTT), 79–80
glycohemoglobin (hemoglobin $A_{1c}$), 80–81
goiter disease:
   thyroid function tests, 108, 109
   thyroid scan, 299, 300
gold compounds:
   platelet count, 66
   white blood cell count, 65
gonorrhea cultures, 130, 140–43
gout:
   joint tap, 364, 365
   uric acid, 111
Graves' disease:
   thyroid antibodies, 109
   thyroid function test, 109
   thyroid scan, 300
growth, subnormal:
   chromosomal analysis, 61
   growth hormone, 81
growth hormone (HGH, somatotropin), 81
GTT (glucose tolerance test), 79–80
gum disease:
   dental x-rays, 262, 264
   platelet count, 65

hair, excessive body, *see* hirsutism
hair analysis, 381–82
hallucinations:
   digoxin monitoring, 70
   toxicology screening, 110
haloperidol: prolactin, 96
Hashimoto's thyroiditis:
   thyroid antibodies, 109
   thyroid function tests, 109
hay fever: allergy testing, 371
HBcAb (hepatitis B core antibody), 138
HBsAb (hepatitis B surface antibody), 138
HBsAg (hepatitis B surface antigen), 137–38
HCG (human chorionic gonadotropin), 93–94
HCT (hematocrit), 35, 37, 61–62
headache:
   barbiturate monitoring, 70
   body temperature measurement, 397
   carbon monoxide, 57
   cerebral arteriogram, 238
   CT scan, 257

ophthalmoscopy, 333
   sinus x-ray, 277
   spinal tap, 367–68
head injury:
   bicarbonate, 52
   CT scan, 257
   electroencephalogram, 375
   ophthalmoscopy, 333
   skull x-ray, 277–78
healthy people, medical tests for, 449–62
hearing difficulties:
   aminoglycoside monitoring, 69, 70
   audiometry, 382–84
   home ear examination, 409–12
heart attack:
   acid phosphatase, 42
   body temperature measurement, 399
   CPK, 151–52
   dexamethasone suppression test, 69
   infarct imaging, 170–71
   lactic acid, 86
   LDH, 151, 152
   SGOT, 101, 151, 152
   urinary blood, 120
   white blood cell count, 64
   white blood cell differential, 65
heart attack enzymes, 151–52
heartbeat, rapid: thyroid function tests, 108
heartbeats, irregular:
   digoxin monitoring, 70
   electrocardiogram, 154
   Holter monitoring, 158, 159–69
   phenytoin monitoring, 71
   potassium, 92, 93
   quinidine monitoring, 71
   toxicology screening, 110
heartburn: upper gastrointestinal series, 281
heart disease, 147–74
   abdominal tap, 363
   apexcardiogram, 161
   arterial blood gases (ABGs), 51
   carbon monoxide, 57
   cardiac blood pool imaging, 171–73
   coronary arteriography, 162–67
   echocardiogram, 160–61
   electrocardiogram, 93, 153–60
   Holter monitoring, 155, 158–60
   infarct imaging, 170–71
   magnetic resonance imaging, 386
   phonocardiogram, 161
   pulse measurement, 402

thallium scan, 167–69
heart failure:
    urinary protein, 119
    urine casts, 123
    *see also* congestive heart failure
heart murmur: antistreptolysin-O (ASO) titer, 136
heart size and shape: chest x-ray, 253
heatstroke: body temperature measurement, 399
hematocrit (HCT), 35, 37, 61–62
hematuria, 119–20, 427
    cystoscopy, 322
    intravenous pyelogram, 269
    pelvic ultrasound, 308
hemochromatosis, *see* iron overload
hemoglobin (Hgb), 35, 62–63
    urinary, 119–20, 427
hemoglobin $A_{1c}$ (glycohemoglobin), 80–81
hemoglobin electrophoresis, 62, 81–82, 105
hemoglobin S (sickle-cell) test, 105–6
hemolytic anemia, *see* anemia, hemolytic
hemophilia: partial thromboplastin time, 91
hemoptysis:
    bronchogram, 249–51
    bronchoscopy, 315
    chest x-ray, 251–53
    laryngoscopy, 329
    lymph node biopsy, 356
hemorrhaging:
    abdominal tap, 363
    arteriogram, 237, 240
    CT scan, 257, 259
    lactic acid, 86
    platelet count, 65
    pleural tap, 367
    serum protein, 104
    spinal tap, 370
    *see also* gastrointestinal bleeding
heparin: partial thromboplastin time, 90
hepatic necrosis: ammonia, 48
hepatitis:
    alkaline phosphatase, 46
    alpha-fetoprotein, 47
    amylase, 48
    bilirubin, 53, 120
    cholesterol, 150
    hepatitis virus tests, 137–38
    liver biopsy, 352
    liver/spleen scan, 295
    SGOT, 101, 152

urobilinogen, 121
hepatitis A virus antibody (anti-HAV), 137
hepatitis B core antibody (HBcAb), 138
hepatitis B surface antibody (HBsAb), 138
hepatitis B surface antigen (HbsAg), 137–38
hepatoma, *see* liver cancer
hepatomegaly: liver/spleen scan, 294
herpes:
    Tzanck test, 144
    vaginal self-examination, 177
    viral cultures, 133, 143–44
heterophil test, 138–39
hexosaminidase A and B, serum, 107
Hgb (hemoglobin), 35, 62–63
    urinary, 119–20, 427
HGH (growth hormone, somatotropin), 81
hiatal hernia:
    upper gastrointestinal endoscopy, 341
    upper gastrointestinal series, 280, 283
hip pain:
    arthroscopy, 312
    joint tap, 364
hirsutism:
    cortisol, 66
    testosterone, 108
His bundle electrocardiography, 167
histamine: growth hormone, 81
histocompatibility testing, 54, 82–83
hives: allergy testing, 371
HLA (human leukocyte antigen), 82–83
hoarseness:
    laryngoscopy, 329
    lymph node biopsy, 356
Hodgkin's disease:
    body scan, 292
    body temperature measurement, 399
    bone marrow examination, 346, 348
    CT scan, 254
    lymph node biopsy, 357
    mediastinoscopy, 333
Holter monitoring, 155, 158–60
home medical tests, 393–448
homovanillic acid (HVA), 58–59
hotness, feelings of: thyroid function tests, 108
"hot spot" myocardial imaging, 170–71
HPRL (lactogenic hormone), 95–96
human chorionic gonadotropin (HCG), 93–94
human growth hormone (HGH, somatotropin), 81

human leukocyte antigen (HLA), 82−83
hunger: glucose, 80
HVA (homovanillic acid), 58−59
hydantoin derivatives:
    immunoglobulins, 83
    white blood cell count, 65
hydatidiform moles: human chorionic
    gonadotropin, 94
hydralazine:
    aldosterone levels, 45
    antinuclear antibodies, 50
hydrocephalus: CT scan, 259
hydrochlorothiazide:
    estriol, 73
    estrogens, 74
hyperbilirubinemia: bilirubin, 53
hypercalcemia: calcium, 56
hypercalciuria:
    calcium, 56
    kidney stone analysis, 86
hyperkalemia: potassium, 93
hypernatremia: sodium, 106
hyperparathyroidism:
    acid phosphatase, 42
    calcium, 55
    parathyroid hormone, 90
    phosphorus, 92
hypertension:
    aldosterone, 45
    catecholamines, 58−59
    glucose, 79
    home monitoring, 413−18
    intravenous pyelogram, 269
    ophthalmoscopy, 333, 335
    renin, 96
hyperthyroidism:
    carbon monoxide, 57
    folic acid, 75
    glucose, 79, 117
    magnesium, 89
    prolactin, 95
    pulse measurement, 402
    radioactive iodine uptake test, 300
    serum protein electrophoresis, 105
    thyroid function tests, 108, 109
    thyroid scan, 299
    white blood cell differential, 65
hyperuricemia: uric acid, 111
hyperventilation:
    arterial blood gases, 51
    carbon dioxide, 57

    chloride, 60
    urine pH, 116
hypocalcemia: calcium, 56
hypoglycemia:
    adrenocortioctropic hormone, 43
    gastrin, 78
    glucose, 78−80
hypogonadism: follicle-stimulating hormone,
    76
hypokalemia: potassium, 93
hyponatremia: sodium, 106
hypoparathyroidism:
    calcium, 56
    parathyroid hormone, 90
    prolactin, 95
hypothyroidism:
    glucose, 79
    radioactive iodine uptake test, 300
    thyroid function tests, 108, 109
hysterosalpingogram, 202−4
hysteroscopy, 202


ice water test, 374−75
idiopathic thrombocytopenia purpura: platelet
    count, 66
immune system tests:
    antinuclear antibodies, 50
    direct Coombs test, 49−50
    indirect Coombs test, 49−50
immunoglobulins, 83−84
immunosuppression:
    bone marrow examination, 346
    white blood cell differential, 65
impedance audiometry, 384
impedance plethysmography (IPG), 384−85
impedometer testing, 201
impotence, see erection problems
incontinence:
    cystometrogram, 373−74
    cystourethrogram, 260, 262
    stress incontinence test, 375
Inderal, see propranolol
indirect (unconjugated) bilirubin, 52−53
indirect Coombs test, 49−50
indomethacin (Indocin):
    alkaline phosphatase, 46
    amylase, 48
    D-xylose absorption test, 72
    prothrombin time, 96
    SGOT, 102

SGPT, 102
   white blood cell differential, 65
infarct imaging, 170−71
infections:
   acid phosphatase, 42
   antibody tests, 136−40
   CT scan, 257
   cultures, 126−33
   ferritin, 75
   glucose, 79
   lactic acid, 86
   platelet count, 66
   sedimentation rate, 100, 101
   serum protein, 104
   *see also specific infections*
infertility, female, 201−2
   chromosomal analysis, 61
   endometrial biopsy, 185, 186−87
   follicle-stimulating hormone, 76
   hysterosalpingogram, 202−4
   laparoscopy, 325
   luteinizing hormone, 88−89
infertility, male, 201−2
   chromosomal analysis, 61
   follicle-stimulating hormone, 76, 225
   luteinizing hormone, 88−89, 225
   postcoital test, 201, 223
   semen analysis, 201, 221−23
   testicular biopsy, 225−26
   testosterone, 108, 225
inflammatory disorders:
   platelet count, 66
   serum protein electrophoresis, 104, 105
   white blood cell differential, 65
   *see also specific diseases*
informed choice, 21
insulin:
   catecholamines, 59
   glucose, 79, 117
   growth hormone, 81
   phosphorus, 92
   potassium, 93
intestinal infections: stool cultures, 129, 130
intestinal obstructions:
   amylase, 48
   carbon dioxide, 57
intoxication tests:
   blood alcohol (ethanol), 44−45
   breath, 44
intradermal test, 371, 372−73
intravenous (IV) cholangiogram, 268

intravenous pyelogram (IVP), 269−72
IPG (impedance plethysmography), 384−85
iron (total iron-binding capacity, TIBC), 84−85
iron deficiency, *see* anemia, iron-deficiency
iron overload:
   ferritin, 74−75
   total iron-binding capacity, 84
irrational behavior: toxicology screening, 110
irritability:
   glucose, 79
   magnesium, 89
isocarboxazid (Marplan): D-xylose absorption test, 72
isoniazid:
   alkaline phosphatase, 46
   antinuclear antibodies, 50
   SGOT, 102
   SGPT, 102
   white blood cell count, 64−65
   white blood cell differential, 65
itching:
   lymph node biopsy, 356
   salicylate monitoring, 71
   self-test for pinworms, 447−48
IVP (intravenous pyelogram), 269−72

jaundice:
   abdominal ultrasound, 305
   alkaline phosphatase, 46
   bilirubin, 52−53, 120
   cholescintigraphy, 291
   CT scan, 254
   endoscopic retrograde cholangiopancreatogram, 342
   gallbladder x-rays, 266
   intravenous cholangiogram, 268
   liver biopsy, 351
   SGOT, 101
   SGPT, 102
   urobilinogen, 121
jock itch, fungal tests, 135
joint pain and swelling:
   arthrogram, 243−44
   arthroscopy, 243, 312−15
   ASO titer, 136
   joint tap, 99, 363−65
   sedimentation rate, 100
   x-rays, 264−65
joint tap (aspiration), 99, 363−65

kanamycin:
  ammonia levels, 48
  BUN, 111
  urine cells, 122
karotype (chromosomal analysis), 60–61, 212
keloids: skin biopsy, 358
ketones, 38–39, 85, 86, 118, 426
kidney biopsy, 348–50
kidney disease:
  abdominal tap, 363
  abdominal ultrasound, 306
  acid phosphatase, 42
  aldosterone, 45
  antistreptolysin-O titer, 136
  arterial blood gases, 51
  bicarbonate, 42
  BUN, 110
  calcium, 56
  chloride, 60
  creatinine, 67–68
  creatinine clearance, 67–68
  CT scan, 254
  cystometrogram, 374
  D-xylose absorption test, 72
  gastrin, 78
  intravenous pyelogram, 269–72
  kidney biopsy, 348–50
  magnetic resonance imaging, 386
  pericardial tap, 174
  phosphorus, 92
  renal scan, 297–99
  renin, 96–97
  sedimentation rate, 101
  serum osmolality, 103
  serum protein electrophoresis, 104, 105
  sodium, 106
  uric acid, 111
  urinary blood, 120
  urinary protein, 118
  urine casts, 123
  urine cells, 122
  urine glucose, 117
  urine pH, 116
  urine specific gravity, 115
kidney failure:
  carbon dioxide, 57
  magnesium, 89
  potassium, 93
  uric acid, 111
  white blood cell count, 64
kidney scan, 297–99

kidney stones:
  abdominal x-ray, 233, 234
  BUN, 110
  calcium, 55
  CT scan, 254
  cystoscopy, 325
  intravenous pyelogram, 269, 272
  kidney stone analysis, 85–86
  renal scan, 297
  retrograde ureteropyelography, 325
  uric acid, 111
  urinary crystals, 123
  urine cells, 122
  urine pH, 116, 426
kidney tumors:
  urinary blood, 120
  urine cells, 122
kiss test, 390
Klinefelter's syndrome: chromosomal analysis, 61
knee joint pain and swelling:
  arthrogram, 243–44
  arthroscopy, 243, 312–15
  joint tap, 364
  x-rays, 165
KUB, 233–34

laboratory error, 28
lactic dehydrogenase (LDH), 151, 152
lactogenic hormone (HPRL), 95–96
lactulose: ammonia levels, 48
laparoscopy, 202, 205, 325–28
laryngoscopy, 329–31
Lasix:
  uric acid, 111
  white blood cell differential, 65
laxatives:
  potassium, 93
  serum protein, 104
LDH (lactic dehydrogenase), 151, 152
lead, 87–88
lead poisoning: hair analysis, 381
leg swelling:
  Doppler ultrasound, 309
  impedance plethysmography, 384–85
  lymphangiogram, 272
  venogram, 284
LE prep (lupus erythematosus cell test), 50
lethargy:
  calcium, 55
  potassium, 92

sodium, 106
leukemia:
  body temperature measurement, 399
  bone marrow examination, 346, 348
  ferritin, 75
  lactic acid, 86
  LDH, 152
  peripheral blood smear, 66
  platelet count, 66
  serum protein, 104
  uric acid, 111
  urinary protein, 119
  white blood cell count, 64
  white blood cell differential, 65
leukocyte dipsticks, 428, 429, 430
leukocytosis: white blood cell count, 64
leukopenia: folic acid, 75
levodopa:
  glucose, 79
  growth hormone, 81
  ketones, 85
  uric acid, 112
LH (luteinizing hormone), 76, 88–89, 225
Librium, *see* chlordiazepoxide
licorice:
  aldosterone, 45
  carbon dioxide, 57
  plasma renin activity, 97
ligament injuries:
  arthroscopy, 314
  x-rays, 265
light, sensitivity to: magnesium, 89
lightheadedness: hematocrit, 62
lipase, 88
lithium:
  glucose, 79
  monitoring of, 70–71
  thyroid function tests, 109
liver biopsy, 351–53
liver cancer:
  alkaline phosphatase, 46
  alpha-fetoprotein (AFP), 47
  body scan, 293
  SGPT, 102
liver disease:
  abdominal tap, 363
  abdominal ultrasound, 305
  aldosterone, 45
  alkaline phosphatase and, 45–46
  amylase, 48
  arterial blood gases, 51

bicarbonate, 52
bilirubin, 53, 120–21
BUN, 110, 111
carcinoembryonic antigen, 59
cholescintigraphy, 292
cholesterol, 150
CT scan, 254, 256
endoscopic retrograde
    cholangiopancreatogram, 342
estrogens, 74
ferritin, 75
glucose, 79, 117
hematocrit, 62
LDH, 152
liver biopsy, 351–53
liver/spleen scan, 293–95
percutaneous transhepatic cholangiogram,
    268–69
potassium, 93
prothrombin time, 96
rheumatoid factor, 99
serum protein, 104
serum protein electrophoresis, 104, 105
SGOT, 101, 102, 152
SGPT, 102
urobilinogen, 121
liver/spleen scan, 293–95
Lou Gehrig's disease, *see* amyotropic lateral
    sclerosis
lower gastrointestinal series, 245–48
lower limb venography, 283–85
LS-spine (lumbosacral) films, 278–80
lumbar myelogram, 275–77
lumbar puncture, 146, 367–70
lumbosacral (LS-spine) films, 278–80
lung biopsy, 317, 318, 353–55
lung cancer:
  body scan, 293
  bronchoscopy, 315, 318
  chest x-ray, 251–53
  CT scan, 254
  lung biopsy, 317, 318, 353–55
  mediastinoscopy, 331–33
lung disease:
  bicarbonate, 52
  bronchoscopy, 129, 249, 250, 315–19
  carbon dioxide, 56
  carbon monoxide, 57
  carcinoembryonic antigen, 59
  hematocrit, 62
  lung biopsy, 317–18

lung disease (*cont'd*)
  lung scan, 241, 295–97
  mediastinoscopy, 331–33
  pleural tap, 365–67
  pulmonary arteriography, 242
  pulmonary function tests, 387–89
lung scans, 241, 295–97
lupus erythematosus, systemic (SLE):
  antinuclear antibodies, 50
  direct Coombs tests, 49
  joint tap, 365
  histocompatibility testing, 83
  kidney biopsy, 350
  rheumatoid factor, 99
  white blood cell differential, 65
lupus erythematosus cell test (LE prep), 50
luteinizing hormone (LH), 76, 88–89, 225
lymphangiogram, 272–74
lymph node biopsy, 356–57
lymphoma (lymphatic cancer):
  body scan, 292, 293
  lymphangiogram, 272, 274
  lymph node biopsy, 357
  mediastinoscopy, 333
  serum protein electrophoresis, 105
  *see also* Hodgkin's disease

macular degeneration: Amsler Grid test, 407, 408
magnesium, 89
magnetic resonance imaging (MRI), 385–87
malabsorptive disorders:
  cholesterols, 150
  D-xylose absorption test, 72
  folic acid, 75
  magnesium, 89
  Schilling test, 100
  serum protein, 104
  upper gastrointestinal series, 283
malaise:
  body temperature measurement, 397
  carbon monoxide, 57
  potassium, 93
malaria:
  peripheral blood smear, 66
  white blood cell differential, 65
male PAP (prostatic acid phosphatase) test, 42–43
malignant melanoma: skin biopsy, 359
malnutrition:
  BUN, 110

cholesterol, 150
D-xylose absorption test, 72
glucose, 79
magnesium, 89
  serum protein, 104
mammogram, 189–92
MAO inhibitors:
  barbiturate monitoring, 70
  glucose, 79
maple syrup urine disease: urine odor, 115
Marplan, *see* isocarboxazid
match test, 418, 419, 420
maximum midexpiratory flow (MMEF), 389
maximum voluntary ventilation (MVV), 389, 418, 419–21
MCH (mean corpuscular hemoglobin), 63
MCHC (mean corpuscular hemoglobin concentration), 63–64
MCV (mean corpuscular volume), 63–64
mean corpuscular hemoglobin (MCH), 63
mean corpuscular hemoglobin concentration (MCHC), 63–64
mean corpuscular volume (MCV), 63–64
mediastinoscopy, 331–33
Mediterranean anemia, *see* thalassemia
mefenamic acid: prothrombin time, 96
melanoma: skin biopsy, 358
memory loss: cerebral arteriogram, 238
meningitis:
  spinal tap, 370
  white blood cell count, 64
menstrual irregularities:
  cortisol, 66
  endometrial biopsy, 185–87
  estrogens, 74
  follicle-stimulating hormone, 76
  pregnancy testing, 94
  prolactin, 95
mental retardation: chromosomal analysis, 61
meperidine: lipase, 88
meprobamate (Equanil, Miltown):
  dexamethasone suppression test, 69
  estriol, 73
  estrogens, 74
  platelet count, 66
mercury poisoning: hair analysis, 381
metabolic acidosis:
  arterial blood gases, 51
  lactic acid, 86
metabolic alkalosis: arterial blood gases, 51
methadone: immunoglobulins, 83

methenamine mandelate: estriol, 73
methicillin:
   BUN, 111
   carbon dioxide, 57
   urine cells, 122
methimazole: prothrombin time and, 96
methotrexate:
   folic acid, 75
   immunoglobulins, 83
methyl alcohol: carbon dioxide, 57
methyldopa (Aldomet):
   alkaline phosphatase, 46
   antibody screening tests, 49–50
   creatinine, 68
   glucose, 79
   growth hormone, 81
   prolactin, 96
   SGOT, 102
   SGPT, 102
   uric acid, 112
methylprednisone: immunoglobulins, 83
microsomal antibodies, 109
Miltown, see meprobamate
MMEF (maximum midexpiratory flow), 389
moles:
   human chorionic gonadotropin, 94
   skin biopsy, 358
mongolism, see Down's syndrome
mononucleosis, infectious:
   bilirubin, 53
   heterophil test, 138–39
   mono spot, 138–39
   rheumatoid factor, 99
   SGOT, 101, 152
   SGPT, 102
morphine:
   alkaline phosphatase, 46
   amylase, 48
   lipase, 88
   SGOT, 102
   SGPT, 102
mouth, dryness in: salivary gland scan, 301
MRI (magnetic resonance imaging), 385–87
mucus method, 196, 197, 198–99, 200, 201
multiple myeloma:
   acid phosphatase, 42
   Bence Jones protein, 119
   bone biopsy, 346
   bone marrow examination, 346
   bone scan, 288
   calcium, 56

sedimentation rate, 101
serum protein, 104
serum protein electrophoresis, 104
uric acid, 111
urinary protein, 119
multiple sclerosis: cystometrogram, 374
mumps:
   amylase, 48
   follicle-stimulating hormone, 76
muscle diseases:
   catecholamines, 59
   urinary blood, 120
muscle injuries: CPK, 152
muscle pain:
   aldosterone, 45
   parathyroid hormone, 90
muscles, soft and flabby: barbiturate
      monitoring, 70
muscle spasms and twitches:
   bicarbonate, 52
   calcium, 55
   chloride, 60
   electromyogram, 377
   magnesium, 89
   parathyroid hormone, 90
   potassium, 93
muscular dystrophy:
   CPK, 152
   electromyogram, 379
   nerve conduction studies, 379
muscular weakness:
   aldosterone, 45
   potassium, 92, 93
MVV (maximum voluntary ventilation), 389,
      418, 419–21
myasthenia gravis:
   electromyogram, 379
   histocompatibility testing, 83
   nerve conduction studies, 379
mycoplasma infections: gold agglutinins, 137
myelogram, 272–74, 368
myeloma:
   serum protein electrophoresis, 105
   see also multiple myeloma
myocardial perfusion imaging, 167–69

Na (sodium), 106–7
narcotics:
   alkaline phosphatase, 46
   amylase, 48
   bilirubin, 53

narcotics (*cont'd*)
   body temperature measurement, 399
   immunoglobulins, 83
   SGOT, 102
   SGPT, 102
   toxicology screening, 109–10
   *see also specific drugs*
Nardil, *see* phenelzine
nausea:
   abdominal x-ray, 233
   alkaline phosphatase, 46
   digoxin monitoring, 70
   glucose, 79
   heart attack enzymes, 151
   lipase, 88
   potassium, 93
   pregnancy testing, 94
   salicylate monitoring, 71
   SGOT, 101
   SGPT, 102
Nembutal, *see* pentobarbital
neomycin:
   ammonia levels, 48
   cholesterol, 150
nephrosis: urine casts, 123
nephrotic syndrome:
   serum protein electrophoresis, 104, 105
   urine casts, 123
nerve conduction studies, 377–79
nervousness:
   glucose, 79, 80
   thyroid function tests, 108
neural tube defects, fetal: alpha-fetoprotein, 47
neurofibromas: skin biopsy, 358
nicotinic acid:
   glucose, 79, 117
   growth hormone, 81
night sweats: lymph node biopsy, 356
nitrite dipsticks, 428, 429, 430–31
NMR (nuclear magnetic resonance), 385–87
nocturnal penile tumescence (NPT) stamp test, 219–21
noise, sensitivity to: magnesium, 89
noradrenaline (norepinephrine), 58–59
normal test values, 27–29
nose bleeds: platelet count, 65
NPT (nocturnal penile tumescence) stamp test, 219–21
nuclear magnetic resonance (NMR), 385–87
nuclear scans, 286–302

   bone, 287–89
   brain, 289–90
   gallbladder and biliary tract, 290–92
   gallium, 292–93
   liver/spleen, 293–95
   lung, 241, 295–97
   renal, 297
   salivary gland, 301
   testicular, 301
   thyroid, 299–301
   vein, 302
numbness:
   brain scan, 289
   cerebral arteriogram, 238
   Doppler ultrasound, 309
   electromyogram, 377
   spinal tap, 367

obesity:
   cortisol, 66
   glucose, 79
obstetric (fetal) ultrasound, 205–8, 211
occlusal dental x-rays, 262, 263
occlusive impedance phlebography, 384–85
OCG (oral cholecystogram), 266–68
open laparoscopy, 328
ophthalmoscopy (funduscopy), 333–35
optic nerve degeneration: ophthalmoscopy, 335
oral cholecystogram (OCG), 266–68
oral contraceptives:
   alkaline phosphatase, 46
   bilirubin, 53
   calcium, 56
   cholesterol, 150
   cortisol, 66
   estrogens, 74
   folic acid, 75
   glucose, 79
   immunoglobulins, 83
   luteinizing hormone, 89
   serum protein, 104
   SGOT, 102
   SGPT, 102
   thyroid function tests, 109
oral hypoglycemic drugs: glucose, 79
osteoarthritis: joint tap, 365
osteomalacia:
   alkaline phosphatase, 46
   calcium, 56
osteomyelitis, *see* bone infection

osteoporosis:
  calcium, 55
  spine films, 280
osteosarcoma: bone biopsy, 346
ova and parasite test, 130
ovarian cancer:
  alpha-fetoprotein (AFP), 47
  carcinoembryonic antigen, 59
  culdocentesis, 204–5
ovarian disorders:
  culdocentesis, 204–5
  estrogens, 74
  follicle stimulating hormone, 76
  laparoscopy, 328
  luteinizing hormone, 88–89
  pelvic ultrasound, 307–9
  progesterone, 95
ovulation:
  fertility awareness, 195–201
  white blood cell differential, 65
oxalates: acid phosphatase, 42
oxyphenbutazone: prothrombin time, 96

Paget's disease:
  acid phosphatase, 42
  alkaline phosphatase, 46
pallor: hematocrit, 62
pancreatic cancer:
  abdominal ultrasound, 306
  alpha-fetoprotein, 47
  amylase, 48
  CT scan, 254, 256
pancreatic duct obstructions: endoscopic
    retrograde cholangiopancreatogram, 342
pancreatic tumors:
  abdominal ultrasound, 306
  gastrin, 78
pancreatitis:
  abdominal tap, 363
  abdominal ultrasound, 306
  amylase, 48
  carcinoembryonic antigen, 59
  CT scan, 256
  lipase, 88
  magnesium, 89
  SGOT, 102, 152
  triglyceride, 148
panographic dental x-rays, 262, 263
Papanicolaou (Pap) smear, 179–83
PAP (prostatic acid phosphatase) test, male,

42–43
para-aminosalicylic acid (PAS):
  prothrombin time, 96
  urinary protein, 119
  urobilinogen, 121
paraldehyde: carbon dioxide, 57
paralysis:
  CT scan, 257
  Doppler ultrasound, 309
  electromyogram, 377
  nerve conduction studies, 377
  potassium, 93
  spinal tap, 367
parasitic infections:
  lymphangiogram and, 272
  ova and parasite test, 130
  white blood cell count, 64
  white blood cell differential, 65
parathyroid disease:
  acid phosphatase, 42
  calcium, 55–56
  magnesium, 89
  parathyroid hormone, 90
parathyroid hormone (PTH), 55, 89–90, 92
Parkinson's disease: cystometrogram, 374
partial thromboplastin time (PTT), 90–91
patch tests, 371, 372–73
peak expiratory flow rate (PEFR), 418–19,
    420
PEFR (peak expiratory flow rate), 418–19,
    420
pelvic inflammatory disease (PID):
  gonorrhea cultures, 141
  sedimentation rate, 101
pelvic pain:
  laparoscopy, 325–28
  magnetic resonance imaging, 386
  sedimentation rate, 100
pelvic ultrasound, 307–9
penicillin:
  alkaline phosphatase, 46
  antibody screening tests, 49–50
  antinuclear antibodies, 50
  platelet count, 66
  SGOT, 102
  SGPT, 102
  urinary protein, 119
  white blood cell differential, 65
penicillin G: potassium, 93
penile discharges: gonorrhea cultures, 141
pentobarbital (Nembutal) monitoring, 70

percutaneous transhepatic cholangiogram, 268–69
perfusion lung scan, 295–97
periapical dental x-rays, 262, 263
pericardial biopsy, 174
pericardial effusion: pericardial tap, 173–74
pericardial tap (pericardiocentesis), 173–74
peripheral blood smear, 66
peritoneal tap, 362–63
permanent sections, 344
personality changes, sudden: toxicology screening, 110
PFT (pulmonary function tests), 387–89, 418–21
phenazopyridine (Pyridium):
    bilirubin, 121
    estriol, 73
    estrogens, 74
    glucose, 79
    ketones, 85, 118
    urobilinogen, 121
phenelzine (Nardil): D-xylose absorption test, 72
Phenergan, see promethazine
phenobarbital:
    dexamethasone suppression test, 69
    monitoring, 70
phenolphthalein:
    estriol, 73
    glucose, 79
phenothiazides: glucose, 79
phenothiazines:
    bilirubin, 121
    catecholamines, 59
    follicle-stimulating hormone, 76
    growth hormone, 81
    estriol, 73
    estrogens, 74
    pregnancy testing, 94
    prolactin, 96
    urine glucose, 117
    urobilinogen, 121
phenylbutazone:
    alkaline phosphatase, 46
    immunoglobulins, 83
    platelet count, 66
    prothrombin time, 96
    SGOT, 102
    SGPT, 102
    urine cells, 122
phenylketonuria (PKU) screening, 91

phenytoin (Dilantin, diphenylhydantoin):
    bilirubin, 53
    cholesterol, 150
    cortisol, 66
    dexamethasone suppression test, 69
    folic acid, 75
    glucose, 79
    immunoglobulins, 83
    monitoring, 71
    prothrombin time, 96
    thyroid function tests, 109
pheochromocytoma: catecholamines, 58
phlebitis, see thrombophlebitis
phlebography, ascending contrast, 283–85
phonocardiogram, 161
phosphorus, 55, 91–92
PID, see pelvic inflammatory disease
pinworms, self-test for, 447–48
pituitary gland disease:
    progesterone, 95
    prolactin, 95
    serum osmolality, 103
    testosterone, 108
PKU (phenylketonuria) screening, 91
plasma, blood, 35
plasma renin activity (PRA), 97
platelet (thrombocyte) count, 35, 65–66
pleural effusion:
    chest x-ray, 253
    pleural tap, 365–67
pleural tap, 365–67
pneumoencephalography, 257
pneumonia:
    body temperature measurement, 399
    carbon dioxide, 56
    chest x-ray, 251–53
    cold agglutinins, 137
    lung scan, 297
    sputum culture, 128
    white blood cell count, 64
polio:
    electromyogram, 379
    nerve conduction studies, 379
polycythemia:
    hematocrit, 62
    hemoglobin, 62
    platelet count, 66
    red blood cell count, 63
polymyositis: rheumatoid factor, 99
portacaval shunt: ammonia levels, 48
postcoital test, 201, 223

postural proteinuria: urinary protein, 119
potassium, 70, 92–93
PRA (plasma renin activity), 97
precocious puberty:
  cortisol, 66
  follicle-stimulating hormone, 76
  testosterone, 108
predictive value of tests, 26–27
pregnancy:
  adrenocorticotropic hormone, 43
  ammonia, 48
  calcium, 56
  cortisol, 66
  direct Coombs test, 49
  estriol, 73
  estrogens, 74
  folic acid, 75
  glucose, 79
  gonorrhea cultures, 141
  herpes cultures, 143
  ketones, 118
  platelet count, 66
  progesterone, 95–96
  prolactin, 95
  Rh antibody titer, 49, 53–55
  rubella tests, 139
  sedimentation rate, 100, 101
  serum protein, 104
  serum protein electrophoresis, 105
  toxoplasmosis tests, 139–40
  urinary protein, 119
  white blood cell differential, 65
  x-rays, 228
  see also fetal testing; toxemia of pregnancy
pregnancy, ectopic:
  amylase, 48
  culdocentesis, 204–5
  fetal ultrasound, 205, 208
  laparoscopy, 328
pregnancy testing, 38, 93–94, 205, 207
  home, 431–34
pregnanediol test, 95
primaquine: white blood cell count, 65
primidone: barbiturate monitoring, 70
probenecid (Benemid):
  glucose, 79
  uric acid, 111
procainamide: antinuclear antibodies, 50
procaine: urobilinogen, 121
proctosigmoidoscopy, 245, 248, 319, 335–38
progesterone, 76, 94–96

aldosterone, 45
estriol, 73
estrogens, 74
follicle-stimulating hormone, 76
luteinizing hormone, 89
pregnancy, 95–96
progestins: thyroid function tests, 109
prolactin, 95–96
promethazine (Phenergan): pregnancy testing,
  94
propranolol (Inderal):
  alkaline phosphatase, 46
  glucose, 79
  growth hormone, 81
  SGOT, 102
  SGPT, 102
propylthiouracil: prothrombin time, 96
prostate cancer:
  acid phosphatase, 42–43, 223–24
  prostate biopsy, 223–25
  testosterone, 108
prostate disorders:
  cystoscopy, 322
  cystourethrogram, 260–62
  pelvic ultrasound, 308
  urine cells, 122
prostatic acid phosphatase (male PAP), 42–
  43
protein, serum, 56, 103–5
protein, urinary, 118–19, 426–27
protein electrophoresis, 103, 104–5, 370
prothrombin time (PT), 96
pseudogout: joint tap, 365
pseudohyperparathyroidism: parathyroid
  hormone, 90
psoriasis: histocompatibility testing, 83
PT (prothrombin time), 96
PTH (parathyroid hormone), 55, 89–90, 92
PTT (partial thromboplastin time), 90–91
puberty, delayed: chromosomal analysis, 61
pulmonary arteriography (angiography), 241–
  242
pulmonary artery catheterization, 167
pulmonary embolism:
  acid phosphatase, 42
  chest x-ray, 241
  lactic acid, 86
  LDH, 152
  lung scan, 241, 295–97
  pulmonary arteriography, 241–42
  SGOT, 101–2, 152

pulmonary fibrosis:
   lung biopsy, 355
   pulmonary function tests, 387, 388
pulmonary function tests (PFT), 387–89,
   418–21
pulse measurement, 400–403
punch biopsy, 357–58
pyelogram, intravenous (IVP), 269–72
pyelonephritis:
   BUN, 110
   creatinine clearance, 68
   renal scan, 297
   urine casts, 123
   urine cells, 122
Pyridium, see phenazopyridine

quinidine:
   monitoring, 71
   platelet count, 66
   prothrombin time, 96
quinine: prothrombin time, 96

radiation:
   follicle-stimulating hormone, 76
   growth hormone, 81
   immunoglobulins, 83
   platelet count, 66
   thyroid function tests and, 109
   uric acid, 111
   white blood cell differential, 65
radioactive iodine (RAI) uptake test, 109,
   299–301
radioallergosorbent test (RAST), 372, 373
radioimmunoassay (RIA), 94
random specimen, urine, 38
rape: acid phosphatase, 42–43
rapid plasma reagin (RPR), 144–46
RAST (radioallergosorbent test), 372, 373
RBC (red blood cell) count, 35, 63
rectal bleeding: sigmoidoscopy, 336
rectal cancer:
   anoscopy, 335–38
   carcinoembryonic antigen, 59
rectal pain: sigmoidoscopy, 336
red blood cell (RBC) count, 35, 63
red blood cell indices, 35, 63–64
reflexes, decreased: potassium, 93
regurgitation: upper gastrointestinal series,
   280
renal artery stenosis: dexamethasone
   suppression test, 69

renal biopsy, 348–50
renal calculi analysis, 85–86
renal disease, see kidney disease
renal scan, 297–99
renin, 96–97
reserpine: prolactin, 96
respiratory acidosis:
   arterial blood gases, 51
   bicarbonate, 52
respiratory alkalosis:
   arterial blood gases, 51
   bicarbonate, 52
resting heart rate measurement, 400
restlessness:
   glucose, 80
   salicylate monitoring, 71
reticulocyte count, 63, 98
retinopathy: ophthalmoscopy, 335
retrograde cystourethrography, 260–62
retrograde ureteropyelography, 325
Reye's syndrome: ammonia, 48
RF (rheumatoid factor), 50, 98–99
Rh antibody titer, 49, 53–57
rheumatic fever:
   antistreptolysin-O titer, 136
   sedimentation rate, 101
rheumatoid arthritis, see arthritis, rheumatoid
rheumatoid factor (RF), 50, 98–99
RIA (radioimmunoassay), 94
rib fractures: chest x-ray, 251, 253
rickets: alkaline phosphatase, 46
rifampin: barbiturate monitoring, 70
ringworm: fungal tests, 135
RPR (rapid plasma reagin), 144–46
rubella antibody testing, 139

salicylates:
   barbiturate monitoring, 70
   urine cells, 122
   see also aspirin
salivary glands, swelling of: amylase, 48
salivary gland scan, 301
salt: lithium monitoring, 71
salt-losing syndrome: aldosterone levels, 45
sarcoma: body scan, 293
scabies test, 135
scarlet fever: throat cultures, 131
Schilling test, 99–100
Schiotz method, 379–80
scleroderma: rheumatoid factor, 99

sclerotic disorders: slit-lamp examination, 335
scratch test, 371, 372–73
screening tests, 22–23
scrotal scan, 301
secobarbital monitoring, 70
second opinions, 28
second-voided (double-voided) urine
    specimen, 38–39, 79, 117
secretin: gastrin, 78
sedimentation rate, 100–101
seizures:
    brain scan, 289
    electroencephalogram, 375, 377
    theophylline monitoring, 72
    *see also* convulsions
semen analysis, 201, 221–23
senna:
    estriol, 73
    estrogens, 74
sensation, loss of: CT scan, 257
sensitivity of tests, 26, 27
septicemia: white blood cell count, 64
serologic testing, 35
serum glutamic oxalacetic transaminase
    (SGOT), 101–2, 151, 152
serum glutamic pyruvic transaminase (SGPT),
    102
serum osmolality, 103
serum protein, 56, 103–5
serum protein electrophoresis, 103, 104–5
sexual desire, male, decreased: prolactin, 95
sexual development, abnormal:
    chromosomal analysis, 61
    cortisol, 66
    estrogens, 74
    testosterone, 108
sexually transmitted disease tests, 140–46
SGOT (serum glutamic oxalacetic
    transaminase), 101–2, 151, 152
SGPT (serum glutamic pyruvic transaminase),
    102
shakiness: theophylline monitoring, 72
shave biopsy, 358
shock:
    arterial blood gases, 51
    lactic acid, 86
    serum protein, 104
    urine casts, 123
    urine volume, 113
shoulder pain and swelling:
    arthrogram, 243–44

arthroscopy, 312
    joint tap, 364
sickle-cell anemia, *see* anemia, sickle-cell
sickle-cell (hemoglobin S) test, 105–6
sigmoidoscopy, 319, 335–38
Simmonds' disease: glucose, 79
sinus x-ray, 277, 278
skin, bluish tinge to: salicylate monitoring, 71
skin, dry, thyroid function tests, 108
skin, hyperpigmentation of: cortisol, 66
skin biopsy, 61, 357–59
skin cultures, 132–33
skin diseases:
    body temperature measurement, 397
    white blood cell differential, 65
skin rash:
    allergy testing, 371
    antinuclear antibodies, 50
    antistreptolysin-O titer, 136
    body temperature measurement, 397
    platelet count, 65
skin tests:
    allergy, 371–73
    tuberculin, 133–35
skull x-rays, 277–78
SLE, *see* lupus erythematosus, systemic
sleep disturbances: prolactin, 96
sleepiness: carbon monoxide, 57
slit-lamp examination, 335
small bowel follow-through, 280, 282, 283
sneezing, allergy testing, 371
sodium (Na), 106–7
sodium bicarbonate:
    lithium monitoring, 71
    urinary protein, 119
    urobilinogen, 121
somatotropin (HGH, growth hormone), 81
sorbitol: lactic acid, 86
sore throats:
    home throat cultures, 438–40
    throat cultures, 130–31, 141–42
spasms, *see* muscle spasms and twitches
specificity of tests, 26, 27
speech, slurred: cerebral arteriogram, 238
spina bifida:
    alpha-fetoprotein, 47, 212
    amniocentesis, 209, 212
spinal abnormalities:
    CT scan, 254, 256
    myelogram, 275–77
    spine x-rays, 278–80

spinal cord injury:
  cystometrogram, 374
  electromyogram, 377
  magnetic resonance imaging, 386
  nerve conduction studies, 377
spinal tap, 146, 367–70
spine x-rays, 278–80
spironolactone:
  adrenocorticotropic hormone, 43
  cortisol, 66
  potassium, 93
spleen disorders:
  abdominal ultrasound, 305–6
  CT scan, 254, 256
  hematocrit, 62
  laparoscopy, 328
  liver/spleen scan, 293–95
  platelet count, 66
sprue: folic acid, 75
sputum, blood in, see hemoptysis
sputum cultures, 128–29
squamous-cell carcinoma: skin biopsy, 358
starvation:
  BUN, 110
  carbon dioxide, 57
  glucose, 79
  ketones, 85, 118
  serum protein electrophoresis, 105
  urine pH, 116
Stein-Leventhal syndrome: luteinizing
    hormone, 88
Stelazine:
  estrogens, 74
  pregnancy testing, 94
stenosis, heart valve: echocardiogram, 161
steroid drugs:
  adrenocorticotropic hormone, 43
  arterial blood gases, 51
  bicarbonate, 52
  bilirubin, 53
  carbon dioxide, 56
  chloride, 60
  estriol, 73
  estrogens, 74
  follicle-stimulating hormone, 76
  luteinizing hormone, 89
  plasma renin activity, 97
  platelet count, 66
  prothrombin time, 96
  sodium, 106
  see also corticosteroids

stomach cancer:
  alpha-fetoprotein, 47
  body scan, 293
  gastrin, 78
stomach tumors: gastrin, 77, 78
stool cultures, 129–30
stool guaiac, 443–45
strep infections:
  antistreptolysin-O titer, 136–37
  throat cultures, 130–31
stress:
  adrenocorticotropic hormone, 43
  catecholamines, 58, 59
  cortisol, 66
  gastrin, 77, 78
  growth hormone, 81
  ketones, 85, 118
  prolactin, 96
  pulse measurement, 402
  white blood cell count, 64
  white blood cell differential, 65
stress incontinence test, 375
stress test, 155–57
stress thallium scan, 167–69
stroke:
  body temperature measurement, 399
  carotid angiogram, 238
  CT scan, 259
  Doppler ultrasound, 310
  echocardiogram, 160
stupor:
  chloride, 60
  sodium, 106
  toxicology screening, 110
sugar, see glucose
sulfasoxazole: urinary protein, 119
sulfobromophthalein: ketones, 85
sulfonamides:
  alkaline phosphatase, 46
  barbiturate monitoring, 70
  platelet count, 66
  SGOT, 102
  SGPT, 102
  thyroid function tests, 109
  urinary crystals, 123
  urine cells, 122
  urobilinogen, 121
suprapubic (bladder) tap, 41
surgery: white blood cell count, 64
swallowing difficulties:
  laryngoscopy, 329

lymph node biopsy, 356
  upper gastrointestinal endoscopy, 338
  upper gastrointestinal series, 280, 281
sweating:
  glucose, 79, 80
  heart attack enzymes, 151
  hematocrit, 62
  infarct imaging, 170
  lactic acid, 86
  potassium, 93
  salicylate monitoring, 71
  sodium, 106
  urine specific gravity, 115
sweat test, 60, 107, 389–90
synovial biopsy, 365
synovial fluid analysis (joint tap), 99, 363–65
syphilis:
  FTA-ABS, 144–46
  protein electrophoresis, 370
  rheumatoid factor, 99
  RPR, 144–46
  spinal tap, 370
  VDRL, 144–46
systemic lupus erythematosus, see lupus
    erythematosus, systemic

T₃ uptake, 108–9
T₄, 108–9
Talwin: amylase, 48
tangent screen exam, 392
tape test, 447–48
taps, 362–70
  abdominal, 362–63
  amniocentesis, 47, 61, 208–12
  joint, 99, 363–65
  pleural, 365–67
  spinal, 367–70
Tay-Sachs screening, 107
temporal arteritis: sedimentation rate, 101
testicular abnormalities:
  follicle-stimulating hormone, 76
  testicular biopsy, 225–26
  testicular scan, 301
  testicular self-examination, 218–19
testicular biopsy, 225–26
testicular cancer:
  alpha-fetoprotein, 47
  body scan, 293
  testicular self-examination, 218–19
  testosterone, 108
testicular scan, 301

testicular tumors:
  estrogens, 74
  follicle-stimulating hormone, 76
  human chorionic gonadotropin, 94
  testosterone, 108
testosterone, 108, 225
  luteinizing hormone, 89
tetracycline:
  alkaline phosphatase, 46
  antinuclear antibodies, 50
  cholesterol, 150
  estriol, 73
  estrogens, 74
  SGOT, 102
  SGPT, 102
  urinary blood, 120
thalassemia:
  fetoscopy, 213
  hemoglobin electropheresis, 82
  red blood cell indices, 64
thallium scan, 167–69
theophylline:
  bilirubin, 53
  monitoring, 72
thermography, 192
thiazide diuretics:
  ammonia levels, 48
  amylase, 48
  calcium, 56
  cholesterol, 150
  creatinine, 68
  glucose, 79, 117
  platelet count, 66
  potassium, 93
  uric acid, 111
  see also chlorothiazide diuretics
thirst, excessive: lithium monitoring, 71
thoracentesis, 365–67
thoracic myelogram, 275–77
thoracic spine films, 278–80
Thorazine, see chlorpromazine
throat cultures, 130–31, 141–42
  home, 438–40
thrombocyte (platelet) count, 35, 65–66
thrombocytopenia:
  bone marrow examination, 346, 348
  folic acid, 75
  platelet count, 66
thrombophlebitis:
  acid phosphatase, 42
  Doppler ultrasound, 309–10

thrombophlebitis (cont'd)
vein scan, 302
venogram and, 283–85
thrush:
fungal tests, 135
throat cultures, 131
thyroid antibodies, 109
thyroid biopsy, 359–61
thyroid cancer:
thyroid biopsy, 359–61
thyroid scan, 299, 301
thyroid disease:
sedimentation rate, 101
thyroid biopsy, 359–61
thyroid function tests, 108–9
thyroid scan, 199, 299–301
thyroid ultrasound, 109, 306–7
see also specific diseases
thyroid hormones: prothrombin time, 96
thyroid scan, 109, 299–301
thyroid-stimulating hormone (TSH), 109
thyroid ultrasound, 109, 306–7
TIBC (total iron-binding capacity), 84–85
timed specimens, urine, 39
tine (tuberculin skin) test, 133–35
tingling: electromyogram, 377
tiredness:
hematocrit, 62
thyroid function tests, 108
titers, 136–40
tobramycin:
BUN, 111
monitoring, 69, 70
tolbutamide, urinary protein, 119
tomography, 253–60
tongue, sore: folic acid, 75
tonometry, 379–81
tonsillitis:
home throat culture, 438–40
white blood cell count, 64
toxemia of pregnancy:
uric acid, 111
urinary protein, 119
toxicology screening, 109–10
toxoplasmosis tests, 139–40
tracheal aspiration, 129
tracheal tap, 129
transcutaneous coronary artery angioplasty, 167
transillumination, 192
transtracheal aspiration, 129

trauma:
hematocrit, 62
serum protein electrophoresis, 105
urinary hemoglobin, 120
urine casts, 123
treadmill test, 155–57
tremors:
lithium monitoring, 71
thyroid function tests, 108
triamterene: glucose, 79
trichomoniasis:
ova and parasite test, 130
wet mount, 177–78
tricyclic antidepressants:
alkaline phosphatase, 46
prolactin, 96
SGOT, 102
SGPT, 102
triglycerides, blood, 148–50
TSH (thyroid-stimulating hormone), 109
tube feeding, prolonged: ammonia levels, 48
tuberculin skin (tine) test, 133–35
tuberculosis, 127
chest x-ray, 251–53
liver biopsy, 352
lung biopsy, 355
lymph node biopsy, 357
mediastinoscopy, 333
rheumatoid factor, 99
sedimentation rate, 101
sputum cultures, 129, 135
tuberculin skin test, 133–35
white blood cell differential, 65
Tuinal, see amobarbital
tumors:
abdominal tap, 363
arteriogram, 237
body scan, 292–93
CT scan, 254, 257, 259
see also specific tumors
Turner's syndrome:
chromosomal analysis, 61
follicle-stimulating hormone, 76
luteinizing hormone, 88
twitches, see muscle spasms and twitches
Tylenol: white blood cell differential, 65
typhoid fever: stool cultures, 130
Tzanck test, 144

UGI (upper gastrointestinal series), 248, 280–283

ulcers:
    amylase, 48
    gastrin, 77
    upper gastrointestinal endoscopy, 338, 341
    upper gastrointestinal series, 281, 283
ultrasound, 303–10
    abdominal, 304–6
    Doppler, 207, 208, 309–10
    pelvic, 307–9
    thyroid, 109, 306–7
unconjugated (indirect) bilirubin, 52–53
unconsciousness: carbon monoxide, 57, 58
unnecessary testing, 22
upper gastrointestinal endoscopy, 338–42
upper gastrointestinal (UGI) series, 248, 280–283
urethral disorders:
    cystoscopy, 322–25
    cystourethrogram, 260–62
    retrograde ureteropyelography, 325
urethritis:
    urine cells, 122
    urine cultures, 132
uric acid, 111–12
urinalysis, 37–41, 112–23, 131
    home, 62, 421–28
urinary bacteria, 123
urinary catheterization, 41
urinary tract bleeding: platelet count, 65
urinary tract infections:
    cystometrogram, 374
    cystoscopy, 323
    cystourethrogram, 260–62
    leukocyte dipsticks, 428, 429, 430
    nitrite dipsticks, 428, 429, 430–31
    self-testing, 428–31
    urinary blood, 120
    urine cells, 122
    urine clarity, 113
    urine color, 114
    urine cultures, 131–32, 428–29, 430, 431
    urine odor, 115
    urine pH, 116
    urine volume, 113
urination, frequent:
    cystoscopy, 323
    lithium monitoring, 71
    urine cultures, 131
urination, painful:
    body temperature measurement, 397
    cystoscopy, 323

gonorrhea cultures, 141
    urine cultures, 131
urine, blood in, see hematuria
urine casts, 122–23
urine collection procedures, 38–41
    bladder (suprapubic) tap, 41
    clean-catch midstream specimen, 39–40, 132
    first morning specimen, 38
    for infants, 41
    random specimen, 38
    second-voided (double-voided) specimen, 38–39
    timed specimen, 39
    urinary catheterization, 41
urine color and clarity, 113–14, 425
urine crystals, 123
urine cultures, 131–32, 428–29
urine dilution test, 116
urine glucose, 116–18, 426
urine odor, 114–15
urine output, decreased:
    barbiturate monitoring, 70
    potassium, 93
    salicylate monitoring, 71
urine pH, 116, 425–26
urine specific gravity, 115–16, 425
urine volume, 112–13
urobilinogen, 121, 427–28
uterine cancer:
    body scan, 293
    carcinoembryonic antigen, 59
uterine disorders:
    culdoscopy, 328
    laparoscopy, 325, 328
    pelvic ultrasound, 307–9

vabra aspiration, 187
vaginal bleeding: platelet count, 65
vaginal infections:
    fungal tests, 135
    gonorrhea cultures, 140
    ova and parasite test, 135
    vaginal self-examination, 177
    wet mount, 177, 178
vaginal self-examination, 175–77
Valium, see diazepam
vanillylmandelic acid (VMA), 58–59
VDRL (Venereal Disease Research Laboratory), 144–46
vectorcardiogram, 155

vein scan, 302
venogram, 283–85
ventilation lung scan, 295–97
ventricular puncture, 370
vertebral arteriogram, 237–40
vertebral radiography, 278–80
viral cultures, 133, 143–44
viral infections: white blood cell differential, 65
virilization: testosterone, 108
vision, loss of:
    CT scan, 257
    Doppler ultrasound, 309
vision tests, 390–92, 403–9
visual disturbance:
    aminoglycoside monitoring, 69, 70
    cerebral arteriogram, 238
    glaucoma testing, 379–81
    home vision tests, 403–9
    ophthalmoscopy, 333–35
    salicylate monitoring, 71
visual field test, 392
vitamin A:
    cholesterol, 150
    prothrombin time, 96
vitamin $B_3$: cholesterol, 150
vitamin $B_{12}$ absorption (Schilling test), 99–100
vitamin $B_{12}$ deficiency:
    folic acid, 75
    hematocrit, 62
    platelet count, 66
    red blood cell indices, 64
    vitamin $B_{12}$ testing, 124
    white blood cell differential, 65
vitamin $B_{12}$ testing, 123–24
vitamin C:
    bilirubin, 53, 121
    creatinine, 68
    folic acid, 75
    glucose, 79
    uric acid, 112
    urinary blood, 120
    urinary crystals, 123
    urine pH, 116
    urobilinogen, 121
vitamin D, excessive:
    calcium, 56
    phosphorus, 92
vitamin D deficiency:
    calcium, 56

parathyroid hormone, 90
    phosphorus, 92
VMA (vanillylmandelic acid), 58–59
vocal chord disorders: laryngoscopy, 329–31
voice, change in: laryngoscopy, 329
vomiting:
    abdominal x-ray, 233
    alkaline phosphatase, 46
    arterial blood gases, 51
    bicarbonate, 52
    body temperature measurement, 397
    carbon dioxide, 56, 57
    chloride, 60
    digoxin monitoring, 70
    glucose, 79
    hematocrit, 62
    ketones, 85, 118
    lipase, 88
    lithium monitoring, 71
    phosphorus, 92
    potassium, 93
    serum protein, 104
    SGOT, 101
    SGPT, 102
    sodium, 106
    upper gastrointestinal endoscopy, 338
    urine color, 113
    urine pH, 116
    urine specific gravity, 115
    urine volume, 112, 113
Von Gierke's disease: glucose, 79
von Willebrand's disease: partial thromboplastin time, 91

warfarin (Coumadin):
    prothrombin time, 96
    thyroid function tests, 109
    urine cells, 122
warts: skin biopsy, 358
WBC (white blood cell count), 35, 64–65
weakness:
    Bence Jones protein, 119
    brain scan, 289
    calcium, 55
    cerebral arteriogram, 238
    chloride, 60
    cortisol, 66
    Doppler ultrasound, 309
    D-xylose absorption test, 72
    electromyogram, 377, 379

glucose, 79, 80
hematocrit, 62
lithium monitoring, 71
magnesium, 89
nerve conduction studies, 377, 379
potassium, 93
sodium, 106
weight gain: thyroid function tests, 108
weight loss:
  body temperature measurement, 397
  D-xylose absorption test, 72
  ketones, 118
  lymph node biopsy, 356
  sedimentation rate, 100
  thyroid function tests, 108
wet mount, 177–79
white blood cell count (WBC), 35, 64–65
white blood cell differential, 35, 64–65
whooping cough: throat cultures, 131
wound cultures, 132–33
wrist pain:
  arthroscopy, 312
  joint tap, 364

xanthomatosis: triglyceride, 148
xeromammography, 190–92

xerostomia: salivary gland scan, 301
x-rays, 227–85
  abdominal, 233–34
  arteriogram, cardiac, 162–67
  arteriogram, cerebral, 237–40
  arteriogram, general, 234–37
  arteriogram, pulmonary, 241–42
  arthrogram, 243–45
  barium enema, 245–48
  bronchogram, 249–51
  chest, 241, 251–53
  CT scans, 253–60
  cystourethrogram, 26–62
  dental, 262–64
  extremity, 264–65
  gallbladder, 266–69
  intravenous pyelogram, 269–72
  lymphangiogram, 272–74
  myelogram, 275–77
  sinus, 277, 278
  skull, 277–78
  spine, 278–80
  upper gastrointestinal series, 280–83
  venogram, 283–85

Zollinger-Ellison syndrome: gastrin, 78

# About the Authors

**D**avid Sobel received his M.D. degree from the University of California, San Francisco and completed a Masters of Public Health degree and a residency in General Preventive Medicine at the School of Public Health, University of California, Berkeley. He is now Regional Director of Patient Education and Health Promotion for the Kaiser Permanente Medical Care Program in Northern California and Chief of Preventive Medicine, Kaiser Permanente Medical Center in San Jose, California. He also serves as Medical Director of The Institute for the Study of Human Knowledge.

Dr. Sobel's interests include medical self-care, patient education, preventive medicine, behavioral medicine, and psychosocial factors in health. He is contributing editor to the publication *Medical Self-Care*, author of *To Your Health*—a lay health guide—and editor of the book *Ways of Health: Holistic Approaches to Ancient and Contemporary Medicine*. He has worked as a "TV doctor" on a weekly news program and has appeared as a frequent guest on "Hour Magazine," a nationally syndicated daytime television show. His work in the media has earned awards from the American Heart Association and the American Film Festival.

**T**om Ferguson received his M.D. from the Yale University School of Medicine. While still a medical student, he founded the magazine *Medical Self-Care*, which the Wilson Library Journal recently ranked as the nation's "outstanding" health magazine. He is the editor of *Medical Self-Care* and a contributing editor to *Prevention*. He also writes regularly on health topics for *Esquire* and *American Health*. His previous book was *Medical Self-Care: Access to Health Tools* (New York, Summit Books/Simon & Schuster, Inc., 1980).

Dr. Ferguson has served on the Advisory Board of the California Governor's Wellness Council, and has received the Distinguished Achievement Award from the Educational Press Association of America and the Lifetime Extension Award for his reporting "on the rapidly expanding area of self-help in health and medicine." He lives in Austin, Texas, and lectures widely on self-care and the future of health care.